Patient Education for Children, Teens, and Parents

3rd Edition

DATE DUE

American Academy of Pediatrics
141 Northwest Point Blvd
Elk Grove Village, IL 60007-1098

Library of Congress Control Number: 2006922507
ISBN-13: 978-1-58110-231-4
ISBN-10: 1-58110-231-3
MA0360

The recommendations in this publication do not indicate an exclusive course of treatment or serve as a standard of medical care. Variations, taking into account individual circumstances, may be appropriate.

Introduction

Studies have shown that information handouts are effective educational tools and are an excellent means to reinforce verbal instructions. In the short term, handouts help to lessen parent anxiety, increase patient and parent compliance, and reduce the number of unnecessary telephone calls and office visits. Long-term benefits include increased knowledge of development, enhanced parent-child relationships, and increased parental self-confidence.

To support your efforts at effective patient and parent teaching, the American Academy of Pediatrics (AAP) has compiled more than 150 patient education handouts into this handy reusable manual. This compendium includes the same information as our printed brochures and fact sheets. A Spanish-language version with identical features and content is also available (part number MA0361), as well as both English and Spanish versions on the AAP *Patient Education Online* Web site (available Fall 2006 at **http://patiented.aap.org**). For more information about these patient education products and others, please visit the AAP Bookstore at **www.aap.org/bookstore.**

The manual is divided into 11 sections: Common Illnesses and Conditions; Newborns, Infants, and Toddlers; Developmental Issues; Nutrition and Fitness; Safety and Prevention; Adolescents and School-aged Children; Behavioral and Psychosocial Issues; Sexual Health and Sexuality; Substance Abuse Issues; Immunization Information; and Promoting Pediatric Care. Within each section, the handouts are arranged alphabetically by topic. A list of handouts is included at the beginning of the manual, and a helpful index can be found at the end of the manual. Also included is a handout checklist for use by parents and patients to indicate which handouts they would like to receive. A copy of the checklist can then be placed in a patient's chart as a patient education record.

The pages of this manual are perforated and 3-hole punched. You may remove pages for duplication, then store the originals in a binder for future use. A copyright line is included on each page. Permission to duplicate the pages for noncommercial purposes is granted, and no additional or special permission is needed to copy and distribute the materials to your patients. There is space on most of the handouts for you to insert your practice information and personalized patient instructions.

Table of Contents

Table of Contents

SECTION FIVE

Safety and Prevention

SECTION SIX

Adolescents and School-aged Children

SECTION SEVEN

Behavioral and Psychosocial Issues

SECTION EIGHT

Sexual Health and Sexuality

Below is a listing of publications available from the American Academy of Pediatrics. Please check the publications that you would like to receive, and give this form to your health care professional.

Common Illnesses and Conditions

- ☐ Acne—How to Treat and Control It
- ☐ ADHD and Your School-aged Child
- ☐ ADHD—What About Medicines for ADHD? Questions From Teens Who Have ADHD
- ☐ ADHD—What Is ADHD Anyway? Questions From Teens
- ☐ Allergies in Children
- ☐ Anemia and Your Young Child: Guidelines for Parents
- ☐ Asthma and Your Child
- ☐ Bronchiolitis and Your Young Child
- ☐ Catheterization—What is Clean Intermittent Catheterization?
- ☐ The Chickenpox Vaccine
- ☐ Constipation and Your Child
- ☐ Corticosteroids—Inhaled and Intranasal Corticosteroids and Your Child
- ☐ Croup and Your Young Child
- ☐ Diarrhea and Dehydration
- ☐ Ear—Acute Ear Infection and Your Child
- ☐ Ear—Middle Ear Fluid and Your Child
- ☐ Eyes—Your Child's Eyes
- ☐ Febrile Seizures
- ☐ Fever and Your Child
- ☐ *Haemophilus influenzae* type b
- ☐ Head Lice: Every Parent's Concern
- ☐ Headaches—Important Information for Teens Who Get Headaches
- ☐ Hepatitis B
- ☐ Hepatitis C
- ☐ Hip Dysplasia (Developmental Dysplasia of the Hip)
- ☐ Imaging Tests: A Look Inside Your Child's Body
- ☐ Infections—Common Childhood Infections
- ☐ Influenza—The Flu (Influenza)
- ☐ Lyme Disease
- ☐ Meningococcal Disease—Information for Teens and College Students
- ☐ Pneumococcal Infection and Vaccine
- ☐ Respiratory Syncytial Virus
- ☐ Sinusitis and Your Child
- ☐ Sleep Apnea and Your Child
- ☐ Sleep Problems in Children
- ☐ Tonsils and the Adenoid
- ☐ Urinary Tract Infections in Young Children

Newborns, Infants, and Toddlers

- ☐ Baby Bottle Tooth Decay—How to Prevent It
- ☐ Baby Walkers
- ☐ Bedwetting
- ☐ Breastfeeding Your Baby: Getting Started
- ☐ Car Safety Seats: A Guide for Families
- ☐ Car Safety Seats—One-Minute Car Safety Seat Check-up
- ☐ Car Safety Seats—Safe Transportation of Children With Special Needs: A Guide for Families
- ☐ Child Care—Choosing Child Care: What's Best for Your Family?
- ☐ Circumcision: Information for Parents
- ☐ Diaper Rash
- ☐ Hearing—Newborn Hearing Screening and Your Baby
- ☐ Premature Infants—Early Arrival: Information for Parents of Premature Infants
- ☐ Shaken Baby Syndrome—Prevent Shaken Baby Syndrome
- ☐ SIDS: Important Information for Parents
- ☐ Sun Exposure—Fun in the Sun: Keep Your Baby Safe
- ☐ Thumbs, Fingers, and Pacifiers
- ☐ Toilet Training
- ☐ Uncircumcised Penis—Care of the Uncircumcised Penis

Developmental Issues

- ☐ Autism—Understanding Autism Spectrum Disorders (ASDs): An Introduction
- ☐ Developmental Delays—Is Your One-Year-Old Communicating With You?
- ☐ Developmental Milestones—Your Child's Growth: Developmental Milestones
- ☐ Learning Disabilities: What Parents Need to Know
- ☐ Reading—Helping Your Child Learn to Read

Nutrition and Fitness

- ☐ Calcium and You
- ☐ Fitness—Encourage Your Child to Be Physically Active
- ☐ Nutrition—Feeding Kids Right Isn't Always Easy: Tips for Preventing Food Hassles
- ☐ Nutrition—Growing Up Healthy: Fat, Cholesterol, and More
- ☐ Nutrition—Right From the Start: ABCs of Good Nutrition for Young Children
- ☐ Nutrition—Starting Solid Foods
- ☐ Nutrition—What's to Eat?: Healthy Foods for Hungry Children
- ☐ Sports and Your Child
- ☐ Teen Health—Get Fit, Stay Healthy

Safety and Prevention

- ☐ Air Bag Safety
- ☐ Anesthesia and Your Child
- ☐ Antibiotics and Your Child
- ☐ Blood Transfusions—Safety of Blood Transfusions
- ☐ Choking Prevention and First Aid for Infants and Children
- ☐ Dental Health—A Guide to Children's Dental Health
- ☐ Driving Safety—The Teen Driver: Guidelines for Parents
- ☐ Environmental Hazards—Your Child and the Environment
- ☐ Fire Safety—Keep Your Family Safe: Fire Safety and Burn Prevention at Home

Patient Request Form

- [ ] Head Injuries—Minor Head Injuries in Children
- [ ] Home Safety Checklist
- [ ] Lawn Mower Safety
- [ ] Lead Screening for Children
- [ ] Medications—A Guide to Your Child's Medicines
- [ ] Playground Safety
- [ ] Poison—Protect Your Child From Poison
- [ ] Repellents—A Parent's Guide to Insect Repellents
- [ ] Smoking—Dangers of Secondhand Smoke
- [ ] Toy Safety
- [ ] Trampolines
- [ ] Water Safety—A Parent's Guide to Water Safety

Adolescents and School-aged Children

- [ ] Adolescents—Tips for Parents of Adolescents
- [ ] College Students—Health Care for College Students: What Your Pediatrician Wants You to Know
- [ ] Lactose Intolerance and Your Child
- [ ] Puberty—Ready or Not Expect Some Big Changes
- [ ] School Health Centers and Your Child
- [ ] School Health—Students With Chronic Health Conditions: Guidance for Families, Schools, and Students
- [ ] Teen Health—For Today's Teens: A Message From Your Pediatrician

Behavioral and Psychosocial Issues

- [ ] Adoption: Guidelines for Parents
- [ ] Communication—Healthy Communication With Your Child
- [ ] Depression/Suicide—Surviving: Coping With Adolescent Depression and Suicide: Guidelines for Parents
- [ ] Discipline and Your Child
- [ ] Divorce and Children
- [ ] Eating Disorders: Anorexia and Bulimia
- [ ] Emotional Needs—Responding to Children's Emotional Needs During Times of Crisis: Information for Parents
- [ ] Gambling: Not a Safe Thrill
- [ ] Media History
- [ ] Media—Medicine and the Media
- [ ] Media Ratings—The Ratings Game: Choosing Your Child's Entertainment
- [ ] Media—Understanding the Impact of Media on Children and Teens
- [ ] Mental Health—Your Child's Mental Health: When to Seek Help and Where to Get Help
- [ ] Sibling Relationships
- [ ] Single Parenting
- [ ] Television and the Family
- [ ] Temper Tantrums: A Normal Part of Growing Up

Sexual Health and Sexuality

- [ ] Breast Self-Exam
- [ ] Emergency Contraception
- [ ] Gay, Lesbian, and Bisexual Teens: Facts for Teens and Their Parents
- [ ] Gay, Lesbian, or Bisexual Parents: Information for Children and Parents
- [ ] HIV/AIDS—Know the Facts About HIV and AIDS
- [ ] The Pelvic Exam
- [ ] Sexual Abuse—Child Sexual Abuse: What It Is and How to Prevent It
- [ ] Sexuality—Deciding to Wait
- [ ] Sexuality—Making Healthy Decisions About Sex
- [ ] Sexuality—Talking to Your Teen About Sex
- [ ] Sexuality—Talking With Your Young Child About Sex
- [ ] Testicular Self-Exam

Substance Abuse Issues

- [ ] Alcohol: Your Child and Drugs
- [ ] Cocaine: Your Child and Drugs
- [ ] Drugs—Testing Your Teen for Illicit Drugs: Information for Parents
- [ ] Inhalant Abuse: Your Child and Drugs: Guidelines for Parents
- [ ] Marijuana: Your Child and Drugs
- [ ] Steroids: Play Safe, Play Fair
- [ ] Substance Abuse Prevention
- [ ] Tobacco—The Risks of Tobacco Use: A Message to Parents and Teens
- [ ] Tobacco—Smokeless Tobacco: Guidelines for Teens
- [ ] Tobacco: Straight Talk for Teens

Immunization Information

- [ ] Chickenpox Vaccine (Vaccine Information Sheet)
- [ ] Diphtheria, Tetanus, & Pertussis Vaccines (Vaccine Information Sheet)
- [ ] *Haemophilus Influenzae* Type b (Hib) Vaccine (Vaccine Information Sheet)
- [ ] Hepatitis B Vaccine (Vaccine Information Sheet)
- [ ] Immunization Schedule—Recommended Immunization Schedule for Children and Adolescents Who Start Late or Who Are More Than 1 Month Behind—United States, 2006
- [ ] Immunization Schedule—Recommended Childhood and Adolescent Immunization Schedule—United States, 2006
- [ ] Immunizations: What You Need to Know
- [ ] Influenza—Inactivated Influenza Vaccine (Vaccine Information Sheet)
- [ ] Influenza—Live, Intranasal Influenza Vaccine (Vaccine Information Sheet)
- [ ] Measles, Mumps, & Rubella Vaccines (Vaccine Information Sheet)
- [ ] Meningococcal Vaccines (Vaccine Information Sheet)
- [ ] Pneumococcal Conjugate Vaccine (Vaccine Information Sheet)
- [ ] Polio Vaccine (Vaccine Information Sheet)
- [ ] Tetanus and Diphtheria Vaccine (Td) (Vaccine Information Sheet)

Promoting Pediatric Care

- [ ] Pediatric Care—How Special Is Your Child?
- [ ] Pediatric Care—You and Your Pediatrician
- [ ] Pediatric Subspecialists

Common Illnesses and Conditions

acne—how to treat and control it

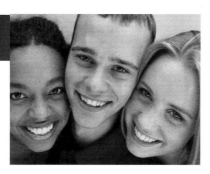

Got **ZITS**? You're not alone.

Almost **all teens get them** at one time or another. It's called *acne*. Whether your case is mild or severe, **there are things you can do to keep it under control.** Read on to find out how.

What causes acne?

During puberty, your skin gets oilier and you sweat more. This can cause pimples. There are many myths about what causes acne, but there are really only **3 main causes.**

1. **Hormones.** You get more of them during puberty. Certain hormones, called *androgens,* trigger the oil glands on the face, back, and upper chest to begin producing oil. This can cause acne in some people.

2. **Heredity.** Acne can run in families. If your mom or dad had acne as a teen, there may be a chance that you'll get it too.

3. **Plugged oil ducts.** Small whiteheads or blackheads can form when the oil ducts in your skin get plugged. They can turn into the hard and bumpy pimples of acne.

What *doesn't* cause acne?

Don't let people tell you it's your fault. It's not. Acne is not caused by

- **Food.** Even though soft drinks, chocolate, and greasy foods aren't really good for you, they don't cause acne.

- **Dirt.** That black stuff in a blackhead is not dirt. A chemical reaction in the oil duct turns it black. No matter how much you wash your face, you can still get acne.

- **Contact with people.** You can't catch acne from or give acne to another person.

- **Your thoughts.** Thinking about sex won't cause acne.

Don't make it worse

You might think it helps, but **don't**

- **Pop or pinch your zits.** All this does is break open the lining of the oil ducts and make them more red and swollen. This can also cause scars.

- Scrub your skin too hard—it irritates the skin. Other things that can irritate the skin are headbands, hats, and chin straps.

- Use **greasy makeup** or **oily hair products.** These can block oil ducts and make acne worse.

- **Get stressed out.** Sometimes stress and anxiety can cause pimples. Try to keep your stress down by getting enough sleep and having time to relax.

Other things that can make acne worse

- **Medicines.** If you have to take a prescription medicine, **ask your pediatrician** if it can cause pimples.

- *Changes in hormones.* Some girls get more pimples before and during their periods. This is caused by changes in the levels of hormones.

What can I do?

The bad news—There's no cure for acne. The good news—It usually clears up as you get older. In the meantime, there are a few things you can do to **help keep those zits under control.**

First Steps: Benzoyl peroxide lotion or gel—the most effective acne treatment you can get without a prescription. It helps kill bacteria in the skin, unplug oil ducts, and heal pimples. There are a lot of different brands and different strengths (2.5%, 5%, or 10%). The gel may dry out your skin and make it redder than the lotion, so try the lotion first.

How to use benzoyl peroxide

- *Start slowly*—only once a day with a 5% lotion. After a week, try using it twice a day (morning and night) if your skin isn't too red or isn't peeling.

- Don't just dab it on top of your pimples. **Apply a thin layer** to the entire area where pimples may occur. Avoid the skin around your eyes.

- If your acne isn't better **after 4 to 6 weeks**, try a 10% lotion or gel. Use it once a day at first and then try twice a day if doesn't irritate your skin.

Next Steps: Stronger treatments—If benzoyl peroxide doesn't get your zits under control, your pediatrician may prescribe

- **A retinoid to be used on the skin** (like Retin A, Differin, and other brands). This comes in a cream or gel and helps unplug oil ducts. It must be used *exactly* as directed. Try to stay out of the sun (including tanning salons) when taking this medicine. Retinoids can cause your skin to peel and turn red.

- **Antibiotics,** in **cream, lotion, solution,** or **gel** form, may be used for "inflammatory" acne (when you have red bumps or pus bumps).

- **Antibiotics,** in **pill** form, may be used if the treatments used on the skin don't help.

- **Isotretinoin** (Accutane and other brands) is a very strong medicine taken as a pill. It's **only used for severe acne that hasn't responded** to any other treatment. Because it's such a powerful drug, it must *never be taken just before or during pregnancy.* There is a danger of severe or even fatal deformities to unborn babies. Patients who take this medicine must be carefully supervised by a doctor knowledgeable about its usage, such as a pediatric dermatologist or other expert in treating acne. Isotretinoin should be used cautiously (and only with careful monitoring by a dermatologist and psychiatrist) in patients with a history of depression. Don't be surprised if your doctor requires a negative pregnancy test, some blood tests, and a signed consent form before prescribing isotretinoin.

No matter what treatment you use, remember

- **Be patient.** Give each treatment enough time to work. It may take 3 to 6 weeks or longer before you see a change.

- **Be faithful.** Follow your program **every day.** Don't stop and start each time your skin changes.

- **Follow directions.** Not using it correctly is the most common reason why treatments fail.

- ***Only use your medicine.*** Doctors prescribe medicine specifically for particular patients. What's good for a friend may not be good for you.

- **Don't overdo it.** Too much scrubbing makes skin worse. Too much benzoyl peroxide or topical retinoid creams can make your face red and scaly. Too much oral antibiotic may cause side effects.

- **Don't worry** about what other people think. It's no fun having acne, and some people may say hurtful things about it. Try not to let it bother you. Remember, most teens get some acne at some point. Also remember that ***it's only temporary,*** and there are ***a lot of treatment options*** to keep it under control.

Acne and birth control pills

Birth control pills can be useful for treating young women with acne. However, taking birth control pills and other medicines may make both less effective. If you are on the Pill, talk with your pediatrician about how it might affect your acne.

From your doctor

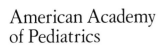

American Academy of Pediatrics

DEDICATED TO THE HEALTH OF ALL CHILDREN™

The American Academy of Pediatrics is an organization of 60,000 primary care pediatricians, pediatric medical subspecialists, and pediatric surgical specialists dedicated to the health, safety, and well-being of infants, children, adolescents, and young adults.

American Academy of Pediatrics
Web site—www.aap.org

Copyright © 2006
American Academy of Pediatrics, Updated 3/06

ADHD and Your School-aged Child

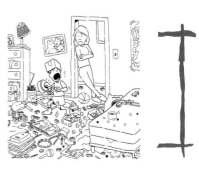

Attention-deficit/hyperactivity disorder (ADHD) is a condition of the brain that makes it hard for children to control their behavior. It is one of the most common chronic conditions of childhood. All children have behavior problems at times. Children with ADHD have frequent, severe problems that interfere with their ability to live normal lives.

A child with ADHD may have one or more of the following behavior symptoms:

- **Inattention** — Has a hard time paying attention, daydreams, is easily distracted, is disorganized, loses a lot of things.
- **Hyperactivity** — Seems to be in constant motion, has difficulty staying seated, squirms, talks too much.
- **Impulsivity** — Acts and speaks without thinking, unable to wait, interrupts others.

How can I tell if my child has ADHD?

Your pediatrician will assess whether your child has ADHD using standard guidelines developed by the American Academy of Pediatrics. Keep in mind the following:

- These guidelines are for children 6 to 12 years of age. It is difficult to diagnose ADHD in children who are younger than this age group.
- The diagnosis is a process that involves several steps. It requires information about your child's behavior from you, your child's school, and/or other caregivers.
- Your pediatrician also will look for other conditions that have the same types of symptoms as ADHD. Some children have ADHD and another (coexisting) condition, e.g., conduct disorder, depression, anxiety, or a learning disability.
- There is no proven test for ADHD at this time.

If your child has ADHD, the symptoms will

- Occur in more than one setting, such as home, school, and social settings.
- Be more severe than in other children the same age.
- Start before your child reaches 7 years of age.
- Continue for more than six months.
- Make it difficult to function at school, at home, and/or in social settings.

What does treatment for ADHD involve?

As with other chronic conditions, families must manage the treatment of ADHD on an ongoing basis. In most cases, treatment for ADHD includes the following:

1. **A long-term management plan.** This will have:
   - **Target outcomes** (behavior goals, e.g., better school work)
   - **Follow-up activities** (e.g., medication, making changes that affect behavior at school and at home)
   - **Monitoring** (checking the child's progress with the target outcomes)
2. **Medication.** For most children, stimulant medications are a safe and effective way to relieve ADHD symptoms.
3. **Behavior Therapy.** This focuses on changing the child's environment to help improve behavior.
4. **Parent Training.** Training can give parents specific skills to deal with ADHD behaviors in a positive way.
5. **Education.** All involved need to understand what ADHD is.
6. **Teamwork.** Treatment works best when doctors, parents, teachers, caregivers, other health care professionals, and the child work together.

It may take some time to tailor your child's treatment plan to meet his needs. Treatment may not fully eliminate the ADHD-type behaviors. However, most school-aged children with ADHD respond well when their treatment plan includes both stimulant medications and behavior therapy.

Is there a cure for ADHD?

There is no proven cure for ADHD at this time. The cause of ADHD is unclear. Research is ongoing to learn more about the role of the brain in ADHD and the best ways to treat the disorder. Many good treatment options are available. The outlook for children who receive treatment for ADHD is encouraging.

As a parent, you play a very important part in providing effective treatment for your child.

For further information *ask your pediatrician about* "Understanding ADHD: Information for Parents About Attention-Deficit/Hyperactivity Disorder," *a new booklet from the American Academy of Pediatrics.*

This information is based on the American Academy of Pediatrics' policy statements *Diagnosis and Evaluation of the Child with Attention-Deficit/Hyperactivity Disorder,* published in the May 2000 issue of *Pediatrics,* and *Treatment of the School-Aged Child with Attention-Deficit/Hyperactivity Disorder,* published in the October 2001 issue of *Pediatrics. Parent Pages* offer parents relevant facts that explain current policies about children's health.

The information contained in this publication should not be used as a substitute for the medical care and advice of your pediatrician. There may be variations in treatment that your pediatrician may recommend based on individual facts and circumstances.

American Academy of Pediatrics

DEDICATED TO THE HEALTH OF ALL CHILDREN™

The American Academy of Pediatrics is an organization of 60,000 primary care pediatricians, pediatric medical subspecialists, and pediatric surgical specialists dedicated to the health, safety, and well-being of infants, children, adolescents, and young adults.

American Academy of Pediatrics
Web site—www.aap.org

Copyright © 2001
American Academy of Pediatrics

what about medicines for ADHD?
questions from teens who have ADHD

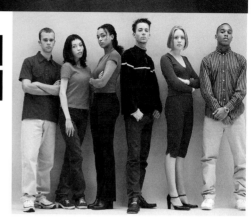

Q: What can I do besides taking medicines?

A: Medicines and **behavior therapies** are the only treatments that have been shown by scientific studies to work consistently for ADHD. Medicines are prescribed by a doctor, while behavior therapies usually are done with a counselor. These 2 treatments are probably best used together, but you might be able to do well with one or the other. You *can't rely on other treatments* such as biofeedback, allergy treatments, special diets, vision training, or chiropractic because there isn't enough evidence that shows they work.

Counseling may help you learn how to cope with some issues you may face. And there are things **YOU** can do to help yourself. For example, *things that may help you stay focused* include using a daily planner for schoolwork and other activities, making to-do lists, and even getting enough sleep.

Q: How can medicines help me?

A: There are several different ADHD medicines. They work by causing the brain to have more *neurotransmitters* in the right places. Neurotransmitters are chemicals in the brain that help us focus our attention, control our impulses, organize and plan, and stick to routines. Medicines for ADHD *can help you focus your thoughts and ignore distractions* so that you can reach your full potential. They also can help you control your emotions and behavior. Check with your pediatrician.

Q: Are medicines safe?

A: For most teens with ADHD, stimulant medicines are safe and effective if taken as recommended. However, like most medicines, there **could be side effects.** Luckily, the side effects tend to happen early on, are usually mild, and don't last too long. If you have any side effects, tell your pediatrician. Changes may need to be made in your medicines or their dosages.

- **Most common side effects** include decreased appetite or weight loss, problems falling asleep, headaches, jitteriness, and stomachaches.
- **Less common side effects** include a bad mood as medicines wear off (called the rebound effect) and facial twitches or tics.

Q: Will medicines change my personality?

A: Medicines won't change who you are and should not change your personality. If you notice changes in your mood or personality, *tell your pediatrician.* Occasionally when medicines wear off, some teens become more irritable for a short time. An adjustment of the medicines by your pediatrician may be helpful.

Q: Will medicines affect my growth?

A: Medicines will **not** keep you from growing. Significant growth delay is a very rare side effect of some medicines prescribed for ADHD. Most scientific studies show that taking these medicines has little to no long-term effect on growth in most cases.

Q: Do I need to take medicines at school?

A: There are 3 types of medicines used for teens with ADHD: *short acting* (immediate release), *intermediate acting,* and *long acting.* You can avoid taking medicines at school if you take the intermediate- or long-acting kind. Long-acting medicines usually are taken once in the morning or evening. Short-acting medicines usually are taken every 4 hours.

Q: Does taking medicines make me a drug user?

A: No! Although you may need medicines to help you stay in control of your behavior, medicines used to treat *ADHD do not lead to drug abuse. In fact, taking medicines as prescribed by your pediatrician and doing better in school may help you avoid drug use and abuse.* (But **never** give or share your medicines with anyone else.)

Q: Will I have to take medicines **forever**?

A: In most cases, ADHD continues later in life. Whether you need to keep taking medicines as an adult **depends on your own needs. The need for medicines may change over time.** Many adults with ADHD have learned how to **succeed in life** without medicines by using behavior therapies.

The information contained in this publication should not be used as a substitute for the medical care and advice of your pediatrician. There may be variations in treatment that your pediatrician may recommend based on individual facts and circumstances.

The persons whose photographs are depicted in this publication are professional models. They have no relation to the issues discussed. Any characters they are portraying are fictional.

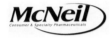

Supported by a grant from McNeil Consumer & Specialty Pharmaceuticals and partially funded by the CHADD National Resource Center on AD/HD.

From your doctor

American Academy of Pediatrics

DEDICATED TO THE HEALTH OF ALL CHILDREN™

The American Academy of Pediatrics is an organization of 60,000 primary care pediatricians, pediatric medical subspecialists, and pediatric surgical specialists dedicated to the health, safety, and well-being of infants, children, adolescents, and young adults.

American Academy of Pediatrics
Web site—www.aap.org

Copyright © 2005
American Academy of Pediatrics

what is ADHD anyway? questions from teens

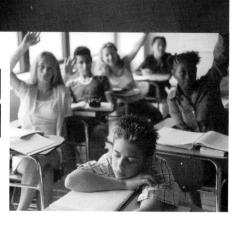

Attention-deficit/hyperactivity disorder

(ADHD) is a condition of the brain that **makes it difficult for people to concentrate.** The following are quick answers to some common questions:

Q: What causes ADHD?

A: There isn't just one cause. Research shows that

- **ADHD is a medical condition** caused by small changes in how the brain works. It seems to be related to 2 chemicals in your brain called *dopamine* and *norepinephrine.* These chemicals help send messages between nerve cells in the brain—especially those areas of the brain that control attention and activity level.

- **ADHD most often runs in families.**

- In a few people with ADHD, being *born prematurely* or being *exposed to alcohol during the pregnancy* can contribute to ADHD.

- Immunizations and eating too much sugar **do NOT cause** ADHD. And there **isn't enough evidence that shows** allergies and food additives cause ADHD.

Q: How can you tell if someone has ADHD?

A: You can't tell if someone has ADHD just by looks. People with ADHD don't look any different, but *how they act may make them stand out* from the crowd. Some people with ADHD are very hyperactive (they move around a lot and are not able to sit still) and have behavior problems that are obvious to everyone. Other people with ADHD are quiet and more laid back on the outside, but on the inside struggle with schoolwork and other tasks. They are distracted by people and things around them when they try to study; they may have trouble organizing schoolwork or forget to turn in assignments.

Q: Can ADHD cause someone to act up or get in trouble?

A: Having ADHD can cause you to struggle in school or have problems controlling your behavior. Some people may say or think that your struggles and problems are because you are bad, lazy, or not smart. **But they're wrong.** It's important that you get help so your impulses don't get you into serious trouble.

Q: Don't little kids who have ADHD outgrow it by the time they are teens?

A: Often kids with the hyperactive kind of ADHD get less hyperactive as they get into their teens, but usually they still have **a lot of difficulty paying attention,** remembering what they have read, and getting their work done. They may or may not have other behavior problems. Some kids with ADHD have never been hyperactive at all, but usually their attention problems also continue into their teens.

Q: If I have trouble with homework or tests, do I have ADHD?

A: There could be many reasons why a student struggles with schoolwork and tests. **ADHD could be one reason.** It may or may not be, but your pediatrician is the best person to say for sure. Kids with ADHD often say it's hard to concentrate, focus on a task (for example, schoolwork, chores, or a job), manage their time, and finish tasks. This could explain why they may have trouble with schoolwork and tests. Whatever the problem, **there are many people willing to help you.** You need to find the approach that works best for you.

Q: Does having ADHD mean a person is not very smart?

A: Absolutely not! People who have trouble paying attention may have problems in school, but that doesn't mean they're not smart. In fact, some people with ADHD are very smart, *but may not be able to reach their potential in school until they get treatment.*

ADHD is a common problem. Teens with ADHD have the potential to do well in school and live a normal life with the right treatment.

Q: Is it just a guy thing?

A: ADHD is **more common in guys than girls.** About 3 times more guys than girls are diagnosed with ADHD. But **more girls are being identified with ADHD.**

Q: What do I do if I think I have ADHD?

A: Don't be afraid to talk with your parents or other adults that you trust. Together you can meet with your pediatrician and find out if you really have ADHD. If you do, **your pediatrician will help you** learn how to live with ADHD and find ways to deal with your condition.

The information contained in this publication should not be used as a substitute for the medical care and advice of your pediatrician. There may be variations in treatment that your pediatrician may recommend based on individual facts and circumstances.

The persons whose photographs are depicted in this publication are professional models. They have no relation to the issues discussed. Any characters they are portraying are fictional.

From your doctor

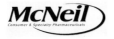

Supported by a grant from McNeil Consumer & Specialty Pharmaceuticals and partially funded by the CHADD National Resource Center on AD/HD.

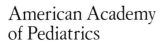

American Academy of Pediatrics

DEDICATED TO THE HEALTH OF ALL CHILDREN™

The American Academy of Pediatrics is an organization of 60,000 primary care pediatricians, pediatric medical subspecialists, and pediatric surgical specialists dedicated to the health, safety, and well-being of infants, children, adolescents, and young adults.

American Academy of Pediatrics
Web site — www.aap.org

Copyright © 2005
American Academy of Pediatrics

Allergies in Children

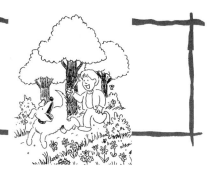

You probably know a child who has asthma or allergies. Perhaps it is your own child. Asthma, hay fever, hives, and eczema are familiar words for most of us. In fact, in the United States over 35 million adults and children have these allergy-related problems.

Allergies can be as minor as sneezing and itching. For some children, however, allergies can become very serious or even life-threatening. Whether minor or serious, allergies can be prevented and controlled. The more you understand about allergies and asthma—the symptoms, causes, and treatments—the better prepared you will be to help improve the quality of life for you and your child.

What is an allergy?

An allergy happens when the human body's natural defense system (the immune system) overreacts to an otherwise harmless substance (like pollen). There are many ways in which an allergy can exhibit itself:

- **Asthma** is when airways swell and air passages in the lungs become narrow. This may be triggered by an allergic reaction, although nonallergic triggers can be involved.
- **Allergic rhinitis** is an allergic reaction mainly in the nasal passages. It can occur in one or more "seasons" (seasonal allergic rhinitis or **"hay-fever"**) or all year long (perennial allergic rhinitis).
- **Eczema** (atopic dermatitis) is a chronic, itchy rash, most commonly found in young children. It may be made worse by certain allergies.
- **Hives** (urticaria) are itchy welts that may be due to allergies, viral infections, or unknown causes. Certain foods, viral infections, and medications are most likely to cause hives.
- **Contact dermatitis** can be just a skin irritation or an allergic reaction. The allergic type is an itchy skin rash caused by touching, rubbing, or coming into contact with things like poison ivy, chemicals, or household detergents.
- **Food allergy** is an allergic reaction to food that can range from stomach-ache, to skin rash, to a serious respiratory and medical emergency.

What causes allergies?

The causes of allergies are not fully understood. Children get allergies from coming into contact with allergens. Allergens can be inhaled, eaten, injected (from stings or medicine), or they can come into contact with the skin. Some of the more common allergens are:

- pollens
- molds
- house dust mites
- animal dander and saliva (cat, dog, horse, rabbit)
- chemicals used in industry
- some foods and medicines
- venom from insect stings

The tendency to have allergies is often passed on in families. For example, if a parent has an allergy problem, there is a higher than normal chance that his or her child also will have allergies. This risk increases if both parents are allergic.

How can I tell an allergy from a cold?

The symptoms of an allergy include:

- an itchy runny nose, with thin, clear nasal discharge and/or a stuffy nose
- itchy watery eyes
- repeated attacks of sneezing and itching of the nose, eyes, or skin that last for weeks or months
- no fever
- often seasonal (spring, summer, fall before frost)

Cold symptoms include:

- stuffy nose
- nasal discharge that is usually clear initially but can turn colored and thick
- a duration of 3 to 10 days, with or without fever
- occasional sneezing
- absence of itching

When do allergies in children first show up?

A few children show signs of allergic reactions during infancy. Other children experience their first problems during adolescence. The first signs of eczema often occur in the first few years of life. Children with asthma and hay fever usually start to show signs during preschool or at least by early grade school. For some children, allergies lessen around the time of puberty. Others will continue to have problems into adult years.

Do drug treatments help?

There are many good medicines to treat allergies and asthma. Some, like antihistamines, are available over-the-counter. They may help relieve many of the symptoms of hay fever and eczema, especially itching, sneezing, and runny nose. Other kinds of medications must be prescribed by your pediatrician. Both allergy and asthma medicines may have side effects. Some antihistamines may cause sleepiness, sometimes interfering with mental tasks. Decongestants (like pseudoephedrine) and oral asthma medications (like albuterol) may make your child irritable. Before using any medication you should talk to your pediatrician and carefully read the warnings listed on the label. If any of these medicines fail to relieve the symptoms, or if side effects interfere with rest, school, or play, you should call your pediatrician. Your child may need a different medication or dose.

When does my child need to see an allergist?

In some cases, avoiding the cause of the allergy or using medicines may not control allergic symptoms. If this happens, your pediatrician may recommend that you see a *pediatric allergist,* a doctor who specializes in hay fever, asthma, eczema, and other allergy-related diseases. The allergist will most likely:

- look for unsuspected triggers for your child's allergic disease
- suggest ways to avoid the cause of your child's allergic symptoms
- give you a specific medication plan to follow

Allergy shots may be recommended. These shots contain small but gradually increasing amounts of the substances to which your child is allergic. This binds the antibodies that cause the allergic symptoms so your child is less sensitive to these substances. Allergy shots are not effective for food allergies. Staying away from the substance that causes trouble is best. Only a small number of children require allergy shots.

How can I help my child?

If you know your child has an allergy, you can try to prevent a problem with the following measures:

- Keeping windows closed during the pollen season, especially on windy days when dust and pollen blow around and in the morning when some pollen counts are highest
- Keeping the house clean and dry to reduce mold and dust mites
- Keeping the household free of pets and indoor plants
- Avoiding foods or other substances known to cause allergic reactions in your child
- Preventing anyone from smoking anywhere near your child, especially in your home and car

You can help your child live a happy, healthy life by working closely with your pediatrician to prevent problems and by using recommended medications. Your pediatrician also can tell you about simple environmental precautions to take and help you decide if your child needs to see an allergy specialist.

The information contained in this publication should not be used as a substitute for the medical care and advice of your pediatrician. There may be variations in treatment that your pediatrician may recommend based on individual facts and circumstances.

Milk allergy

Everyone has heard of children who are allergic to ordinary cow's milk. However, milk allergy is rare. Only 1 child in 100 is truly allergic to cow's milk.

If you suspect your baby has a milk allergy, talk to your pediatrician. Be sure to mention if there is a family history of allergy. Contact your pediatrician or go to the emergency room *right* away if your child:

- Has difficulty with breathing
- Turns blue
- Is pale or weak
- Has swelling in the head and neck area
- Has bloody diarrhea

The best way to prevent a milk allergy is to breastfeed your baby for as long as possible. Very few breastfed babies develop milk allergy. This is especially important if anyone in the immediate family is allergy-prone. When you introduce other foods to your baby, do it gradually (a new one at 1- or 2-week intervals). Watch for the signs of allergy.

If you cannot breastfeed, you may need to use a milk substitute. Talk to your pediatrician about the best milk substitute for your child.

Common allergies

Condition	Triggers	Symptoms
Asthma	A wide range of things can trigger an asthma attack. These include cigarette smoke, viral infections, pollen, dust mites, furry animals, cold air, changing weather conditions, exercise, and even stress.	Coughing, wheezing, difficult breathing; coughing with activity or exertion; chest tightness.
Hay Fever	Pollen from trees, grasses, or weeds.	Stuffy nose, sneezing, and a runny nose; breathing through the mouth because of stuffy nose; rubbing or wrinkling the nose and facial grimacing to relieve nasal itch; watery, itchy eyes; redness or swelling in and under the eyes.
Food allergies	Any foods, but the most common are eggs, peanuts, milk (see information on milk allergies), nuts, soy, fish, wheat, peas, and shellfish.	Vomiting, diarrhea, hives, eczema, difficult breathing, and possibly a drop in blood pressure (shock).
Eczema (atopic dermatitis)	Sometimes made worse by food allergies, contact with allergens (pollen, dust mites, furry animals), irritants, sweating.	A patchy, dry, red, itchy rash that often occurs in the creases of the arms, legs, and neck; however, in infants it often starts on the cheeks, behind the ears, and on the thighs.
Hives	Viral infections, food allergies, and drugs (such as aspirin, penicillin, or sulfa) but cause is often unknown.	Itchy, mosquito-bite-like skin patches that are more red or pale than the surrounding skin. Hives may be found on different parts of the body and do not stay at the same spot for more than a few hours.
Contact dermatitis	Contact with a plant substance such as poison ivy or oak, household detergents and cleansers, and chemicals in some cosmetics and perfumes.	Itchy, red, raised patches that may blister if severe. Most of these patches are confined to the areas of direct contact with the allergen.

American Academy
of Pediatrics

DEDICATED TO THE HEALTH OF ALL CHILDREN™

The American Academy of Pediatrics is an organization of 60,000 primary care pediatricians, pediatric medical subspecialists, and pediatric surgical specialists dedicated to the health, safety, and well-being of infants, children, adolescents, and young adults.

American Academy of Pediatrics
Web site— www.aap.org

Anemia and Your Young Child
Guidelines for Parents
Adapted from *Caring for Your Baby and Young Child: Birth to Age 5.*

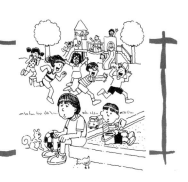

Anemia is a condition that is sometimes found in young children. It can make your child feel cranky, tired, and weak. Though these symptoms may worry you, most cases of anemia are easily treated. This brochure explains the different types of anemia and its causes, symptoms, and treatments.

What is anemia?

Anemia is a condition that occurs when there are not enough red blood cells or hemoglobin to carry oxygen to the other cells in the body. The body's cells need oxygen to survive. Your child may become anemic for any of the following reasons:

- Her body does not produce enough red blood cells.
- Her body destroys or loses (through bleeding) too many red blood cells.
- There is not enough hemoglobin in her red blood cells. *Hemoglobin* is a special pigment that makes it possible for the red blood cells to carry oxygen to all the cells of the body, and to carry waste material (carbon dioxide) away.

Types of anemia

Iron-deficiency anemia is the most common type of anemia in young children. It is caused by a lack of iron in the diet. The body needs iron to produce hemoglobin. If there is too little iron, there will not be enough hemoglobin in the red blood cells. Infants who are given cow's milk too early (before 1 year of age) often develop anemia because there is very little iron in cow's milk. Also, it is hard for young infants to digest cow's milk. Cow's milk can irritate a young infant's bowel and cause slight bleeding. This bleeding lowers the number of red blood cells, and can result in anemia.

A lack of other nutrients in the diet can also cause anemia. Too little folic acid can lead to anemia, though this is very rare. It is most often seen in children fed on goat's milk, which contains very little folic acid. Rarely, too little vitamin B12, vitamin E, or copper can also cause anemia.

Blood loss can also cause anemia. Blood loss can be caused by illness or injury. In rare cases, the blood does not clot properly. This can cause a newborn infant to bleed heavily from his circumcision or a minor injury. Because newborns often lack vitamin K, which helps the blood clot, infants generally get a vitamin K injection right after birth.

Hemolytic anemia occurs when the red blood cells are easily destroyed. *Sickle-cell anemia*, a very severe hemolytic anemia, is most common in children of African heritage. Sickle-cell anemia is caused by an abnormal hemoglobin. Children with sickle-cell anemia may suffer many "crises" or periods of great pain, and need to be hospitalized. *Thalassemia*, another hemolytic anemia, is most common in children of Mediterranean or East Asian origin. If you have a history of sickle-cell anemia or thalassemia in your family, make sure you tell your pediatrician so that your child is tested for it.

Signs and symptoms of anemia

Anemia causes the following signs and symptoms:

- Pale, gray, or "ashy" skin (also, the lining of the eyelids and the nail beds may look less pink than normal)
- Irritability
- Mild weakness
- Tiring easily

Children with severe anemia may have the following additional signs and symptoms:

- Shortness of breath
- Rapid heart rate
- Swollen hands and feet

Also, a newborn with hemolytic anemia may become jaundiced (turn yellow), although many newborns are mildly jaundiced and do not become anemic.

Children who lack iron in their diets may also eat strange things such as ice, dirt, clay, and cornstarch. This behavior is called "pica." It is not harmful unless your child eats something toxic, such as lead paint chips. Usually the pica stops after the anemia is treated and as the child grows older.

If your child shows any of these symptoms or signs, see your pediatrician. A simple blood count can diagnose anemia in most cases.

Treatment for anemia

Since there are so many different types of anemia, it is very important to identify the cause before beginning any treatment. Do not try to treat your child with vitamins, iron, or other nutrients or over-the-counter medications unless your pediatrician recommends it. This is important because such treatment may mask the real cause of the problem. This could delay a proper diagnosis.

If the anemia is due to a lack of iron, your child will be given an iron-containing medication. This comes in a drop form for infants, and liquid or tablet forms for older children. Your pediatrician will determine how long your child should take the iron medication by checking her blood regularly. Do not stop giving the medication until your pediatrician tells you it is no longer needed.

Iron medications are extremely poisonous if too much is taken. Iron is one of the most common causes of poisoning in children under 5 years of age. Keep this and all medication out of the reach of small children.

Following are a few tips concerning iron medication:

- Do not give iron with milk. Milk blocks the absorption of iron.
- Vitamin C increases iron absorption. You might want to follow the dose of iron with a glass of orange juice.
- Liquid iron can turn the teeth a grayish-black color. Have your child swallow it quickly and then rinse her mouth with water. You also may want to brush your child's teeth after every dose of iron. Tooth-staining by iron looks bad, but it is not permanent.
- Iron can cause the stools to become a dark black color. Do not be worried by this change.

Preventing anemia

Iron-deficiency anemia and other nutritional anemias can be prevented easily. Make sure your child is eating a well-balanced diet by following these suggestions:

- Do not give your baby cow's milk until he is over 12 months old.
- If your child is breast-fed, give him foods with added iron, such as cereal, when you begin feeding him solid foods. Before then, he will get enough iron from the breast milk. However, feeding him solid foods with too little iron will decrease the amount of iron he gets from the milk.
- If you formula-feed your baby, give him formula with added iron.
- Make sure your older child eats a well-balanced diet with foods that contain iron. Many grains and cereals have added iron (check labels to be sure). Other good sources of iron include egg yolks, red meat, potatoes, tomatoes, molasses, and raisins. Also, to increase the iron in your family's diet, use the fruit pulp in juices, and cook potatoes with the skins on.

With proper treatment, your child's anemia should improve quickly. Be sure to contact your pediatrician if you think your child might be anemic.

The information contained in this publication should not be used as a substitute for the medical care and advice of your pediatrician. There may be variations in treatment that your pediatrician may recommend based on individual facts and circumstances.

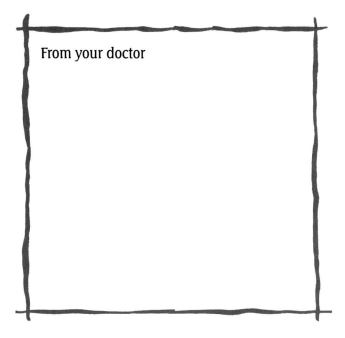

From your doctor

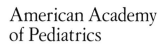

American Academy of Pediatrics

DEDICATED TO THE HEALTH OF ALL CHILDREN™

The American Academy of Pediatrics is an organization of 60,000 primary care pediatricians, pediatric medical subspecialists, and pediatric surgical specialists dedicated to the health, safety, and well-being of infants, children, adolescents, and young adults.

American Academy of Pediatrics
Web site — www.aap.org

Copyright © 1997
American Academy of Pediatrics

Asthma and Your Child

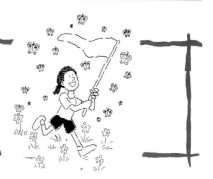

Asthma is a chronic disease of the breathing tubes that carry air to the lungs. These airways become narrow and their linings become swollen, irritated, and inflamed. In patients with asthma, the airways are always irritated and inflamed, even though symptoms are not always present. The degree and severity of airway irritation varies over time. One of the most important goals of asthma treatment is to control the irritation in the airways.

Read on to learn more about who gets asthma, symptoms, diagnosis, triggers, and treatment as well as how to communicate with your child's school.

Who gets asthma?

Asthma is the most common serious chronic disease of childhood. It is the leading cause of school absence for chronic disease. In the United States, nearly 5 million children have asthma. It can cause lots of sickness and result in hospital stays and even death. The number of children with asthma is increasing, and the amount of illness caused by asthma may also be increasing in some parts of the country. The reasons for these increases are not exactly known.

Recent studies suggest that how often and how early a child has certain exposures can influence the development of asthma. For example, children who come from large families, live with pets, or attend child care often in the first year of life are actually *less* likely to develop asthma.

Studies have also shown that a child's exposure to infections early in life can affect whether he develops allergies or asthma. Some infections seem to decrease the risk of developing asthma, whereas one infection, respiratory syncytial virus (RSV), increases the risk during childhood.

What are symptoms of asthma?

Symptoms of asthma can be different for each person. They can appear quickly or develop slowly. Some children have symptoms of asthma often enough that they have to take medicine every day. Other children may need medicine just once in a while.

A cough may be the first and sometimes only asthma symptom. Other symptoms may include

- Difficulty breathing
- Wheezing
- Shortness of breath
- Tightness in the chest
- Decreased exercise tolerance

How is asthma diagnosed?

It's often difficult, especially in young children, to diagnose asthma. After a careful physical exam, your pediatrician will need to ask you specific questions about your child's health. The information that you provide will help your pediatrician determine if your child has asthma.

- Does your child have symptoms such as wheezing, coughing, or shortness of breath?

- How often do the symptoms occur and how bad do they get?
- Is your child missing school or unable to participate in sports or other activities because of breathing problems?
- Is coughing or wheezing keeping your child up at night?
- What triggers the symptoms?
- When do the symptoms get worse (for example, with colds, allergens, exercise)?
- Is there a history of chronic runny nose or eczema?
- Which medicines have been tried? Did they help?
- Is there any family history of allergies or asthma?

If your child is old enough (usually older than 5 or 6 years), your pediatrician may also test your child's lung function. One way to do this is with a *spirometer*. This device measures the amount of air blown out of the lungs. Your pediatrician may also want to test your child's lung function after giving her some asthma medicine.

Some children don't feel better after using medicines. If medicines don't work, tests may be given to check for other conditions that can make asthma worse or have the same symptoms as asthma. These conditions include allergic rhinitis (hay fever), sinusitis (sinus infection), gastroesophageal reflux disease (heartburn), vocal cord dysfunction (spasms of the vocal cords or voice box), and obesity.

Keep in mind that asthma can be a complicated disease to diagnose, and the results of airway function testing may be normal even if your child has asthma. For some children, the tendency to wheeze with infections goes away as they get older and their lungs grow.

What are asthma triggers?

Certain things cause asthma *attacks* or make asthma worse. These are called *triggers*. Some common asthma triggers are

1. **Allergens** (Things to which your child might be allergic. Nearly all children with asthma have allergies, and allergies can be a major cause of asthma symptoms.)
   - House dust mites
   - Animal dander
   - Cockroaches
   - Mold
   - Pollens
2. **Infections of the lungs and sinuses**
   - Viral infections
   - Other infections such as pneumonia or sinus infections
3. **Irritants in the environment** (air that you breathe)
   - Cigarette and other smoke
   - Air pollution
   - Cold or dry air
   - Odors, fragrances, chemicals in sprays, and cleaning products

- Unventilated space heaters (gas or kerosene) and fireplaces
- Odors and gases released from new carpets, furniture, or materials in new buildings
4. **Exercise** (About 80% of people with asthma develop wheezing, coughing, and a tight feeling in the chest when they exercise.)

These triggers can be found in your home, your child's school, child care, and relatives' homes.

How is asthma treated?

The goal of asthma treatment is to reduce symptoms so children can fully participate in normal physical activities. This can be done by avoiding asthma triggers and providing asthma medicine. It's also important to prevent emergency department visits and hospital stays because of asthma attacks. If your child experiences asthma symptoms more than once or twice per week, let your pediatrician know.

Avoiding triggers

While you can't make your home completely allergen- or irritant-free, there are things you can do to reduce your child's exposure to triggers. This will help decrease symptoms as well as the need for asthma medicines. The following tips may help:
- **Don't smoke.** Also, don't let anyone else smoke in your home or car.
- **Reduce exposure to dust mites.** If your child is allergic to dust mites, cover your child's mattress and pillows with special allergy-proof covers, wash his bedding in hot water every 1 to 2 weeks, remove stuffed toys from the bedroom, and vacuum and dust often. If possible, use a dehumidifier or remove carpeting in the bedroom. Bedrooms in basements should not be carpeted.
- **Reduce exposure to pet allergens.** If your child is allergic to furry pets, remove the pets from the home. If this isn't possible, keep the pets out of your child's bedroom and wash them often. Consider a high-efficiency particulate air (HEPA) filter in the bedroom and if possible, remove carpeting.
- **Control cockroaches.** If you have a roach problem, always use the least toxic methods to control them. For example, you should repair holes in walls or other entry points, set roach traps, and avoid leaving out exposed food, water, or garbage. Avoid bug sprays and bombs as these could trigger an asthma attack. If these measures fail, you may need to consult a licensed exterminator.
- **Prevent mold.** Mold in homes is often caused by excessive moisture indoors. This can result from water damage caused by flooding, leaky roofs, leaking pipes, or excessive humidity. Repair any sources of water leakage. Control indoor humidity by using exhaust fans in the bathrooms and kitchen and adding a dehumidifier in areas with high humidity. The Environmental Protection Agency (EPA) currently recommends cleaning existing mold with detergent and water (though there may be debris that can continue to contribute to allergic reactions). Some materials such as wallboards with mold have to be replaced.
- **Reduce pollen exposure.** If you child is allergic to pollen, use an air conditioner in your child's bedroom, with the fresh air vent closed, and leave doors and windows closed during high pollen times. (Seasons with high pollen counts vary by region. Check with your allergist, local newspaper, or the Internet for local pollen counts.)
- **Reduce indoor irritants.** Use unscented cleaning products and avoid mothballs, room deodorizers, and scented candles.
- **Check air quality reports.** When the air quality is very poor, keep your child indoors. Check weather forecasts or the Internet for air quality reports.

Using medicines

Asthma is different in every child, and symptoms can change over time. Your pediatrician will decide which asthma medicine is best for your child based on the severity and frequency of symptoms and your child's age. Children with asthma whose symptoms occur once in a while are given medicines only for short periods. Children with asthma whose symptoms occur more often need to take controller medicines every day.

Sometimes it's necessary to take several medicines at the same time to control and prevent symptoms. Your pediatrician may give your child several medicines at first, to get the asthma symptoms under control, and then decrease the medicines as needed. Your pediatrician may also recommend a peak flow meter for your child to use at home to monitor lung function. This can help you make decisions about changing therapy or follow the effects of changes made by your pediatrician.

It usually helps to have an *asthma management plan* written down so you can refer to it from time to time. Such a plan should contain information on daily medicines your child takes as well as instructions on what to do for symptoms. A plan should also be provided to your child's school or child care. Asthma medicines come in a variety of forms, including the following:
- Metered-dose inhalers (MDIs)
- Dry powder inhalers (DPIs)
- Liquids that can be used in nebulizers
- Pills

Inhaled forms are preferred because they deliver the medicine directly to the air passages with minimal side effects.

There are 2 groups of asthma medicines: quick-relief medicines and controller medicines.

Quick-relief medicines

Quick-relief medicines are for short-term use to open up narrowed airways and help relieve the feeling of tightness in the chest, wheezing, and breathlessness. They can also be used to prevent exercise-induced asthma. These medicines are taken only on an as-needed basis. The most common quick-relief medicine is albuterol. Your pediatrician may also recommend having an oral corticosteroid medicine (pill or liquid) available should your child have a moderate to severe asthma attack.

Exercise and asthma

Physical activity is important for your child's physical and mental health. Children with asthma should be able and encouraged to participate completely in physical education, sports, and other activities in school.

Exercise can often trigger symptoms in children with asthma. It can almost always be prevented with the use of quick-relief medicines taken 10 to 15 minutes before exercise. If it occurs often, however, it may mean your child's asthma isn't under control. Proper asthma control can make a great difference in your child's ability to exercise normally. It is important for parents to speak to their child's physical education teachers and coaches about their child's asthma management.

Controller medicines

Controller medicines are used on a daily basis to control asthma and reduce the number of days or nights that your child has symptoms. Controller medicines are not used for relief of symptoms. Children with symptoms more than twice per week or who wake up more than twice per month should be on controller medicines.

Controller medicines include the following:
- Inhaled steroids
- Long-acting bronchodilators
- Combination products that contain inhaled steroids and long-acting bronchodilators
- Leukotriene receptor antagonists (only available in oral form)
- Other inhaled medicines such as cromolyn or nedocromil
  Inhaled corticosteroids are the preferred controller medicine for all ages. When used in recommended doses, they are safe for most children. In your child's case, however, your pediatrician may recommend another type of controller medicine.

Devices to help deliver asthma medicines

Medicines for asthma can be given to your child using a variety of devices including the following:
- **Nebulizer.** This may be used with very young children. This device uses an air compressor and cup to change liquid medicine into a mist that can be inhaled through a mouthpiece or mask. Controller medicines and quick-relief medicines can be given this way.
- **Metered-dose inhaler.** This is the most commonly used device for asthma medicines. Spacers, with an attached mask or mouthpiece, should be used to help make it easier to use MDIs. They should always be used with inhaled steroids.
- **Dry powder inhaler.** This device is available for some medicines. You don't need to coordinate pressing with breathing with a DPI, but its use still requires some training. It may have less taste and often has a built-in counter to help keep track of doses taken and doses left.

Because there are several different inhalers on the market, your pediatrician will suggest the one that is best for your child. There are important differences in the way they are used and amounts of medicines they deliver to the airways. You and your child will be taught how to use the inhaler, but your child's technique should be checked regularly to make sure she is getting the right dose of medicine.

inhaler

Peak flow meter

To help monitor asthma, your child may need to use a *peak flow meter.* This is a handheld device that measures how fast a person can blow air out of the lungs. Asthma treatment plans using peak flow meters use 3 zones—green, yellow, and red, like traffic lights—to help you decide if your child's asthma is doing well or getting worse. Peak flow rates *decrease* (the numbers on the

scale go down) when your child's asthma is getting worse or out of control. Peak flow rates *increase* (the numbers on the scale go up) when the asthma treatment is working and the airways are opening up.

When to use the peak flow meter (if your pediatrician has recommended one)

Check your child's asthma using the peak flow meter at the following times:
- Every morning before he takes any medicines.
- If your child's symptoms worsen or he has an asthma attack. Check the peak flow rate before and after using medicines for the attack. This will help you to see if the medicines are working.
- Other times during the day, if your pediatrician suggests.

Keep in mind, there are differences in peak flow rate measurements at different times of the day. These differences are minimal when asthma is well controlled. Increasing differences may be an early sign of worsening asthma. Also, children of different sizes and ages have different peak flow rate measurements.

Keep a record of your child's peak flow numbers each day. This will help you and your pediatrician see how your child's asthma is doing. Bring this record with you when you visit your pediatrician.

Asthma and schools

Children spend many hours at school. That is why it is so important that asthma symptoms are well managed while they are there. It's also important that you are aware of your child's symptoms and any problems with how your child's asthma is managed in school.

The following are other things to keep in mind:
- **Communicate.** Good communication is important to asthma care and management in school. You might want to meet with your child's teachers, the school nurse, and coaches at the beginning of the school year. The school needs to know about your child's asthma, how severe it is, what medicines your child takes, and what to do in an emergency. This communication can be helped by having your pediatrician complete an asthma action plan for the school, as well as a medicine permission form that includes whether your child should be allowed to carry and use her own inhaler. You should also sign a release at school and your pediatrician's office to allow the exchange of medical information between you, the school, and your pediatrician. Ask the school about its policies on how your child will get access to her medicines and how they deal with emergencies, field trips, and after-school activities. The school should also inform you about any changes or problems with your child's symptoms while she is at school.
- **Keep a peak flow meter at school.** Peak flow meters can be helpful for school staff in determining the severity of an asthma attack.
- **Check for triggers at school.** The environment at school is as important as the environment at home. Use the *How Asthma-Friendly Is Your School?* checklist to check your child's school and classroom. This checklist is available on the National Heart, Lung, and Blood Institute Web site at www.nhlbi.nih.gov/health/public/lung/asthma/friendhi.htm.

Coping with asthma at school

Talk with your child about how well his asthma is being managed in school. Also talk with your child's teachers, school nurse, coaches, and other school personnel about how well your child is coping with asthma in school.

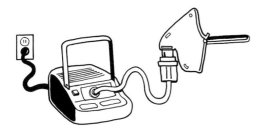

The following are some problems students with asthma may face at school:

- **Missing school** because of asthma symptoms or doctor visits.
- **Avoiding school or school activities.** Work with your pediatrician and school personnel to encourage your child to participate in school activities.
- **Not taking medicine before exercise.** Your child may avoid going to the school office or nurse's office to use his inhaler before exercise. Schools that allow children to carry their inhalers with them can help avoid this problem. This is a good idea only if your child always remembers to take his medicine and knows how to take it properly.

Remember

Asthma is a complicated yet treatable condition. By using medicines, avoiding triggers and environments that can cause asthma attacks, and carefully managing symptoms, children with asthma can lead normal and healthy lives.

The following are some things to keep in mind:

- If you are concerned your child may have asthma, talk with your pediatrician. Your pediatrician may test your child's airway function. It is important to remember that asthma is a complicated disease to diagnose, and the results of airway function testing may be normal even if your child has asthma.
- Decreasing your child's exposure to triggers will help decrease symptoms and the need for asthma medicines.
- There is no one magic medicine that controls all asthma. Sometimes several medicines need to be taken at the same time to control and prevent symptoms. Your pediatrician will choose the best medicines for your child and talk with you about when to use them.
- To help control asthma, your child may need to use a peak flow meter.
- It's important that asthma symptoms are well managed while your child is at school.

If you have any questions about your child's health, symptoms of asthma, or how your child's asthma is being managed, talk with your pediatrician.

Source: American Academy of Pediatrics, Section on Allergy and Immunology: *Pediatric Asthma Speaker's Kit.* Elk Grove Village, IL: American Academy of Pediatrics; 2003

The information contained in this publication should not be used as a substitute for the medical care and advice of your pediatrician. There may be variations in treatment that your pediatrician may recommend based on individual facts and circumstances.

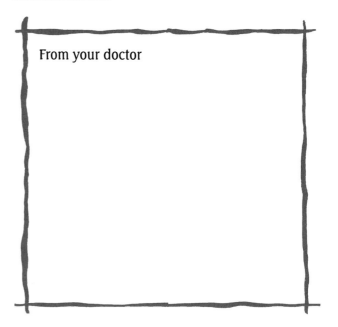

From your doctor

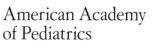

American Academy of Pediatrics

DEDICATED TO THE HEALTH OF ALL CHILDREN™

The American Academy of Pediatrics is an organization of 60,000 primary care pediatricians, pediatric medical subspecialists, and pediatric surgical specialists dedicated to the health, safety, and well-being of infants, children, adolescents, and young adults.

American Academy of Pediatrics
Web site — www.aap.org

Copyright © 2005
American Academy of Pediatrics

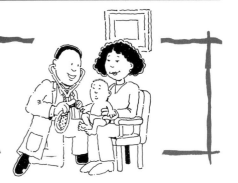

Bronchiolitis and Your Young Child

Bronchiolitis is a common respiratory illness among infants. One of its symptoms is trouble breathing, which can be scary for parents and children. Read more to learn about bronchiolitis, its causes, signs and symptoms, how to treat it, and how to prevent it.

What is bronchiolitis?

Bronchiolitis is an infection that causes the small breathing tubes of the lungs (bronchioles) to swell. This blocks airflow through the lungs, making it hard to breathe. It occurs most often in infants because their airways are smaller and more easily blocked. Bronchiolitis is not the same as *bronchitis,* which is an infection of the larger, more central airways that typically causes problems in adults.

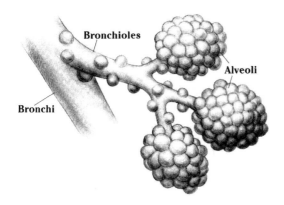

What causes bronchiolitis?

Bronchiolitis is caused by one of several viruses. *Respiratory syncytial virus* (RSV) is the most likely cause from October through March. Other viruses can also cause bronchiolitis.

Infants with RSV infection are more likely to get bronchiolitis. Most adults and many children with RSV infection only get a cold, while others may have wheezing and difficulty breathing. RSV is spread by contact with an infected person's mucus or saliva. It often spreads through families and child care centers. (See "How can you prevent your baby from getting bronchiolitis?")

What are the signs and symptoms of bronchiolitis?

Bronchiolitis often starts with signs of a cold, such as a runny nose, mild cough, and fever. After a day or two, the cough may get worse and the infant will begin to breathe faster. The following signs may mean that the infant is having trouble breathing:

- He may widen his nostrils and squeeze the muscles under his rib cage to try to get more air in and out of his lungs.
- When he breathes, he may grunt and tighten his stomach muscles.

- He will make a high-pitched whistling sound, called a wheeze, each time he breathes out.
- He may have trouble drinking because he may have trouble sucking and swallowing.
- If it gets very hard for him to breathe, you may notice a bluish tint around his lips and fingertips. This tells you that his airways are so blocked that there is not enough oxygen getting into his blood.

If your baby shows any of these signs of troubled breathing, call your pediatrician.

Your child may become dehydrated if he cannot comfortably drink fluids. Call your pediatrician if your baby develops any of the following signs of dehydration:

- Drinking less than normal
- Dry mouth
- Crying without tears
- Urinating less often than normal

Bronchiolitis may cause more severe illness in children who have a chronic illness. If you think your child has bronchiolitis *and* your child has any of the following conditions, call your pediatrician:

- Cystic fibrosis
- Congenital heart disease
- Chronic lung disease (seen in some infants who were on breathing machines or respirators as newborns)
- Immune deficiency disease (like acquired immunodeficiency syndrome [AIDS])
- Organ or bone marrow transplant
- A cancer for which he is receiving chemotherapy

Can bronchiolitis be treated at home?

There is no specific treatment for RSV or the other viruses that cause bronchiolitis. Antibiotics are not helpful because they treat illnesses caused by bacteria, not viruses. However, you can try to ease your child's symptoms.

To relieve a stuffy nose

- **Thin the mucus** using saline nose drops recommended by your pediatrician. *Never use nonprescription nose drops that contain any medicine.*
- **Clear your baby's nose** with a suction bulb. Squeeze the bulb first. Gently put the rubber tip into one nostril, and slowly release the bulb. This suction will draw the clogged mucus out of the nose. This works best when your baby is younger than 6 months.

To relieve fever

- **Give your baby acetaminophen.** (Follow the recommended dosage for your child's age.) Do not give your baby aspirin because it has been associated with Reye syndrome, a disease that affects the liver and brain. Check with your pediatrician first before giving any other cold medicines.

To prevent dehydration

- **Make sure your baby drinks lots of fluid.** She may want clear liquids rather than milk or formula. She may feed more slowly or not feel like eating because she is having trouble breathing.

How will your pediatrician treat bronchiolitis?

If your baby is having mild to moderate trouble breathing, your pediatrician may try using a drug that opens up the breathing tubes. This may help some infants.

Some children with bronchiolitis need to be treated in a hospital for breathing problems or dehydration. Breathing problems may need to be treated with oxygen and medicine. Dehydration is treated with a special liquid diet or intravenous (IV) fluids.

In very rare cases when these treatments aren't working, an infant might have to be put on a respirator. This usually is only temporary until the infection is gone.

How can you prevent your baby from getting bronchiolitis?

Although there is no way to prevent RSV and bronchiolitis, there are some steps you can take to help prevent the spread of infections, including the following:

- Make sure everyone washes their hands before touching your baby.
- Keep your baby away from anyone who has a cold, fever, or runny nose.
- Avoid sharing eating utensils and drinking cups with anyone who has a cold, fever, or runny nose.

If you have questions about the treatment of bronchiolitis, call your pediatrician.

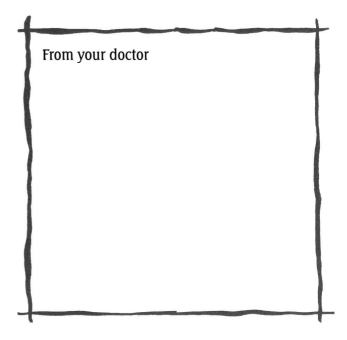

From your doctor

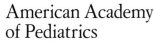
American Academy of Pediatrics
DEDICATED TO THE HEALTH OF ALL CHILDREN™

The American Academy of Pediatrics is an organization of 60,000 primary care pediatricians, pediatric medical subspecialists, and pediatric surgical specialists dedicated to the health, safety, and well-being of infants, children, adolescents, and young adults.
American Academy of Pediatrics
Web site—www.aap.org
Copyright © 2005
American Academy of Pediatrics

What is Clean Intermittent Catheterization?

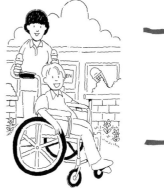

If your child cannot empty his or her bladder completely, or has a problem with urine leakage, your child may need to start a catheterization program. These problems are commonly seen in children with spina bifida, spinal cord injuries, or some urinary tract defects.

Clean intermittent catheterization (CIC) is a technique used to remove urine from the bladder. This is done by placing a thin, flexible tube (catheter) through the urethra into the bladder to drain the urine.

This brochure will help you understand the basics of CIC. It includes instructions for girls and boys. It does not take the place of one-to-one teaching. Contact your pediatrician, doctor, or nurse practitioner if you have any questions.

Why is CIC important?

Urine is the waste product that is produced by the kidneys. The bladder is the container in the body that holds the urine until it is emptied. The human body needs to empty its bladder of urine several times a day. The bladder can be drained by urinating or by using a catheter.

If your child needs CIC, your doctor will tell you how often your child's bladder should be emptied. It can be as often as every 2 to 4 hours depending on your child's condition.

CIC is especially important for the following reasons:

- **Reduces accidents.** It lets your child empty his bladder so he has fewer accidents. Older children may no longer need to wear diapers. It helps stop the odor and skin problems that come from being wet with urine.
- **Reduces the risk of urinary tract infections.** Emptying the bladder regularly reduces the risk of urinary tract infections caused by bacteria that stay in the bladder too long.
- **Reduces the risk of reflux.** Reflux is a condition where urine from the bladder goes back up to the kidneys. This can cause serious kidney damage.

What supplies are needed?

It is best to have all of your supplies organized and ready when you need them. Keep the following items in a clean, dry container such as a plastic shoe box or cosmetic case.

- **Catheters.** Your doctor will give you a prescription for the appropriate catheter size for your child.
- **Disposable wipes or a washcloth.** Your child's genitalia will need to be cleaned before CIC.
- **Lubricant.** Use only a water-soluble lubricant. You can buy the lubricant at pharmacies or drug stores. Do not use oil-based lubricants such as petroleum jelly because they do not dissolve in water.
- **Container.** You may need a container to drain the urine into if you are not doing the catheterizations on the toilet, or if you need to keep a record of how much your child drains.
- **Syringe.** You will need a syringe for cleaning the catheter.

CIC for girls

- First wash your hands with soap and water, then dry them. You also can use a waterless cleaner, such as an antibacterial cleanser that does not require water.
- Next have your box of supplies within easy reach.
- Place your daughter on her back or position her on the toilet or in her wheelchair. You should practice CIC in the position you will be using most often. If she is on the toilet, separate her legs widely enough to be able to clearly see her urethra. If she is doing her catheterizations herself, she will practice identifying her urethra by touch. When your daughter is learning to catheterize herself, she can use a mirror to see where her urethra is located.

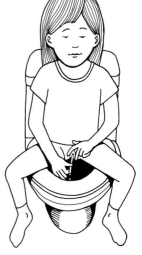

- Clean your daughter's genitalia with a washcloth or disposable wipe.
- Separate the labia and wipe thoroughly from front to back.
- Place a generous amount of the water-soluble lubricant on the end of the catheter with the holes.
- Place the other end of the catheter into a container or let it drain into the toilet.
- Find your daughter's urethra (see picture below). Gently insert the lubricated end of the catheter into the urethra about 2 to 3 inches. It may become slightly more difficult to insert just prior to entering the bladder. That is because a muscle called the sphincter sits at the opening of the bladder and is naturally tightly contracted. The sphincter will relax as you continue to gently insert the catheter until you reach the bladder and see urine flow.
- Once the catheter is in the bladder, hold it there until the urine flow stops. Then move the catheter slightly, or insert it a little more, to see if the flow continues. Gently press on your daughter's lower abdomen with your hand or ask your daughter to lean forward to be certain there is no more urine in the bladder.
- Slowly remove the catheter, holding your finger at the tip or pinching the catheter end before removing the final portion. Pull catheter out in a downward movement to prevent backflow of urine.
- Wash your hands. Clean and store your catheter as directed.

When to call your doctor

Call your doctor if your child is having any of the following problems or symptoms of a urinary tract infection:

- Fever
- Abdominal or back pain
- Pain or burning during CIC
- Less urine than usual from CIC
- Frequent need to urinate or catheterize
- Leaking of urine between catheterizations (more than usual)
- Cloudy or hazy urine with a strong odor
- Bloody urine

CIC for boys

- First wash your hands with soap and water, then dry them. You also can use a waterless cleaner, such as an antibacterial cleanser that does not require water.
- Next have your box of supplies within easy reach.
- Place your son on his back or, if it is easier for both of you, have him sit on the toilet or in his wheelchair. If he is doing his own catheter- ization, he may stand or sit on the toilet or in his wheelchair.
- Clean the tip of his penis with a wash- cloth or disposable wipes in a circular motion starting at the center and working outward. If your son is uncircumcised, pull back the foreskin so that the tip of his penis is visible before cleansing.
- Place a generous amount of the water- soluble lubricant on the end of the catheter with the holes.
- Place the other end of the catheter into a container or let it drain into the toilet.
- Hold your son's penis upright. Gently insert the lubricated end of the catheter into the urethra (see picture below) about 4 to 6 inches until urine begins to flow. You may need to lower the penis as you continue to insert the catheter. It may become more difficult to advance the catheter as you get closer to the bladder. Do not worry, this is normal. Continue to gently insert the catheter with steady pressure until you feel the catheter slip into the bladder. Once urine flow begins, insert the catheter about an inch farther to allow the urine to flow better.
- Hold the catheter in place until the urine flow stops. You may gently press on your son's lower abdomen or ask him to squeeze his abdominal muscles or lean forward to be sure the bladder is empty.

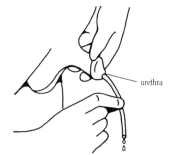

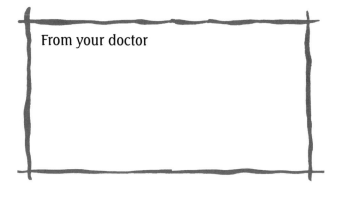
urethra

- Remove the catheter once the urine flow stops completely. Hold your finger over the end of the catheter while removing it. This will prevent any urine in the tube from dripping out.
- If your son is uncircumcised, gently replace the foreskin over the end of his penis by pushing it forward.
- Wash your hands. Clean and store your catheter as directed.

Cleaning your supplies

It is very important that you keep your child's CIC supplies clean. Make sure you wash your hands often and well whenever you perform CIC. If you are using disposable catheters, throw the catheters away after each use.

If you have reusable catheters (metal or latex-free), then you should wash them with soap and water after each use. You can use a syringe to squirt soapy water and plain water through the catheters. Rinse them completely and allow them to dry. After they are dry, store them in a plastic bag, traveling toothbrush holder, or any other clean container.

Throw catheters away as soon as they become brittle or lose their flexibility, or the holes become rough.

Remember

It may take a while to get used to doing CIC, but keep in mind that as you and your child become more used to this process, it will become easier. Talk with your child about CIC to explain exactly what you are doing. If your child is not doing CIC on his own, explain that when he is old enough he should be able to do CIC without your help. Encourage your child to be independent. And remember, it is natural for you or your child to have questions. Feel free to talk with your doctor about any questions or problems that you or your child are having with CIC. Eventually CIC can help make things easier and better for you and your child.

The information contained in this publication should not be used as a substitute for the medical care and advice of your pediatrician. There may be variations in treatment that your pediatrician may recommend based on individual facts and circumstances.

From your doctor

American Academy of Pediatrics
DEDICATED TO THE HEALTH OF ALL CHILDREN™

The American Academy of Pediatrics is an organization of 60,000 primary care pediatricians, pediatric medical subspecialists, and pediatric surgical specialists dedicated to the health, safety, and well-being of infants, children, adolescents, and young adults.
American Academy of Pediatrics
Web site—www.aap.org
Copyright © 2003
American Academy of Pediatrics

© 2007 American Academy of Pediatrics

The Chickenpox Vaccine

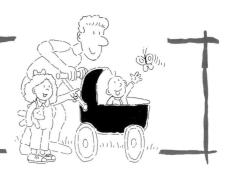

Chickenpox can be itchy and uncomfortable for your child. It was one of the most common childhood illnesses before the chickenpox vaccine was recommended routinely for infants. Anyone who hasn't received the vaccine can get chickenpox if exposed, but it occurs most often in children 6 to 10 years of age. It's also called varicella.

The most obvious sign of chickenpox is a rash of tiny, itchy blisters. Often symptoms are mild. In some cases, symptoms can be severe, especially for newborns, teens, and adults. This is why the chickenpox vaccine is important. It's one way you can protect your child from getting chickenpox.

Read more to learn about chickenpox and the chickenpox vaccine.

What are the symptoms of chickenpox?

First, a rash of tiny blisters develops on your child's scalp and body. Over 3 to 4 days this rash spreads to the face, arms, and legs. Your child may have between 250 to 500 small, itchy blisters or just a few. After 2 to 4 days, the first blisters usually dry up. Then they scab over and finally heal. Tiny sores and scars may develop. If your child scratches the blisters, they can become infected.

Your child also may have a fever and other symptoms including

- Coughing
- Fussiness
- Loss of appetite
- Headaches

How is chickenpox spread?

Chickenpox is very contagious. It's only spread from humans. After your child is exposed to the virus that causes chickenpox, it can take 10 to 21 days before symptoms appear. Your child is contagious 1 to 2 days before the rash starts and for up to 5 days after the rash appears. Your child will have to stay home from child care or school until she is no longer contagious.

The chickenpox virus may be spread

- Through the air when an infected person coughs or sneezes
- By direct contact with the fluid from broken blisters of an infected person
- By direct contact with sores from a person with shingles

Children and adults have a high risk of getting chickenpox if they have never received the chickenpox vaccine and someone at home or school has chickenpox.

How is chickenpox treated?

Acyclovir can help make the symptoms of chickenpox less severe if taken within 24 hours after the start of the rash. Most children don't need this medicine. Your pediatrician may prescribe it if your child has eczema or asthma, or is a teen.

The following are things you can do at home:

- **Remind your child not to scratch.** If your child scratches the blisters before they are able to heal, they can become infected, can turn into small sores, and may leave scars.
- **Trim your child's nails.** You can help prevent other infections by keeping your child's fingernails trimmed.
- **Relieve the itch.** An oatmeal bath may help ease the itch. Oatmeal baths are available without a prescription.
- **Reduce a fever.** Acetaminophen may help reduce your child's fever. Call your pediatrician if your child's fever lasts longer than 4 days or rises above 102°F after the third day of having chickenpox, or if your child becomes dehydrated. Let your pediatrician know if the rash gets very red, warm, or tender. Your child may have an infection that needs other treatment.

Never give aspirin or other salicylates (medicines used to reduce pain or fever) to your child unless your pediatrician says it's OK. Aspirin has been linked to Reye syndrome, a disease that affects the liver and brain, especially when given to children with chickenpox or the flu (influenza).

Can chickenpox cause other problems?

Most healthy children who get chickenpox won't have any problems. Before the vaccine was available, each year in the United States about 9,000 people were hospitalized for chickenpox and about 90 people died from the disease.

The most common problem from chickenpox is a bacterial infection of the skin. Two other problems are pneumonia and encephalitis (an inflammation of the brain). The following groups are at higher risk of developing these problems:

- People who have weak immune systems and get sick easily
- Infants younger than 1 year
- Teens and adults
- Newborns whose mothers had chickenpox around the time of delivery
- Premature infants whose mothers have not had chickenpox
- Children with eczema and other skin conditions
- Children taking salicylates

When adults get chickenpox, the disease is usually more severe. For example,

- Adults often develop pneumonia.
- Adults are almost 10 times more likely to be hospitalized than children younger than 14 years.
- Adults are more than 20 times more likely to die from chickenpox.
- If a pregnant woman gets chickenpox, her unborn baby may have problems.

When should my child get the chickenpox vaccine?

The American Academy of Pediatrics recommends 1 dose of the chickenpox vaccine for all healthy children between 12 and 18 months of age who have not had chickenpox. The chickenpox vaccine may be given to your child at the same time as other vaccines. Ask your pediatrician about when your child should get the vaccine if your child hasn't received it by 18 months of age.

Why should I vaccinate my child?

Most children who get the chickenpox vaccine don't get chickenpox. If a vaccinated child does get it, the symptoms are generally much milder (for example, fewer sores and a low fever or no fever). In fact, the disease may be so mild that the sores look like insect bites. Also, a vaccinated child may get well faster.

Aside from the health benefits, vaccinating your child could save you time and money. In general, a child with chickenpox may need to miss up to 9 days of school; parents may need to miss work to care for their child.

Is the chickenpox vaccine safe?

Many studies show the chickenpox vaccine is safe and effective. Because the chickenpox vaccine was licensed in 1995, millions of doses of vaccine have been given to children in the United States. Research is being done to see how long the vaccine protects and if a person will need a booster shot in the future.

In general, side effects from the chickenpox vaccine are mild and include
- Redness, soreness, or swelling where the shot was given
- Tiredness
- Fussiness
- Fever
- Nausea

A few children develop a rash at the spot where the shot was given or on other parts of the body. This can occur up to 1 month after the shot and can last for several days.

Who should NOT get the vaccine?

Although the chickenpox vaccine is safe for healthy children, it's not safe for the following people:
- Children with weakened immune systems
- Children with severe allergies to gelatin or the antibiotic neomycin
- Pregnant women

If you are concerned, ask your pediatrician if the chickenpox vaccine is safe for your child.

What is shingles?

Once someone has had chickenpox, the virus stays in the body of the infected person forever. About 10% to 20% of all people who have had chickenpox develop shingles. Clusters of blister-like sores develop and last for 2 to 3 weeks. People with shingles usually feel numbness and itching or severe pain. Anyone can get shingles, but it usually occurs in adults older than 50 years.

The information contained in this publication should not be used as a substitute for the medical care and advice of your pediatrician. There may be variations in treatment that your pediatrician may recommend based on individual facts and circumstances.

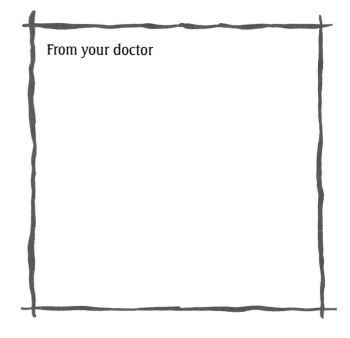

From your doctor

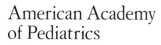

American Academy
of Pediatrics

DEDICATED TO THE HEALTH OF ALL CHILDREN™

The American Academy of Pediatrics is an organization of 60,000 primary care pediatricians, pediatric medical subspecialists, and pediatric surgical specialists dedicated to the health, safety, and well-being of infants, children, adolescents, and young adults.

American Academy of Pediatrics
Web site — www.aap.org

Copyright © 2005
American Academy of Pediatrics

Constipation and Your Child

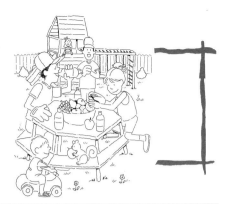

Bowel patterns vary from child to child just as they do in adults. What's normal for your child may be different from what's normal for another child. Most children have bowel movements 1 or 2 times a day. Other children may go 2 to 3 days or longer before passing a normal stool.

If your child doesn't have daily bowel movements, you may worry that she is constipated. But if she is healthy and has normal stools without discomfort or pain, this may be her normal bowel pattern.

Children with constipation have stools that are hard, dry, and difficult or painful to pass. These stools may occur daily or may be less frequent. Although constipation can cause discomfort and pain, it's usually temporary and can be treated.

Constipation is a common problem in children. It's one of the main reasons children are referred to a specialist called a *pediatric gastroenterologist*. Read more to learn about constipation and its causes, symptoms, and treatments, as well as ways to prevent it.

What causes constipation?

Constipation frequently occurs for a variety of reasons.
- **Diet.** Changes in diet, or not enough fiber or fluid in your child's diet, can cause constipation. (See "Getting enough fiber in your diet.")
- **Illness.** If your child is sick and loses his appetite, a change in his diet can throw off his system and cause him to be constipated. Constipation may be a side effect of some medicines. Constipation may result from certain medical conditions (such as hypothyroidism or low thyroid).
- **Withholding.** Your child may withhold his stool for different reasons. He may withhold to avoid pain from passing a hard stool—it can be even more painful if your child has a bad diaper rash. Or he may be dealing with issues about independence and control—this is common between the ages of 2 and 5 years. Your child also may withhold because he simply doesn't want to take a break from play. Your older child may withhold when he's away from home, at camp or school, because he's embarrassed or uncomfortable using a public toilet.
- **Other changes.** In general, any changes in your child's routine (such as traveling, hot weather, or stressful situations) may affect his overall health and how his bowels function.

If constipation isn't treated, it may get worse. The longer the stool stays inside the lower intestinal track, the larger, firmer, and drier it becomes. Then it becomes more difficult and painful to pass the stool. Your child may hold back his stool because of the pain. This creates a vicious cycle.

What are the symptoms of constipation?

Symptoms of constipation may include the following:
- Many days without normal bowel movements
- Hard stools that are difficult or painful to pass
- Abdominal pain (stomachaches, cramping, nausea)
- Rectal bleeding from tears called *fissures*

What is encopresis?

If your child withholds her stools, she may produce such large stools that her rectum stretches. She may no longer feel the urge to pass a stool until it is too big to be passed without the help of an enema, laxative, or other treatment. Sometimes only liquid can pass around the stool and leaks out onto your child's underwear. The liquid stool may look like diarrhea, confusing both parent and pediatrician, but it's not. This problem is called *encopresis*.

- Soiling (See "What is encopresis?")
- Poor appetite
- Cranky behavior

You also may notice your child crossing her legs, making faces, stretching, clenching her buttocks, or twisting her body on the floor. It may look like your child is trying to push the stool out but instead she's really trying to hold it in.

How is constipation treated?

Constipation is treated in different ways. Your pediatrician will recommend a treatment based on your child's age and how serious the problem is. If your child's case is severe, he may need a special medical test, such as an x-ray. In most cases, no tests are needed.

Treatment of babies. Constipation is rarely a problem in younger infants. It may become a problem when your baby starts solid foods. Your pediatrician may suggest adding more water or juice to your child's diet.

Treatment of older children. When a child or teen is constipated, it may be because his diet doesn't include enough high-fiber foods and water. Your pediatrician may suggest adding more high-fiber foods to your child's diet, and encourage him to drink more water. These changes in your child's diet will help get rid of abdominal pain from constipation.

Severe cases. If your child has a severe case of constipation, your pediatrician may prescribe medicine to soften or remove the stool. *Never give your child laxatives or enemas unless your pediatrician says it's OK; laxatives can be dangerous to children if not used properly.* After the stool is removed, your pediatrician may suggest ways you can help your child develop good bowel habits to prevent stools from backing up again.

How can constipation be prevented?

Because each child's bowel patterns are different, become familiar with your child's normal bowel patterns. Make note of the usual size and consistency of her stools. This will help you and your pediatrician determine when constipation occurs and how severe the problem is. If your child doesn't have normal bowel movements every few days, or is uncomfortable when stools are passed, she may need help in developing proper bowel habits.

Getting enough fiber in your diet

The American Academy of Pediatrics recommends that children between the ages of 2 and 19 years eat a daily amount of fiber that equals their age plus 5 grams of fiber. For example, 7 grams of fiber is recommended if your child is 2 years old (2 plus 5 grams).

The following are some high-fiber foods:

Food	Grams of Fiber
Fruits	
Apple with skin (medium)	3.5
Pear with skin	4.6
Peach with skin	2.1
Raspberries (1 cup)	5.1
Vegetables Cooked	
Broccoli (1 stalk)	5.0
Carrots (1 cup)	4.6
Cauliflower (1 cup)	2.1
Beans Cooked	
Kidney beans (½ cup)	7.4
Lima beans (½ cup)	2.6
Navy beans (½ cup)	3.1
Whole Grains Cooked	
Whole-wheat cereal (1 cup flakes)	3.0
Whole-wheat bread (1 slice)	1.7

You can...

- Encourage your child to drink plenty of water and eat more high-fiber foods.
- Help your child set up a regular toilet routine.
- Encourage your child to be physically active. Exercise along with a balanced diet provides the foundation for a healthy, active life.

Remember

If you are concerned about your child's bowel movements, talk with your pediatrician. A simple change in diet and exercise may be the answer. If not, your pediatrician can suggest a plan that works best for your child.

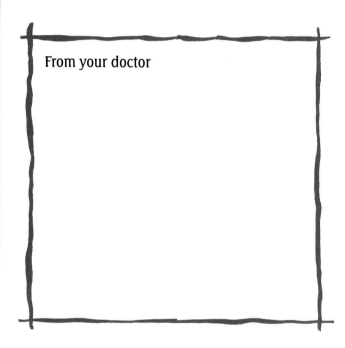

From your doctor

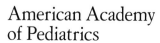

American Academy of Pediatrics

DEDICATED TO THE HEALTH OF ALL CHILDREN™

The American Academy of Pediatrics is an organization of 60,000 primary care pediatricians, pediatric medical subspecialists, and pediatric surgical specialists dedicated to the health, safety, and well-being of infants, children, adolescents, and young adults.

American Academy of Pediatrics
Web site — www.aap.org

Copyright © 2005
American Academy of Pediatrics

Inhaled and Intranasal Corticosteroids and Your Child

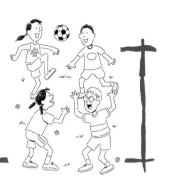

If your child has asthma or allergic rhinitis (hay fever), your pediatrician may prescribe a *corticosteroid,* also commonly referred to as a *steroid.* These medicines are the best available to decrease the swelling and irritation (inflammation) that occurs with persistent asthma or allergy. They are not the same as the *anabolic steroids* that are used illegally by some athletes to build muscles.

In general, corticosteroids are safe and have few side effects if used correctly and as recommended by your pediatrician. Millions of children have safely taken steroids to help their noses and lungs, some for many years in a row. However, you may still have concerns about steroids. Read on about the benefits and risks of this kind of medicine.

What are corticosteroids?

Corticosteroid medicine can be useful in reducing inflammation in the body. It's medicine based on cortisol. Cortisol is a substance that your body makes to control many of its functions.

The medicine works in 2 ways. *Systemic corticosteroids* must go through the body to treat the inflammation. *Inhaled* or *intranasal corticosteroids* go directly to where the inflammation is.

What will be prescribed?

Your pediatrician will decide which medicine is best for your child.

Systemic corticosteroids

May be given for a short period if your child has a bad asthma attack. In some cases, these medicines can save lives.

Form—Your child may take a pill, tablet, or liquid. Medicine may also be given by a shot or through the vein (IV).

Inhaled corticosteroids

May be given to prevent or control asthma symptoms. Inflammation inside the bronchial tubes of the lungs is felt to be an important cause of asthma. Inhaled corticosteroids work by decreasing this inflammation. Inhaled corticosteroids are the most effective long-term medicine for the control and prevention of asthma. They can reduce asthma symptoms, and your child may not need to take as many other medicines. Inhaled corticosteroids also can improve sleep and activity and prevent asthma attacks.

Form—Medicine is breathed in through an inhaler.

Intranasal corticosteroids

May be given to prevent or control a runny nose and congestion from allergies. Intranasal corticosteroids work very well in treating allergy symptoms, and your child may not need to take as many other allergy medicines.

Form—Medicine is sprayed into the nose.

Are corticosteroids safe?

In general, corticosteroids are safe and work well if the medicine is taken as recommended by your pediatrician. However, as with all medicines, you should know about the possible side effects. There are far fewer risks with inhaled or intranasal corticosteroids than with the side effects of systemic corticosteroids because much less medicine is given. The amount of medicine given in a systemic corticosteroid can be 10 to 100 times more.

Systemic corticosteroids

Side effects can be seen when a child is on this type of steroid for a short period. Side effects can include behavior change, increased appetite, acne, thrush (a yeast infection in the mouth), stomach upset, or trouble sleeping. These all go away when the medicine is stopped. More serious side effects can happen if this medicine is used often or for 2 weeks or longer. They include cataracts (clouding of the lens of the eye), weight gain, worsening of diabetes, bone thinning, slowing of growth, reduced ability to fight off infections, stomach ulcers, and high blood pressure.

Inhaled corticosteroids

There are few side effects, and they are much less common and less serious than those that occur from long-term systemic use. They may include a yeast infection in the mouth or hoarseness. The risk can be reduced using a spacer or holding chamber, rinsing the mouth after use, or using the lowest dose needed.

Intranasal corticosteroids

Side effects are not common. They may include irritation of the nose, or feeling that something is "running down the throat" at the time the nose spray is used. Occasionally, a child can have nosebleeds from using the spray. If this occurs, stopping the nose spray for a few days often allows the child to be able to restart the medicine and continue using it.

What about my child's growth?

Recent studies have shown that inhaled corticosteroids for asthma may slow down growth in some children during the first year of treatment, but this is only temporary. These children ended up with their normal expected heights as adults.

To reduce the risk of any side effects, your pediatrician will prescribe the lowest dose needed to control the symptoms. Your child's height will also be measured regularly during office visits.

Remember

Corticosteroids are the most powerful medicines available to reduce your child's asthma and allergy symptoms. They can greatly improve the overall quality of your child's life. All experts agree that the benefits of corticosteroids, when used correctly, are greater than the possible risks. Your pediatrician will make sure that they are given as safely as possible. If you have any questions or concerns about these medicines, talk with your pediatrician.

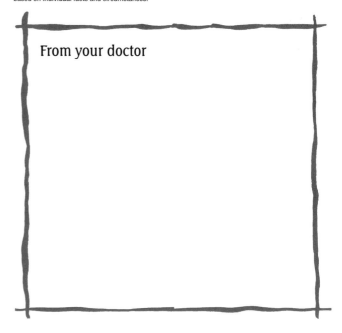

From your doctor

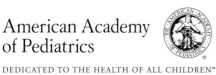

American Academy of Pediatrics

DEDICATED TO THE HEALTH OF ALL CHILDREN™

The American Academy of Pediatrics is an organization of 60,000 primary care pediatricians, pediatric medical subspecialists, and pediatric surgical specialists dedicated to the health, safety, and well-being of infants, children, adolescents, and young adults.

American Academy of Pediatrics
Web site—www.aap.org

Copyright © 2006
American Academy of Pediatrics

Croup and Your Young Child

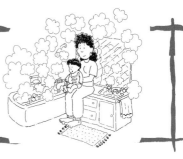

Croup is a common illness in young children. It can be scary for parents as well as children. This brochure explains the different types of croup and the causes, symptoms, and treatments.

What is croup?

Croup is an infection that causes a swelling of the voice box (larynx) and windpipe (trachea), making the airway just below the vocal cords become narrow. This makes breathing noisy and difficult.

Most children get infectious croup once or twice, and some children get croup whenever they have a respiratory illness. Children are most likely to get croup between 6 months and 3 years of age. After age 3, it is not as common because the windpipe is larger and swelling is less likely to get in the way of breathing. Croup can occur at any time of the year, but it is more common in the winter months.

Different types of croup

- *Viral croup* is the most common and is the result of a viral infection in the voice box and windpipe. This kind of croup often starts with a cold that slowly turns into a barking cough. Your child's voice will become hoarse and her breathing will get noisier. She may make a coarse musical sound each time she breathes in, called *stridor*. Most children with viral croup have a low fever, but some have temperatures up to 104°F.
- *Spasmodic croup* is usually caused by a mild upper respiratory infection or allergy. It can be scary because it comes on suddenly in the middle of the night. Your child may go to bed with a mild cold and wake up in a few hours, gasping for breath. He will be hoarse and have stridor when he breathes in. He also may have a cough that sounds like a seal barking. Most children with spasmodic croup do not have a fever. This type of croup can reoccur. It is probably similar to asthma and often responds to asthma medicines.

As your child's effort to breathe increases, he may stop eating and drinking. He also may become too tired to cough, although you will hear the stridor more with each breath. The danger with croup accompanied by stridor is that the airway will keep swelling. If this happens, it may reach a point where your child cannot breathe at all.

Stridor is common with mild croup, especially when a child is crying or moving actively. But if a child has stridor while resting, it can be a sign of severe croup.

Treatment

If your child wakes up in the middle of the night with croup, take her into the bathroom. Close the door and turn the shower on the hottest setting to let the bathroom steam up. Sit in the steamy bathroom with your child. Within 15 to 20 minutes, the warm, moist air should help her breathing. (She still will have the barking cough, though.)

For the rest of that night (and 2 to 3 nights after), try to use a cold-water vaporizer or humidifier in your child's room. Sometimes another attack of croup will occur the same night or the next. If it does, repeat the steam treatment in the bathroom. Steam almost always works. If it does not, take your child outdoors for a few minutes. Inhaling moist, cool night air may help open the air passages so that she can breathe more freely. If that does not help, call your pediatrician. If your child's breathing becomes a serious struggle or if your child looks blue, call for emergency medical services. (In most areas, dial 911.)

Never try to open your child's airway with your finger. Breathing is being blocked by swollen tissue out of your reach, so you cannot clear it away. Besides, putting your finger in your child's throat will only upset her. This can make her breathing even more difficult. For the same reasons, do not force your child to throw up. If she does vomit, hold her head down and then quickly sit her back up once she is finished.

Treating with medication

If your child has viral croup and is not breathing better after the steam treatment, your pediatrician may prescribe a steroid medication to reduce swelling. Steroids can be inhaled, taken by mouth, or given by injection. Treatment with a few doses of steroids should do no harm. For spasmodic croup, your pediatrician may recommend a bronchodilator to help your child's breathing.

Antibiotics, which treat bacteria, are not helpful because croup is almost always caused by a virus or allergy. Cough syrups are of little use too, because they do not affect the larynx or trachea, where the infection is located. These also may get in the way of your child coughing up the mucus from the infection.

If you are concerned that your child has croup, call your pediatrician even if it is the middle of the night. Also, listen closely to your child's breathing. Call for emergency medical services immediately if he

- Makes a whistling sound that gets louder with each breath
- Cannot speak or make verbal sounds for lack of breath
- Seems to be struggling to get a breath
- Has a bluish mouth or fingernails
- Has stridor when resting
- Drools or has extreme difficulty swallowing saliva

In the most serious cases, your child will not be getting enough oxygen into his blood. If this happens, he may need to go into the hospital. Luckily, these severe cases of croup do not occur very often.

Other infections

Another cause of stridor, barking cough, and serious breathing problems is acute epiglottitis (also known as supraglottitis). This is a dangerous infection with symptoms that can be a lot like those of croup. Luckily, the infection is less common now because there is a vaccine to protect against its cause, a bacterium called *Haemophilus influenzae* type b (Hib).

Acute epiglottitis usually affects children 1 to 5 years old and comes on suddenly with a high fever. Your child may seem very sick. She may have to sit up to be able to breathe. She also may drool because she cannot swallow the saliva in her mouth. If not treated, this disease could lead to complete blockage of your child's airway. If your pediatrician suspects acute epiglottitis, your child will go into the hospital for treatment with antibiotics. She will need a tube in her windpipe to help her breathe. Call your pediatrician immediately if you think your child has epiglottitis.

To protect against acute epiglottitis, your child should get the first dose of the Hib vaccine when she is 2 months old. This vaccine will also protect against meningitis (a swelling in the covering of the brain). Since the Hib vaccine has been available, the number of cases of acute epiglottitis and meningitis has decreased.

When croup persists or recurs frequently, your child may have some narrowing of the airway that is not related to an infection. This may be a problem that was present when your child was born, or one that developed later. If your child has persistent or recurrent croup, your pediatrician may refer you to a specialist for further evaluation.

Croup is a common illness during childhood. Although most cases are mild, croup can become serious and prevent your child from breathing. Contact your pediatrician if you suspect your child has croup. He or she will make sure your child is evaluated and treated properly.

The information contained in this publication should not be used as a substitute for the medical care and advice of your pediatrician. There may be variations in treatment that your pediatrician may recommend based on individual facts and circumstances.

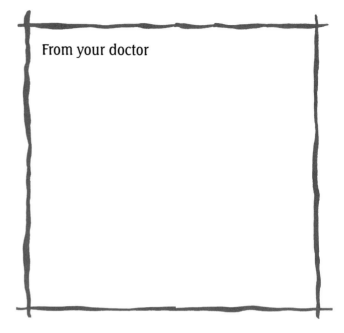

From your doctor

American Academy of Pediatrics

DEDICATED TO THE HEALTH OF ALL CHILDREN™

The American Academy of Pediatrics is an organization of 60,000 primary care pediatricians, pediatric medical subspecialists, and pediatric surgical specialists dedicated to the health, safety, and well-being of infants, children, adolescents, and young adults.

American Academy of Pediatrics
Web site — www.aap.org

Copyright © 1996
American Academy of Pediatrics, Updated 1/01

Diarrhea and Dehydration

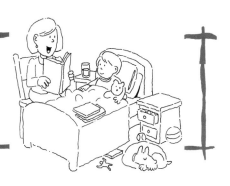

What is diarrhea?

Diarrhea is the passage of watery stools.

What causes diarrhea?

Most diarrhea in children is caused by one of several diarrhea-causing viruses and gets better by itself within a week. Although there can be many causes of diarrhea, the treatment suggested here is appropriate for acute illness (sudden onset, short lasting), which occurs most commonly.

A child with viral diarrhea has a fever and often starts the illness with some vomiting. Shortly after these symptoms appear, the child develops diarrhea. Often children with viral diarrhea "feel bad," but do not act ill.

You should call your pediatrician if your child is less than 6 months of age or has any of the following:

- blood in stool
- frequent vomiting
- abdominal pain
- urinates less frequently (wets fewer than 6 diapers per day)
- no tears when crying
- loss of appetite for liquids
- high fever
- frequent diarrhea
- dry, sticky mouth
- weight loss
- extreme thirst

It is not necessary to call your pediatrician if your child *continues* to look *well* even though there may be:

- frequent or large stools
- lots of intestinal gas
- green or yellow stools

How long will the diarrhea last?

Most of the time mild diarrhea lasts from 3 to 6 days. Occasionally a child will have loose stools for several days longer. As long as the child acts well and is taking adequate fluids and food, loose stools are not a great concern.

Mild illness and diet

Most children should continue to eat a normal diet including formula or milk while they have mild diarrhea. Breastfeeding should continue. If your baby seems bloated or gassy after drinking cow's milk or formula, call your pediatrician to discuss a temporary change in diet.

Special fluids for mild illness

These are not usually necessary for children with mild illness.

Moderate illness

Children with moderate diarrhea can be cared for easily at home with close supervision, special fluids, and your pediatrician's advice. Your pediatrician will recommend the amount and length of time that special fluids should be used. Later, a normal diet can be resumed. Some children are not able to tolerate cow's milk when they have diarrhea and it may be temporarily removed from the diet by your pediatrician. Breastfeeding should continue.

Special fluids for moderate illness

Special fluids (called electrolyte solutions) have been designed to replace water and salts lost during diarrhea. These are extremely helpful for the home management of mild to moderately severe illness. Do not try to prepare these special fluids yourself. Use only commercially available fluids—brand-name and generic brands are equally effective. Your pediatrician or pharmacist can tell you what products are available.

If a child is not vomiting, these fluids can be used in very generous amounts until the child starts making normal amounts of urine again.

Severe illness

If your child develops the warning signs of illness listed on the first page, he or she may require IV fluids in the emergency department for several hours to correct dehydration. Usually hospitalization is not necessary. Immediately seek your pediatrician's advice for the appropriate care if symptoms of severe illness occur.

Commonly asked questions:

Q. Should a child with diarrhea be fasted?
A. Absolutely not! Once she is rehydrated, let the child eat as much or as little of the usual diet as she wants. If she is vomiting, offer small amounts of liquids frequently.

Q. What about soft drinks, juices, or boiled skim milk?
A. A child with mild diarrhea can have regular fluids. But, if there is enough diarrhea to make your child thirsty, he must have special fluids (see Special fluids for moderate illness). Soft drinks, soda pop, soups, juices, sports drinks, and boiled skim milk have the wrong amounts of sugar and salt and may make your child sicker.

Q. What about anti-diarrhea medicines?
A. These medicines are not useful in most cases of diarrhea and can sometimes be harmful. Never use them unless they are recommended by your pediatrician.

Q. Which therapy is best?
A. Because diarrhea is so common, there are many different home remedies that have been tried through the years. Some of these old ideas may not be effective and some may actually make things worse. The recommendations in this brochure are based on the best information available at this time. If you have any questions about them, please check with your pediatrician

Reminder–do's and don'ts

DO

- Watch for signs of dehydration which occur when a child loses too much fluid and becomes dried out. Symptoms of dehydration include a decrease in urination, no tears when baby cries, high fever, dry mouth, weight loss, extreme thirst, listlessness, and sunken eyes.
- Keep your pediatrician informed if there is any significant change in how your child is behaving.
- Report if your child has blood in his stool.
- Report if your child develops a high fever (more than 102°F or 39°C).
- Continue to feed your child if she is not vomiting. You may have to give your child smaller amounts of food than normal or give your child foods that do not further upset his or her stomach.
- Use diarrhea replacement fluids that are specifically made for diarrhea if your child is thirsty.

DON'T

- Try to make special salt and fluid combinations at home unless your pediatrician instructs you and you have the proper instruments.
- Prevent the child from eating if she is hungry.
- Use boiled milk or other salty broth and soups.
- Use "anti-diarrhea" medicines unless prescribed by your pediatrician.

The information contained in this publication should not be used as a substitute for the medical care and advice of your pediatrician. There may be variations in treatment that your pediatrician may recommend based on individual facts and circumstances.

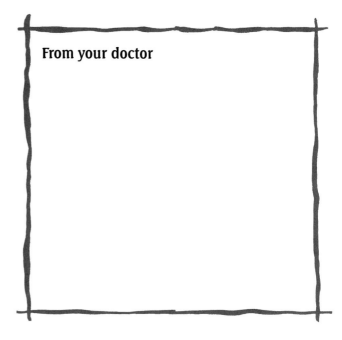

From your doctor

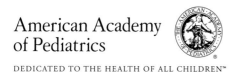

American Academy of Pediatrics

DEDICATED TO THE HEALTH OF ALL CHILDREN™

The American Academy of Pediatrics is an organization of 60,000 primary care pediatricians, pediatric medical subspecialists, and pediatric surgical specialists dedicated to the health, safety, and well-being of infants, children, adolescents, and young adults.
American Academy of Pediatrics
Web site — www.aap.org
Copyright © 1996
American Academy of Pediatrics, Reaffirmed 7/04

Acute Ear Infections and Your Child

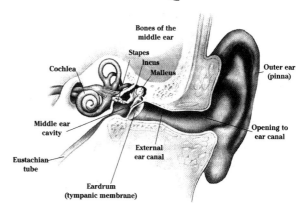

Next to the common cold, an ear infection is the most common childhood illness. In fact, most children have at least 1 ear infection by the time they are 3 years old. Most of the time, ear infections clear up without causing any lasting problems.

Read more to learn about the symptoms, treatments, and possible complications of *acute otitis media,* a common infection of the middle ear.

How do ear infections develop?

The ear has 3 parts—the outer ear, middle ear, and inner ear. A small tube (eustachian tube) connects the middle ear to the back of the nose. When a child has a cold, nose or throat infection, or allergy, the eustachian tube can become blocked, causing a buildup of fluid in the middle ear. If bacteria or a virus infects this fluid, it can cause swelling and pain in the ear. This type of ear infection is called *acute otitis media.*

Often after the symptoms of acute otitis media clear up, fluid remains in the ear. Acute otitis media then develops into another kind of ear problem called *otitis media with effusion (middle ear fluid).* This condition is harder to detect than acute otitis media because except for the fluid and usually some mild hearing loss, there are often no other noticeable symptoms. This fluid may last several months and, in most cases, disappears on its own. The child's hearing then returns to normal.

Is my child at risk for developing an ear infection?

Risk factors for developing childhood ear infections include

- **Age.** Infants and young children are more likely to get ear infections than older children. The size and shape of an infant's eustachian tube makes it easier for an infection to develop. Ear infections occur most often in children between 3 months and 3 years of age. Also, the younger a child is at the time of the first ear infection, the greater the chance he will have repeated infections.
- **Family history.** Ear infections can run in families. Children are more likely to have repeated middle ear infections if a parent or sibling also had repeated ear infections.
- **Colds/allergies.** Colds often lead to ear infections. Children in group child care settings have a higher chance of passing their colds to each other because they are exposed to more viruses from the other children. Allergies that cause stuffy noses can also lead to ear infections.
- **Tobacco smoke.** Children who breathe in someone else's tobacco smoke have a higher risk of developing health problems, including ear infections.
- **Bottle-feeding.** Babies who are bottle-fed, especially while they are lying down, get more ear infections than breastfed babies. If you bottle-feed your child, hold his head above the stomach level during feedings. This helps keep the eustachian tubes from being blocked.

Cross-Section of the Ear

How can I reduce the risk of an ear infection?

Two things you can do to help reduce your child's risk of getting an ear infection are

- Breastfeed instead of bottle-feed. Breastfeeding may decrease the risk of frequent colds and ear infections.
- Keep your child away from tobacco smoke, especially in your home or car. Also, vaccines against bacteria (such as pneumococcal vaccine) and viruses (such as influenza vaccine) may reduce the number of ear infections in children with frequent infections.

What are the symptoms of an ear infection?

Your child may have many symptoms during an ear infection. Talk with your pediatrician about the best way to treat your child's symptoms.

- **Pain.** The most common symptom of an ear infection is pain. Older children can tell you that their ears hurt. Younger children may only seem irritable and cry. You may notice this more during feedings because sucking and swallowing may cause painful pressure changes in the middle ear.
- **Loss of appetite.** Your child may have less of an appetite because of the ear pain.
- **Trouble sleeping.** Your child may have trouble sleeping because of the ear pain.
- **Fever.** Your child may have a temperature ranging from 100°F (normal) to 104°F.
- **Ear drainage.** You might notice yellow or white fluid, possibly blood-tinged, draining from your child's ear. The fluid may have a foul odor and will look different from normal earwax (which is orange-yellow or reddish-brown). Pain and pressure often decrease after this drainage begins, but this doesn't always mean that the infection is going away. If this happens it's not an emergency, but your child will need to see your pediatrician.

© 2007 American Academy of Pediatrics

Causes of ear pain

There are other reasons besides an ear infection why your child's ears may hurt. The following can cause ear pain:

- An infection of the skin of the ear canal, often called "swimmer's ear"
- Blocked or plugged eustachian tubes from colds or allergies
- A sore throat
- Teething or sore gums

- **Trouble hearing.** During and after an ear infection, your child may have trouble hearing for several weeks. This occurs because the fluid behind the eardrum gets in the way of sound transmission. This is usually temporary and clears up after the fluid from the middle ear drains away.

How are ear infections treated?

Because pain is often the first and most uncomfortable symptom of ear infection, it's important to help comfort your child by giving her pain medicine. Acetaminophen or ibuprofen are over-the-counter pain medicines that may help decrease much of the pain. Be sure to use the right dosage for your child's age and size. *Don't give aspirin to your child.* It has been associated with Reye syndrome, a disease that affects the liver and brain. There are also ear drops that may relieve ear pain for a short time. Ask your pediatrician whether these drops should be used. There is no need to use over-the-counter cold medicines (decongestants and antihistamines), because they don't help clear up ear infections.

Not all ear infections require antibiotics. Some children who don't have a high fever and aren't severely ill may be observed without antibiotics. In most cases, pain and fever will improve in the first 1 to 2 days.

If your child is younger than 2 years, has drainage from the ear, has a fever higher than 102.5°F, seems to be in a lot of pain, is unable to sleep, isn't eating, or is acting ill, it's important to call your pediatrician. If your child is older than 2 years and your child's symptoms are mild, you may wait a couple of days to see if she improves.

Your child's ear pain and fever should go away within 2 to 3 days of their onset. If your child's condition doesn't improve within 2 days, call your pediatrician. Your pediatrician may wish to see your child and may prescribe an antibiotic, if one wasn't given initially. If an antibiotic was already started, your child may need a different antibiotic. Be sure to follow your pediatrician's instructions closely.

If an antibiotic was prescribed, make sure your child finishes the entire prescription. If you stop the medicine too soon, some of the bacteria that caused the ear infection may still be present and cause an infection to start all over again.

As the infection starts to clear up, your child might feel a "popping" in the ears. This is a normal sign of healing. Children with ear infections don't need to stay home if they are feeling well, as long as a child care provider or someone at school can give them their medicine properly, if needed. If your child needs to travel in an airplane, or wants to swim, contact your pediatrician for specific instructions.

Signs of hearing problems

Because your child can have trouble hearing without other symptoms of an ear infection, watch for the following changes in behavior (especially during or after a cold):

- Talking more loudly or softly than usual
- Saying "huh?" or "what?" more than usual
- Not responding to sounds
- Having more trouble understanding language in noisy rooms
- Listening with the TV or radio turned up louder than usual

If you think your child may have difficulty hearing, call your pediatrician. Being able to hear and listen to others talk helps a child learn speech and language. This is especially important during the first few years of life.

Are there complications from ear infections?

Although it's very rare, complications from ear infections can develop, including the following:

- An infection of the inner ear that causes dizziness and imbalance (labyrinthitis)
- An infection of the skull behind the ear (mastoiditis)
- Scarring or thickening of the eardrum
- Loss of feeling or movement in the face (facial paralysis)
- Permanent hearing loss

It's normal for children to have several ear infections when they are young—even as many as 2 separate infections within a few months. Most ear infections that develop in children are minor. Recurring ear infections may be a nuisance, but they usually clear up without any lasting problems. With proper care and treatment, ear infections can usually be managed successfully. But, if your child has one ear infection after another for several months, you may want to talk about other treatment options with your pediatrician.

The information contained in this publication should not be used as a substitute for the medical care and advice of your pediatrician. There may be variations in treatment that your pediatrician may recommend based on individual facts and circumstances.

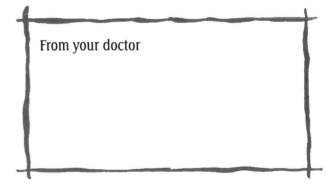

From your doctor

American Academy
of Pediatrics

DEDICATED TO THE HEALTH OF ALL CHILDREN™

The American Academy of Pediatrics is an organization of 60,000 primary care pediatricians, pediatric medical subspecialists, and pediatric surgical specialists dedicated to the health, safety, and well-being of infants, children, adolescents, and young adults.

American Academy of Pediatrics
Web site — www.aap.org

Copyright © 2004
American Academy of Pediatrics

Middle Ear Fluid and Your Child

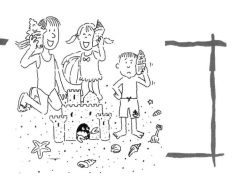

The *middle* ear is the space, usually filled with air, behind the eardrum. When a child has middle ear fluid (otitis media with effusion), it means that a watery or mucous-like fluid has collected in the middle ear. *Otitis media* means *middle ear inflammation,* and *effusion* means *fluid.*

Middle ear fluid is **not** the same as an ear infection. An ear infection occurs when middle ear fluid is infected with viruses, bacteria, or both, often during a cold. Children with middle ear fluid have no signs or symptoms of infection. Most children don't have fever or severe pain, but may have mild discomfort or trouble hearing. About 90% of children get middle ear fluid at some time before age 5.

Read more to learn about the causes, symptoms, risk reduction, testing, and treatments for middle ear fluid, as well as how middle ear fluid may affect your child's learning.

What causes middle ear fluid?

There is no one cause for middle ear fluid. Often your pediatrician may not know the cause. Middle ear fluid could be caused by

- A past ear infection
- A cold or flu
- Blockage of the eustachian tube (a small tube that connects the middle ear to the back of the nose)

What are the symptoms of middle ear fluid?

Many healthy children with middle ear fluid have little or no problems. They often get better on their own. Often middle ear fluid is found at a regular checkup. Ear discomfort, if present, is usually mild. Your child may be irritable, rub his ears, or have trouble sleeping. Other symptoms include hearing loss, changes in behavior, loss of balance, clumsiness, and repeated ear infections. You may notice your child sitting closer to the TV or turning the sound up louder than usual. Sometimes it may seem like your child isn't paying attention to you.

Talk with your pediatrician if you are concerned about your child's hearing.

Can middle ear fluid affect my child's learning?

Some children with middle ear fluid are at risk for delays in speaking or may have problems with learning or schoolwork. Children at risk may include those with

- Permanent hearing loss not caused by middle ear fluid
- Speech and language delays or disorders
- Developmental delay of social and communication skills disorders (for example, autism-spectrum disorders)
- Syndromes that affect cognitive, speech, and language delays (for example, Down syndrome)

Keep a record of your child's ear problems

Write down your child's name, pediatrician's name and number, date and type of ear problem or infection, treatment, and results. This may help your pediatrician find the cause of the middle ear fluid.

- Craniofacial disorders that affect cognitive, speech, and language delays (for example, cleft palate)
- Blindness or visual loss that can't be corrected

If your child is at risk and has ongoing middle ear fluid, her hearing, speech, and language should be checked out right away.

How can I reduce the risk of middle ear fluid?

Children who live with smokers, attend group child care, or use pacifiers have more ear infections. Because some children who have middle ear infections later get middle ear fluid, you may want to

- Keep your child away from tobacco smoke.
- Keep your child away from children who are sick.
- Throw away pacifiers or limit to daytime use (if your child is older than 1 year).

Are there special tests to check for middle ear fluid?

Two tests that can check for middle ear fluid are a *pneumatic otoscope* and *tympanometry.* A pneumatic otoscope is the best test for middle ear fluid. With this tool, the pediatrician looks at the eardrum. Tympanometry is another test for middle ear fluid. Tympanometry shows how well the eardrum moves. An eardrum with fluid behind it doesn't move as well as a normal eardrum. Your child must sit still for both tests; the tests are painless.

Because these tests don't check hearing level, a hearing test may be given, if needed. Hearing tests measure how well your child hears. Although hearing tests don't test for middle ear fluid, they can measure if the fluid is affecting your child's hearing level. The type of hearing test given depends on your child's age and ability to listen.

How can middle ear fluid be treated?

Middle ear fluid can be treated in many ways. Treatment options include observation and tube surgery or adenoid surgery. Because a treatment that works for one child may not work for another, your pediatrician can help you decide what treatment is best for your child. If one treatment doesn't work, another treatment can be tried. Ask your pediatrician about the costs, advantages, and disadvantages of each treatment.

When should middle ear fluid be treated?

Your pediatrician will decide if treatment is needed based on several factors including the following:

- If your child is at risk (see "Can middle ear fluid affect my child's learning?")
- How long your child has had middle ear fluid
- The amount of hearing loss or other problems caused by the fluid

What treatments are not recommended?

A number of treatments are not recommended for young children with middle ear fluid.

- **Medicines** not recommended include decongestants and antihistamines; prolonged, frequent, or low-dose courses of antibiotics; and steroid nasal sprays.
- **Surgical treatments** not recommended include myringotomy (draining of fluid without placing a tube) and tonsillectomy (removal of the tonsils). If your pediatrician suggests one of these surgeries, it may be for another medical reason. Ask your pediatrician why your child needs the surgery. If you are still unsure, you may want to talk to another doctor.

What about other treatment options?

No recommendation can be made regarding complementary and alternative medicine treatments, including herbal medicines, for middle ear fluid. There isn't enough evidence showing that these treatments work. Some of these treatments have major risks.

No recommendation can be made regarding allergy management treatments for middle ear fluid. There isn't enough evidence showing a cause-and-effect relationship between allergy and middle ear fluid. Also, the benefits of treatment are uncertain, there are major potentially harmful effects, and treatments can be expensive.

The information contained in this publication should not be used as a substitute for the medical care and advice of your pediatrician. There may be variations in treatment that your pediatrician may recommend based on individual facts and circumstances.

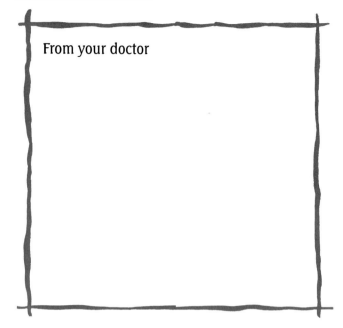

From your doctor

American Academy
of Pediatrics

DEDICATED TO THE HEALTH OF ALL CHILDREN™

The American Academy of Pediatrics is an organization of 60,000 primary care pediatricians, pediatric medical subspecialists, and pediatric surgical specialists dedicated to the health, safety, and well-being of infants, children, adolescents, and young adults.

American Academy of Pediatrics
Web site—www.aap.org

Copyright © 2004
American Academy of Pediatrics, Updated 5/04

© 2007 American Academy of Pediatrics

Your Child's Eyes

Adapted from *Caring for Your Baby and Young Child: Birth to Age 5*

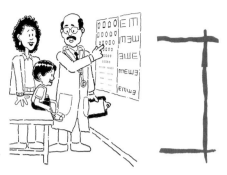

Eye exams by your pediatrician are an important way to identify problems with your child's vision. Problems that are found early have a better chance of being treated successfully. Read on to find out more about your child's vision, including signs of vision problems and information on various eye conditions.

How vision develops

A baby's vision develops very quickly during the first year of life.
- At birth babies don't have normal adult vision, but they can see.
- Newborns can respond to large shapes and faces as well as bright colors.
- By 3 to 4 months most infants can focus clearly on a wide variety of smaller objects. Some babies can even tell the difference between colors (especially red and green).
- By 4 months a baby's eyes should be straight (well aligned) and should work together to allow the development of depth perception (binocular vision).
- By 12 months a child's vision reaches normal adult levels.

Keep in mind that vision doesn't develop exactly on the same schedule in all infants, but the overall pattern of development is the same. Because visual development is so quick during the first year, early detection of visual problems is critical so that permanent visual damage doesn't occur. Because vision continues to develop even after the first year, regular eye exams by your pediatrician remain important to identify problems that may arise later in childhood.

Warning signs for infants

(up to 1 year of age)

Babies older than 3 months should be able to follow or "track" an object, like a toy or ball, with their eyes as it moves across their field of vision. If your baby can't make steady eye contact by this time or seems unable to see, let your pediatrician know. Before 4 months of age most infants occasionally cross their eyes. However, eyes that cross all the time or one eye that turns out is usually abnormal and is another reason to seek your pediatrician's advice.

Warning signs for preschool children

If your child's eyes become misaligned (strabismus), let your pediatrician know right away. However, vision problems such as a lazy eye (amblyopia) may have no warning signs, and your child may not complain of vision problems. Thus, it's important at this time to have your child's vision checked. There are special tests to check your child's vision.

Warning signs at any age

No matter how old your child is, if you spot any one of the following, let your pediatrician know:
- Eyes that look crossed, turn out, or don't focus together
- White, grayish-white, or yellow-colored material in the pupil
- Eyes that flutter quickly from side-to-side or up-and-down

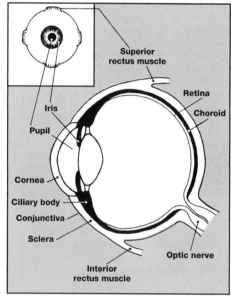

- Bulging eye(s)
- Persistent eye pain, itching, or discomfort
- Redness in either eye that doesn't go away in a few days
- Pus or crust in either eye
- Eyes that are always watery
- Drooping eyelid(s)
- Excessive rubbing or squinting of the eyes
- Eyes that are always sensitive to light
- Any change in the eyes from how they usually look

When should your child's eyes be checked?

Vision screening is a very important way to identify vision problems. During an exam the doctor looks for eye disease and checks to see if the eyes are working properly. Children with a family history of childhood vision problems are more likely to have eye problems themselves.

The American Academy of Ophthalmology and the American Academy of Pediatrics recommend that children have their eyes checked by a pediatrician at the following ages:

Newborn.
All infants before discharge from the hospital should have their eyes checked in the newborn nursery for infections, defects, cataracts, or glaucoma. This is especially true for premature infants, infants who were given oxygen, and infants with multiple medical problems.

By 6 months of age.
Pediatricians should screen infants at their well-baby visits to check for proper eye health, vision development, and alignment of the eyes.

At 3 to 4 years of age.
All children should have their eyes and vision checked for any abnormalities that may cause problems with later development.

At 5 years of age and older.
Your pediatrician should check your child's vision in each eye separately every year. If a problem is found during routine eye exams, your pediatrician may have your child see an eye doctor trained and experienced in the care of children's eye problems. Your pediatrician can advise you on eye doctors in your area.

Learning disabilities

Learning disabilities are quite common in childhood years and have many causes. The eyes are often suspected but are almost never the cause of learning problems. So-called vision therapy is unlikely to improve a learning disability. Thus, your pediatrician may refer your child for an evaluation by an educational specialist to find the exact cause.

Specific eye problems

Astigmatism.
An irregularly shaped cornea that can cause blurred vision. It's often treated with glasses if it causes blurred vision.

Blepharitis (swollen eyelids).
An inflammation in the oily glands of the eyelid. This usually results in swollen eyelids and excessive crusting of the eyelashes. It's usually treated with warm compresses and washing the eyelids with baby shampoo. Antibiotics may be needed if there's an infection.

Blocked tear ducts.
In some infants the eyes overflow with tears and collect mucus. Gentle massage of the tear duct can help relieve the blockage. If that doesn't work, a tear duct probing procedure or surgery may be needed.

Cataract.
A clouding of the lens of the eye. Most cataracts must be surgically removed. Cataracts in infants and children are rare and are usually not related to cataracts in adults.

Chalazion.
A firm, painless bump on the eyelid due to a blocked oil gland. It may resolve on its own or be treated with eye drops or warm compresses. In some cases, surgery may be needed.

Corneal abrasion (scratched cornea).
A scratch of the front surface of the eye (the cornea). It can be very painful, and the eyes usually tear and are also sensitive to light. It's usually treated with antibiotic drops or ointment and occasionally an eye patch.

Droopy eyelids (ptosis).
When the eyelids are not as open as they should be. This is caused by weakness in the muscle that opens the eyelid. If severe, it can interfere with vision and need surgery.

Falsely misaligned eyes (pseudostrabismus).
Caused by a wide nasal bridge or extra folds of skin between the nose and eye—the eyes look cross-eyed.

Farsightedness (hyperopia).
Difficulty seeing close objects. A small degree of farsightedness is normal in infants and children. If it becomes severe or causes the eyes to cross, glasses are needed.

Glaucoma.
A condition in which the pressure inside the eye is too high. If left untreated, glaucoma can cause blindness. Warning signs are extreme sensitivity to light, tearing, persistent pain, an enlarged eye, cloudy cornea, and lid spasm. Glaucoma in childhood usually needs surgery.

Lazy eye (amblyopia).
Reduced vision from lack of use in an otherwise normal eye. It's often caused by poor focusing or misalignment of the eyes. It's usually treated by applying a patch or special eye drops to the "good" eye. Other treatments commonly include glasses or eye muscle surgery for strabismus.

Misaligned eyes (strabismus).
When one eye turns inward, upward, downward, or outward. This is caused by eye muscles that are too tight. It's usually treated with glasses or, in some cases, surgery.

Nearsightedness (myopia).
Difficulty seeing far away objects. Nearsightedness is very rare in babies, but becomes more common in school-aged children. Glasses are used to correct blurred distance vision. Once nearsighted, children do not usually outgrow the condition.

Pinkeye (conjunctivitis).
A reddening of the white part of the eye, usually due to infections, allergies, or irritation. Signs include tearing, discharge, and the feeling that there's something in the eye. Depending on its cause, pinkeye is often treated with eye drops or ointment. Frequent hand washing can limit the spread of eye infections to other family members and classmates.

Stye (hordeolum).
A painful, red bump on the eyelid due to an infected oil or sweat gland. It's often treated with warm compresses and antibiotic drops or ointment.

The information contained in this publication should not be used as a substitute for the medical care and advice of your pediatrician. There may be variations in treatment that your pediatrician may recommend based on individual facts and circumstances.

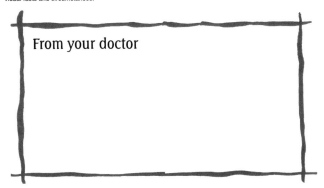

From your doctor

American Academy of Pediatrics

DEDICATED TO THE HEALTH OF ALL CHILDREN™

The American Academy of Pediatrics is an organization of 60,000 primary care pediatricians, pediatric medical subspecialists, and pediatric surgical specialists dedicated to the health, safety, and well-being of infants, children, adolescents, and young adults.

American Academy of Pediatrics
Web site—www.aap.org

Copyright © 2005
American Academy of Pediatrics

Febrile Seizures

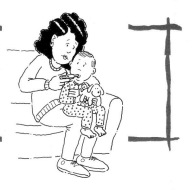

In some children, fevers can trigger seizures. Febrile seizures occur in 2% to 5% of all children between the ages of 6 months and 5 years. Seizures, sometimes called "fits" or "spells," are frightening, but they usually are harmless. The information in this brochure will help you understand febrile seizures and what happens if your child has one.

What is a febrile seizure?

A febrile seizure usually happens during the first few hours of a fever. The child may look strange for a few moments, then stiffen, twitch, and roll his eyes. He will be unresponsive for a short time, his breathing will be disturbed, and his skin may appear a little darker than usual. After the seizure, the child quickly returns to normal. Seizures usually last less than 1 minute but, although uncommon, can last for up to 15 minutes.

Febrile seizures rarely happen more than once within a 24-hour period. Other kinds of seizures (ones that are not caused by fever) last longer, can affect only one part of the body, and may occur repeatedly.

What do I do if my child has a febrile seizure?

If your child has a febrile seizure, act immediately to prevent injury.

- Place her on the floor or bed away from any hard or sharp objects.
- Turn her head to the side so that any saliva or vomit can drain from her mouth.
- Do not put anything into her mouth; she will not swallow her tongue.
- Call your pediatrician.

Will my child have more seizures?

Febrile seizures tend to run in families. The risk of having seizures with other episodes of fever depends on the age of your child. Children younger than 1 year of age at the time of their first seizure have about a 50% chance of having another febrile seizure. Children older than 1 year of age at the time of their first seizure have only a 30% chance of having a second febrile seizure.

Will my child get epilepsy?

Epilepsy is a term used for multiple and recurrent seizures. Epileptic seizures are not caused by fever. Children with a history of febrile seizures are at only a slightly higher risk of developing epilepsy by age 7 than children who have not had febrile seizures.

Are febrile seizures dangerous?

While febrile seizures may be very scary, they are harmless to the child. Febrile seizures do not cause brain damage, nervous system problems, paralysis, mental retardation, or death.

How are febrile seizures treated?

If your child has a febrile seizure, call your pediatrician right away. He or she will want to examine your child in order to determine the cause of your child's fever. It is more important to determine and treat the cause of the fever rather than the seizure. A spinal tap may be done to be sure your child does not have a serious infection like meningitis, especially if your child is younger than 1 year of age.

In general, physicians do not recommend treatment of a simple febrile seizure with preventive medications. However, this should be discussed with your pediatrician. In cases of prolonged or repeated seizures, the recommendation may be different.

Anti-fever drugs like acetaminophen and ibuprofen can help lower a fever, but they do not prevent febrile seizures. Your pediatrician will talk to you about the best ways to take care of your child's fever.

If your child has had a febrile seizure, do not fear the worst. These types of seizures are not dangerous to your child and do not cause long-term health problems. If you have concerns about this issue or anything related to your child's health, talk to your pediatrician.

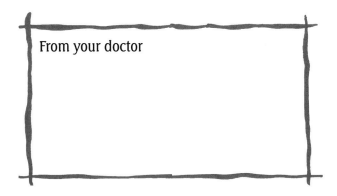

From your doctor

American Academy of Pediatrics

DEDICATED TO THE HEALTH OF ALL CHILDREN™

The American Academy of Pediatrics is an organization of 60,000 primary care pediatricians, pediatric medical subspecialists, and pediatric surgical specialists dedicated to the health, safety, and well-being of infants, children, adolescents, and young adults.

American Academy of Pediatrics
Web site — www.aap.o

Copyright © 1999
American Academy of Pediatrics

Fever and Your Child

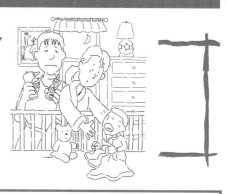

If your child has a fever, it is probably a sign that her body is fighting an infection. When your child becomes ill because of a virus or bacteria, her body may respond by increasing body temperature. It is important to remember that, except in the case of heat stroke, fever itself is not an illness—only a symptom of one. Fever itself also is not a sign that your child needs an antibiotic.

Many conditions, such as an ear infection, a common cold, the flu, a urinary tract infection, or pneumonia, may cause a child to develop a fever. In some cases, medication, injury, poison, or an extreme level of overactivity may produce a fever. An environment that is too hot may result in heat stroke, a potentially dangerous rise in body temperature. It is important to look for the cause of the fever.

Fevers are generally harmless and help your child fight infection. They can be considered a good sign that your child's immune system is working and the body is trying to rid itself of the infection.

The main purpose for treating fever is to help your child feel better. Reducing her temperature may make her more comfortable until the illness that has caused the fever has been treated or, more likely, run its course.

What is a fever?

A fever is a body temperature that is higher than normal. Your child's normal body temperature varies with his age, general health, activity level, the time of day, and how much clothing he is wearing. Everyone's temperature tends to be lower early in the morning and higher between late afternoon and early evening. Body temperature also will be slightly higher with strenuous exercise.

Most pediatricians consider any thermometer reading above **100.4°F (38°C)** a sign of a fever. This number may vary depending on the method used for taking your child's temperature. If you call your pediatrician, say which method you used.

Signs and symptoms of a fever

If your child has a fever, her heart and breathing rates naturally will speed up. You may notice that your child feels warm. She may appear flushed or perspire more than usual. Her body also will require more fluids.

Some children feel fine when they have a fever. However, most will have symptoms of the illness that is causing the fever. Your child may have an earache,

When to call your pediatrician right away

Call your pediatrician immediately if your child has a fever and
- Looks very ill, is unusually drowsy, or is very fussy
- Has been in an extremely hot place, such as an overheated car
- Has additional symptoms such as a stiff neck, severe headache, severe sore throat, severe ear pain, an unexplained rash, or repeated vomiting or diarrhea
- Has a condition that suppresses immune responses, such as sickle-cell disease or cancer, or is taking steroids
- Has had a seizure
- Is younger than 2 months of age and has a rectal temperature of 100.4°F (38°C) or higher

What if my child has a febrile seizure?

In some young children, fever can trigger seizures. These are usually harmless. However, they can be frightening. When this happens, your child may look strange for a few minutes, shake, then stiffen, twitch, and roll his eyes.
- Place him on the floor or bed, away from any hard or sharp objects.
- Turn his head to the side so that any saliva or vomit can drain from his mouth.
- Do not put anything into his mouth.
- Call your pediatrician.

Your pediatrician should always examine your child after a febrile seizure, especially if it is his first one. It is important to look for the cause of the febrile seizure.

a sore throat, a rash, or a stomachache. These signs can provide important clues as to the cause of your child's fever.

Managing a mild fever

A child older than 6 months of age who has a temperature below 101°F (38.3°C) probably does not need to be treated for fever, unless the child is uncomfortable. Observe her behavior. If she is eating and sleeping well and is able to play, you may wait to see if the fever improves by itself.

In the meantime,
- Keep her room comfortably cool.
- Make sure that she is dressed in light clothing.
- Encourage her to drink fluids such as water, diluted fruit juices, or a commercially prepared oral electrolyte solution.
- Be sure that she does not overexert herself.

Over-the-counter medications for fever

There are also medications you can give your child to reduce his temperature if he is uncomfortable. Both **acetaminophen** and **ibuprofen** are safe and effective in proper doses. Be sure to follow the correct dosage and medication schedule for your child. Remember, any medication can be dangerous if you give your child too much.

Ibuprofen should only be used for children older than 6 months of age. It should not be given to children who are vomiting constantly or are dehydrated. *Do not use aspirin to treat your child's fever. Aspirin has been linked with side effects such as an upset stomach, intestinal bleeding, and, most seriously, Reye syndrome.*

If your child is vomiting and unable to take medication by mouth, your pediatrician may recommend a rectal suppository for your child. Acetaminophen suppositories can be effective in reducing fever in a vomiting child.

Read the label on all medications to make sure that your child receives the right dose for his age and weight. To be safe, talk to your pediatrician before giving your child any medication to treat fever if he is younger than 2 years of age.

How to take your child's temperature

While you often can tell if your child is warmer than usual by feeling his forehead, only a thermometer can tell if he has a fever and how high the temperature is. There are several types of thermometers and methods for taking your child's temperature.

Mercury thermometers should not be used. The American Academy of Pediatrics (AAP) encourages parents to remove mercury thermometers from their homes to prevent accidental exposure to this toxin.

Rectal: If your child is younger than 3 years of age, taking his temperature with a rectal digital thermometer provides the best reading.

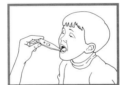

- Clean the end of the thermometer with rubbing alcohol or soap and water. Rinse it with cool water. Do not rinse with hot water.
- Put a small amount of lubricant, such as petroleum jelly, on the end.
- Place your child belly down across your lap or on a firm surface. Hold him by placing your palm against his lower back, just above his bottom.
- With the other hand, turn on the thermometer switch and insert the thermometer 0.5" to 1" into the anal opening. Hold the thermometer in place loosely with 2 fingers, keeping your hand cupped around your child's bottom. Do not insert the thermometer too far. Hold in place for about 1 minute, until you hear the "beep." Remove the thermometer to check the digital reading.

Oral: Once your child is 4 or 5 years of age, you may prefer taking his temperature by mouth with an oral digital thermometer.

- Clean the thermometer with lukewarm soapy water or rubbing alcohol. Rinse with cool water.

- Turn on the switch and place the sensor under his tongue toward the back of his mouth. Hold in place for about 1 minute, until you hear the "beep." Check the digital reading.
- For a correct reading, wait at least 15 minutes after your child has had a hot or cold drink before putting the thermometer in his mouth.

Ear: Tympanic thermometers, which measure temperature inside the ear, are another option for older babies and children.

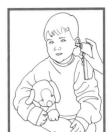

- Gently put the end of the thermometer in the ear canal. Press the start button. You will get a digital reading of your child's temperature within seconds.
- While it provides quick results, this thermometer needs to be placed correctly in your child's ear to be accurate. Too much earwax may cause the reading to be incorrect.

Underarm (Axillary): Although not as accurate, if your child is older than 3 months of age, you can take his underarm temperature to see if he has a fever.

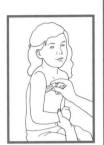

- Place the sensor end of either an oral or rectal digital thermometer in your child's armpit.
- Hold his arm tightly against his chest for about 1 minute, until you hear the "beep." Check the digital reading.

Other methods for taking your child's temperature are available. They are not recommended at this time. Ask your pediatrician for advice.

Sponging

Your pediatrician may recommend that you try sponging your child with lukewarm water in cases such as the following:
- Your child's temperature is above 104°F (40°C).
- She is vomiting and unable to take medication.
- She has had a febrile seizure in the past (see "What if my child has a febrile seizure?").

Sponging may reduce your child's temperature as water evaporates from her skin. Your pediatrician can advise you on this method.

Do not use cold water to sponge your child, as this could cause shivering. That could increase her temperature. Never add alcohol to the water. Alcohol can be absorbed into the skin or inhaled, causing serious problems such as a coma.

Usually 5 to 10 minutes in the tub is enough time for a child's temperature to start dropping. If your child becomes upset during the sponging, simply let her play in the water. If she is still bothered by the bath, it is better to remove her even if she has not been in long enough to reduce her temperature. Also remove her from the bath if she continues to shiver because shivering may increase body temperature.

Do not try to reduce your child's temperature to normal too quickly. This could cause the temperature to rebound higher.

Be sure to call your pediatrician if your child still "acts sick" once her temperature is brought down, or if you feel that your child is very sick. Also call if the fever persists for
- More than 24 hours in a child younger than 2 years of age
- More than 3 days in a child 2 years of age or older

The information contained in this publication should not be used as a substitute for the medical care and advice of your pediatrician. There may be variations in treatment that your pediatrician may recommend based on individual facts and circumstances.

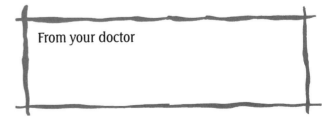

From your doctor

American Academy of Pediatrics

DEDICATED TO THE HEALTH OF ALL CHILDREN™

The American Academy of Pediatrics is an organization of 60,000 primary care pediatricians, pediatric medical subspecialists, and pediatric surgical specialists dedicated to the health, safety, and well-being of infants, children, adolescents, and young adults.

American Academy of Pediatrics
Web site — www.aap.org

Copyright © 2001
American Academy of Pediatrics

Haemophilus influenzae type b

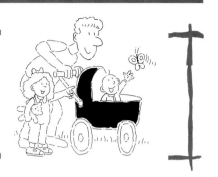

The continued occurance of preventable childhood diseases emphasizes the necessity of vaccination for all children. Regular medical care includes vaccinations, which are an important part of your child's total health care.

This brochure explains why it's important to make sure your child is vaccinated on time. Without protection provided by the Hib conjugate vaccines (*Haemophilus influenzae* type b conjugate vaccines), your child could suffer from serious illnesses that could have been prevented.

What is this disease?

Haemophilus influenzae type b is a germ (or bacterium) that can cause several kinds of dangerous infections in children. It is very different from the "flu" (influenza virus).

Why are the *H influenzae* vaccines so important for infants?

These vaccines provide protection during the first years of life, when it is easiest for your child to get *H influenzae* type b infection. When children are fully immunized with the *H influenzae* type B vaccine, they are protected against the illnesses caused by the *H influenzae* type b germ.

Without timely immunizations, your child faces the risk of becoming very sick with serious diseases such as:

- Meningitis, a serious infection of the covering of the brain and spinal cord. Before the vaccine was used, *H influenzae* type b was the most common cause of bacterial meningitis in the United States. It caused about 12,000 cases of meningitis each year in children younger than 5 years of age—especially in babies 6 to 12 months old. Of those children infected, 1 in 20 died from this disease, and 1 in 4 developed permanent brain damage.
- Epiglottitis, a dangerous throat infection that can cause a child to choke to death if not treated immediately.
- Pneumonia and serious infections in the blood, bones, joints, skin, and the covering of the heart.

When should my child get the Hib conjugate vaccines?

The immunization schedule will vary depending on which vaccine your child receives and at what age the series was started. The American Academy of Pediatrics (AAP) recommends that your child receive two or three doses of the vaccine between 2 to 6 months of age and a booster dose at 12 to 15 months. Your child's pediatrician will tell you about the different Hib vaccines available and the recommended immunization schedule for each.

Are there side effects to Hib conjugate vaccines?

Most children have no side effects with the Hib conjugate vaccines. There have been no serious reactions linked to these vaccines. Those side effects that sometimes occur are mild and temporary. The possible side effects include:

- Soreness, swelling, or redness where the shot was given
- A mild to moderate fever
- Fussiness

These symptoms may begin within 24 hours after the shot is given and usually go away within 48 to 72 hours.

Talk to your pediatrician about the possible reactions to these immunizations and when to call his or her office for more details. As with any medical problems, call your doctor promptly if you are concerned.

Other information...

Your pediatrician can tell you more about other vaccines your child needs to stay healthy.

Immunizations have provided protection for children for years—but the vaccines only work if *you* make sure your child gets immunized.

Remember…your child's health depends on it!

Immunization is just one important part of preventive health care for children. The American Academy of Pediatrics, representing the nation's pediatricians, is dedicated to working toward a better future for our children. Join us by making sure your children receive the best possible health care.

The information contained in this publication should not be used as a substitute for the medical care and advice of your pediatrician. There may be variations in treatment that your pediatrician may recommend based on individual facts and circumstances.

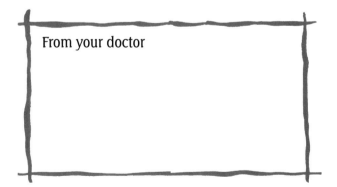

From your doctor

American Academy of Pediatrics

DEDICATED TO THE HEALTH OF ALL CHILDREN™

The American Academy of Pediatrics is an organization of 60,000 primary care pediatricians, pediatric medical subspecialists, and pediatric surgical specialists dedicated to the health, safety, and well-being of infants, children, adolescents, and young adults.

American Academy of Pediatrics
Web site—www.aap.org

Copyright © 1997
American Academy of Pediatrics, Updated 11/98

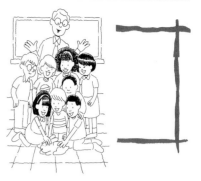

Head Lice:
Every Parent's Concern

Head lice are a common problem and concern among many parents. If your child is in school or attends child care you will probably receive a note at some point reporting a case of head lice in your child's classroom. Every year in the United States, 6 to 12 million school-aged children get head lice.

Fortunately, head lice are not a serious medical problem, and they do not carry any diseases.

Anyone can get head lice. Despite what many people may think, head lice are not a sign of poor hygiene or an unclean home environment.

It can be difficult to tell if your child has an active case of head lice. That is why it is important for parents to be informed. Parents should know what head lice are and what to do if their child gets them.

Correctly identifying and treating the problem can save children from unnecessary embarrassment and days lost from school.

What are lice?

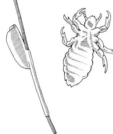

Head lice are insects found only on human hair. They feed on human blood—much like mosquitoes. Adult head lice have cigar-shaped bodies. Across their middles are small indentations. They are about 2 mm to 3 mm long (about the size of a sesame seed). Their bodies have dark and light areas, which help them blend in with the color of the hair.

Head lice lay eggs and attach them to hair close to the scalp. The eggs and their shell casings are called *nits*. They are attached with a gluelike substance that holds them in place until they hatch. The empty eggshells remain attached to the hair and are not easily removed.

Newly hatched lice are called *nymphs*. It only takes about 12 days for nymphs to reach adulthood. Adult lice only live about 28 days, but the females can lay up to 10 eggs a day, starting a new generation of lice.

How do children get head lice?

Close, head-to-head contact is the primary way head lice spread from one child to another. However, because head lice are crawling insects that do not fly or hop from head to head, contact must be quite close for the lice to spread. Head lice can also be spread from sharing items such as combs, brushes, and hats, although this is a less likely way for them to spread.

Despite what many people think, the length of hair and how often it is brushed or shampooed do not affect the spread of head lice.

Who gets head lice?

Head lice affect everyone. It makes little difference where children live or to which ethnicity they belong, although head lice are less common in black children in the United States (most likely due to the shape of their hair shafts).

In addition, girls seem to get head lice more often than boys. This is probably due to the way girls and boys play. Girls tend to play close together while boys are often more active and play farther apart.

Symptoms of head lice

The most common symptom of head lice is itching, especially behind the ears or at the back of the neck. However, an itchy scalp may also be a symptom of other conditions such as eczema, dandruff, or allergic reactions to hair products.

Head lice are often difficult to find. A positive diagnosis of an active case of head lice can only be made if you find live lice. Nits can remain on the hair for months but do not indicate an active infestation.

How to check for head lice

To check your child for head lice, follow these steps

- Seat your child in a brightly lit room, in an area where you can easily examine the head from different angles.
- Part the hair and look at your child's scalp. Nits will look like small white or yellow-brown specks. They will be firmly attached to the hair. Nits may be easier to see at the hairline at the back of the neck or behind the ears. Live lice will move quickly away from the light.
- Comb through your child's hair in small sections using a fine-tooth comb. After each comb-through, wipe the comb on a wet paper towel. Examine the scalp, comb, and paper towel carefully.

You may need to use a magnifying glass. It is often difficult to tell the difference between dandruff or other hair debris and nits. However, dandruff is much easier to comb out of the hair while nits are much harder to remove.

Treatment for head lice

In the past, the only way to get rid of head lice was to comb them out or, in some cases, shave the child's head. Today, chemical treatments for head lice are available and can be found at your local drug or discount store. Most of these products contain 1% permethrin as a cream rinse, which has proven to be a very effective treatment for head lice. Although head lice treatments also are available by prescription, they are not usually the first choice for treating head lice.

In general, there are 3 steps in treating head lice. Because it is possible for head lice to show resistance to these treatments, see your pediatrician if you have followed these steps but your child still has live lice.

Step 1: Kill the lice.

Head lice treatments come in a variety of forms such as shampoo, cream rinse, gel, and mousse. Most need to be applied to dry hair because wet hair can dilute the chemicals in the treatment. Keep the treatment on the hair for the full amount of time recommended by the manufacturer. While lice treatments are effective at killing live lice, they may not always kill all of the eggs. For this reason, a second treatment is usually necessary 7 to 10 days after the first treatment.

Step 2: Comb out the nits.

This step is not necessary to prevent lice from spreading; however, it may make you and your child feel better knowing the nits are removed. It may also prevent your child from being misdiagnosed with an active case of head lice. And it will help prevent your child from becoming reinfested from any eggs that were not killed at first.

Nits can be combed out after the treatment has been applied to the hair. Many products include a special comb. Carefully read the directions that come with the treatment for proper combing instructions.

Combing out the nits often takes a great deal of time and patience. During this step you may want to give your child something to do, such as a book to read.

Continue to check your child's hair daily for 2 weeks after treatment. If you still see nits in your child's hair, use a fine-tooth comb (or try using your fingernail) to remove them.

Step 3: Prevent lice from spreading.

You do not need to throw away any items belonging to your child, but you may want to follow these prevention tips

- Wash your child's clothes, towels, hats, and bed linens in hot water and dry on high heat.
- Soak combs and brushes in boiling hot water for 5 to 10 minutes.
- Vacuum furniture, carpeting, car seats, and other fabrics that your child was in contact with 24 to 48 hours before treatment.
- Items that your child has been in very close contact with that cannot be washed, such as stuffed animals or toys, can be placed in a plastic bag for 2 weeks (by which time any live lice would die).
- Do not spray pesticides in your home because they can expose your family to dangerous chemicals.
- Check other members of your household for lice and, if present, treat these persons and manage their personal items as outlined previously.

Remember that live lice cannot live more than 24 to 48 hours off the head, so extraordinary cleaning measures are usually not necessary. It is better to spend the time properly treating the child with head lice.

Home remedies

You may have heard of home remedies that involve "washing" your child's hair with thick or oily substances such as petroleum jelly, mayonnaise, tub margarine, herbal oils, or olive oil and leaving it on the hair overnight (the child sleeps wearing a shower cap). The theory is that coating the hair with these substances will smother the lice. These remedies have not been scientifically proven to work. However, they certainly won't hurt your child. Home treatments that should be avoided include coating your child's hair with any toxic or highly flammable substances such as gasoline or kerosene, or using products that are intended for use on animals.

Remember

While having head lice may be embarrassing to you or your child, it does not put your child at risk for any serious health problems. If your child has head lice, work quickly to treat the condition and prevent the lice from spreading. You may need to repeat the treatment to ensure all the lice are gone. If you are unsure about how to detect head lice, suspect your child has lice, have tried to treat a case of head lice only to have them return, or have additional questions about treating head lice, call your pediatrician.

Head lice and school

Some schools routinely check students for lice. This can be very time consuming and cause children to miss valuable classroom time. Also, it is only effective if the person doing the checking knows what live head lice look like. An inexperienced person can mistake other scalp conditions for lice.

If you have been told that your child has head lice, and you can't find any, ask your school nurse or pediatrician for help—this way you will know what you are looking for next time. Remember that if your child has recently been treated for lice and only has nits remaining, further treatment is not necessary—just pick out the nits. If they are more than half an inch from the scalp, they are no longer alive. However, if they are closer, they could hatch and cause another infestation.

Healthy children should not be excluded from, or allowed to miss, school because of head lice. Most cases of head lice begin a month or more before they are discovered. Therefore it makes little sense to remove the child once the lice have been found. Instead, children with head lice could remain in class, but be discouraged from close or direct head contact with others. Otherwise, some children can end up missing weeks of school because of head lice.

In addition, many schools have "no nit" policies that do not allow children to return to school until all visible nits are gone. These policies are not effective because the presence of nits is not the same as having an active case of head lice. Also, because nits are often difficult to remove, some can remain in the hair for months. As a result, "no nit" policies often lead to unnecessary treatments, missed school, and loss of work for parents. For more information on the American Academy of Pediatrics' position on "no nit" policies, visit our Web site at www.aap.org.

The information contained in this publication should not be used as a substitute for the medical care and advice of your pediatrician. There may be variations in treatment that your pediatrician may recommend based on individual facts and circumstances.

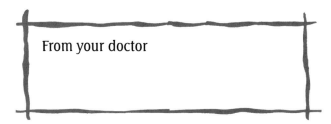

From your doctor

American Academy
of Pediatrics

DEDICATED TO THE HEALTH OF ALL CHILDREN™

The American Academy of Pediatrics is an organization of 60,000 primary care pediatricians, pediatric medical subspecialists, and pediatric surgical specialists dedicated to the health, safety, and well-being of infants, children, adolescents, and young adults.

American Academy of Pediatrics
Web site—www.aap.org

Copyright © 2003
American Academy of Pediatrics

Important Information for Teens Who Get Headaches

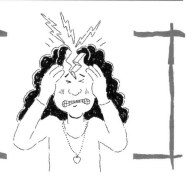

A headache is not a disease, but it may indicate that something is wrong. Headaches are common among teenagers and generally are not serious. In fact, 50% to 75% of all teens report having at least one headache per month. However, more frequent headaches can be upsetting and worrisome for you and your family. The most common headaches for teenagers are tension headaches and migraines. Sometimes these problems may be associated with health concerns that require a visit to your pediatrician.

What causes headaches?

Headaches are most commonly caused by:

Illness—Headaches often are a symptom of other illnesses. Viral infections, strep throat, allergies, sinus infections, and urinary tract infections can be accompanied by headaches. Fever may also be associated with headaches.

Skipping meals—Even if you're trying to lose weight, you still need to eat regularly. Fad diets can make you hungry and also can give you a headache. Not getting enough fluids—which leads to dehydration—also may cause a headache.

Drugs—Alcohol, cocaine, amphetamines, diet pills, and other drugs may give you a headache.

Often headaches are triggered by sleep problems, minor head injuries, or certain foods (dairy products, chocolate, food additives like nitrates, nitrites, and monosodium glutamate).

Sometimes, headaches can also be caused by prescribed medication, such as birth control pills, tetracycline for acne, and high doses of vitamin A.

Less commonly, headaches can be caused by a dental infection or abscess, and jaw alignment problems (TMJ syndrome). Although headaches are only rarely caused by eye problems, pain around the eyes—which can feel like a headache—can be caused by eye muscle imbalance or not wearing glasses that have been prescribed for you.

Only in **very** rare cases are headaches a symptom of a brain tumor, high blood pressure, or other serious problem.

Types of headaches

Tension headaches often feel like a tight band is around your head. The pain is dull and aching and usually will be felt on both sides of your head, but may be in front and back as well.

Pressure at school or at home, arguments with parents or friends, having too much to do, and feeling anxious or depressed can all cause a headache.

Migraines often are described as throbbing and usually are felt on only one side of your head, but may be felt on both. A migraine may make you feel light-headed or dizzy, and/or make your stomach upset. You may see spots or be sensitive to light, sounds, and smells. If you get migraines, chances are one of your parents or other family members also have had this problem.

A third, less common, type of headache is called a **psychogenic** headache. Psychogenic headaches are similar to tension headaches, but the cause is an emotional problem such as depression. Signs of depression include loss of energy, poor appetite or overeating, loss of interest in usual activities, change in sleeping patterns (trouble falling asleep, waking in the middle of the night or too early in the morning), and difficulty thinking or concentrating.

When should I see the pediatrician?

If you are worried about your headaches—or if this problem begins to disrupt your school, home, or social life—see your pediatrician. Other signs that may mean you should visit your pediatrician include:

Head injury—Headaches from a recent head injury should be checked right away—especially if you were knocked out by the injury.

Seizures/convulsions—Any headaches associated with seizures or fainting require immediate attention.

Frequency—You get more than one headache a week.

Degree of pain—Headache pain is severe and prevents you from doing activities you want to do.

Time of attack—Headaches that wake you from sleep or occur in early morning.

Visual difficulties—Headaches that cause blurred vision, eye spots, or other visual changes.

Other associated symptoms—If fever, vomiting, stiff neck, toothache, or jaw pain accompany your headache, you may require an examination—including laboratory or x-ray tests.

How are headaches treated?

Whichever type of headache you get, and whatever the cause, your pediatrician can explain why you get headaches and how they can be controlled. Be sure to ask any questions you may have.

If you get tension headaches or mild migraines, your pediatrician may suggest an aspirin or an aspirin substitute, such as acetaminophen or ibuprofen, and rest. If you get more severe headaches or classic migraines (when you have a visual disturbance called an "aura"), prescription medicine may be required. Your pediatrician may suggest that you keep a **headache diary** to help pinpoint information about what is causing the headaches. A headache diary helps you keep track of the following: when headaches occur, how long they last, what you were doing when the headaches start, what you had eaten, how much sleep you have had, and what seems to make the headaches better or worse.

If what you eat seems to trigger your headaches, your pediatrician will suggest that you eliminate certain foods from your diet. If stress is the culprit, your doctor can help you cope by suggesting special treatments such as relaxation exercises. Headaches that are caused by an emotional or psychological problem may require additional visits to your pediatrician or to other health care professionals to get to the cause of the problem. Sometimes entire families need counseling to eliminate the stress that is causing headaches.

It's important to know that, whatever the cause, headache pain is real. More importantly, with your pediatrician's help, you can identify the source of your headaches and get this problem under control.

The information contained in this publication should not be used as a substitute for the medical care and advice of your pediatrician. There may be variations in treatment that your pediatrician may recommend based on individual facts and circumstances.

From your doctor

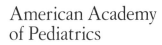

American Academy of Pediatrics

DEDICATED TO THE HEALTH OF ALL CHILDREN™

The American Academy of Pediatrics is an organization of 60,000 primary care pediatricians, pediatric medical subspecialists, and pediatric surgical specialists dedicated to the health, safety, and well-being of infants, children, adolescents, and young adults.

American Academy of Pediatrics
Web site — www.aap.org

Copyright © 1991
American Academy of Pediatrics

Hepatitis B

Hepatitis B is a liver disease caused by the hepatitis B virus (HBV). Lifelong HBV infection can lead to liver cancer or scarring of the liver (cirrhosis).

There are more than 1 million people in the United States living with lifelong HBV infection. Anyone can get infected with HBV, including your child.

The hepatitis B vaccine is the best way to protect your child from being infected. Read more to learn about how HBV is spread and why this vaccine is so important.

How is hepatitis B virus spread?

HBV often is spread by blood or body fluids. Exposure to these fluids can happen in the following ways:
- During birth (if the mother has HBV)
- Sharing personal items like razors or toothbrushes with an infected person
- Having unprotected sex with an infected person
- Injecting or "shooting" drugs using a needle with infected blood

Some children also may become infected with HBV while living in the same household as a person with a lifelong form of the infection. It is unknown how or why this happens.

Why is my child at risk?

You may feel your child will never be exposed to HBV in any of these ways. However, keep the following facts in mind:
- One third of people who are infected with HBV in the United States don't know how they got it.
- Some people with HBV may not even know they are infected.
- Not everyone with HBV, especially children, feels or looks sick.
- Nearly half of the more than 5,000 adult Americans who die from hepatitis B each year caught their infection in childhood.

People with HBV can pass it to others who aren't protected. Without the hepatitis B vaccine, 1 out of every 20 Americans could become infected. Vaccinating your child against this virus will protect her now and when she is older and exposed to more people.

Is the hepatitis B vaccine safe?

The vaccine is very safe. No serious reactions have been linked to this vaccine. Side effects are usually mild and include fussiness or soreness where the shot was given. Symptoms usually go away within 48 to 72 hours. Keep in mind, getting the vaccine is much safer than getting the disease.

When should my child get the hepatitis B vaccine?

Your child needs at least 3 doses of hepatitis B vaccine to be fully protected. The doses are usually given
- At birth
- At 1 to 4 months of age
- At 6 to 18 months of age

Premature babies and newborns with other illnesses may need to have their first dose delayed. Newborns who don't get the vaccine at birth should get all 3 doses by 18 months of age.

If a mother tests positive for HBV, her child must be vaccinated as soon as possible (preferably within 12 hours of birth). The second dose can be given at 1 month of age, and the final dose by 6 months of age.

Older children or teens who have not been immunized and anyone living with a person who is infected by HBV should receive 3 doses of the vaccine to protect against infection.

It's important that your child get all 3 doses. More than 95% of children who receive all the recommended doses of the vaccine are fully protected against the illnesses caused by HBV.

Who should *not* get the vaccine?

In rare cases, there are children who should ***not*** get the vaccine, including
- Children with severe allergies to yeast. Yeast, which is used to make bread, also is used to make the hepatitis B vaccine.
- Children who had a severe reaction to a previous dose of the vaccine.
- Children who are more than mildly sick on the day the vaccination is scheduled. These children may need to wait until they are feeling better. However, children with minor colds, an upset stomach, or a temperature lower than 100.5°F can safely receive the hepatitis B vaccine.

Remember

Immunizations have protected children for years—but vaccines only work if your child is immunized. It only takes 3 doses of the hepatitis B vaccine to protect your child for a lifetime.

The information contained in this publication should not be used as a substitute for the medical care and advice of your pediatrician. There may be variations in treatment that your pediatrician may recommend based on individual facts and circumstances.

American Academy
of Pediatrics

DEDICATED TO THE HEALTH OF ALL CHILDREN™

The American Academy of Pediatrics is an organization of 60,000 primary care pediatricians, pediatric medical subspecialists, and pediatric surgical specialists dedicated to the health, safety, and well-being of infants, children, adolescents, and young adults.

American Academy of Pediatrics
Web site—www.aap.org

Copyright © 2005
American Academy of Pediatrics

Hepatitis C

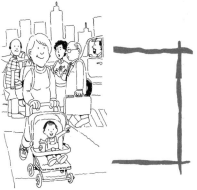

About 4 million Americans are infected with Hepatitis C virus (HCV), and many do not even know it. Anyone can get infected with HCV, including children.

Parents need to be aware of HCV because some groups of children are at risk of infection. Read on to find out more about HCV, the symptoms of infection, how HCV is spread, who is at risk, long-term effects, and treatments.

What is HCV?

Hepatitis C virus is a virus that can cause liver disease. Although most people recover from the initial phase of HCV infection, up to 80% of them may develop evidence of chronic liver infection that may lead to much more serious liver problems and possibly death. Hepatitis C virus is the cause of approximately 10,000 deaths each year in the United States.

What are the symptoms of HCV infection?

Infection with HCV usually begins as nothing more than a mild flulike illness (although many babies and children show no symptoms). Some people may experience one or more of the following:

- Flulike symptoms (body aches, fever, diarrhea, or nausea)
- Extreme tiredness
- Lack of appetite or weight loss
- Dark yellow urine
- Light, clay-colored bowel movements
- Stomach pain, especially in the upper right side of the abdomen
- Jaundice (a yellowing of the eyes and skin)

Infants with HCV infection also may have an enlarged liver or spleen, grow more slowly, or fail to gain weight.

If your child has some of the symptoms of HCV infection, contact your pediatrician. Be sure to tell your pediatrician if your child has been exposed to anyone with HCV. To diagnose HCV infection, your pediatrician will examine your child and test your child's blood for the virus.

How is HCV spread?

Hepatitis C virus cannot be spread by touching, hugging, or kissing. Therefore, children with HCV infection can participate in all normal childhood activities and should not be excluded from child care centers or schools. However, because it can be spread through contact with blood, parents of children with HCV infection should make sure household items such as toothbrushes, razors, nail clippers, or other items that may contain small amounts of blood, are not shared.

Hepatitis C virus also can be spread through sexual contact. Infected teens and young adults should be strongly advised to avoid having sex. If they are going to have sex, they need to use latex condoms to prevent the spread of HCV. Drinking alcohol also should be avoided by anyone with HCV infection because alcohol can speed up liver damage.

Protection from HCV infection

Adults and teens can protect themselves from HCV infection by making healthy lifestyle choices and *avoiding* the following:

- Having unprotected sex or sexual contact with multiple partners
- Using drugs (injecting drugs, sharing needles or other drug paraphernalia, or sniffing cocaine)
- Getting tattoos or body piercings with tools that are not sterilized

Who is at risk for HCV infection?

Those most at risk for HCV infection include the following:

- Anyone who received a blood transfusion before July 1992 or clotting concentrates derived from blood plasma before 1987, particularly children who were born premature and may have received one or more unscreened blood transfusions before July 1992
- Children who may have received solid organ transplants before July 1992
- Children who may have received extended hemodialysis for kidney disease
- Children who have used injected street drugs
- Babies born to mothers infected with HCV (Up to 5% of these infants may become infected themselves. This occurs at the time of birth, and there is no treatment that can prevent this from happening.)
- Children who have evidence of liver disease (hepatitis) but do not have hepatitis A or B virus infection
- Children adopted from mothers who may have been at risk for HCV (ie, intravenous drug users)
- Anyone who took medicines called Gammagard or Polygam between April 1993 and February 1994

The good news is that infants infected with HCV at birth often remain healthy during the first few years of life. However, more studies are needed to find out if these infants will have problems from the infection as they grow older. Research also shows that mothers infected with HCV can continue to breastfeed without risking harm to their babies.

What are the long-term effects of HCV infection?

In some children, HCV infection can lead to persistent liver disease in the form of cirrhosis or scarring of the liver. Cirrhosis occurs when the liver cells die and are replaced by scar tissue and fat. The liver eventually stops working and can no longer remove wastes from the body. Infants who develop cirrhosis of the liver because of chronic HCV infection may require a liver transplant to survive. Children infected with HCV also are at risk for developing other serious liver diseases, including liver cancer.

How is HCV infection treated?

There are a variety of medicines available for adults with HCV infection, however none of them have been approved for use in children. Vitamin supplements may be prescribed, and many infected infants are given phenobarbital, a drug used to control seizures, that also stimulates liver function. Infant formulas containing fats that are more easily digested than those in standard formulas also may be recommended. Children whose HCV infection has already caused liver damage should see a pediatric gastroenterologist or hepatologist experienced in treating liver disorders.

Hope for treatment is on the horizon. Recent medical advances may result in the testing of several new drugs for HCV infection within the next few years.

Living with HCV infection

People with HCV infection often live many years without symptoms. Many don't know they have the disease until they start to have symptoms of more advanced liver problems. Children and adolescents with HCV infection should be immunized against hepatitis A and B because infection with those other hepatitis viruses will make HCV infection much worse. At the present time, there is no vaccine to prevent hepatitis C.

Medical scientists are working hard on developing medicines to help people with HCV infection. Learning about HCV and helping your child make healthy lifestyle choices will help protect your child from getting HCV infection.

If you feel your child or adolescent may have HCV infection or may have been exposed to the virus, talk to your pediatrician.

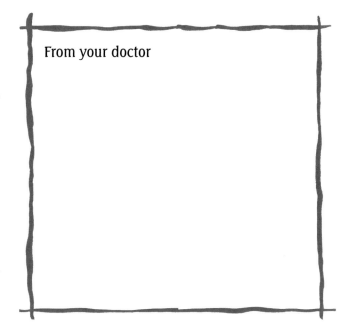

From your doctor

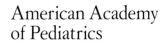

American Academy of Pediatrics

DEDICATED TO THE HEALTH OF ALL CHILDREN™

The American Academy of Pediatrics is an organization of 60,000 primary care pediatricians, pediatric medical subspecialists, and pediatric surgical specialists dedicated to the health, safety, and well-being of infants, children, adolescents, and young adults.

American Academy of Pediatrics
Web site—www.aap.org

Copyright © 2003
American Academy of Pediatrics

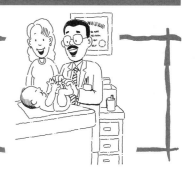

Hip Dysplasia
(Developmental Dysplasia of the Hip)

Hip dysplasia (developmental dysplasia of the hip) is a condition in which a child's upper thighbone is dislocated from the hip socket. It can be present at birth or develop during a child's first year of life.

Hip dysplasia is not always detectable at birth or even during early infancy. In spite of careful screening of children for hip dysplasia during regular well-child exams, a number of children with hip dysplasia are not diagnosed until after they are 1 year old.

Hip dysplasia is rare. However, if your baby is diagnosed with the condition, quick treatment is important.

What causes hip dysplasia?
No one is sure why hip dysplasia occurs (or why the left hip dislocates more often than the right hip). One reason may have to do with the hormones a baby is exposed to before birth. While these hormones serve to relax muscles in the pregnant mother's body, in some cases they also may cause a baby's joints to become too relaxed and prone to dislocation. This condition often corrects itself in several days, and the hip develops normally. In some cases, these dislocations cause changes in the hip anatomy that need treatment.

Who is at risk?
Factors that may increase the risk of hip dysplasia include
- Sex—more frequent in girls
- Family history—more likely when other family members have had hip dysplasia
- Birth position—more common in infants born in the breech position
- Birth order—firstborn children most at risk for hip dysplasia

Detecting hip dysplasia
Your pediatrician will check your newborn for hip dysplasia right after birth and at every well-child exam until your child is walking normally.

During the exam, your child's pediatrician will carefully flex and rotate your child's legs to see if the thighbones are properly positioned in the hip sockets. This does not require a great deal of force and will not hurt your baby.

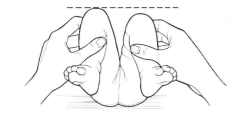

Your child's pediatrician also will look for other signs that may suggest a problem, including
- Limited range of motion in either leg
- One leg is shorter than the other
- Thigh or buttock creases appear uneven or lopsided

If your child's pediatrician suspects a problem with your child's hip, you may be referred to an orthopedic specialist who has experience treating hip dysplasia.

Treating hip dysplasia
Early treatment is important. The sooner treatment begins, the simpler it will be. In the past parents were told to double or triple diaper their babies to keep the legs in a position where dislocation was unlikely. *This practice is not recommended.* The diapering will not prevent hip dysplasia and will only delay effective treatment. Failure to treat this condition can result in permanent disability.

If your child is diagnosed with hip dysplasia before she is 6 months old, she will most likely be treated with a soft brace (such as the Pavlik harness) that holds the legs flexed and apart to allow the thighbones to be secure in the hip sockets.

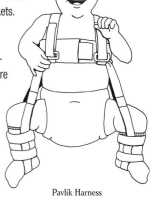

Pavlik Harness

The orthopedic consultant will tell you how long and when your baby will need to wear the brace. Your child also will be examined frequently during this time to make sure that the hips remain normal and stable.

In resistant cases or in older children, hip dysplasia may need to be treated with a combination of braces, casts, traction, or surgery. Your child will be admitted to the hospital if surgery is necessary. After surgery, your child will be placed in a hip spica cast for about 3 months. A hip spica cast is a hard cast that immobilizes the hips and keeps them in the correct position. When the cast is removed, your child will need to wear a removable hip brace for several more months.

Remember
If you have any concerns about your child's walking, talk with his pediatrician. If the cause is hip dysplasia, prompt treatment is important.

The information contained in this publication should not be used as a substitute for the medical care and advice of your pediatrician. There may be variations in treatment that your pediatrician may recommend based on individual facts and circumstances.

American Academy of Pediatrics
DEDICATED TO THE HEALTH OF ALL CHILDREN™

The American Academy of Pediatrics is an organization of 60,000 primary care pediatricians, pediatric medical subspecialists, and pediatric surgical specialists dedicated to the health, safety, and well-being of infants, children, adolescents, and young adults.
American Academy of Pediatrics
Web site—www.aap.org
Copyright © 2003
American Academy of Pediatrics

Imaging Tests: A Look Inside Your Child's Body

If your pediatrician isn't sure what the cause of your child's illness or injury is, imaging tests may be needed. Imaging tests are used to "look" inside the body. They can help diagnose injuries and illnesses from broken bones to cancer. Some tests can even find problems before symptoms appear. Read this handout to learn more about imaging tests.

Who gives imaging tests?

Radiologists are doctors trained to give imaging tests. They also study the results and make diagnoses. Some radiologists have special training and a lot of experience working with children. If your child needs an imaging test, your pediatrician will refer you to a radiologist. The radiologist will share the results with your pediatrician. In some cases, a technician (not a doctor) gives the test. The technician usually cannot give you any information about your child's test. The radiologist needs to see the test results before any information can be shared.

What types of imaging tests are there?

X-rays

X-rays can help diagnose many illnesses. During an x-ray, electromagnetic waves (a form of light) pass through the body and create an image on film. This image is called an *x-ray* or *radiograph*. X-rays are usually used to see bones, muscles or organs (like the heart or liver), and air inside the body. Metal objects also can be seen.

X-rays can be done on most parts of the body. For example, chest x-rays can reveal pneumonia or a collapsed lung, an enlarged heart, or rib fractures. Arm or leg x-rays can show broken bones or other bone problems.

Time: Each x-ray takes only a few seconds, like a picture taken with a camera. Results may be ready during your visit or may take several days.

Radiation: X-rays expose the body to very small amounts of radiation, but only to the areas of the body being studied.

Pain: None.

Cost/availability: Low cost; widely available.

Before the test: Nothing special needs to be done before the test.

During the test: The body part to be examined is placed between the x-ray machine and the x-ray film. Other parts of the body may be covered with a lead-lined apron to reduce radiation exposure. The machine is turned on, and a picture is taken. Patients must keep very still for the image to be clear. Young children may need special straps to keep them still during the test. If you can stay with your child, you will be given a lead-lined apron to wear.

Isn't radiation dangerous?

There are different types of radiation, including ultraviolet rays from the sun, microwaves, radio waves, and ionizing radiation (like from x-rays and other imaging tests). While too much radiation can harm or kill living tissue, the amount of radiation in most imaging tests is generally very safe. In fact, no harm has been shown from the levels of radiation used in the imaging tests described here. Imaging machines have improved over the years, decreasing the amount of radiation used. Most people are exposed to more radiation from the environment than from these tests.

Radiologists take special steps to reduce radiation exposure during a test. For example, they only x-ray the body parts that need to be x-rayed and use lead aprons to cover other parts of the body not being studied. If you're still concerned, keep in mind that the benefits of imaging tests are greater than the risk of radiation.

Fluoroscopy

Fluoroscopy is a type of x-ray that creates a real-time "x-ray movie" of the inside of the body. An x-ray beam placed on a specific area of the body creates images that are shown on a TV-like monitor.

Fluoroscopy is mainly used to diagnose illness of the stomach and intestines, lungs and airway, or bladder. Fluoroscopy is also used to help guide instruments or devices into the body, such as a catheter for feeding tubes.

Time: About 5 to 20 minutes.

Radiation: Higher than x-rays, but it depends on how long the test lasts. For most studies, the fluoroscopy camera is only on when needed to keep radiation doses as low as possible.

Pain: None, but preparing before the test may be unpleasant.

Cost/availability: More expensive than x-rays; widely available.

Before the test: For some types of fluoroscopy tests patients may need to fast, drink only liquids, or have an enema. Sometimes a contrast material (a fluid that shows things in the body that are hard to see without it) is injected or given by mouth. If the child cannot drink it, a tube may need to be placed through the mouth to the stomach. (Placement of the feeding tube is very safe and is only uncomfortable for a short time. The use of the feeding tube can shorten the time it takes to do the test. Less time can reduce your child's exposure to radiation.)

During the test: The room is darkened, and the area of the body being examined is placed between the x-ray and fluoroscopy screen. Images of the body are then sent to a monitor where they can be seen in motion.

Computed tomography or CT scan

A CT scan is a special type of x-ray that uses computers to create detailed images of the body. A rotating x-ray tube that surrounds the patient takes pictures of organs and tissues from many angles. Hundreds of images can be created in a short time.

A CT scan is very useful because it can create more detailed pictures than an ordinary x-ray. It is often used to find tumors, infections, or evidence of injury in different parts of the body.

Time: A CT scan only takes a few seconds. Results can take a few hours to 24 hours, depending on where it's done.

Radiation: Higher than x-rays but lower than the dose from fluoroscopy.

Pain: None, unless the child will need an injection of a contrast material. This must be done through a vein (IV) in the arm.

Cost/availability: High cost; widely available.

Before the test: A contrast material may need to be injected or taken by mouth.

During the test: The patient lies on a narrow table that slides in and out of the CT scanner. The x-ray tube rotates around the patient, sending information to a computer that forms the images. Young patients may need to be sedated for a CT scan.

Magnetic resonance imaging (MR imaging or MRI)

An MRI uses a large and powerful magnet, radio waves, and a computer to create very detailed images of the inside of the body.

An MRI is very helpful in studying the brain and spinal cord, the soft tissues of the body, and the joints. An MRI is often used to detect birth defects, inflammation, infection, tumors, and injury.

Time: About 30 to 60 minutes. Results are usually ready within 24 hours.

Radiation: None.

Pain: None, but patients may need an injection of a contrast material and an IV. Also, some patients may feel cramped in the machine (open MRI machines are available in some areas). During scanning, loud humming and knocking will be heard. Small children may be frightened by these noises.

Cost/availability: High cost; not available everywhere.

Before the test: Younger children may need to be sedated before the test. All metal objects need to be removed before the test. Internal items like pacemakers, hearing aids, or insulin pumps may not be allowed in the MRI scanner room and may mean your child can't have an MRI.

During the test: The patient lies on a table that slides into the scanner (a narrow tunnel that holds the magnet). It's important that the patient stay very still. Inside the scanner, the patient will hear a fan and feel air blowing. Because the machine can be noisy, patients are given earphones. Some centers have headphones that your child can use to listen to music during the exam.

Ultrasound (sonography)

Ultrasound uses sound waves to create images of the body. The sound waves enter the body, and the returning echoes are captured as images. These images are called *sonograms, echocardiograms (heart echo),* or *ultrasound scans.*

What if my child needs to be sedated?

Your child may need to stay still for some imaging tests. If your child moves during the test, the image will be blurred, and the test may need to be redone. To keep this from happening, some children may need a sedative to help them relax and stay still.

If your child will be sedated, you may be asked to do the following **before the test:**

- Don't give your child anything to eat or drink for 3 to 8 hours.
- Limit how much sleep your child gets. This will help your child to fall asleep during the test.
- Let your pediatrician or radiologist know if your child is ill, has a fever, or is very congested on the day of the test. The exam may need to be rescheduled.

Ultrasound tests can help diagnose illnesses of the kidneys, bladder, and uterus; the heart (called an *echocardiography*); as well as the liver, spleen, gallbladder, and pancreas. Ultrasound is also used to look at the brains of young infants, especially premature babies. It is best used for looking at parts of the body that are either solid (like the liver) or fluid-filled (like the gallbladder). Ultrasound doesn't produce clear images of organs filled with gas or air (such as lungs) or with hard surfaces, such as the inside of bones.

Time: 15 minutes to 1 hour.

Radiation: None.

Pain: None.

Cost/availability: Moderate cost; widely available.

Before the test: In some cases, patients may need to fast or drink more water before the test.

During the test: First, a special jelly or oil is put on the skin. Next, a hand-held device called a *transducer* is moved back and forth over the area being examined. The transducer creates sound waves (that can't be heard or felt) that are reflected back to the machine. A computer creates images from the sound waves.

Nuclear imaging

A *nuclear imaging scan* (sometimes called *radionuclide scanning*) shows the structure of a body part as well as how it works. Before the scan, a radioactive substance called a *tracer* is injected or given by mouth. A machine called a *gamma camera* used outside the body then detects the rays of energy given off by the tracer, and an image is created and shown on a computer screen.

Organs including the kidneys, liver, heart, lungs, and brain are often studied using this test. Bone imaging may show trauma, infection, or a tumor even before any problems are seen with x-rays.

Time: Between 15 minutes and 1 hour. Most results take 1 to 3 days.

Radiation: Less radiation than from fluoroscopy or CT. The tracer loses its radioactivity within 24 hours, leaving the body in the urine or stool. For most nuclear medicine studies, the amount of radiation in the urine or stool is not harmful for the child or those exposed to the urine or stool.

Pain: None, but patients may need the tracer injected and an IV. With some exams, a catheter may need to be placed into the bladder.

Cost/availability: Moderate cost; often available wherever CT or MRI is available.

Before the test: The tracer is usually given by mouth or through an injection. Patients may need to fast or drink a lot of water before some nuclear imaging scans. Young children may need to be sedated.

During the test: After the tracer is in place, the patient lies on a scanning table. The camera is then moved slowly over the body. Images are created and displayed on a computer.

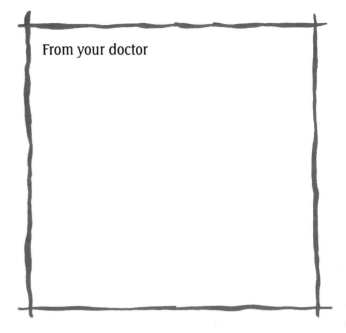

From your doctor

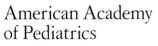

American Academy of Pediatrics

DEDICATED TO THE HEALTH OF ALL CHILDREN™

The American Academy of Pediatrics is an organization of 60,000 primary care pediatricians, pediatric medical subspecialists, and pediatric surgical specialists dedicated to the health, safety, and well-being of infants, children, adolescents, and young adults.

American Academy of Pediatrics
Web site — www.aap.org

Copyright © 2006
American Academy of Pediatrics

Common Childhood Infections

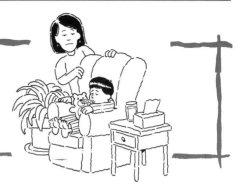

Every child gets sick at some point. While you can't always stop this from happening, you can at least help your child feel better if you know the signs and symptoms of the most common childhood infections. Read on to learn more about common childhood infections—signs and symptoms, treatments, and when to call your pediatrician.

Bronchiolitis

Bronchiolitis is a viral infection that causes the small breathing tubes (bronchioles) of the lungs to swell. This blocks air flow through the lungs, making it hard to breathe. It occurs most often in infants because their airways are smaller and more easily blocked. *Bronchiolitis* is not the same as *bronchitis,* an infection of the larger airways that typically causes severe and chronic problems in adults.

Signs and Symptoms: Bronchiolitis often starts with signs of a cold, such as a runny nose, mild cough, and fever. After a day or two the cough may get worse and your infant will begin to breathe faster.

Treatment: Give your infant acetaminophen if he has a fever. Make sure your infant drinks a lot of fluids.

Call your pediatrician if your child stops taking fluids or has a lot of trouble breathing. He may need to go to the hospital for oxygen, fluids, or medicine to help him breathe.

Colds

Most children have from 8 to 10 colds in their first 2 years of life. Most colds come and go and rarely lead to anything worse. There is no cure for the common cold, but you can try to ease your child's symptoms. Colds are caused by viruses and they are not affected by antibiotics.

Signs and Symptoms: A child with a cold will sneeze and have watery eyes; a cough; and a stuffy, runny nose. Your child may be cranky, especially if she also has a mild fever or a headache. Colds usually last about a week. Any fever should appear at the start of the cold and then go away.

Treatment: See "How can I make my child feel better?"

Call your pediatrician if any of the following occur:

- Fever lasting for more than 2 to 3 days
- Worsening symptoms after a week of illness

What are the causes of infection?

Most infections in children are caused by viruses. A virus can't be treated with antibiotics. Instead, the body gets rid of the virus on its own. Other times, an infection can be caused by bacteria. While some bacteria can live in the body without causing any harm, they can cause infections when they move to parts of the body where they don't belong. Infections caused by certain bacteria are treated with antibiotics.

Can I prevent my child from getting sick?

Though there is no way to keep your child away from germs, there are some steps you can take to help prevent them from spreading, including

- Make sure everyone washes his or her hands. Regular hand washing helps prevent the spread of germs.
- Keep your child away from anyone who has a cold, fever, or runny nose.
- Avoid sharing eating utensils, drinking cups, toothbrushes, wash-cloths, or towels with anyone who has a cold, fever, or runny nose.
- Wash dishes and utensils in hot, soapy water.
- Don't smoke around your child.

- A hard time drinking fluids or breathing
- Ear pain
- Blue lips or nails
- Extreme sleepiness or crankiness

Croup

Croup is caused by viruses. A child with croup will have noisy and difficult breathing due to a swelling of the voice box (larynx) and windpipe (trachea).

Signs and Symptoms: Your child may go to bed with a runny nose and mild cough, but wake up during the night with a cough that sounds like a seal's bark. Breathing may become noisy and difficult, a condition called *stridor.* Your child may or may not have a fever.

Treatment: Most cases of croup can be taken care of at home. Often a cool-mist vaporizer may help your child breathe better. If not, fill your bathroom with steam from the tub or shower. Bring your child into the bathroom and let him breathe in the steam for a few minutes. Keep a close eye on your child so that he doesn't get too warm or burn himself with the hot water. Sit with your child on your lap, and read a short story to pass the time. Another thing that might help him breathe better is taking him outside to inhale the cool night air.

Call your pediatrician if your child's breathing doesn't get better. If your child gets irritable or very cranky, these may be signs that he isn't getting enough oxygen. Your child may need medicine to help him breathe. The medicine may be inhaled, taken by mouth, or given by injection. In severe cases, your child may need to stay in the hospital until he can breathe better.

Ear infection

Most children have at least one ear infection by the time they are 3 years old. Most of the time, ear infections clear up without causing any lasting problems. Occasionally, a cold or flu causes a build-up of fluid in the ear. If bacteria or a virus infects this fluid, it can cause swelling and pain in the ear. This type of ear infection is called *acute otitis media.* Often after the symptoms of acute otitis media clear up, fluid remains in the ear. It then develops into another ear condition called *otitis media with effusion (middle ear fluid).*

Signs and Symptoms: The most common symptom is ear pain. Your child may have less appetite, trouble sleeping, fever, or ear drainage that is yellow or white, possibly blood-tinged. Pain often decreases after this drainage, but your child still will need to see the pediatrician.

Treatment: To treat your child's ear pain, the first symptom of an ear infection, give your child acetaminophen or ibuprofen. Ask your pediatrician for the right dosage for your child's age and size. There are also ear drops that may help ease the pain for a short time. There's no need to use over-the-counter cold medicines (decongestants and antihistamines). If the ear pain or fever doesn't go away after 2 to 3 days, call your pediatrician. Your pediatrician may wish to see your child and prescribe an antibiotic. If so, be sure to give your child the full dose for the whole time it's prescribed so the infection doesn't return. It's common for fluid to remain, even after the pain and fever have gone.

Call your pediatrician if your child is younger than 2 years, has drainage from the ear that looks like blood or pus, has a fever higher than 102.5°F, seems to be in a lot of pain, is unable to sleep, isn't eating, or is acting ill.

Flu (Influenza)

The flu is caused by a virus and usually occurs between January and March. Unlike a cold, the flu can last a week or longer and children usually feel much sicker. Stomach upsets and vomiting are also common with the flu. Your child usually will feel the worst during the first 2 or 3 days.

Signs and Symptoms: Flu symptoms include the following:

- A sudden fever (temperature usually above 101°F)
- Chills and shakes with the fever
- Extreme tiredness
- Headache and body aches
- Dry, hacking cough
- Sore throat
- Vomiting and stomach pain (stomach flu)
- Stuffy, runny nose

There usually are no serious problems from the flu. However, sometimes an ear infection, a sinus infection, or even pneumonia may develop. Talk with your pediatrician if your child's ear hurts, her cough persists, or her fever lasts beyond 3 to 4 days.

Signs of infection in an infant

Infections can be especially dangerous in a child younger than 2 months. **Call your pediatrician** right away if your infant develops any of the following symptoms:

- Not eating well
- Poor color
- Lack of energy
- Weak cry
- Rectal temperature of 100.4°F or higher
- Trouble breathing
- Unusual fussiness
- Sleeping more than usual
- Vomiting or diarrhea

How will my pediatrician help?

When your child is sick, your pediatrician will let you know what the best treatment is for your child. In some cases, all you may need to do is make sure your child gets plenty of rest and eats a balanced diet. (See "How can I make my child feel better?") Other times, your child may need medicine. Most infections can be treated at home. However, if an infection becomes severe, your child may need to see the pediatrician and, rarely, go to the hospital.

Treatment: See "How can I make my child feel better?" In children older than 1 year, type A flu can be treated with antiviral drugs. If these medicines are given in the first day or two of the illness they can help your child get better faster. In some cases, these medicines can be taken before exposure to the flu to prevent illness. Extra rest and a lot of fluids also can make your child feel better.

There are safe and effective **vaccines** to protect against the flu. Healthy children 6–23 months of age should get a flu shot each fall, as should everyone in the household of a child this age. Children with health problems that make it risky for them to get the flu also should get flu vaccine each fall. When flu vaccine is in short supply, children 6–23 months of age and children with chronic health problems will get it first.

Call your pediatrician if your child experiences any of the following:

- Hard time breathing
- Blue lips or nails
- A cough that just will not go away (for more than 1 week)
- Pain in the ear
- Continued or new onset of fever after 3 to 4 days of illness

Impetigo

Impetigo is a skin infection that can spread on the skin quickly. It also can spread to other people if they touch the infected skin. This infection is caused by strep or staph bacteria. It's most common in warm weather and often appears on the face, but may be found anywhere on the body.

Signs and Symptoms: Impetigo looks like a rash with yellow, oozing, or crusty blisters.

Treatment: Most cases of impetigo can be treated with an antibiotic. The antibiotic is taken by mouth or put on the skin in ointment form.

Call your pediatrician if the skin around the sores becomes red or has red streaks, or if your child develops a fever or has urine that looks red or brown.

Pinkeye (Conjunctivitis)

Pinkeye is an inflammation of the thin tissue covering the white part of the eye and the inside of the eyelids. It can affect one or both eyes. There are different kinds, including bacterial, viral, allergic, or chemical (for example, chlorine in a swimming pool). Bacterial or viral infections are contagious and can spread easily in school or child care.

Signs and Symptoms: When a child has pinkeye, one or both eyes are watery, itchy, and red. The undersides of the eyelids may be irritated, and there may be a white discharge coming from one or both eyes.

Treatment: Your pediatrician may prescribe antibiotic drops or ointment if it's a bacterial infection. Be sure to use all of the medicine to keep the infection from coming back. A warm cloth placed on the eyes may also help your child's eyes feel better.

Call your pediatrician if your child has eye irritation or eye pain with a high fever, sluggishness, or more severe swelling and redness around the eye. These could be signs of a more serious infection. Because not all pinkeye infections are contagious, your pediatrician will let you know if your child can still go to school or child care.

Pneumonia

Pneumonia is an infection of the lungs. It often occurs a few days after the start of a cold. Most cases of pneumonia are mild. Pneumonia is caused by viruses or bacteria.

Signs and Symptoms: The symptoms vary based on the cause and severity of the illness. A child may have a cough, mild fever, less of an appetite, and less energy. If one of the more severe types of pneumonia develops, your child suddenly may have shaking chills; a high fever (102.5°F); chest pain; and difficult, rapid breathing. A cough may not develop until later. Your pediatrician may need an x-ray to make sure that pneumonia is the cause of the symptoms.

Treatment: Most cases of pneumonia can be treated safely at home. The fever that occurs with pneumonia caused by a virus may be treated with acetaminophen or ibuprofen. Bronchodilators may help if there is wheezing. Pneumonia caused by bacteria tends to have more severe symptoms and is treated with antibiotics.

Call your pediatrician if your child's symptoms are severe or if your child is very young. He may need to go to the hospital for treatment.

Sinusitis

When a child has a cold, the sinuses around the nose often get stuffy and swollen. The sinuses may also fill with fluid. Sometimes this fluid gets infected with bacteria. When this happens, your child has a sinus infection. Sinusitis usually develops after your child has had a cold for at least 10 to 14 days.

Signs and Symptoms

- Nasal discharge for more than 10 days after a cold
- Fever
- A cough that lasts more than 14 days after a cold
- Tenderness in the face
- Headaches

Treatment: Sinusitis that goes with a cold usually resolves by itself. Antibiotics may be prescribed to clear up your child's sinusitis. Home treatments, such as taking a steamy shower, placing a humidifier in your child's room, and using a saline nasal spray, may help to drain the blocked sinuses.

Call your pediatrician if your child's symptoms don't get better after 3 to 4 days of treatment, your child has severe head or face pain, or your child has a sudden high fever.

Strep throat

Strep usually develops in children older than 3 years. It's caused by streptococcal bacteria.

Signs and Symptoms: Strep causes a sore throat, fever, and swollen glands in the neck. (If there is also a sandpaper-like skin rash on the body, the condition is called *scarlet fever*.) Because many viruses can cause the same symptoms as strep, your pediatrician will need to test for strep. To do this, he will do a rapid strep test and may obtain a culture.

Treatment: Because strep throat may lead to rheumatic fever, it's treated with antibiotics. After 24 to 36 hours of antibiotic treatment, your child is no longer contagious and should start to feel better. Remember to have your

---

How can I make my child feel better?

There is no "cure" for infections caused by a virus, but there are things you can do to help your child feel better until the virus runs its course. The following are ways you can try to ease your child's symptoms:

To relieve stuffy nose

- **Thin the mucus** using saline nose drops. Ask your pediatrician which ones to use. *Never use nonprescription nose drops that contain any medicine.*
- **Clear your baby's nose** with a suction bulb. Squeeze the bulb first, then gently put the rubber tip into one nostril and slowly release the bulb. This suction will draw the clogged mucus out of the nose. This works best for babies younger than 6 months.
- **Use a cool-mist humidifier** in your child's room. This helps to moisten the air and clear your child's nasal passages. Be sure to clean the humidifier often.

To relieve fever

- **Give your child acetaminophen or ibuprofen.** Ask your pediatrician for the right dosage for your child's age and size. Don't give aspirin to your child because it has been associated with Reye syndrome, a disease that affects the liver and the brain. Check with your pediatrician first before giving any other cold medicines.

To prevent dehydration

- **Make sure your child drinks a lot of fluids.** He may want clear liquids rather than milk or formula. He may eat more slowly or not feel like eating because he is having a hard time breathing.

---

child finish all the medicine. If you stop treatment too early, the infection may come back and problems may develop.

Call your pediatrician if your child's fever returns or she has a hard time breathing.

Sty

A sty is an infection in a gland of the eyelid. Sties are not very contagious. Once your child has had a sty, he is more likely to get one again.

Signs and Symptoms: Tenderness, swelling, and redness on the eyelid are the most common signs of a sty.

Treatment: To ease the pain and discomfort of a sty, place a warm cloth on the eyelid 3 to 4 times a day until signs of the infection are gone.

Call your pediatrician if the warm cloth treatments don't work. An antibiotic ointment may be prescribed. In some cases, your pediatrician may refer your child to an eye doctor who can drain the sty surgically.

Urinary tract infection

Urinary tract infections (UTIs) are found in children from infancy through the teen years. A UTI occurs in the kidney or bladder and is caused by bacteria. X-rays and other tests, including urine tests, are often needed to help find the cause of the UTI.

Signs and Symptoms: A child with a UTI will have painful and frequent urination, and sometimes fever, vomiting, stomach pain, and back pain. In young children, fever or irritability may be the only clues.

Treatment: UTIs are treated with antibiotics. Be sure to use all of the medicine to keep the infection from coming back.

Call your pediatrician if your child's urine looks pink, red, or brown, or if your child has a fever or severe back pain.

Vomiting and diarrhea

Vomiting and diarrhea are the reasons many parents call the pediatrician. These illnesses usually are caused by viruses that infect the intestines, but sometimes they are caused by bacteria. They usually last only about a day or two but can last up to a week in some cases.

Signs and Symptoms

- Frequent and uncontrollable loose, watery stools
- Vomiting
- Stomach pain, cramping

Treatment: If your child is throwing up, your pediatrician may tell you to not give food and fluid for a few hours. You then can give your child small sips of clear fluids, later followed by easy-to-digest foods. This will help prevent more vomiting, which can lead to dehydration. Children younger than 2 years should not be given medicine for diarrhea unless your pediatrician tells you it's OK.

Call your pediatrician if your child has any of the following signs of dehydration:

- No tears
- Dry diaper or no urination for 6 hours
- Dry mouth, skin, or lips
- Sunken eyes
- Less energy or activity
- Less alert
- Sunken soft spot on head (for infants)

Most cases of dehydration can be treated by giving your child fluids. However, if dehydration is severe, your child may need special solutions by mouth or an intravenous (IV) tube inserted to get fluids into her veins. To reduce the chance of dehydration, call your pediatrician early if your child has vomiting or diarrhea that won't go away.

Remember

If any of these illnesses or infections develop, call your pediatrician. Most important, if the illness or infection doesn't seem to go away, or seems to get worse, call your pediatrician.

The information contained in this publication should not be used as a substitute for the medical care and advice of your pediatrician. There may be variations in treatment that your pediatrician may recommend based on individual facts and circumstances.

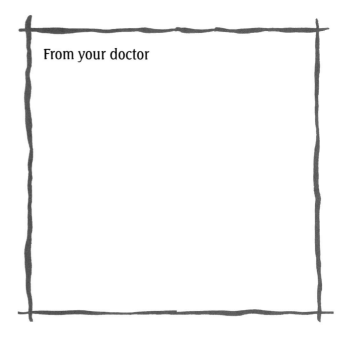

From your doctor

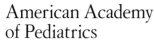

American Academy of Pediatrics

DEDICATED TO THE HEALTH OF ALL CHILDREN™

The American Academy of Pediatrics is an organization of 60,000 primary care pediatricians, pediatric medical subspecialists, and pediatric surgical specialists dedicated to the health, safety, and well-being of infants, children, adolescents, and young adults.

American Academy of Pediatrics
Web site—www.aap.org

Copyright © 2005
American Academy of Pediatrics, Updated 2/05

The Flu (Influenza)

The flu (influenza)—every child gets it at some time or another. What is the flu? Can it be prevented? Should my child get a flu shot or immunization? These are a few of the most common questions parents have about the flu. Read more to learn about this illness.

What is the flu?

The flu is an illness caused by a virus. There are 3 different flu viruses—types A, B, and C. Types A (the most common) and B (usually milder) cause outbreaks of the flu.

Each year the flu is slightly different because there are many different types of flu viruses. The flu season most commonly occurs between January and March. People can be infected several times during their lifetime because the virus changes.

The flu can last a week or even longer. Your child usually will feel the worst during the first 2 or 3 days. Flu symptoms include

- A sudden fever (temperature usually above 101°F)
- Chills and shakes with the fever
- Extreme tiredness
- Headache and body aches
- Dry, hacking cough
- Sore throat
- Vomiting and belly pain
- Stuffy, runny nose

There usually are no serious complications from the flu. However, sometimes an ear infection, a sinus infection, or even pneumonia may develop. Talk with your pediatrician if your child's ear hurts, his cough persists, or his fever lasts beyond 3 to 4 days.

How the flu is spread

The flu is spread from person to person in the following ways:

- Direct hand-to-hand contact
- Indirect contact (eg, if your child touches a contaminated surface like a toy or doorknob and then touches her eyes, nose, or mouth)
- Virus droplets passed through the air from coughing or sneezing

The flu spreads very easily, especially to preschool- and school-aged children and adults who spend time with children. The virus usually spreads during the first several days of the illness.

Treatment

In children older than 1 year, type A flu can be treated with antiviral drugs if given in the first day or two of the illness. This can speed recovery. Under some circumstances, antiviral drugs can be taken before exposure to the flu and prevent illness. This is particularly important for children with serious health problems who haven't had the flu shot. Antibiotics can be used to fight bacterial infections but have *no* effect on viruses, including flu viruses. Extra rest and lots of fluids also can help your child feel better.

Caution

Don't give aspirin to your child for the flu. An increased risk of developing Reye syndrome (an illness that can seriously affect the liver and brain) is associated with aspirin use during bouts of the flu.

If your child is uncomfortable because of fever, acetaminophen may help him feel better. Check first with your pediatrician before giving your child any other medicines, including over-the-counter cold and cough medicines.

Prevention

Good hygiene is the best way to prevent the flu from spreading to other family members. If your child has the flu, the following will help prevent its spread:

- Teach your child to cover her mouth and nose with a tissue or her sleeve, but not with her hands, when coughing or sneezing. If your child is old enough, teach her how to blow her nose properly.
- Use tissues for runny noses and to catch sneezes. Throw them in the trash after each use.
- Avoid kissing your child on or around the mouth or face, though she will need plenty of hugs while she's sick.
- Make sure everyone washes his or her hands before and after coming into close contact with someone with the flu.
- Wash dishes and utensils in hot, soapy water or the dishwasher.
- Don't let children share pacifiers, cups, utensils, washcloths, or towels. Never share toothbrushes.
- Use disposable paper cups in the bathroom and kitchen.
- Disinfect. Viruses can live for more than 30 minutes on doorknobs, toilet handles, countertops, and even toys. Use a disinfectant or soap and hot water to keep these areas clean.
- Don't smoke around your child. Children who are exposed to tobacco smoke cough and wheeze more and have a harder time getting over the flu.

Flu shot

There are safe and effective vaccines to protect against the flu. They are particularly recommended for children with health problems that make it risky for them to get the flu. This includes children with the following:

- Heart disease
- Lung disease, including asthma
- Immune problems, such as human immunodeficiency virus (HIV) infection
- Blood diseases
- Cancer
- Chronic kidney disease
- Metabolic diseases, such as diabetes
- Long-term aspirin ltherapy, such as with rheumatoid arthritis

Healthy children 6–23 months of age are recommended to get a flu shot each fall, as is everyone in the household of a child of this age. Your pediatrician can recommend what's best for your child.

For children younger than 9 years, the vaccine requires 2 immunizations or shots given 1 month apart the first year it's given. After that, only 1 dose is needed each year. The best time to get the flu vaccine is in October to early December before the flu season starts. Vaccination should begin earlier (eg, September) for those needing 2 shots.

Because the strains of flu virus are different every year, a new flu vaccine is developed each year. The vaccine is made from killed flu viruses and helps the immune system fight the flu. Most children are immune within 2 weeks of getting the vaccine. Side effects usually are minor and include soreness at the site of the injection and a low-grade fever. The flu shot can't cause the flu.

Side effects

Even though there are few side effects from the vaccine, production of the vaccine involves the use of eggs. If your child has had a serious allergic reaction to eggs or egg products, he should be skin tested before getting the vaccine. If skin testing confirms hypersensitivity to eggs, the vaccine usually shouldn't be given.

Flu or cold?

Both the flu and colds are caused by viruses and share many of the same symptoms, but there are differences. A child with a common cold usually has less of a fever and only mild coughing. Children with the flu usually feel much sicker and achy and are miserable. Also, the flu tends to strike more quickly than a cold. Stomach upsets and vomiting are more common with the flu than with a cold. Children who have colds usually have enough energy to play and keep up with their normal day-to-day routines. The flu, on the other hand, keeps most children in bed for several days.

When to call your pediatrician

An older child with the flu usually doesn't need to see the pediatrician unless the condition becomes more serious. If your child is 3 months of age or younger, however, call your pediatrician if she has a fever. For a child older than 3 months who has been exposed to the flu, call your pediatrician if your child experiences any of the following:

- Difficulty breathing
- Blue lips or nails
- A cough that just will not go away (for more than 1 week)
- Pain in the ear
- Continued or new onset of fever after 3 to 4 days of illness

If your child seems extremely sick or her condition doesn't improve, call your pediatrician.

Nasal spray flu vaccine

Scientists have developed a nasal spray flu vaccine. Unlike the flu vaccine given by injection, it's made from living but weakened (attenuated) flu viruses. Live attenuated influenza vaccine (trade name FluMist) is the first live-virus flu vaccine approved in the United States. It's approved only for *healthy* children 5 years and older and healthy adults aged 18 to 49 years, and shouldn't be given to children who have asthma.

Note: Products are mentioned for informational purposes only and do not imply an endorsement by the American Academy of Pediatrics.

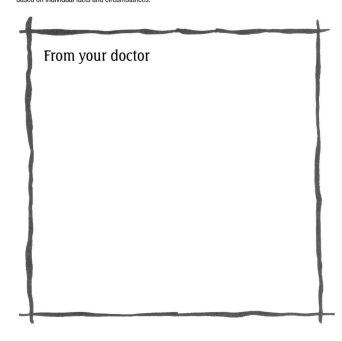

From your doctor

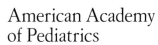

American Academy
of Pediatrics

DEDICATED TO THE HEALTH OF ALL CHILDREN™

The American Academy of Pediatrics is an organization of 60,000 primary care pediatricians, pediatric medical subspecialists, and pediatric surgical specialists dedicated to the health, safety, and well-being of infants, children, adolescents, and young adults.

American Academy of Pediatrics
Web site—www.aap.org

Copyright © 2004
American Academy of Pediatrics, Updated 4/04

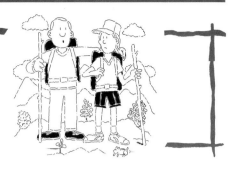

Lyme Disease

Lyme disease is an important public health problem in some areas of the United States. Since its discovery in Lyme, CT, in 1975, thousands of cases of the disease have been reported across the United States and around the world. By knowing more about the disease and how to prevent it, you can help keep your family safe from the effects of Lyme disease.

What is Lyme disease?

Lyme disease is an infection caused by a bacteria called a *spirochete*. The disease is spread to humans by the bites of deer ticks infected with this bacteria. Deer ticks are tiny black-brown creatures. They live in forests or grassy, wooded, marshy areas near rivers, lakes, or oceans. Many people who have been infected with Lyme disease were bitten by deer ticks while hiking or camping, during other outdoor activities, or even while spending time in their own backyards, from the late spring to early fall.

Where is Lyme disease most common?

Deer ticks that are infected with Lyme disease live in areas that have very low and high seasonal temperatures and high humidity. In the United States, Lyme disease is more common in the following regions:

- **Northeast** (Connecticut, Delaware, Maine, Maryland, Massachusetts, New Hampshire, New Jersey, New York, Pennsylvania, Rhode Island, and Vermont)
- **North central states** (Michigan, Minnesota, and Wisconsin)
- **West Coast** (California)

How will I know if my child has Lyme disease?

The first and most obvious symptom of Lyme disease is a rash that begins as a pink or red circle several inches in diameter. This is where your child was bitten. It may appear from 3 to 30 days *after* the bite occurred and expand over time. Some people may have a single circle, while others may have many. Most people who develop the rash won't feel anything, but for others the rash may hurt, itch, burn, or feel warm to the touch. The rash most commonly appears on the head, neck, groin, thighs, trunk, and armpits.

Along with the rash, other symptoms may include
- Headache
- Chills
- Fever
- Fatigue
- Swollen glands, usually in the neck or groin
- Aches and pains in the muscles or joints

If your child develops the rash with or without any of these symptoms, call your pediatrician.

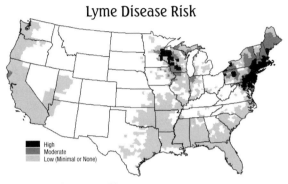

Lyme Disease Risk

- ■ High
- ▨ Moderate
- ░ Low (Minimal or None)

How serious is Lyme disease?

For most people, Lyme disease can be easily recognized and treated. If left untreated, Lyme disease can get worse. In very rare cases, there is a late stage of Lyme disease that can cause problems to joints, vision, facial muscles, and the nervous system.

How is Lyme disease treated?

Lyme disease is treated with antibiotics (usually penicillin, a cephalosporin, or a tetracycline) prescribed by your pediatrician. The antibiotics are usually taken by mouth, but also can be given intravenously (directly into the bloodstream through a vein) in more severe cases. Both early and late stages of the disease can be treated with antibiotics.

How can I prevent Lyme disease?

The Lyme disease vaccine is no longer sold. It was available for people 15 to 70 years of age.

If you live or work in a region where Lyme disease is a problem, or if you visit such an area, the following are ways to protect your family from the ticks that carry the disease:

- **Avoid places where ticks live.** Whenever possible, avoid shaded, moist areas likely to be infested with ticks.
- **Cover arms and legs.** Have your child wear a long-sleeved shirt and tuck his pants into his socks.
- **Wear a hat** to help keep ticks away from the scalp. Keep long hair pulled back.
- **Wear light-colored clothing** to make it easier to spot ticks.
- **Wear enclosed shoes or boots.** Avoid wearing sandals in an area where ticks may live.
- **Use insect repellent.** Products with *DEET* are effective against ticks and can be used on the skin. However, large amounts of DEET can be harmful to your child if it is absorbed through the skin. Look for products that contain no more than 30% DEET. Wash the DEET off with soap and water when your child returns indoors. Products with *permethrin* can be used on clothing, but *cannot* be applied to the skin.

Ticks and how to remove them

Ticks do not fly, jump, or drop from trees. They hide in long grass and small trees, bushes, or shrubs waiting for an animal or person to brush by. Then they attach themselves to the animal or person's skin. When a tick is found on a person or pet, try to remove as much of it as possible using the following steps:

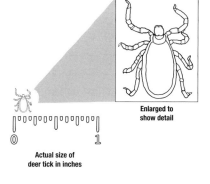

Enlarged to show detail

Actual size of deer tick in inches

1. **Grasp the tick as close to the skin as possible** with fine-tipped tweezers. Be careful not to squeeze the tick's body.
2. **Slowly pull the tick away from the skin.**
3. **After the tick is out, clean the bitten area** with rubbing alcohol or other first aid ointment.

- **Stay on cleared trails whenever possible.** Avoid wandering from a trail or brushing against overhanging branches or shrubs.
- **After coming indoors, check for ticks.** This will only take a couple minutes. Ticks often hide behind the ears or along the hairline. It usually takes more than 48 hours for a person to become infected with the bacteria, so removing any ticks soon after they have attached themselves is very effective for reducing the chances of becoming infected.

Keep in mind, ticks can be found right in your own backyard, depending on where you live. Keeping your yard clear of leaves, brush, and tall grass may reduce the number of ticks. Ask a licensed professional pest control expert about other steps you can take to reduce ticks in your yard.

Remember

If you live in or plan to visit an area where Lyme disease has become a problem, it's important to take steps to avoid being bitten by deer ticks. If you have any questions about the disease, talk with your pediatrician.

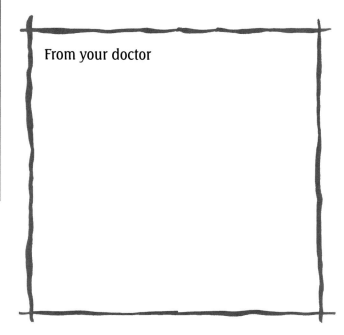

From your doctor

American Academy of Pediatrics

DEDICATED TO THE HEALTH OF ALL CHILDREN™

The American Academy of Pediatrics is an organization of 60,000 primary care pediatricians, pediatric medical subspecialists, and pediatric surgical specialists dedicated to the health, safety, and well-being of infants, children, adolescents, and young adults.

American Academy of Pediatrics
Web site—www.aap.org

Copyright © 2004
American Academy of Pediatrics

meningococcal disease— information for teens and college students

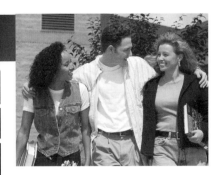

Certain teens and college students have a higher risk of getting meningococcal disease, and it can be deadly. *Read on* to learn more about this serious illness and **how to protect** yourself.

What is meningococcal disease?

Meningococcal disease is caused by bacteria. Many people carry meningococcal bacteria in their throats but never get the disease. However, in a few people it can lead to 2 common forms of the disease: *meningoccemia* and *meningitis.* Meningococcal disease can affect the blood (meningoccemia) and/or brain and spinal cord (meningitis). It can be **life-threatening** unless diagnosed and treated early.

Each year in the United States about 2,500 people get meningococcal disease. While it can strike anybody, the greatest risk in teens occurs between 15 and 18 years of age. Also, students entering college and planning to live in dorms are at a higher risk than other people of the same age. *It's easy for infections to spread in crowded dorms* or in enclosed areas where students often meet to smoke and drink alcohol.

Symptoms and Signs

The symptoms and signs of meningococcal disease often are mistaken for other less serious illnesses like the flu. **Common symptoms** include

- High **fever** (over 101.4°F)
- A flat, pink to red to purple **rash** mainly on the lower arms and legs, including the hands and feet, with small bruises or bleeding under the skin
- **Nausea**
- **Vomiting**
- Generalized muscle **aches**
- Sudden, severe **headache**
- **Confusion**
- **Sensitivity** to light
- **Stiff neck** along with headache and sensitivity to light (can signal the meningitis form of the illness and should never be ignored)

It's **important to get medical treatment right away.** Meningoccemia or meningitis can **get worse very quickly,** even within a few hours from the start of symptoms. If untreated, the disease can be fatal (up to 20% of teens die) or cause kidney failure, hearing loss, limb amputation, or lifelong problems with the nervous system.

Treatment

Meningococcal disease is treated with **antibiotics.** When given shortly after the start of symptoms, these antibiotics may prevent the disease from getting worse.

Because this infection spreads to others very easily, anyone with several hours of close contact with a person with meningococcal disease should contact their physician and also should be given an antibiotic to help prevent meningococcal disease. Ideally, this antibiotic should be given within 24 hours of the diagnosis of meningococcal disease.

Vaccination

The best protection from meningococcal disease for certain teens and college students who will be living in dorms is to be vaccinated. Safe and effective **vaccines are available** to prevent meningococcal disease caused by 3 of the 4 most common types of meningococcal bacteria found in teens. However, the vaccination provides protection against only about two thirds of the cases of meningococcal infections. Although mild side effects, like redness and swelling at the injection site or a slight fever, can occur from the vaccination, these are considered uncommon and usually go away on their own in a few days. Serious allergic reactions to the vaccine are **extremely rare.**

Who should be vaccinated?

- **11- to 12-year-olds** at their annual visit to the pediatrician
- Students entering **high school or 15-year-olds** (whichever comes first)
- Students about to start college and planning to **live in a dorm**

Students who already received a meningococcal vaccine in the last 3 years don't need to be vaccinated, but they should check with their pediatrician to be sure.

Take care of yourself

If you are 11 to 12 years old, it's important that you **see your pediatrician for your annual checkup.** You may need a booster of vaccines besides the one against meningococcal disease (such as the vaccines that prevent tetanus and diphtheria). At the same visit your pediatrician can give you advice about keeping healthy.

If you are a student about to start college, here are some health tips

- Reduce your risk of getting meningitis by *staying away from smoking, drinking alcohol, excessive stress, and exposure to upper respiratory infections.*
- **Strengthen your immune system** by living a healthy lifestyle that includes enough sleep, exercise, and a balanced diet.

- Avoid sharing eating utensils or drinking glasses, cover your mouth when you cough or sneeze, and wash your hands often.
- Get familiar with your college's **student health services.** Find out who to call or where to go if you get sick.
- Remember that *your pediatrician* is available to answer any questions you may have about your health.

The information contained in this publication should not be used as a substitute for the medical care and advice of your pediatrician. There may be variations in treatment that your pediatrician may recommend based on individual facts and circumstances.

The persons whose photographs are depicted in this publication are professional models. They have no relation to the issues discussed. Any characters they are portraying are fiictional.

From your doctor

American Academy
of Pediatrics

DEDICATED TO THE HEALTH OF ALL CHILDREN™

The American Academy of Pediatrics is an organization of 60,000 primary care pediatricians, pediatric medical subspecialists, and pediatric surgical specialists dedicated to the health, safety, and well-being of infants, children, adolescents, and young adults.

American Academy of Pediatrics
Web site—www.aap.org

Copyright ©2002
American Academy of Pediatrics, Updated 5/05

Pneumococcal Infection and Vaccine

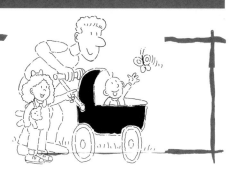

Pneumococcus is a type of bacteria that can attack different parts of the body and cause many serious infections including

- Meningitis (brain)
- Bacteremia (blood stream)
- Pneumonia (lungs)
- Sinusitis (sinus membranes)
- Otitis media (ears)

These infections can be dangerous to very young children, the elderly, and people with certain high-risk health conditions.

Pneumococcal infection

What is pneumococcal infection?

Pneumococcal bacteria live naturally in humans in the back of the nose. Many people carry the bacteria and never get sick. In fact, being a carrier helps boost one's natural immunity to the disease. Others are not immune and can get very sick from the infections caused by the bacteria.

Pneumococcal infections occur most often during the winter months. They spread from person to person the same way a cold or the flu spreads — by droplets passed through the air from coughing or sneezing, and through direct contact such as touching unwashed hands or kissing. The disease may spread quickly, especially in places where there are a lot of children, like child care centers and preschools.

Very young children do not have fully developed immune systems. This makes them more at risk from bacterial infections like pneumococcus. In addition, pneumococcal infections can be life threatening for people with certain health problems such as

- HIV infection or other immune system disorders
- Sickle-cell disease
- White cell cancers like leukemia or lymphoma
- Chronic lung, heart, or kidney disease
- A removed spleen or one that doesn't work properly
- Bone marrow or organ transplants

Common pneumococcal infections and their symptoms

Bacteremia and meningitis

Pneumococcal bacteremia and *pneumococcal meningitis* occur when pneumococcal bacteria get into the bloodstream and/or the central nervous system. Bacteremia is the presence of bacteria in the blood. Meningitis is an infection of the thin lining and blood vessels that cover the brain and spinal cord. Symptoms of meningitis include

- High fever
- Stiff neck
- Headache
- Vomiting

- Extreme tiredness and/or irritability
- Loss of appetite

Pneumonia

Pneumococcal pneumonia is a chest infection in which the lungs become filled with fluid. Symptoms of pneumonia include

- Cough that may bring up thick yellow-green or bloody mucus
- High fever
- Shortness of breath or chest pain
- Extreme tiredness
- Hard and rapid breathing

Sinusitis

Sinusitis occurs when the membranes lining the air-filled pockets in the bone of the face (sinuses) swell. The sinus cavities may fill with fluid. Symptoms of sinusitis include

- Pressure behind the eyes
- Pain in the face
- Trouble breathing through the nose
- Postnasal drip or prolonged runny nose
- Fever
- Toothache

Otitis media

Otitis media is an infection of the middle ear. Young children commonly develop middle ear infections when they have colds, the flu, or other viral respiratory infections. Symptoms of an ear infection include

- Ear pain (very young children may pull at their ears because of the pain)
- Fever
- Restlessness or irritability
- Crying
- Runny nose

Diagnosis and treatment of pneumococcal infections

Your pediatrician will be able to tell if your child has a pneumococcal infection by your child's symptoms, a physical examination, and looking at your child's medical history. X-rays, blood tests, and sometimes a spinal tap also may be done to confirm pneumococcal infection in your child.

Prompt treatment with antibiotics is usually effective. In addition, your child may need bed rest and a lot of fluids. In some cases, your child may need to be hospitalized.

Unfortunately, some strains of the pneumococcal bacteria are developing resistance to the antibiotics usually used to kill them. This means that other antibiotics must be used. Your pediatrician will let you know which antibiotic is best for your child.

Prevention of pneumococcal infections

- Teach your children to wash their hands regularly with soap and water. This helps prevent the spread of infection.
- Avoid dust, tobacco smoke, and other substances that may interfere with breathing and make children more likely to get sick.

Pneumococcal vaccine

A vaccine now offers infants and young children protection against pneumococcal infections. It is most effective against the major pneumococcal diseases — bacteremia, meningitis, and pneumonia. The vaccine is minimally effective in preventing otitis media and sinusitis. Pneumococcal vaccine is safe and can be given as a separate injection at the same time as other immunizations.

Who should receive the vaccine?

The American Academy of Pediatrics recommends that all children younger than 2 years of age receive the Heptavalent Pneumococcal Conjugate Vaccine (PCV7 or Prevnar). A series of doses may be given at 2, 4, 6, and 12 to 15 months of age. A "catch-up" immunization schedule is available for children who get a late start.

Some children between the ages of 2 and 5 years who have certain health problems also need pneumococcal vaccine because they are at higher risk of getting serious infections. Two types of vaccines may be given to children in that group. Your pediatrician can explain which vaccine is best for your child.

Pneumococcal vaccines may be given to some children 5 years of age and older, although the risk associated with pneumococcal infections is much lower in older children.

Are there side effects to pneumococcal vaccines?

Most children have no side effects with pneumococcal vaccines. Those side effects that do occur are mild and temporary. The possible side effects include

- Soreness, swelling, and redness where the shot was given
- A mild-to-moderate fever
- Fussiness

These symptoms may begin within 24 hours after the shot and usually go away within 48 to 72 hours.

Talk to your pediatrician to see if your child should be vaccinated for pneumococcal infection and about the possible reactions to these immunizations.

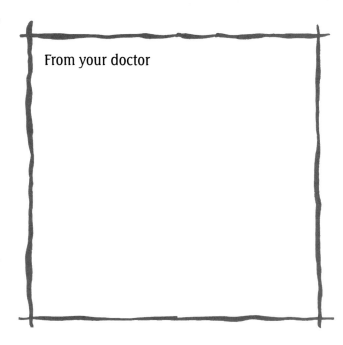

From your doctor

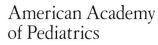

American Academy of Pediatrics

DEDICATED TO THE HEALTH OF ALL CHILDREN™

The American Academy of Pediatrics is an organization of 60,000 primary care pediatricians, pediatric medical subspecialists, and pediatric surgical specialists dedicated to the health, safety, and well-being of infants, children, adolescents, and young adults.

American Academy of Pediatrics
Web site—www.aap.org

Copyright © 2000
American Academy of Pediatrics

Respiratory Syncytial Virus

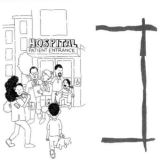

Respiratory syncytial virus (RSV) infects almost all children at least once before they are 2 years old. Most of the time this virus only causes minor cold-like symptoms. However, for some babies infection can be more dangerous.

For certain infants who are extremely preterm (infants born before 32 weeks of pregnancy) or who are born with severe heart disease or severe lung disease, RSV infection can be especially serious. Preterm infants often have underdeveloped lungs and may have difficulty fighting an RSV infection once they become infected.

Each year, about 125,000 children are hospitalized in the United States with RSV infection, and approximately 500 of these children will die. In the first 2 years of life, RSV is the leading cause of pneumonia and bronchiolitis (a swelling of the small airways), and may be associated with wheezing.

Who is at risk?

Infants born prematurely and term infants younger than 6 weeks of age are at increased risk for developing serious RSV infection. Young children with medical conditions, such as chronic lung disease, serious heart conditions, or problems with their immune system, including problems due to cancer or organ transplants, also are at risk.

When and how is RSV spread?

Respiratory syncytial virus infection occurs most often from late fall to early spring. Most illness occurs between November and April, although there may be seasonal variation by region. Respiratory syncytial virus occurs only in humans and is highly contagious. The virus can live for several hours on a surface such as a countertop, table, or playpen, or on unwashed hands. Respiratory syncytial virus is spread by direct or close physical contact, which includes touching or kissing an infected person, or contact with a contaminated surface.

What are the symptoms of RSV?

For most healthy children the symptoms of RSV resemble the common cold and include
- Runny nose
- Coughing
- Low-grade fever

However, signs of more serious infection may include
- Difficult or rapid breathing
- Wheezing
- Irritability and restlessness
- Poor appetite

How can I protect my child from RSV?

There are important steps you can take to prevent exposure to RSV and other viruses, especially in the first few months of your child's life. These precautions include
- Make sure everyone washes their hands before touching your baby.
- Keep your baby away from anyone who has a cold, fever, or runny nose.
- Keep your baby away from crowded areas like shopping malls.
- Keep your baby away from tobacco smoke. Parents should not expose their infants and young children to secondhand tobacco smoke, which increases the risk of and complications from severe viral respiratory infections.
- For high-risk infants, participation in child care should be restricted during RSV season whenever possible.
- All high-risk infants and their contacts should be immunized against influenza beginning at 6 months of age.

There are medications that your pediatrician may prescribe that could reduce the risk of developing serious RSV infection. These medications are used only for the small number of babies who are in the highest risk groups for hospitalization. The American Academy of Pediatrics has developed specific criteria for use of these medications. You should consult with your pediatrician regarding specific details on who is at highest risk and which high-risk infants are most likely to benefit from receipt of these medications.

How is RSV infection treated?

Most cases of RSV infection are mild and disappear on their own within 5 to 7 days. However, if your baby is experiencing severe respiratory symptoms, your pediatrician may use a nasal secretion test to determine the cause of the infection. If your child needs to be hospitalized, your pediatrician will discuss the best management for your child.

Call your pediatrician right away if your infant shows any of the signs of serious RSV infection. Prompt supportive treatment is especially important if your child is at high risk for developing serious RSV infection.

The information contained in this publication should not be used as a substitute for the medical care and advice of your pediatrician. There may be variations in treatment that your pediatrician may recommend based on individual facts and circumstances.

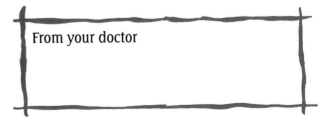

From your doctor

American Academy
of Pediatrics

DEDICATED TO THE HEALTH OF ALL CHILDREN™

The American Academy of Pediatrics is an organization of 60,000 primary care pediatricians, pediatric medical subspecialists, and pediatric surgical specialists dedicated to the health, safety, and well-being of infants, children, adolescents, and young adults.

American Academy of Pediatrics
Web site — www.aap.org

Copyright © 2003
American Academy of Pediatrics, Updated 8/03

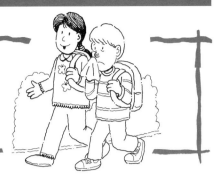

Sinusitis and Your Child

Sinusitis is an inflammation of the lining of the nose and sinuses. It is a very common infection in children.

Viral sinusitis usually accompanies a cold. Allergic sinusitis may accompany allergies such as hay fever. Bacterial sinusitis is a secondary infection caused by the trapping of bacteria in the sinuses during the course of a cold or allergy.

Fluid inside the sinuses

When your child has a viral cold or hay fever, the linings of the nose and sinus cavities swell up and produce more fluid than usual. This is why the nose gets congested and is "runny" during a cold.

Most of the time the swelling disappears by itself as the cold or allergy goes away. However, if the swelling does not go away, the openings that normally allow the sinuses to drain into the back of the nose get blocked and the sinuses fill with fluid. Because the sinuses are blocked and cannot drain properly, bacteria are trapped inside and grow there, causing a secondary infection. Although nose blowing and sniffing may be natural responses to this blockage, when excessive they can make the situation worse by pushing bacteria from the back of the nose into the sinuses.

Is it a cold or bacterial sinusitis?

It is often difficult to tell if an illness is just a viral cold or if it is complicated by a bacterial infection of the sinuses.

Generally viral colds have the following characteristics:
- Colds usually last only 5 to 10 days.
- Colds typically start with clear, watery nasal discharge. After a day or 2, it is normal for the nasal discharge to become thicker and white, yellow, or green. After several days, the discharge becomes clear again and dries.
- Colds include a daytime cough that often gets worse at night.
- If a fever is present, it is usually at the beginning of the cold and is generally low grade, lasting for 1 or 2 days.
- Cold symptoms usually peak in severity at 3 or 5 days, then improve and disappear over the next 7 to 10 days.

Signs and symptoms that your child may have bacterial sinusitis include:
- Cold symptoms (nasal discharge, daytime cough, or both) lasting more than 10 days *without improving*
- Thick yellow nasal discharge *and* a fever for at least 3 or 4 days in a row
- A severe headache behind or around the eyes that gets worse when bending over
- Swelling and dark circles around the eyes, especially in the morning
- Persistent bad breath along with cold symptoms (However, this also could be from a sore throat or a sign that your child is not brushing his teeth!)

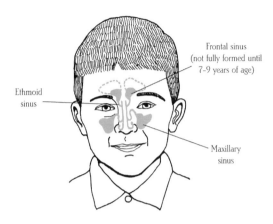

The linings of the sinuses and the nose always produce some fluid (secretions). This fluid keeps the nose and sinus cavities from becoming too dry and adds moisture to the air that you breathe.

In very rare cases, a bacterial sinus infection may spread to the eye or the central nervous system (the brain). If your child has the following symptoms, call your pediatrician immediately:
- Swelling and/or redness around the eyes, not just in the morning but all day
- Severe headache and/or pain in the back of the neck
- Persistent vomiting
- Sensitivity to light
- Increasing irritability

Diagnosing bacterial sinusitis

It may be difficult to tell a sinus infection from an uncomplicated cold, especially in the first few days of the illness. Your pediatrician will most likely be able to tell if your child has bacterial sinusitis after examining your child and hearing about the progression of symptoms. In older children, when the diagnosis is uncertain, your pediatrician may order x-rays or computed tomographic (CT) scans to confirm the diagnosis.

Treating bacterial sinusitis

Following are treatments for bacterial sinusitis and related symptoms:

Sinusitis. If your child has bacterial sinusitis, your pediatrician may prescribe an antibiotic for at least 10 days. Once your child is on the medication, symptoms should start to go away over the next 2 to 3 days—the nasal discharge will clear and the cough will improve. *Even though your child may seem better, continue to give the antibiotics for the prescribed length of time. Ending the medications too early could cause the infection to return.*

If your child's symptoms show no improvement 2 to 3 days after starting the antibiotics, talk with your pediatrician. Your child might need a different medication or need to be re-examined.

Headache or sinus pain. To treat headache or sinus pain, try placing a warm washcloth on your child's face for a few minutes at a time. Pain medications such as acetaminophen or ibuprofen may also help. (However, do not give your child aspirin. It has been associated with a rare but potentially fatal disease called Reye syndrome.)

Nasal congestion. If the secretions in your child's nose are especially thick, your pediatrician may recommend that you help drain them with saline nose drops. These are available without a prescription or can be made at home by adding ¼ teaspoon of table salt to an 8-ounce cup of water. Unless advised by your pediatrician, do not use nose drops that contain medications because they can be absorbed in amounts that can cause side effects.

Placing a cool-mist humidifier in your child's room may help keep your child more comfortable. Clean and dry the humidifier daily to prevent bacteria or mold from growing in it (follow the instructions that came with the humidifier). Hot water vaporizers are not recommended because they can cause scalds or burns.

> **Remember**
>
> If your child has symptoms of a bacterial sinus infection, see your pediatrician. Your pediatrician can properly diagnose and treat the infection and recommend ways to help alleviate the discomfort from some of the symptoms.

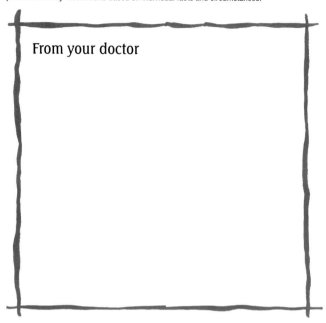

From your doctor

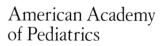

American Academy of Pediatrics

DEDICATED TO THE HEALTH OF ALL CHILDREN™

The American Academy of Pediatrics is an organization of 60,000 primary care pediatricians, pediatric medical subspecialists, and pediatric surgical specialists dedicated to the health, safety, and well-being of infants, children, adolescents, and young adults.

American Academy of Pediatrics
Web site — www.aap.org

Copyright © 2003
American Academy of Pediatrics

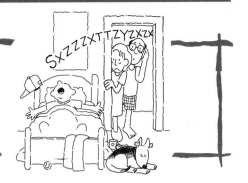

Sleep Apnea and Your Child

Does your child snore a lot? Does he sleep restlessly? Does he have difficulty breathing, or does he gasp or choke, while he sleeps?

If your child has these symptoms, he may have a condition known as sleep apnea.

Sleep apnea is a common problem that affects an estimated 2% of all children, including many who are undiagnosed.

If not treated, sleep apnea can lead to a variety of problems. These include heart, behavior, learning, and growth problems.

How do I know if my child has sleep apnea?

Symptoms of sleep apnea include
- Frequent snoring
- Problems breathing during the night
- Sleepiness during the day
- Difficulty paying attention
- Behavior problems

If you notice any of these symptoms, let your pediatrician know as soon as possible. Your pediatrician may recommend a sleep study—usually an overnight study called a *polysomnogram*. Overnight polysomnograms are conducted at hospitals and major medical centers. During the study, doctors and medical staff will watch your child sleep. Several sensors will be attached to your child to monitor breathing, oxygenation, and brain waves electroencephalogram (EEG).

The results of the study will show whether your child suffers from sleep apnea. Other specialists, such as pediatric pulmonologists, otolaryngologists, neurologists, and pediatricians with specialty training in sleep disorders, may help your pediatrician make the diagnosis.

What causes sleep apnea?

Many children with sleep apnea have larger than normal tonsils and adenoids.

Tonsils are the round, reddish masses on each side of your child's throat. They help fight infections in the body. You can only see the adenoid with an x-ray or special mirror. It lies in the space between the nose and throat.

Large tonsils and adenoid may block a child's airway while she sleeps. This causes her to snore and wake up often during the night. However, not every child with large tonsils and adenoid has sleep apnea. A sleep

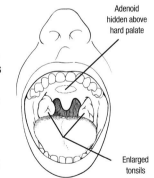

Adenoid hidden above hard palate

Enlarged tonsils

study can tell your doctor whether your child has sleep apnea or if she is simply snoring.

Children born with other medical conditions, such as Down syndrome, cerebral palsy, or craniofacial (skull and face) abnormalities, are at higher risk for sleep apnea. Overweight children are also more likely to suffer from sleep apnea.

How is sleep apnea treated?

The most common way to treat sleep apnea is to remove your child's tonsils and adenoid. This surgery is called a tonsillectomy and adenoidectomy. It is highly effective in treating sleep apnea.

Another effective treatment is nasal continuous positive airway pressure (CPAP), which requires the child to wear a mask while he sleeps. The mask delivers steady air pressure through the child's nose, allowing him to breathe comfortably. Continuous positive airway pressure is usually used in children who do not improve after tonsillectomy and adenoidectomy, or who are not candidates for tonsillectomy and adenoidectomy.

Children who may need additional treatment include children who are overweight or suffering from another complicating condition. Overweight children will improve if they lose weight, but may need to use CPAP until the weight is lost.

Remember
A good night's sleep is important to good health. If your child suffers from the symptoms of sleep apnea, talk with your pediatrician. A proper diagnosis and treatment can mean restful nights and restful days for your child and your family.

The information contained in this publication should not be used as a substitute for the medical care and advice of your pediatrician. There may be variations in treatment that your pediatrician may recommend based on individual facts and circumstances.

From your doctor

American Academy of Pediatrics
DEDICATED TO THE HEALTH OF ALL CHILDREN™

The American Academy of Pediatrics is an organization of 60,000 primary care pediatricians, pediatric medical subspecialists, and pediatric surgical specialists dedicated to the health, safety, and well-being of infants, children, adolescents, and young adults.
American Academy of Pediatrics
Web site—www.aap.org

Copyright © 2003
American Academy of Pediatrics

Sleep Problems in Children
Part I Infants, Toddlers, and Preschoolers

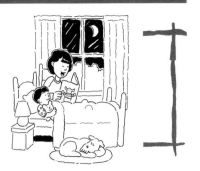

Sleep problems are very common among children during the first few years of life. Problems may include a reluctance to go to sleep, waking up in the middle of the night, nightmares, and sleepwalking. In older children, bed-wetting can also become a challenge.

Children vary in the amount of sleep they need and the amount of time it takes to fall asleep. How easily they wake up and how quickly they can resettle are also different for each child. It is important, however, that as a parent you help your child develop good sleep habits at an early age. The good news is that most sleep problems can be solved and your pediatrician can help.

Infants

Newborn infants have irregular sleep cycles, which take about 6 months to mature. While newborns sleep an average of 16 to 17 hours per day, they may only sleep 1 or 2 hours at a time. As children get older, the total number of hours they need for sleep decreases. However, different children have different needs. It is normal even for a 6 month old to wake up briefly during the night, but these awakenings should only last a few minutes and children should be able to go back to sleep on their own. Here are some suggestions that may help your baby (and you) sleep better at night:

1. **Try to keep her as calm and quiet as possible.** When feeding or changing your baby during the night, avoid stimulating her or waking her up too much so she can easily fall back to sleep.
2. **Don't let your infant sleep as long during the day.** If she sleeps for large blocks of time during the day, she will be more likely to be awake during the night.
3. **Put your baby into the crib at the first signs of drowsiness.** Ideally it is best to let the baby learn to relax and settle herself to sleep. If you make a habit of holding or rocking her until she falls asleep, she may learn to need you to get back to sleep when she wakes up in the middle of the night. This may interfere with her learning to settle herself and fall asleep alone.
4. **Try to avoid putting your baby to bed with a pacifier.** Your baby may get used to falling asleep with it and have trouble learning to settle herself without it. Pacifiers should be used to satisfy the baby's need to suck, not to help a baby sleep. If your baby falls asleep with a pacifier, gently remove it before putting her in bed.

5. **Begin to delay your reaction to infant fussing at 4 to 6 months of age.** Wait a few minutes before you go in to check her, because she will probably settle herself and fall back to sleep in a few minutes anyway. If she continues to cry, check on her, but avoid turning on the light, playing, picking up, or rocking her. If crying continues or begins to sound frantic, wait a few more minutes and then recheck the baby. If she is unable to settle herself, consider what else might be bothering her. She may be hungry, wet or soiled, feverish, or otherwise not feeling well.
6. **Ideally, by a few weeks of age a baby should sleep in a separate room from his parents.**

If your baby is ill, these suggestions should be relaxed. After she feels better, begin to reestablish sleep patterns.

Infant sleep positioning and SIDS
The American Academy of Pediatrics recommends that parents and caregivers place healthy infants on their backs when putting them down to sleep. This is because recent studies have shown an increased incidence of Sudden Infant Death Syndrome (SIDS) in infants who sleep on their stomachs. There is no evidence that sleeping on the back is harmful to healthy infants.

Toddlers and preschoolers

Many parents find their toddler's bedtime one of the hardest parts of the day. It is common for children this age to resist going to sleep, especially if there are older siblings who are still awake. However, remember toddlers and pre-schoolers usually need 10 to 12 hours of sleep each night. If your child's sleeping time does not approach this level, talk to your pediatrician.

Following are some tips to help your toddler develop good sleep habits:

1. **Make sure there is a quiet period before your child goes to bed.** Establish a pleasant routine that may include reading, singing, or a warm bath. A regular routine will help your child understand that it will soon be time to go to sleep. If parents work late hours, it may be tempting to play with their child before bedtime. However, active play just before bedtime may leave the child excited and unable to sleep. Limit television viewing and video game play before bed.

2. **Try to set a consistent schedule** for your child and make bedtime the same time every night. His sleep patterns will adjust accordingly.

3. **Allow your child to take a favorite teddy bear, toy, or special blanket to bed each night.** Such comforting objects often help children fall asleep—especially if they awaken during the middle of the night. Make sure the object is safe. A teddy bear may have a ribbon, button, or other part that may pose a choking hazard for your child. Look for sturdy construction at the seams. Stuffing or pellets inside the stuffed animal may also pose a danger of choking.

4. **Make sure your child is comfortable.** Check the temperature in your child's room. Clothes should not restrict movement. He may like to have a drink of water before bed, have a night-light left on, or the door left slightly open. Try to handle your child's needs before bedtime, so that he doesn't use them to avoid going to bed.

5. **Try to avoid letting your child sleep with you.** This will only make it harder for him to learn to settle himself and fall asleep when he is alone.

6. **Try not to return to your child's room every time he complains or calls out.** A child will quickly learn if you always give in to his requests at bedtime. When your child calls out, try the following:
   - Wait several seconds before answering. Your response time can be longer each time to give your child the message that it is time for sleep. It also gives him the opportunity to fall asleep on his own.
   - Reassure your child that you are there. If you need to go into his room, do not stimulate the child or stay too long.
   - Move farther from your child's bed every time you go to reassure him, until you can do this verbally without entering his room.

The information contained in this publication should not be used as a substitute for the medical care and advice of your pediatrician. There may be variations in treatment that your pediatrician may recommend based on individual facts and circumstances.

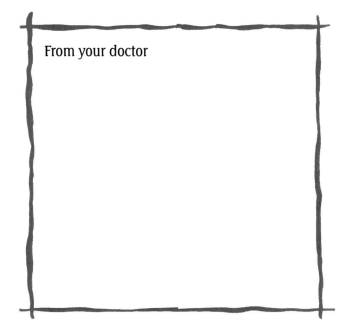

From your doctor

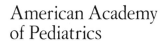

American Academy of Pediatrics

DEDICATED TO THE HEALTH OF ALL CHILDREN™

The American Academy of Pediatrics is an organization of 60,000 primary care pediatricians, pediatric medical subspecialists, and pediatric surgical specialists dedicated to the health, safety, and well-being of infants, children, adolescents, and young adults.

American Academy of Pediatrics
Web site — www.aap.org

Copyright © 2002
American Academy of Pediatrics

Sleep Problems in Children

Part II Common Sleep Problems

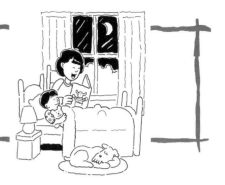

Common sleep problems

For a young child, many things can interrupt a good night's sleep. As a parent, you may be able to prevent some of them.

Nightmares

Nightmares are scary dreams that usually happen during the second half of the night, when dreaming is most intense. This may occur more than once a night. After the nightmare is over, your child may wake up and can tell you what occurred. Children may be crying or fearful after a nightmare but will be aware of your presence. They may have trouble falling back to sleep because they can remember the details of the dream.

How to handle nightmares:
- Go to the child as quickly as possible.
- Assure her that you are there and will not let anything harm her. Allow the child to have the bedroom light on for a short period to reassure her.
- If your child is fearful, comfort and calm her.
- Keep in mind that a nightmare is real to a young child. Listen to her and encourage her to tell you what happened in the dream.
- Once the child is calm, encourage her to go back to sleep.

Night terrors

Night terrors are more severe or frightening than nightmares, but not as common. They occur most often in toddlers and preschoolers. Night terrors come out of the deepest stages of sleep, usually within an hour or so after a child falls asleep. During a night terror, children usually cannot be awakened or comforted. Night terrors may also cause the following:
- Uncontrollable crying
- Sweating, shaking, and fast breathing
- A terrified, confused, and glassy-eyed appearance
- Thrashing around, screaming, kicking, or staring
- Child may not realize anyone is with him
- Child may not appear to recognize you
- Child may try to push you away, especially when you try to restrain him

Night terrors may last as long as 45 minutes, but are usually much shorter. Children seem to fall right back to sleep after a night terror, but they actually have not been awake. Like nightmares, night terrors may occur more often in times of stress or may relate to difficult feelings or fears. However, unlike a nightmare, a child will not remember a night terror.

How to handle night terrors:
- Remain calm. Night terrors are usually more frightening for the parent than for the child.
- Do not try to wake your child.
- Make sure the child does not injure himself. If the child tries to get out of bed, gently restrain him.
- Remember, after a short time, your child will probably relax and sleep quietly again.
- If your child has night terrors, be sure to explain to your baby-sitters what they are and what to do.

Keep in mind that night terrors do not always indicate serious problems. Your child will be more likely to have night terrors when he is overly tired and during periods of stress. Your child can become overly tired when he gives up a daytime nap, wakes up too early, or his nighttime sleep is interrupted. Try to keep your child on a regular sleep schedule or increase the amount of sleep he gets to prevent night terrors. Night terrors usually disappear by the time a child reaches grade school. If they do persist, talk to your pediatrician.

Sleepwalking and sleep talking

Like night terrors, sleepwalking and sleep talking happen when a child is in a deep sleep. While sleepwalking, your child may have a blank, staring face. She may not respond to others and be very difficult to awaken. When your child does wake up, she will probably not remember the episode. Sleepwalking children will often return to bed by themselves and will not even remember that they have gotten out of bed. Sleepwalking can be common, and tends to run in families. It can even occur several times in one night among older children and teenagers. If you have concerns or the condition persists, talk to your child's pediatrician.

How to handle sleepwalking and sleep talking:
- Make sure your child doesn't hurt herself while sleepwalking. Clear the bedroom area of potential hazards that your child could trip over or fall on.
- Lock outside doors so your child cannot leave the house.
- Block stairways so your child cannot go up or down.
- There is no need to try to wake your child when she is sleepwalking or sleep talking. Gently lead her back to bed and she will probably settle down on her own.

Sleepwalking and sleep talking are more likely to occur when your child is overly tired or under stress. Keeping your child's sleep schedule regular may help prevent sleepwalking and sleep talking.

Bed-wetting (also called enuresis)

Nighttime bed-wedding is normal and very common among preschoolers. It affects about 40% of 3 year olds and may run in families. The most common reasons your child may wet the bed include the following:

- A bladder that has not yet developed enough to hold urine for a full night.
- Your child may not yet be able to recognize a full bladder and wake up to use the toilet.
- Stress. Changes in the home, such as a new baby, moving, or a divorce can lead to a sudden case of bed-wetting for a child who has been dry at night in the past.

How to handle bed-wetting:

- Do not blame or punish the child for bed-wetting.
- Have your child use the toilet and avoid drinking large amounts of fluid just before bedtime.
- Until your child can stay dry during the night, put a rubber or plastic cover over the mattress to protect against wetness and odors. Keep the bedding clean.
- If your child is old enough, involve him in handling the problem. Encourage him to help change the wet sheets and covers. This will help teach responsibility and avoid the embarrassment of having other family members know about the problem every time it happens. Do not, however, use this as punishment for the child.
- Talk to your pediatrician about other approaches to bed-wetting, such as rewards for younger children or alarm devices for the older child.

Most importantly, don't pressure your child. Bed-wetting is beyond a child's control and he may only become sad or frustrated if he cannot stop. Set a "no-teasing" rule in the family. Make sure your child understands that bed-wetting is not his fault and it will get better in time.

Teeth grinding

It is also common for children to grind their teeth during the night. Though it produces an unpleasant sound, it is usually not harmful to your young child's teeth. It may be related to tension and anxiety and usually disappears in a short while. However, it may reappear with the next stressful episode.

Give it time

Handling your child's sleep problems may be a challenge and it is normal to become upset at times when a child keeps you awake at night. Try to be understanding. A negative response by a parent can sometimes make a sleep problem worse, especially if it is associated with a stressful situation like divorce, a new sibling, a tragedy in the family, problems at school, or some other recent change in your child's life.

If the problem persists, there may be a physical or emotional reason that your child cannot sleep. If you feel you need additional help, start a sleep diary and discuss the problem with your pediatrician. Keep in mind that most sleep problems are very common, and with time and your pediatrician's help, you and your child will overcome them.

Keeping a sleep diary

It may be helpful for you in preparation for discussing a sleep problem with your pediatrician to keep a sleep diary for your child. Chart the following:

- Where your child sleeps
- How much sleep she normally gets at night
- What time she was put to bed
- What the child needs to fall asleep (favorite toy, blanket, etc)
- The time it takes for her to fall asleep
- The time that you went to bed
- The time awakened during the night
- How long it took to fall back to sleep
- What you did to comfort and console the child
- The time the child woke up in the morning
- The time and length of naps
- Any changes or stresses in the home

Keep in mind that every child is different and no two children may have the same sleep patterns or problems.

The information contained in this publication should not be used as a substitute for the medical care and advice of your pediatrician. There may be variations in treatment that your pediatrician may recommend based on individual facts and circumstances.

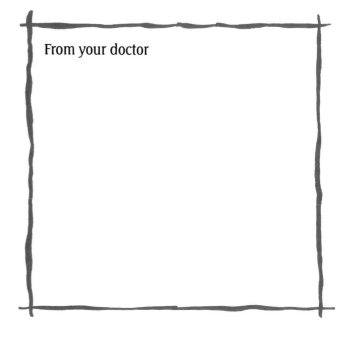

From your doctor

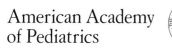

American Academy of Pediatrics

DEDICATED TO THE HEALTH OF ALL CHILDREN™

The American Academy of Pediatrics is an organization of 60,000 primary care pediatricians, pediatric medical subspecialists, and pediatric surgical specialists dedicated to the health, safety, and well-being of infants, children, adolescents, and young adults.

American Academy of Pediatrics
Web site—www.aap.org

Copyright © 2002
American Academy of Pediatrics

Tonsils and the Adenoid

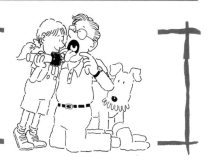

In years past, it was very common for children to have their tonsils and the adenoid taken out. Today, doctors know much more about tonsils and the adenoid and are more careful about recommending removal.

Tonsils and the adenoid: what are they?

The **tonsils** are oval-shaped, pink masses of tissue on both sides of the throat. Tonsils can be different sizes for different children. They can be large or small. There is no "normal" size. You can usually see the tonsils by looking at the back of the mouth with a flashlight. Pressing on the tongue may help, but this makes many children gag. The **uvula**, a fleshy lobe that hangs down in the back of the mouth, should not be mistaken for the tonsils.

The **adenoid** is often referred to as "adenoids." This is incorrect because the adenoid is actually a single mass of tissue. The adenoid is similar to the tonsils and is located in the very upper part of the throat, above the uvula and behind the nose. This area is called the *nasopharynx*. The adenoid can be seen only with special mirrors or instruments passed through the nose.

Both the tonsils and the adenoid are part of your body's defense against infections. Since similar tissues in other parts of the body do the same job, removal of the tonsils or the adenoid does not harm the body's ability to fight infection.

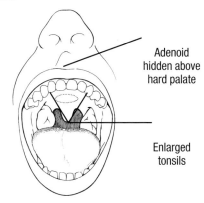

Adenoid hidden above hard palate

Enlarged tonsils

What is tonsillitis?

Tonsillitis is an inflammation of the tonsils usually due to infection. There are several signs of tonsillitis, including:
- Red and swollen tonsils
- White or yellow coating over the tonsils
- A "throaty" voice
- Sore throat
- Uncomfortable or painful swallowing
- Swollen lymph nodes ("glands") in the neck
- Fever

What are the symptoms of an enlarged adenoid?

It is not always easy to tell when your child's adenoid is enlarged. Some children are born with a larger adenoid. Others may have temporary enlargement of their adenoid due to colds or other infections. This is especially common among young children. Constant swelling or enlargement can cause other health problems such as ear and sinus infections. Some signs of adenoid enlargement are:
- Breathing through the mouth instead of the nose most of the time
- Nose sounds "blocked" when the child talks
- Noisy breathing during the day
- Snoring at night

Both the tonsils *and* the adenoid may be enlarged if your child has the symptoms mentioned above, along with any of the following:
- Breathing stops for a short period of time at night during snoring or loud breathing (this is called "sleep apnea").
- Choking or gasping during sleep.
- Difficulty swallowing, especially solid foods.
- A constant "throaty voice," even when there is no tonsillitis.

Treatment

If your child shows any of these signs or symptoms of enlargement of the tonsils or the adenoid, and doesn't seem to be getting better over a period of weeks, talk to your pediatrician. In many children, the tonsils and adenoid become enlarged without obvious infection. They often shrink without treatment.

According to the guidelines of the American Academy of Pediatrics, your pediatrician may recommend surgery for the following conditions:
- Tonsil or adenoid swelling that makes normal breathing difficult (this may or may not include sleep apnea).
- Tonsils that are so swollen that your child has a problem swallowing.
- An enlarged adenoid that makes breathing uncomfortable, severely alters speech and possibly affects normal growth of the face. In this case, surgery to remove only the adenoid may be recommended.
- Your child has repeated ear or sinus infections despite treatment. In this case, surgery to remove only the adenoid may be recommended.
- Your child has an excessive number of severe sore throats each year.
- Your child's lymph nodes beneath the lower jaw are swollen or tender for at least six months, even with antibiotic treatment.

How do I prepare my child for surgery?

Though it is not as common as it once was, some children need to have their tonsils and/or adenoid taken out. If your child needs surgery, make sure he or she knows what will happen before, during, and after surgery. Don't keep the surgery a secret from your child. Surgery can be scary, but it's better to be honest than to leave your child with fears and unanswered questions.

The hospital may have a special program to help you and your child get familiar with the hospital and the surgery. If the hospital allows, try to stay with your child during the entire hospital visit. Let your child know you'll be nearby during the entire operation. Your pediatrician can also help you and your child understand the operation and make it less frightening in the process. A little ice cream afterwards won't hurt either.

The information contained in this publication should not be used as a substitute for the medical care and advice of your pediatrician. There may be variations in treatment that your pediatrician may recommend based on individual facts and circumstances.

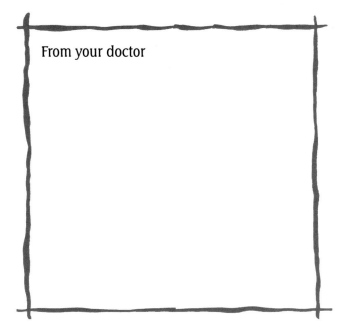

From your doctor

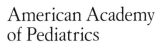

American Academy
of Pediatrics

DEDICATED TO THE HEALTH OF ALL CHILDREN™

The American Academy of Pediatrics is an organization of 60,000 primary care pediatricians, pediatric medical subspecialists, and pediatric surgical specialists dedicated to the health, safety, and well-being of infants, children, adolescents, and young adults.

American Academy of Pediatrics
Web site—www.aap.org

Copyright ©1997
American Academy of Pediatrics, Updated 3/99

Urinary Tract Infections in Young Children

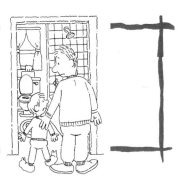

Urinary tract infections (UTIs) are common in young children. UTIs may go untreated because the symptoms may not be obvious to the child or to parents. These infections can lead to serious health problems. From this brochure, parents can learn more about urinary tract infections—what they are, how children get them, and how they are treated.

The Urinary Tract

The urinary tract makes and stores urine. It is made up of the kidneys, ureters, bladder, and the urethra (see illustration). The kidneys produce urine. Urine travels from the kidneys down two narrow tubes called the ureters to the bladder. The bladder is a thin muscular bag that stores urine until it is time to empty urine out of the body. When it is time to empty the bladder, a muscle at the the bottom of the bladder relaxes. Urine then flows out of the body through a tube, called the urethra. The opening of the urethra is at the end of the penis in boys and above the vaginal opening in girls.

Urinary Tract Infections

Normal urine has no germs (bacteria). However, bacteria can get into the urinary tract from two sources: the skin around the rectum and genitals and the bloodstream from other parts of the body. Bacteria may cause infections in any or all parts of the urinary tract, including the following:

- the urethra (called "urethritis")
- the bladder (called "cystitis")
- the kidneys (called "pyelonephritis")

UTIs are common in infants and young children. About 3 percent of girls and 1 percent of boys will have a UTI by 11 years of age. A young child with a high fever and no other symptoms, has a 1 in 20 chance of having a UTI. The frequency of UTIs in girls is much greater than in boys. Uncircumcised boys have slightly more UTIs than those who have been circumcised.

Symptoms

Symptoms of UTIs may include the following:

- fever
- pain or burning during urination
- need to urinate more often, or difficulty getting urine out
- urgent need to urinate, or wetting of underwear or bedding by a child who knows how to use the toilet
- vomiting, refusal to eat
- abdominal pain
- side or back pain
- foul-smelling urine
- cloudy or bloody urine
- unexplained and persistent irritability in an infant
- poor growth in an infant

Diagnosis

If your child has symptoms of a UTI, your pediatrician will do the following:

- ask about your child's symptoms
- ask about any family history of urinary tract problems
- ask about what your child has been eating and drinking (certain foods can irritate the urinary tract and cause similar symptoms)
- examine your child
- get a urine sample from your child

Your pediatrician will need to test your child's urine to see if there are bacteria or other abnormalities. There are several ways to collect urine from a child.

- The preferred method to diagnose a UTI is to place a small tube, called a catheter, through the urethra into the bladder. Urine flows through the tube into a special urine container.
- Another method is to insert a needle through the skin of the lower abdomen to draw urine from the bladder. This is called needle aspiration.
- If your child is very young or not yet toilet trained, the pediatrician may place a plastic bag over the genitals to collect the urine. Since bacteria can contaminate the urine and give a false test result, this method is used only to screen for infection.
- An older child may be asked to urinate into a container.

Your pediatrician will discuss with you the best way to collect your child's urine.

Treatment

UTIs are treated with antibiotics. The way your child receives the antibiotic depends on the severity and type of infection. If your child has a fever or is vomiting and unable to keep fluids down, the antibiotics may be put directly into the bloodstream or muscle using a needle. This is usually done in the hospital. Otherwise, the antibiotics can be given by mouth, as liquid or pills.

UTIs need to be treated right away for the following reasons:

- to get rid of the infection
- to prevent the spread of the infection
- to reduce the chances of kidney damage

Infants and young children with UTIs usually need to take antibiotics for 7 to 14 days, sometimes longer. Make sure your child takes all the medicine your pediatrician prescribes. Do not stop giving your child the medicine until the pediatrician says the treatment is finished, even if your child feels better. UTIs can return if not fully treated.

Follow-up

After your child finishes the antibiotics, your pediatrician may want to test another urine sample to make sure the bacteria are gone. In addition, your pediatrician will want to make sure the urinary tract is normal and that the infection did not cause any damage. Several tests are available to do this, including the following:

Kidney and bladder ultrasound: Uses sound waves to examine the bladder and kidneys.

Voiding cystourethrogram (VCUG): A catheter is placed into the urethra and the bladder is filled with a liquid that can be seen on X-rays.

Intravenous pyelogram: A liquid that can be seen on X-rays is injected into a vein and then travels into the kidneys and bladder.

Nuclear scans: Radioactive materials are injected into a vein to see if the kidneys are normal. There are many kinds of nuclear scans, each giving different information about the kidneys and bladder. The radioactive materials give no more radiation than other kinds of X-rays.

Keep in mind, UTIs are common and most are easy to treat. Early diagnosis and prompt treatment are important because untreated or repeated infections can cause long-term medical problems. Talk to your pediatrician if you suspect that your child might have a UTI.

The information contained in this publication should not be used as a substitute for the medical care and advice of your pediatrician. There may be variations in treatment that your pediatrician may recommend based on individual facts and circumstances.

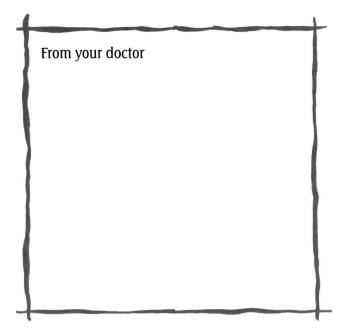

From your doctor

American Academy of Pediatrics

DEDICATED TO THE HEALTH OF ALL CHILDREN™

The American Academy of Pediatrics is an organization of 60,000 primary care pediatricians, pediatric medical subspecialists, and pediatric surgical specialists dedicated to the health, safety, and well-being of infants, children, adolescents, and young adults.

American Academy of Pediatrics
Web site—www.aap.org

Copyright © 1999
American Academy of Pediatrics

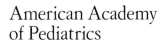

© 2007 American Academy of Pediatrics

Newborns, Infants, and Toddlers

Baby Bottle Tooth Decay—
How to Prevent It

Proper dental care is a lifelong commitment that starts even before your baby's first tooth forms. While daily cleanings and fluoride are important, they alone may not prevent Baby Bottle Tooth Decay (BBTD), a major cause of tooth decay in infants. Baby Bottle Tooth Decay is costly to treat. If left untreated, however, it can quickly destroy the teeth involved. It also can lead to pain, infection, early loss of baby teeth, crooked permanent teeth, and an increased risk of decay in permanent teeth. When you consider the possible dental problems that can result from BBTD and the cost of treating those problems, it is best to prevent BBTD from developing in the first place.

How Does Baby Bottle Tooth Decay Develop?

Baby Bottle Tooth Decay can develop if your child's teeth and gums are in prolonged contact with almost any liquid other than water. This can happen from putting your child to bed with a bottle of formula, milk, juice, soft drinks, sugar water, sugared drinks, etc. Allowing your baby to suck on a bottle or breastfeed for longer than a mealtime, either when awake or asleep, also can cause BBTD.

When liquid from a baby bottle builds up in the mouth, the natural or added sugars found in the liquid are changed to acid by germs in the mouth. This acid then starts to dissolve the teeth (mainly the upper front teeth), causing them to decay. Baby Bottle Tooth Decay can lead to severe damage to your child's baby teeth and also can cause dental problems that affect your child's permanent teeth.

Why Are Baby Teeth Important?

Many parents assume that decay does not matter in baby teeth because the teeth will fall out anyway, but decay in baby teeth poses risks. If your child loses his baby teeth too early because of decay or infection, the permanent teeth will not be ready to replace them yet. Baby teeth act as a guide for the permanent teeth. If baby teeth are lost too early, the teeth that are left may shift position to fill in the gaps. This may not leave any room for the permanent teeth to come in.

What Can I Do to Prevent Baby Bottle Tooth Decay?

Take the following steps to prevent Baby Bottle Tooth Decay:

- Never put your child to bed with a bottle. By 7 or 8 months of age, most children no longer need feedings during the night. Children who drink bottles while lying down also may be more prone to getting ear infections.
- Only give your baby a bottle during meals. Do not use the bottle as a pacifier; do not allow your child to walk around with it or to drink it for extended periods. These practices not only may lead to BBTD, but children can suffer tooth injuries if they fall while sucking on a bottle.
- Teach your child to drink from a cup as soon as possible, usually by 1 year of age. Drinking from a cup does not cause the liquid to collect around the teeth, and a cup cannot be taken to bed. If you are concerned that a cup may be messier than a bottle, especially when you are away from home, use one that has a snap-on lid with a straw or a special valve to prevent spilling.
- If your child must have a bottle for long periods, fill it only with water.

Keeping your baby's mouth clean is also important in preventing tooth decay. After feedings, gently brush your baby's gums and any baby teeth with a soft infant toothbrush.

Start using water and a soft child-sized toothbrush for daily cleanings once your child has seven to eight teeth. By the time your toddler is 2 years of age, you should be brushing her teeth once or twice a day, preferably after breakfast and before bedtime.

Begin using a fluoride toothpaste when you are sure the toothpaste will not be swallowed (usually when your child is around 3 years of age). Use a pea-sized amount of toothpaste to limit the amount your child can swallow. Too much fluoride can be harmful to a child.

Detect Decay Early

Baby Bottle Tooth Decay first shows up as white spots on the upper front teeth. These spots are hard to see at first—even for a pediatrician or dentist—without proper equipment. A child with tooth decay needs to get treatment early to stop the decay from spreading and to prevent lasting damage to the teeth.

If you are concerned that your child may have BBTD, your pediatrician can refer you to a pediatric dentist who will carefully examine your child's teeth for signs of decay.

With the right balance of proper home and professional dental care, your child can grow up to have healthy teeth for a lifetime of smiles.

American Academy
of Pediatrics
DEDICATED TO THE HEALTH OF ALL CHILDREN™

The American Academy of Pediatrics is an organization of 60,000 primary care pediatricians, pediatric medical subspecialists, and pediatric surgical specialists dedicated to the health, safety, and well-being of infants, children, adolescents, and young adults.

American Academy of Pediatrics
Web site — www.aap.org

Copyright ©1995
American Academy of Pediatrics, Updated 9/98

Baby Walkers

- Baby walkers sent an estimated 8,800 children younger than 15 months to the hospital in 1999.
- Thirty-four children died during the years of 1973 through 1998 because of baby walkers.

Children in baby walkers can:

- Roll down the stairs — which often causes broken bones and severe head injuries. This is how most children get hurt in baby walkers.
- Get burned — a child can reach higher when in a walker. A cup of hot coffee on the table, pot handles on the stove, a radiator, a fireplace, or a space heater are all now in baby's reach.
- Drown — a child can fall into a pool, bathtub, or toilet while in a walker.
- Be poisoned — reaching high objects is easier in a walker.

There are no benefits to baby walkers

You may think a walker can help your child learn to walk. But walkers do not help children walk sooner. In fact, walkers can delay normal muscle control and mental development.

Most walker injuries happen while adults are watching. Parents or caregivers simply cannot respond quickly enough. A child in a walker can move more than 3 feet in 1 second! Therefore, walkers are never safe to use, even with close adult supervision. Make sure there are no walkers at home or wherever your child is being cared for. Child care facilities should not allow the use of baby walkers. If your child is in child care at a center or at someone else's home, make sure there are no walkers.

Throw out your baby walkers!

Try something just as enjoyable but safer, such as the following:
- "Stationary walkers" — have no wheels but have seats that rotate, tip, and bounce.
- Playpens — great safety zones for children as they learn to sit, crawl, or walk.
- High chairs — older children often enjoy sitting up in a high chair and playing with toys on the tray.

On July 1, 1997, new safety standards were implemented for baby walkers. Walkers are now made wider so they cannot fit through most doorways, or are made with a braking mechanism to stop them at the edge of a step. But these new walker designs will not prevent all injuries from walkers. They still have wheels, so children can still move fast and reach higher.

The American Academy of Pediatrics and the National Association of Children's Hospitals and Related Institutions have called for a ban on the manufacture and sale of baby walkers with wheels. *Keep your child safe…throw away your baby walker.*

The information contained in this publication should not be used as a substitute for the medical care and advice of your pediatrician. There may be variations in treatment that your pediatrician may recommend based on individual facts and circumstances.

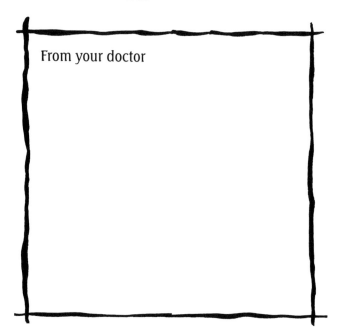

From your doctor

American Academy
of Pediatrics

DEDICATED TO THE HEALTH OF ALL CHILDREN™

The American Academy of Pediatrics is an organization of 60,000 primary care pediatricians, pediatric medical subspecialists, and pediatric surgical specialists dedicated to the health, safety, and well-being of infants, children, adolescents, and young adults.

American Academy of Pediatrics
Web site — www.aap.org

Copyright © 1999
American Academy of Pediatrics

Bedwetting

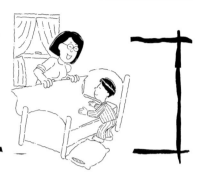

Most children are toilet trained between 2 and 4 years of age. Many children at this age are able to stay dry during the day, but may not be able to stay dry at night until they are older. Between 15% and 30% of 6-year-olds have one episode of bedwetting (also known as enuresis) per month, and as many as 4% or more of 12-year-olds are still wetting their beds some of the time. Like so many things in pediatrics, bedwetting and the issues associated with it have their own developmental time line. Read on to find out more about bedwetting and what can be done about it.

Causes of bedwetting

Although all of the causes of bedwetting are not fully understood, the following are some that are possible:

- Your child is a deep sleeper and does not awaken to the signal of a full bladder.
- Your child's body makes too much urine at night.
- Your child is constipated (this can put pressure on the bladder).
- Your child has a minor illness, is overly tired, or is responding to changes or stresses going on at home.
- There is a family history of bedwetting. (Most children that wet the bed have at least one parent who had the same problem as a child.)
- Your child's bladder is small or not developed enough to hold urine for a full night.
- Your child has an underlying medical problem.

What you can do

Most children wet their beds during toilet training. Even after they stay dry at night for a number of days or even weeks, they may start wetting at night again. If this happens to your child, simply put her back in training pants at night for a while until she is ready to try again. The problem usually disappears as your child gets older. If children reach school age and still have problems wetting the bed, it most likely means they have never developed nighttime bladder control.

If you are concerned about your child's bedwetting or your child expresses concern, talk with your pediatrician. You may be asked the following questions about your child's bedwetting:

- Is there a family history of bedwetting?
- How often and when does your child urinate during the day?
- Have there been any changes in your child's home life such as a new baby, divorce, or new house?
- Does your child drink carbonated beverages, caffeine, citrus juices, or a lot of water before bed?
- Is there anything unusual about how your child urinates or the way the urine looks?

Signs of a medical problem

If your child has been completely toilet trained for 6 months or longer and suddenly begins wetting the bed, talk with your pediatrician. It may be a sign of a medical problem. However, most medical problems that cause bedwetting to recur suddenly have other signs, including

- Changes in how much and how often your child urinates during the day
- Pain, burning, or straining while urinating
- A very small or narrow stream of urine or dribbling that is constant or happens just after urination
- Cloudy or pink urine or bloodstains on underpants
- Daytime and nighttime wetting
- Sudden change in personality or mood
- Poor bowel control
- Urinating after stress (coughing, running, or lifting)
- Certain gait disturbances (problems with walking that may mean an underlying neurologic problem)
- Continuous dampness

If your child has any of these signs, your pediatrician may want to take a closer look at your child's kidneys or bladder. If necessary, your pediatrician will refer you to a pediatric urologist, a doctor who is specially trained to treat children's urinary problems.

Managing bedwetting

Keep the following tips in mind when dealing with bedwetting:

- **Be honest** with your child about what is going on. Let your child know it's not his fault and that he will eventually be able to stay dry all night. Let your child know lots of kids go through this, but no one goes to school and talks about it.
- **Be sensitive** to your child's feelings. If you don't make a big issue out of bedwetting, chances are your child won't, either.
- **Protect the bed.** Until your child stays dry at night, put a plastic cover under the sheets. This protects the mattress from getting wet and smelling like urine.
- **Let your child help.** Encourage your child to help change the wet sheets and covers. This teaches responsibility. It can also keep your child from feeling embarrassed if the rest of the family knows he wet the bed. However, if your child sees this as punishment, it is not recommended.
- **Set a no-teasing rule in your family.** Do not let family members, especially siblings, tease your child. Let them know that it's not his fault.
- **Take steps before bedtime.** Have your child use the toilet and avoid drinking large amounts of fluid just before bedtime.
- **Try to wake him up to use the toilet** (1–2 hours after going to sleep) to help him stay dry through the night.

Reward him for dry nights, but do not punish him for wet ones.

Bedwetting alarms

If your child is still not able to stay dry during the night after using these steps for 1 to 3 months, your pediatrician may recommend using a bedwetting alarm. When a bedwetting alarm senses urine, it sets off an alarm so the child can wake up to use the toilet. When used correctly, it will detect wetness right away and sound the alarm. Be sure your child resets the alarm before going back to sleep.

Bedwetting alarms are successful 50% to 75% of the time. They tend to be most helpful for children who have some dry nights and some bladder control on their own. Ask your pediatrician which type of alarm would be best for your child.

Medicines

Different medicines are available to treat bedwetting. They rarely cure bedwetting, but may help your child, especially in social situations such as sleepovers. However, they are usually a last resort and are not recommended for children younger than 5 years. Also, some of these medicines have side effects. Your pediatrician can tell you more about these medicines and if they are right for your child.

Beware of "cures"

There are many treatment programs and devices that claim they can "cure" bedwetting. Be careful; many of these products make false claims and promises and may be very expensive. Your pediatrician is the best source for advice about bedwetting. Talk with your pediatrician before your child starts any treatment program.

If nothing works

A small number of children who wet the bed do not respond to any treatment. The good news is that bedwetting decreases as the child's body matures. By the teen years, almost all children outgrow bedwetting. Only 1 in 100 adults have problems with bedwetting. Until your older child outgrows bedwetting, she will need a lot of emotional support from your family. Support from a pediatrician or mental health professional also can help.

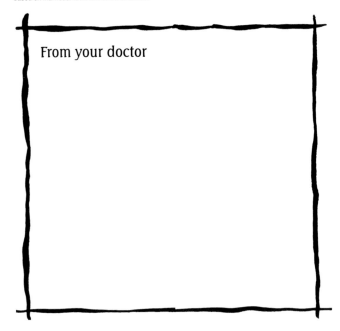

From your doctor

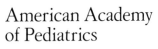

American Academy of Pediatrics

DEDICATED TO THE HEALTH OF ALL CHILDREN™

The American Academy of Pediatrics is an organization of 60,000 primary care pediatricians, pediatric medical subspecialists, and pediatric surgical specialists dedicated to the health, safety, and well-being of infants, children, adolescents, and young adults.

American Academy of Pediatrics
Web site—www.aap.org

Copyright © 2006
American Academy of Pediatrics, Updated 12/05

Breastfeeding Your Baby

Getting Started

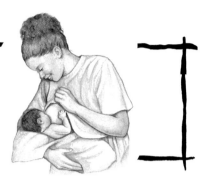

Getting ready for the birth of your baby is an exciting and busy time. One of the most important decisions you will make is how to feed your baby.

Deciding to breastfeed can give your baby the best possible start in life. Breastfeeding benefits you and your baby in many ways. It also is a proud tradition of many cultures.

The following are excerpts from the American Academy of Pediatrics' (AAP) booklet *Breastfeeding Your Baby: Answers to Common Questions*.

Benefits of Breastfeeding

In general, the longer you breastfeed, the greater the benefits will be to you and your baby, and the longer these benefits will last.

Why is breastfeeding so good for my baby?

Breastfeeding is good for your baby because

1. **Breastfeeding provides warmth and closeness.** The physical contact helps create a special bond between you and your baby.
2. **Human milk has many benefits.**
   - It's easier for your baby to digest.
   - It doesn't need to be prepared.
   - It's always available.
   - It has all the nutrients, calories, and fluids your baby needs to be healthy.
   - It has growth factors that ensure the best development of your baby's organs.
   - It has many substances (that formulas don't have) that protect your baby from a variety of diseases and infections. Because of these protective substances, breastfed children are less likely to have
     ~ Ear infections
     ~ Diarrhea
     ~ Pneumonia, wheezing, and bronchiolitis
     ~ Other bacterial and viral infections, such as meningitis

Research also suggests that breastfeeding may help to protect against obesity, diabetes, sudden infant death syndrome (SIDS), and some cancers.

Why is breastfeeding good for me?

Breastfeeding is good for your health because it helps
- Release hormones in your body that promote mothering behavior.
- Return your uterus to the size it was before pregnancy more quickly.
- Burn more calories, which may help you lose the weight you gained during pregnancy.
- Delay the return of your menstrual period to help keep iron in your body.
- Reduce the risk of ovarian cancer and breast cancer.
- Keep bones strong, which helps protect against bone fractures in older age.

How Breastfeeding Works

When you become pregnant, your body begins to prepare for breastfeeding. Your breasts become larger and after your fourth or fifth month of pregnancy, your body is able to produce milk.

What is colostrum?

Colostrum is the first milk your body makes. It's thick with a yellow or orange tint. Colostrum is filled with nutrients your newborn needs. It also contains many substances to protect your baby against diseases and infections.

It's very important for your baby's health to get this early milk, though it may seem like a small amount. Your baby only needs less than 1 tablespoon per feeding on the first day and about 2 tablespoons per feeding on the second day.

What's the difference between *milk coming in* and *let-down*?

Milk coming in and ***let-down*** mean different things, but both are important.
- *Milk comes in* 2 to 5 days after your baby is born. This is when colostrum increases quickly in volume and becomes milky-white transitional milk. Signs that your milk is coming in may be
  ~ Full and tender breasts
  ~ Leaking of milk
  ~ Seeing milk around your baby's mouth
  ~ Hearing your baby swallow when fed

    Breastmilk changes daily and will adjust to your baby's needs for the rest of the time you breastfeed. Because the color or creaminess of the milk can change daily, don't worry about how your milk looks.
- *Let-down* is needed so that your baby can get the colostrum or milk out of the breast. The let-down reflex creates the flow of milk from the back of the breast to the nipple. Let-down occurs each time the baby suckles. Relaxation of the mother and proper latch of the baby are important for triggering let-down. Let-down may also happen between feedings, such as when the breasts are somewhat full or when you hear a baby's cry. The first few times you breastfeed, the let-down reflex may take a few minutes. Afterward, let-down occurs faster, usually within a few seconds. Let-down occurs in both breasts at the same time. It may occur several times during each feeding.

The signs of let-down are different for each woman. Some women feel no sensations, even though breastfeeding is going fine. Other women may experience

~ Strong cramping in the uterus for a few days after delivery when the milk lets down
~ A brief prickle, tingle, or even slight pain in the breast
~ A sudden feeling that breasts are heavier
~ Milk dripping from the breast that's not being used
~ Baby swallowing more milk, or gulping when fed

What is *demand* and *supply?*

The more milk your baby takes from your breast, the more milk you make. This is called *demand and supply* because the more milk your baby demands the more you will supply. Many women with small breasts worry that they won't be able to make enough milk; in general, there's no relationship between breast size and how much milk is produced.

Getting Started

Babies are very alert after they are born and ready to find the breast! The more relaxed and confident you feel, the faster your milk will flow to your baby. Getting comfortable will help you and your baby get started toward a better latch-on.

How soon can I breastfeed?

You can and should breastfeed within the first hour after birth if you and your baby are physically able to do so. After delivery, your baby should be placed on your chest or stomach, skin-to-skin. The early smell and taste of your milk helps your baby learn to nurse. Your breastmilk is all your baby needs. Other liquids, including sugar water and formula, will only lessen the benefits your baby receives from the early breastmilk.

Try to stay with your baby as much as you can. Rooming in with your baby day and night during your hospital stay has been shown to help start breastfeeding and keep it going longer.

What are different breastfeeding positions?

Always take time to get comfortable. Don't be shy about asking for help during the first feedings. It may take a few tries but with a little patience, you and your baby will succeed. The following are 3 breastfeeding positions:

- **Cradle Hold**—The cradle hold is the traditional breastfeeding position. Firmly support your baby's back and bottom. When feeding this way, make sure your baby's entire body is facing your body, not the ceiling.

  - **Clutch Hold**—The clutch, or football, hold is an easy position to hold. If you've had a cesarean delivery, this position may be more comfortable because it keeps the baby's weight off of the stitches.

- **Reclining**—Feeding your baby in a reclining position lets you relax if you've had a cesarean delivery or are tired.

How can I get comfortable while breastfeeding?

A few simple things can help you feel comfortable and relaxed.
- Sit on a comfortable chair, with good back and arm support.
- Lie on your side in bed with your baby facing you. Place pillows to support your back and neck.
- Take deep breaths and picture yourself in a peaceful place.
- Listen to soothing music while sipping a healthy drink.
- Apply moist heat (such as warm wet washcloths) to your breast several minutes before each feeding.
- If your home is very busy, find a quiet place where you won't be disturbed during feedings.
- If you had a cesarean delivery, you may need extra pillows and help with positioning your baby.
- If the baby is properly latched on, the feeding shouldn't hurt.
- Try different breastfeeding positions.

Why is latch-on so important, and how is it done?

A good latch-on means that your baby has opened his mouth wide for the breast, and the baby moves well back onto the breast, taking the areola and nipple far back into his mouth.

Correct latch-on is very important because it
- Makes milk flow better
- Prevents sore nipples
- Keeps your baby satisfied
- Stimulates a good milk supply for baby's weight gain
- Helps to prevent engorged (overly full) breasts

You can help your baby latch on by holding your breast with your free hand. Place your fingers under your breast and rest your thumb lightly on top. Make sure your baby is positioned with his entire body facing you. Your fingers should be well back from the areola so they don't get in the way.

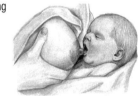

Support your breast and tickle your baby's lower lip with your nipple to stimulate his rooting reflex.

Touching your nipple to the center of your baby's lower lip causes your baby to open his mouth widely. This is called the *rooting reflex*.

As this occurs, pull your baby onto the nipple and areola. Keep in mind that when your baby is correctly positioned, or latched on, your nipple and much of the areola are pulled well into his mouth. Your baby's lips and gums should be around the areola and not just on the nipple. Your baby's chin should be touching your breast; his nose may be touching your breast.

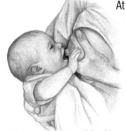

At first you will feel a tugging sensation. You also may feel a brief period of pain. If breastfeeding continues to hurt, pinch, or burn, your baby may not be latched on properly. Break the latch by slipping your finger into the corner of your baby's mouth, reposition, and try again. It can take several tries.

Hospital staff should watch a feeding and make suggestions. If breastfeeding

When your baby's mouth is wide open, bring him quickly, but gently, toward your breast.

continues to hurt, you may need the help of a lactation specialist. Let your pediatrician know if there's a problem.

Beyond the First Feedings

How often should I nurse?

If you and your baby are healthy, breastfeeding is generally most successful when nursing starts within the first hour after delivery. Keep your baby with you as much as you can so that you can respond promptly to signs of hunger. By the second or third day, most babies are more awake and acting hungry, especially at night. Some newborns need to nurse every 1½ hours, while others feed about every 3 hours. Most newborns are hungry at different times, with a long cluster of feeding in the late afternoon or night. Typically, breastfed newborns will feed 8 to 12 or more times per 24 hours (once the milk has come in). If your baby isn't waking on her own during the first few weeks, wake her if 3 to 4 hours have passed since the last feeding. If you are having a hard time waking up your baby for feedings, let your pediatrician know.

What's the best feeding schedule for a breastfed baby?

Feeding schedules are different for every baby, but it's best to start nursing your baby before crying starts. Crying is a late sign of hunger. Whenever possible, use your baby's cues instead of the clock to decide when to nurse. It can be less frustrating for you and your baby if you can learn your baby's early hunger cues. Frequent feedings help stimulate the breasts to produce milk more efficiently.

During a growth spurt (rapid growth), babies will want to nurse all the time. *Remember, this is normal and temporary,* usually lasting about 4 to 5 days. Keep on breastfeeding, and don't give any other liquids or foods.

How long does breastfeeding take?

Each baby feeds differently: some slower, some faster. Some feedings may be longer than others depending on your baby's appetite and the time of day. Some babies may be nursing even though they appear to be sleeping. While some infants nurse for only 10 minutes on one breast, it's quite common for others to stay on one side for much longer. It's generally good to allow your baby to decide when the feeding is over—he will let go and pull back when he is done.

If your baby has fallen asleep at your breast, or if you need to stop a feeding before your baby is done, gently break the suction with your finger. Do this by slipping a finger into your baby's mouth while he is still latched on. Never pull the baby off the breast without releasing the suction.

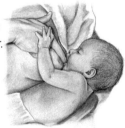

To stimulate both breasts, alternate which breast you offer first. Some women like to keep a safety pin on their bra strap to help remember. While you should try to breastfeed evenly on both sides, many babies seem to prefer one side over the other and nurse longer on that side. When this happens, the breast adapts its milk production to your baby's feedings.

Sliding your finger between the baby's mouth and your breast releases the suction and detaches the baby comfortably, helping you avoid nipple pain.

How can I tell if my baby is hungry?

You will soon get to know your baby's feeding patterns. In addition, babies may want to breastfeed for reasons other than hunger. It's OK for you to offer these "comfort feedings" as another way of meeting your baby's needs.

Nearly all newborns are alert for about 2 hours after delivery and show interest in feeding right away. Let the hospital staff know that you plan to take advantage of this opportunity—it's very important to the breastfeeding process. After 2 hours, many newborns are sleepy and hard to wake for the next day or so.

Watch for the early signs of hunger. This is the time to pick your baby up, gently awaken her, check her diaper, and try to feed her. (See "Early signs of hunger" below.)

Early Signs of Hunger

Your baby starts to let you know when she's hungry by the following early signs or cues:
- Small movements as she starts to awaken
- Whimpering or lip-smacking
- Pulling up arms or legs toward her middle
- Stretching or yawning
- Waking and looking alert
- Putting hands toward her mouth
- Making sucking motions
- Moving fists to her mouth
- Becoming more active
- Nuzzling against your breast

How can I tell if my baby is getting enough milk?

There are several ways you can tell whether your baby is getting enough milk. They include all or some of the following things:
- Your baby has frequent wet and dirty diapers.
- Your baby appears satisfied after feeding.
- Milk is visible during feedings (leaking or dripping).
- Your baby is gaining weight.

Your baby should have several wet or dirty diapers each day for the first few days after delivery. Beginning around the time that your milk comes in, the wet diapers should increase to 6 or more per day. At the same time, stools should start turning green, then yellow. There should be 3 or more stools per 24 hours. Typically, once breastfeeding is going well, breastfed babies have a yellow stool during or after each feeding. As your baby gets older, stools may occur less often, and after a month, may even skip a number of days. If stools are soft, and your baby is feeding and acting well, this is quite normal.

Your baby's feeding patterns are an important sign that he is feeding enough. A newborn may nurse every 1½ to 3 hours around the clock. If you add up all the feedings over the course of the day, your baby should feed at least 8 to 12 times a day.

When feeding well with good latch-on, the infant will suckle deeply, you will hear some swallowing, and the feeding won't be painful. The baby should appear satisfied and/or sleep until time for the next feeding. If your baby sleeps for stretches of longer than 4 hours in the first 2 weeks, wake him for a feeding. If your baby will not waken enough to eat at least 8 times per day, call your pediatrician.

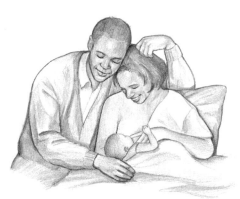

Once breastfeeding is going smoothly, it is simple and convenient. Breastfeeding is the most natural gift that you can give your baby.

Your child will be weighed at each doctor's visit. This is one of the best ways to tell how much milk your baby is getting. The AAP recommends that babies be seen for an office visit (or home visit) between 3 to 5 days of age to check on breastfeeding and baby's weight. During the first week, most infants lose several ounces of weight, but they should be back up to their birth weight by the end of the second week. Once your milk supply is established, your baby should gain between ½ and 1 ounce per day during the first 3 months.

Breastfeeding: A Natural Gift

Breastmilk gives your baby more than just good nutrition. It also provides important substances to fight infection. Breastfeeding has medical and psychological benefits for both of you. For many mothers and babies, breastfeeding goes smoothly from the start. For others, it takes a little time and several attempts to get the process going effectively. Like anything new, breastfeeding takes some practice. This is perfectly normal. If you need help, ask the doctors and nurses while you are still in the hospital, your pediatrician, a lactation specialist, or a breastfeeding support group.

For more information about breastfeeding, read the AAP *New Mother's Guide to Breastfeeding* or visit the AAP Web site at www.aap.org.

Illustrations by Tony LeTourneau

The information contained in this publication should not be used as a substitute for the medical care and advice of your pediatrician. There may be variations in treatment that your pediatrician may recommend based on individual facts and circumstances.

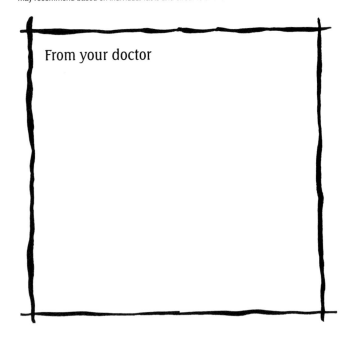

From your doctor

American Academy of Pediatrics

DEDICATED TO THE HEALTH OF ALL CHILDREN™

The American Academy of Pediatrics is an organization of 60,000 primary care pediatricians, pediatric medical subspecialists, and pediatric surgical specialists dedicated to the health, safety, and well-being of infants, children, adolescents, and young adults.

American Academy of Pediatrics
Web site—www.aap.org

Car Safety Seats:
A Guide for Families

Part I 2006 Safety Information

Each year thousands of young children are killed or injured in car crashes. You can help prevent this from happening to your child by always using car safety seats and seat belts correctly. This brochure explains how.

Contents
Which car safety seat is the best?
Rear-facing seats
Important safety rules
Infant-only seats
Convertible seats and features to look for in rear-facing seats
Forward-facing seats
Convertible seats, built-in seats, and combination seats
Travel vests and booster seats
Seat belts
A warning about seat belt adjusters
Installing a car safety seat
Car safety seats and shopping carts
Common questions about car safety seats
Don't leave your child unattended in a car safety seat
Always read and follow manufacturer's instructions

Which car safety seat is the best?
No one seat is the "best" or "safest." The best seat is the one that fits your child's size, is correctly installed, and is used properly every time you drive. When shopping for a car safety seat, keep the following in mind:
- Don't base your decision on price alone. Higher prices can mean added features that may or may not make the seat safer or easier to use. All car safety seats available for purchase in the United States must meet very strict safety standards established and maintained by the federal government.
- When you find a seat you like, try it out. Put your child in it and adjust the harnesses and buckles. Make sure it fits properly and securely in your car. Keep in mind that pictures or displays of car safety seats in stores may not show them being used the right way.

Rear-facing seats
All infants should ride rear-facing until they have reached at least 1 year of age *and* weigh at least 20 pounds. That means that if your baby reaches 20 pounds before her first birthday, she should remain rear-facing until she turns 1.

There are 2 types of rear-facing seats: infant-only seats and convertible seats. Convertible seats can be used rear-facing for infants, and then converted to a forward-facing position once the child is old enough and big enough to do so safely. *(See handout "Car Safety Seats: A Guide for Families, Part II 2006 Product Information" for names of specific seats in these categories.)*

Important safety rules

- Always use a car safety seat. You can start with your baby's first ride home from the hospital.
- Never place a child in a rear-facing car safety seat in the front seat of a vehicle that has a passenger air bag.
- The safest place for all children to ride is in the back seat.
- Set a good example—always wear your seat belt. Help your child form a lifelong habit of buckling up.
- Remember that each car safety seat is different. Read and keep the instructions that came with your seat handy, and follow the manufacturer's instructions at all times.
- Read the owner's manual that came with your car on how to correctly install car safety seats.
- If you need help installing your car safety seat, contact a certified **Child Passenger Safety (CPS) Technician.** To locate and set up an appointment, call toll-free at 866/SEATCHECK (866/732-8243) or visit www.seatcheck.org.

Infant-only seats

- Small and have carrying handles (sometimes come as part of a stroller system).
- Have a built-in harness that covers the child's upper torso.
- Can only be used for infants from birth up to 20 to 30 pounds, depending on model.
- Many come with a detachable base, which can be left in the car. The seat clicks into and out of the base, which means you don't have to install it each time you use it.

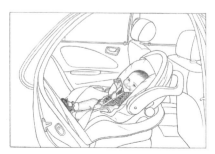

Infant-only car safety seat

Convertible seats (used rear-facing)

- Are used rear-facing for infants from birth to at least 1 year of age and at least 20 to 22 pounds. Can also be used forward-facing by older children. *(See "Forward-facing seats" below.)*
- Have higher rear-facing weight limits than infant-only seats. These are ideal for bigger babies.
- Have the following 3 types of harnesses:
  — **5-point harness**—5 points of attachment: 2 at the shoulders, 2 at the hips, 1 at the crotch
  — **Overhead shield**—A padded tray-like shield that swings down over the child
  — **T-shield**—A padded t-shaped or triangle-shaped shield attached to the shoulder straps

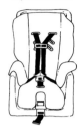

5-point harness

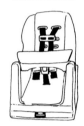

Overhead shield

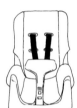

T-shield

Features to look for in rear-facing seats

- **Harness slots.** Look for seats that come with more than one harness slot to give your baby room to grow. The harnesses should be in the slots at or below your baby's shoulders.
- **Adjustable buckles and shields.** Many rear-facing seats have 2 or more buckle positions for growing babies. Many overhead shields can be adjusted as well.
- **Other features.** Angle indicators (built-in angle adjusters that help you get the proper recline) and head support systems are other features that can help you install the seat the right way.

Forward-facing seats

Once your child is at least 1 year of age *and* at least 20 pounds, he can ride forward-facing. However, it is best for him to ride rear-facing until he reaches the highest weight or height limit allowed by the car safety seat. There are many types of seats that can be used forward-facing including convertible seats, built-in seats, combination forward-facing/booster seats, and travel vests. *(See handout "Car Safety Seats: A Guide for Families, Part II 2006 Product Information" for names of specific seats in these categories.)*

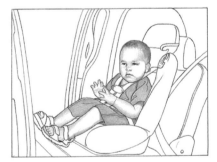

Forward-facing seat

Convertible seats (used forward-facing)

As mentioned previously, convertible seats can also be used forward-facing by children who are at least 1 year of age and weigh at least 20 pounds. However, if you have used your convertible seat rear-facing, you need to make the following 3 adjustments before using it forward-facing:

1. Move the shoulder straps to the slots that are at or *above* your child's shoulders. On many convertible seats, the top harness slots must be used when the seat is in the forward-facing position. Check the instructions to be sure.
2. Move the seat from the reclined to the upright position if required by the manufacturer of the seat.
3. Make sure the seat belt runs through the forward-facing belt path. When converting your seat from rear-facing to forward-facing, carefully follow the car safety seat manufacturer's instructions.

Built-in seats

Built-in seats are available in some cars and vans. Weight and height limits vary. Read your vehicle owner's manual or contact the manufacturer for details about how these seats are used.

Combination forward-facing/booster seats

Some car safety seats combine the features of a forward-facing seat and a booster seat. These seats come with harness straps for children who weigh up to 40 to 65 pounds (depending on the model). Once your child reaches the weight or height limit, you can use the seat as a booster by removing the harness and using your vehicle's lap and shoulder seat belts. Keep in mind that when using the harness straps, the seat can be secured with a lap and shoulder belt or a lap-only belt. However, once you remove the harness, you *must* use a lap and shoulder seat belt. Children must <u>never</u> ride in a booster seat using a lap belt only because serious injury can result.

Travel vests

If your car only has lap belts, a travel vest may be an option. These can also be used for a child who has outgrown his seat with a harness but is not yet ready for a booster seat. *(See handout "Car Safety Seats: A Guide for Families, Part II 2006 Product Information" for names of travel vests.)*

Booster seats

Booster seats do not come with harness straps but are used with the lap and shoulder seat belts in your vehicle, the same way an adult rides. Your child should stay in a car safety seat with a harness as long as possible before

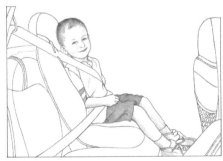

Belt-positioning booster seat

being allowed to ride in a booster seat. You can tell when your child is ready for a booster seat when one of the following is true:

- She reaches the top weight or height allowed for her seat with a harness. (These measurements are listed on labels on the seat and are also included in the instruction booklet that is provided with the car safety seat.)
- Her shoulders are above the harness slots.
- Her ears have reached the top of the seat.

Booster seats are designed to raise your child so that the lap and shoulder seat belts fit properly. This means the lap belt lies low across your child's thighs and the shoulder belt crosses the middle of your child's chest and shoulder. Correct belt fit helps protect the stomach, spine, and head from injury in case of a crash. Both high-back and backless booster seats are available. Booster seats should be used until your child can correctly fit in lap and shoulder seat belts. *(See "Seat belts" below.)*

Seat belts

Your child is ready to use lap and shoulder seat belts when the belts fit properly. This means

- The shoulder belt lies across the middle of the chest and shoulder, not the neck or throat.
- The lap belt is low and snug across the thighs, not the stomach.
- The child is tall enough to sit against the vehicle seat back with her legs bent without slouching and can stay in this position comfortably throughout the trip.

Remember, seat belts are made for adults. If the seat belt does not fit your child correctly, he should stay in a booster seat until the adult seat belts fit him correctly. This is usually when the child reaches about 4' 9" in height and is between 8 and 12 years of age.

Other points to keep in mind when using seat belts

- Never tuck the shoulder belt under the child's arm or behind the back.
- If there's only a lap belt, make sure it's snug and low on the child's thighs, not across the stomach. Try to get a lap and shoulder belt installed in your car by a dealer.
- Never allow children or anyone else to "share" seat belts. All passengers must have their own car safety seats or seat belts.

A warning about seat belt adjusters

There are products on the market that claim to make seat belts fit better. They attach to the seat belt but are not a part of the original belt. These products may actually interfere with proper lap and shoulder belt fit by causing the lap belt to ride too high on the stomach and making the shoulder belt too loose, and may even damage the seat belt itself. No federal standard ensuring the effectiveness and safety of these after-market products has been developed. In addition, most vehicle and car safety seat manufacturers do not recommend their use. Until the National Highway Traffic Safety Administration develops safety standards for these products, the American Academy of Pediatrics (AAP) recommends they not be used. As long as children are riding in the correct car safety seat for their size and age, they do not need to use any additional devices.

Installing a car safety seat

There are 2 main things to remember when installing a car safety seat.

- Your child must be buckled snugly into the seat.
- The seat must be buckled tightly into your vehicle.

Ask yourself the following questions to make sure both are done correctly. If you are not sure, check the instructions that came with your car safety seat, or contact a certified CPS Technician for help.

Is the child buckled into the car safety seat correctly?

- Are you using the correct harness slots?
- Are the harnesses snug?
- Have you placed the plastic harness clip (if your seat comes with one) at armpit level to hold the shoulder straps in place?
- Do the harness straps lie flat?
- Is your baby dressed in clothes that allow the straps to go between the legs? It's OK to adjust the straps to allow for thicker clothes, but make sure the harness still holds the child snugly. Also, remember to tighten the straps again after the thicker clothes are no longer needed.
- Is anything under your baby? Tuck blankets around your baby *after* adjusting the harness straps snugly. Never place them under your baby.
- Is your child slouching down or to the side? If so, pad the sides of the seat and between the crotch with rolled up diapers or blankets.

Is the car safety seat buckled into the vehicle correctly?

- Is the car safety seat facing the right direction for your child's age and weight?
- Is the seat belt routed through the correct belt path?
- Is the seat belt buckled tight? If you can move the seat more than an inch side to side or toward the front of the car, it's not tight enough.
- Is your rear-facing seat reclined enough? Your infant's head should not flop forward. If it does, tilt the car safety seat back a little. Your car safety seat may have a built-in recline adjuster for this purpose. If not, wedge firm padding, such as a rolled towel, under the base.
- Do you need a locking clip? They come with all new car safety seats. If the seat belts in your car move freely even when buckled, you need a locking clip. If you're not sure, check the manual that came with your car. Locking clips are not needed in most newer vehicles and in vehicles with LATCH. *(See "Installation made safer and easier" below for more information.)*
- Some lap belts (especially those found in older vehicles) need a special heavy-duty locking clip. These are only available from the vehicle manufacturer. Check the manual that came with your car for more information.

Installation made safer and easier

Child passenger safety experts have developed several ways to make car safety seat installation safer and easier, including the following:

- **LATCH** (Lower Anchors and Tethers for Children) is an attachment system that makes installing a car safety seat easier by eliminating the need to use seat belts to secure the car safety seat. It includes 2 sets of small bars, called anchors, located in the back seat where the cushions meet. Car safety seats that come with LATCH have a set of attachments that fasten to these vehicle anchors. Nearly all passenger vehicles and all car safety seats made on or after September 1, 2002, come with LATCH. However, unless both your vehicle and the car safety seat have this anchor system, you will still need to use seat belts to secure the car safety seat.

- A **tether** is a strap that attaches a car safety seat to an anchor located on the rear window ledge, the back of the vehicle seat, or on the floor or ceiling of the vehicle. Tethers give extra protection by keeping the car safety seat and the child's head from moving too far forward in a crash or sudden stop. Tethers should not be confused with LATCH attachments; the tether is a longer strap at the top of the seat and LATCH attachments are located at or near the base of the seat.

  All new cars, minivans, and light trucks have been required to have tether anchors since September 2000. Most new forward-facing car safety seats and a few rear-facing car safety seats come with tethers. For older car safety seats, tether kits are available. It is highly recommended that tethers be used because they greatly improve the protection of your child in the event of a crash. Check with the car safety seat manufacturer to find out how you can get a tether for your seat if yours does not have one.

- **Child Passenger Safety (CPS) Technicians** can help you. If you have more questions about installing your car safety seat, a certified CPS Technician may be able to help. A list of certified CPS Technicians is available by state or ZIP code on the National Highway Traffic Safety Administration (NHTSA) Web site at www.nhtsa.dot.gov/people/injury/childps/contacts/. A list of inspection stations—where you can go for help with installation—is available in both English and Spanish at www.seatcheck.org or toll-free at 866/SEATCHECK (866/732-8243). You can also get this information by calling the toll-free NHTSA Auto Safety Hot Line at 888/DASH-2-DOT (888/327-4236), from 8:00 am to 10:00 pm ET, Monday through Friday.

Car safety seats and shopping carts

Many infant-only car safety seats lock into shopping carts, and many stores have shopping carts with built-in infant seats. This may seem safe but your baby could tip over or fall out of the cart. Thousands of children are hurt every year from falling from shopping carts or from the carts tipping over. Instead of placing your baby's car safety seat on the cart, consider using a stroller or frontpack while shopping with your baby.

Common questions about car safety seats

Q: What if my baby is born prematurely?

A: Use a car safety seat without a shield harness. Shields often are too high and too far from the body to fit correctly. A small baby's face could hit a shield in a crash. Premature infants should be observed in their car safety seats while still in the hospital to make sure the reclined position does not cause low heart rate, low oxygen, or breathing problems. If your baby needs to lie flat during travel, use a crash-tested car bed. If possible, an adult should ride in the back seat next to your baby to watch him closely.

Q: What if my baby weighs more than 20 pounds but is not 1 year old yet?

A: Many babies reach 20 pounds well before their first birthday. However, just because your baby weighs more than 20 pounds does not make him ready to ride forward-facing. Look for a convertible seat that can be used rear-facing by children who weigh more than 20 pounds. *(See handout "Car Safety Seats: A Guide for Families, Part II 2006 Product Information" to see which seats have these higher weight limits.)*

Q: What if my child has special health care needs?

A: Children with special health problems may need other restraint systems. Talk about this with your pediatrician. Easter Seals, Inc has car safety seat programs for children with special health care needs. More information is available from Easter Seals, Inc at 800/221-6827. You also can learn more about transporting children with special needs by calling the Automotive Safety Program at 317/274-2977 or by visiting its Web site at www.preventinjury.org. For more information and a list of car safety seats available for children with special needs, see the AAP brochure, *Safe Transportation of Children With Special Needs: A Guide for Families*.

Q: What if my car has air bags?

A: All new cars come equipped with air bags. When used with seat belts, air bags work very well to protect older children and adults. However, air bags are very dangerous to children riding in rear-facing car safety seats and to child passengers who are not properly positioned. If your car has a passenger air bag, infants in rear-facing seats *must ride in the back seat*. Even in a low-speed crash, the air bag can inflate, strike the car safety seat, and cause serious brain and neck injury and death.

  Toddlers who ride in forward-facing car safety seats also are at risk from air bag injuries. **All children up to age 13 years are safest in the back seat.** If you must put an older child in the front seat, slide the vehicle seat back as far as it will go. Make sure your child is properly restrained for his age and size and stays in the proper position at all times. This will help prevent the air bag from striking your child.

  Air bag on/off switches are available in the few cases in which an infant must ride in the front seat. Most families don't need to use the air bag on/off switch. Air bags that are turned off cannot protect other passengers riding in the front seat. Air bag on/off switches only should be used if *all* of the following are true:

- Your child has special heath care needs.
- Your pediatrician recommends constant supervision of your child during travel.
- No other adult can ride in the back seat with your child.

  On/off switches also must be used if you have a vehicle with no back seat or a back seat that is not made for passengers.

Q: What if my car has side air bags?

A: Side air bags improve safety for adults in side impact crashes. However, children who are seated near a side air bag may be at risk for serious injury. Read your vehicle owner's manual for recommendations that apply to your vehicle.

Q: What if my car only has lap belts in the back seat?

A: Lap belts work fine with infant-only, convertible, and forward-facing car safety seats. They cannot be used with booster seats, and they are not the safest way to buckle older children. If your car only has lap belts, use a forward-facing car safety seat with a harness and higher weight limits. *(See handout "Car Safety Seats: A Guide for Families, Part II 2006 Product Information" for a listing of the seats with these higher weight limits.)*

- Check with a car dealer or the manufacturer of your car to see if shoulder belts can be installed.
- Use a travel vest (some can be used with lap belts).
- Consider buying another car with lap and shoulder belts in the back seat.

Q: What if I drive more children than can be buckled safely in the back seat?

A: Avoid having to drive more children than can be buckled safely in the back seat, especially if your car has passenger air bags. However, if necessary, a child in a forward-facing car safety seat with a harness may be the best choice to ride in the front seat. This is because a child who is in a booster seat or using a regular seat belt can easily move out of position and be at greater risk for injuries from the air bag.

Q: Can I use a car safety seat on an airplane?

A: The Federal Aviation Administration (FAA) and the AAP recommend that when flying, children should be securely fastened in car safety seats until 4 years of age, and then should be secured with the airplane seat belts. This will help keep them safe during takeoff and landing or in case of turbulence. Most infant, convertible, and forward-facing seats are certified to be used on airplanes. Booster seats and travel vests are not certified to be used on airplanes. Check the label on your car safety seat and call the car safety seat manufacturer before you travel to be sure your seat meets current FAA regulations.

Q: Can I use a car safety seat that was in a crash?

A: If the car safety seat was in a moderate or severe crash, it needs to be replaced. If the crash was minor, the seat does not automatically need to be replaced. A crash is considered minor if *all* of the following are true:
- The vehicle could be driven away from the crash.
- The vehicle door closest to the car safety seat was not damaged.
- No one in the vehicle was injured.
- The air bags did not go off.
- You can't see any damage to the car safety seat.

  If you are unsure, call the manufacturer of the seat. See the resource section in the handout "Car Safety Seats: A Guide for Families, Part II 2006 Product Information" for manufacturer names and phone numbers.

Q: What about using a used car safety seat?

A: Avoid using used car safety seats, especially if obtained from a yard sale or secondhand (consignment) shop because there is no way to know the seat's history. Also never use a car safety seat that
- **Is too old.** Look on the label for the date it was made. Do not use seats that are more than 10 years old. Many manufacturers recommend that car safety seats only be used for 5 to 6 years from the date of manufacture. Check with the manufacturer to find out how long the company recommends using its seat.
- **Has any visible cracks in the frame of the seat.**
- **Does not have a label with the date of manufacture and model number.** Without these, you cannot check to see if the seat has been recalled.
- **Does not come with instructions.** You need them to know how to use the seat. You can get a copy of the instruction manual by contacting the manufacturer.

Don't leave your child unattended in a car safety seat

Children should never be left alone in a car whether they are in their car safety seats or not. Any of the following can happen when a child is left alone in a vehicle:
- Temperatures can reach deadly levels in minutes, and the child can die of heat stroke.
- He can be strangled by power windows, sunroofs, or accessories.
- He can be taken during a car theft or kidnapped from the vehicle.
- He can knock the vehicle into gear, setting it in motion.

  Don't leave your baby unattended in a car safety seat outside of the vehicle either. When your baby falls asleep in her car safety seat, it can be tempting to bring her inside and leave her alone in the seat, but this can be unsafe. Your baby can fall out of the seat, or the seat can fall over. And remember, placing the car safety seat on a shopping cart is unsafe too. The best place for your baby to sleep is on her back in a safe crib.

- **Is missing parts.** Used car safety seats often come without important parts. Check with the manufacturer to make sure you can get the right parts.
- **Is a shield booster.** Although shield boosters are still around, the AAP recommends against their use. Major injuries have occurred to children in shield boosters. The only time shield boosters should be used is if the shield is removed and the seat is used with a lap and shoulder belt.
- **Was recalled.** You can find out by calling the manufacturer or by contacting the following:
  — **Auto Safety Hot Line:** Toll-free: 888/DASH-2-DOT (888/327-4236), from 8:00 am to 10:00 pm ET, Monday through Friday.
  — **National Highway Traffic Safety Administration (NHTSA)** www-odi.nhtsa.dot.gov/cars/problems/recalls/childseat.cfm

If the seat has been recalled, be sure to follow the instructions to fix it or to get the parts you need. You also may get a registration card for future recall notices from the hotline.

Always read and follow manufacturer's instructions

If you do not have the manufacturer's instructions for your car safety seat, write or call the company's customer service department. A representative will ask you for the model number, name of seat, and date of manufacture. The manufacturer's address and phone number are on the label on the seat.

All products listed on the following pages meet Federal Motor Vehicle Safety Standard 213 as of the date of publication. There may be car safety seats available that are not listed in this brochure. The following information is current as of the date of publication. Before buying a car safety seat, check the manufacturer's instructions for important safety information about proper fitting and use.

Although the American Academy of Pediatrics (AAP) is not a testing or standard-setting organization, this guide sets forth the AAP recommendations based on the peer-reviewed literature available at the time of its publication, and sets forth some of the factors that parents should consider before selecting and using a car safety seat.

The appearance of the name American Academy of Pediatrics (AAP) does not constitute a guarantee or endorsement of the products listed or the claims made. Phone numbers and Web site addresses are as current as possible, but may change at any time.

The information contained in this publication should not be used as a substitute for the medical care and advice of your pediatrician. There may be variations in treatment that your pediatrician may recommend based on individual facts and circumstances.

Illustrations on pages 1 and 2 by Wendy Wray.

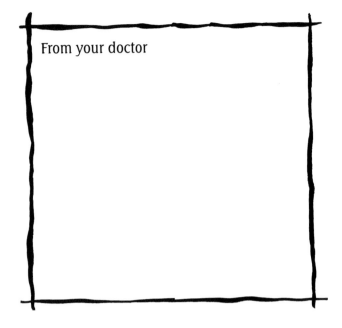

From your doctor

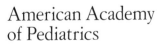

American Academy
of Pediatrics

DEDICATED TO THE HEALTH OF ALL CHILDREN™

The American Academy of Pediatrics is an organization of 60,000 primary care pediatricians, pediatric medical subspecialists, and pediatric surgical specialists dedicated to the health, safety, and well-being of infants, children, adolescents, and young adults.

American Academy of Pediatrics
Web site — www.aap.org

Copyright © 2006
American Academy of Pediatrics

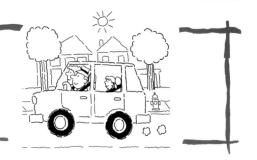

Car Safety Seats:
A Guide for Families
Part II 2006 Product Information

Infant-only seats

Manufacturers names are boldfaced.

Name	Harness Type	Rear-Facing Weight Limits	Height Limits	Price
Baby Trend Latch-Loc Adjustable Back	5-point	5–22 pounds	28½"	$80
Britax Baby Safe	5-point	4–22 pounds	30"	$299.99
Britax Companion	5-point	4–22 pounds	30"	$169.99
Chicco Key Fit Infant Car Seat	5-point	4–22 pounds	30"	$140
Combi Centre/ST/DX/EX	5-point	5–22 pounds	29"	$89–$99
Combi Connection	5-point	5–22 pounds	29"	$199.99
Combi Tyro Infant Car Seat	5-point	22 pounds	29"	$129–$149
Compass Baby I400 LP Infant Car Seat	5-point	4–22 pounds	30"	$100–$140
Cosco Arriva	5-point	5–22 pounds	29"	$40
Eddie Bauer Infant Car Seat	5-point	5–22 pounds	29"	$90–$100
Eddie Bauer Comfort Infant Car Seat	5-point	5–22 pounds	29"	$100
Evenflo Discovery	3-point	5–22 pounds	28"	$50–$60
Evenflo Embrace	5-point	5–22 pounds	28"	$60–$90
Graco Infant Safe Seat	5-point	5–30 pounds	32"	$129–$169
Graco SnugRide	3-point 5-point	5–22 pounds	29"	$69–$120
Peg Perego Primo Viaggio SIP	5-point	22 pounds	30"	$179–$199
Safety 1st Designer 22	5-point	5–22 pounds	29"	$60–$80
Safety 1st First Ride DX	5-point	5–22 pounds	29"	$50
Safety 1st Starter	5-point	5–22 pounds	29"	$60

Convertible seats

Name	Harness Type	Rear-Facing Weight Limits/ Height Limits	Forward-Facing Weight Limits/ Height Limits	Price
Britax Boulevard	5-point	5–33 pounds	20–65 pounds 27"–49"	$289.99
Britax Decathlon	5-point	5–33 pounds	20–65 pounds 27"–49"	$269.99
Britax Roundabout with Latch	5-point	5–33 pounds	20–40 pounds 27"–40"	$199.99
Britax Marathon	5-point	5–33 pounds	20–65 pounds 27"–49"	$249.99
Combi Avatar	5-point	5–30 pounds	20–40 pounds	$179–$199
Cosco Alpha Omega (rear-facing, forward-facing, or booster)	5-point	5–35 pounds 36"	With harness: 22–40 pounds 43" As booster: 40–80 pounds 52"	$140
Cosco Alpha Omega Elite (rear-facing, forward-facing, or booster)	5-point	5–35 pounds 36"	With harness: 20–40 pounds 40" As booster: 30–100 pounds 52"	$150–$160
Cosco Scenera/DX	5-point Overhead shield	5–35 pounds 36"	22–40 pounds 43"	$50–$70
Cosco Touriva/Regal Ride	5-point	5–35 pounds 36"	22–40 pounds 43"	$40–$70
Eddie Bauer 3-in-1 (rear-facing, forward-facing, or booster)	5-point	5–35 pounds 36"	With harness: 22–40 pounds 43" As booster: 40–80 pounds 52"	$170
Eddie Bauer Deluxe 3-in-1 Convertible Car Seat (rear-facing, forward-facing, or booster)	5-point Overhead shield	5–35 pounds 36"	With harness: 20–40 pounds 40" As booster: 30–100 pounds 52"	$170–$180
Evenflo Titan 5	5-point	5–30 pounds	20–40 pounds	$60–$70
Evenflo Tribute 5/DLX	5-point Overhead shield	5–30 pounds	20–40 pounds	$50–$60
Evenflo Triumph 5/DLX	5-point	5–30 pounds	20–40 pounds	$120–$140

Convertible seats, continued

Name	Harness Type	Rear-Facing Weight Limits/ Height Limits	Forward-Facing Weight Limits/ Height Limits	Price
Graco ComfortSport	5-point	30 pounds	20–40 pounds 40"	$69–$120
Lenox TattleTale Smart Child Seat	5-point	5–33 pounds 19"–32"	20–40 pounds 29"–40"	$209–$259
Safety 1st Enspira (rear-facing, forward-facing, or booster)	5-point	5–35 pounds 36"	With harness: 22–40 pounds 43" As booster: 40–80 pounds 52"	$100
Safety 1st Intera (rear-facing, forward-facing, or booster)	5-point	5–35 pounds 36"	With harness: 22–40 pounds 43" As booster: 40–100 pounds 57"	$140
Sunshine Kids Radian Car Seat	5-point	5–33 pounds	65 pounds 49"	$199
Tripleplay Products Sit 'n' Stroll	5-point	5–30 pounds	20–40 pounds	$200

Combination seats (Can be used with 5-point harness or as belt-positioning booster.)

Name	Weight Limits/Height Limits With Harness	Weight Limits/Height Limits as Belt Positioner	Price
Cosco High Back Booster	22–40 pounds 43"	40–80 pounds 52"	$50
Cosco Summit	22–40 pounds 43"	40–100 pounds 52"	$90–$100
Cosco Ventura DX	22–40 pounds 43"	40–80 pounds 52"	$60
Eddie Bauer Comfort High Back Booster, Deluxe	22–40 pounds 43"	40–100 pounds 52"	$80–$120
Eddie Bauer High Back Booster	22–40 pounds 43"	40–80 pounds 52"	$80
Evenflo Express, Chase, Traditions, Vision	20–40 pounds	30–100 pounds 54"	$50–$70
Evenflo Generations, Bolero	20–40 pounds	30–100 pounds 57"	$70–$100
Graco Platinum/Treasured/Ultra CarGo	20–40 pounds 27"–43"	30–100 pounds 35"–54"	$69–$99
Lenox TattleTale Smart Child Seat	20–40 pounds 29"–40"	40–80 pounds 35"–57"	$259
Recaro Young Sport	18–40 pounds 27"–40"	30–80 pounds 37"–59"	$249
Safety 1st Apex 65	20–65 pounds 52"	40–100 pounds 57"	$130
Safety 1st Vantage Point, Surveyor	22–40 pounds 43"	40–100 pounds 52"	$70–$80

Forward-facing toddler seats

Name	Harness Type	Weight Limits	Height Limits	Price
Britax Regent	5-point	22–80 pounds	19"–53"	$239.99
Graco Toddler Safe Seat	5-point	20–40 pounds	27"–43"	$129–$169
SafeGuard Child Seat	5-point	22–65 pounds	57"	$429

Booster seats

Name	Type	Weight Limits	Height Limits	Price
Baby Trend Recaro	High back	30–80 pounds	37"–59"	$349
Britax Bodyguard	High back	40–100 pounds	43"–60"	$129.99
Britax Parkway Booster	High back	30–100 pounds	38"–60"	$99.99
Britax Starriser Comfy	High back	30–80 pounds	33"–53"	$89.99
Combi Dakota	Backless	33–100 pounds	33"–57"	$39–$59
Combi Kobuk	High back	33–100 pounds	33"–57"	$79–$89
Compass Baby B500 LP Folding Booster Car Seat	High back	30–100 pounds	38"–57"	$75–$90
Cosco High Rise, Ambassador	Backless	30–100 pounds	57"	$15–$20
Cosco Protek	High back Backless	30–100 pounds	57"	$30–$40
Cosco Select Ride	High back	40–80 pounds	52"	$30

Booster seats, continued

Name	Type	Weight Limits	Height Limits	Price
Cosco Traveler	High back	30–80 pounds	52"	$20
Cosco Voyager	High back	40–80 pounds	52"	$20–$25
Evenflo Big Kid Deluxe/LX, Everest	High back Backless	30–100 pounds 40–100 pounds	57"	$40–$80
Evenflo Big Kid No Back	Backless	40–100 pounds	57"	$15
Evenflo Sightseer/Barbie/Hot Wheels	High back	30–100 pounds	37"–54"	$30–$40
Graco My CarGo	High back	30–100 pounds	35"–54"	$40
Graco TurboBooster	High back Backless	30–100 pounds 40–100 pounds	38"–57" 40"–57"	$50–$80 $20
LaRoche Grizzly Bear Booster	High back	40–100 pounds	36"–57"	$119
LaRoche Polar Bear Booster	High back	30–100 pounds	33"–57"	$129
LaRoche Teddy Bear Booster	High back	30–80 pounds	33"–54"	$109
Recaro Start	High back	30–80 pounds	59"	$349
Recaro Young Style	High back	30–80 pounds	59"	$149
Safety Angel Ride Ryte	High back Backless	30–100 pounds 40–100 pounds	33"–54"	$70–$75 $45–$48

Travel vests

Name	Weight Limits/Age Limits	Price
E-Z-ON Vest	20–168 pounds	$120
E-Z-ON Modified Vest	20–100 pounds 2–12 years of age	$120–$140
E-Z-ON 86Y Harness	66–168 pounds	$60–$80
E-Z-ON Kid Y Harness (must be used with the Safety Angel Ride Ryte booster)	30–80 pounds	$48–$52
RideSafer Travel Vest	Small vest: 35–60 pounds (3–6 years) Large vest: 50–80 pounds (5–9 years)	$99.99
Safety 1st Tote 'n Go DX	25–40 pounds with harness	$20

Built-in (integrated) seats

Built-in or integrated child safety seats are available on selected models from some motor vehicle manufacturers. Check with the manufacturers for specifics.

Manufacturer phone numbers and Web sites

For more information on the seats listed in this guide, please contact the individual manufacturers.

Baby Trend
800/328-7363
www.babytrend.com

Britax Child Safety
888/427-4829
www.britaxusa.com

Chicco USA
www.chiccousa.com

Combi International
800/992-6624
www.combi-intl.com

Compass Baby
888/899-BABY (888/899-2229)
www.compassbaby.com

Cosco, Inc.
800/544-1108
www.coscojuvenile.com

Eddie Bauer
800/544-1108
www.djgusa.com/eddiebauer

Evenflo Company Inc.
800/233-5921
www.evenflo.com

E-Z-ON Products/Safety Angel
800/323-6598
www.ezonpro.com

Graco
800/345-4109
www.gracobaby.com

IMMI/SafeGuard
800/974-7798
www.safeguardseat.com

Jupiter Industries
800/465-5795
www.jupiterindustries.com

LaRoche Brothers, Inc.
978/632-8638

Lenox Juvenile Group
888/372-0622
www.smartchildseat.com

Peg Perego USA, Inc.
800/671-1701
www.pegperego.com

Recaro of North America
800/8-RECARO
www.recaro-nao.com

Safety 1st
800/544-1108
www.safety1st.com

Safe Traffic Systems, Inc.
847/329 8111
www.safetrafficsystem.com

Sunshine Kids Juvenile Products
888/336-7909
www.skjp.com

TriplePlay Products, LLC
800/829-1625
www.tripleplayproducts.com

Although the American Academy of Pediatrics (AAP) is not a testing or standard-setting organization, this guide sets forth the AAP recommendations based on the peer-reviewed literature available at the time of its publication, and sets forth some of the factors that parents should consider before selecting and using a car safety seat.

The appearance of the name American Academy of Pediatrics (AAP) does not constitute a guarantee or endorsement of the products listed or the claims made. Phone numbers and Web site addresses are as current as possible, but may change at any time.

Prices are approximate and may vary.

The information contained in this publication should not be used as a substitute for the medical care and advice of your pediatrician. There may be variations in treatment that your pediatrician may recommend based on individual facts and circumstances.

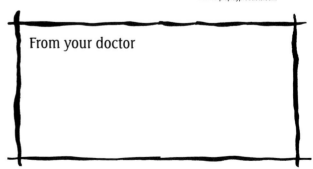

From your doctor

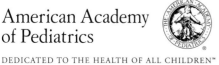

American Academy
of Pediatrics

DEDICATED TO THE HEALTH OF ALL CHILDREN™

The American Academy of Pediatrics is an organization of 60,000 primary care pediatricians, pediatric medical subspecialists, and pediatric surgical specialists dedicated to the health, safety, and well-being of infants, children, adolescents, and young adults.

American Academy of Pediatrics
Web site—www.aap.org

Copyright © 2006
American Academy of Pediatrics

One-Minute Car Safety Seat Check-up

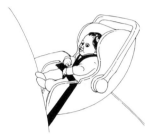

A. Infant-only seat

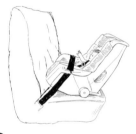

B. Rear-facing convertible seat

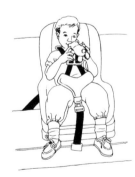

C. Convertible seat turned to face forward

Using a car safety seat correctly makes a big difference. Even the "safest" seat may not protect your child in a crash unless it is used correctly. So take a minute to check to be sure…

►► Does your car have a passenger air bag?

- An infant in a rear-facing seat should NEVER be placed in the front seat of a vehicle that has a passenger air bag.
- The safest place for all children to ride is in the back seat.
- If an older child must ride in the front seat, move the vehicle seat as far back as possible, buckle the child properly, and make sure he stays in the proper position at all times.

►► Is your child facing the right way for weight, height, and age?

- Infants should ride facing the back of the car until they have reached at least 1 year of age **AND** weigh at least 20 pounds (A and B).
- A child who weighs 20 pounds or exceeds the height limit for the car safety seat before she reaches 1 year of age should continue to ride rear-facing in a car safety seat approved for use at higher weights and heights in the rear-facing position.
- A child who weighs more than 20 pounds **AND** is older than 1 year may face forward (C). It is safest for a child to ride rear-facing until she reaches the top weight or height allowed by the seat for use in the rear-facing position.
- Once your child faces forward, she should remain in a car safety seat with a full harness until she reaches the top weight or height allowed by the seat. When changing the convertible seat for use in the forward-facing position, you must make adjustments. Check your car safety seat instructions.

►► Is the harness snug; does it stay on your child's shoulders?

- Harnesses should fit snugly against your child's body. Check the car safety seat instructions on how to adjust the straps.
- The chest clip should be placed at armpit level (C) to keep the harness straps on the shoulders.

►► Has your child grown too tall or reached the top weight limit for the forward-facing seat?

- Children are best protected in a car safety seat with a full harness until they reach the top weight or height limit of the car safety seat.
- Once your child outgrows his car safety seat, use a belt-positioning booster seat to help protect him until he is big enough for the seat belt to fit properly. A belt-positioning booster seat is used with a lap and shoulder belt (D).
- Shield boosters: Although boosters with shields may meet current Federal Motor Vehicle Safety Standards for use by children who weigh 30 to 40 pounds, on the basis of current published peer-reviewed literature, the American Academy of Pediatrics (AAP) does not recommend their use.
- A seat belt fits properly when the shoulder belt crosses the chest, the lap belt is low and snug across the thighs, and the child is tall enough so that when he sits against the vehicle seat back, his legs bend at the knees and his feet hang down.

►► Does the car safety seat fit correctly in your vehicle?

- Not all car safety seats fit in all vehicles.
- When the car safety seat is installed, be sure it does not move side-to-side or toward the front of the car.
- Read the section on car safety seats in the owner's manual for your car.

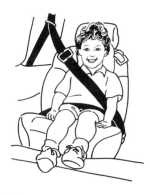

D. Belt-positioning
booster seat

▸▸ Is the seat belt in the right place and pulled tight?

- Route the seat belt through the correct path (check your instructions to make sure), kneel in the seat to press it down, and pull the belt *tight*.
- A convertible seat has 2 different belt paths, 1 for use rear-facing and 1 for use forward-facing.
- Check the owner's manual for your car to see if you need to use a locking clip. Check the car safety seat instructions to see if you need a tether to keep the safety seat secure.

▸▸ Can you use the LATCH system?

- Lower Anchors and Tethers for Children (LATCH) is an anchor system that allows you to install a car safety seat without using a seat belt.
- Most new vehicles and all new car safety seats have these attachments to secure the car safety seat in the vehicle.
- Unless both the vehicle and the car safety seat have this system, seat belts are still needed to secure the car safety seat.

▸▸ Do you have the instructions for the car safety seat?

- Follow them and keep them with the car safety seat. You will need them as your child gets bigger.
- Be sure to send in the registration card that comes with the car safety seat. It will be important in case your car safety seat is recalled.

▸▸ Has your child's car safety seat been recalled?

- Call the Auto Safety Hotline or check the National Highway Traffic Safety Administration (NHTSA) Web site for a list of recalled seats. (See below.)
- Be sure to make any needed repairs to your car safety seat.

▸▸ Has your child's car safety seat been in a crash?

- If so, it may have been weakened and should not be used, even if it looks fine.
- If you must use a secondhand car safety seat, first check its full history. Do not use a car safety seat that has been in a crash, has been recalled, is too old (check with the manufacturer), has any cracks in its frame, or is missing parts. Make sure it has a label from the manufacturer and instructions.
- Call the car safety seat manufacturer if you have questions about the safety of your seat.

Questions?

Ask your pediatrician, a local safety group, or NHTSA. A certified Child Passenger Safety (CPS) Technician can help you use your child's car safety seat correctly. On the NHTSA Auto Safety Hotline or Web site, you may give your ZIP code to find the nearest CPS Technician.

The NHTSA Auto Safety Hotline
888/DASH-2-DOT (888/327-4236) (8:00 am to 10:00 pm ET, Monday through Friday) www.nhtsa.dot.gov/people/injury/childps/

The AAP offers more information in the brochure *Car Safety Seats: A Guide for Families.* Ask your pediatrician about this brochure or visit the AAP Web site at www.aap.org.

Although the American Academy of Pediatrics (AAP) is not a testing or standard-setting organization, this guide sets forth AAP recommendations based on the peer-reviewed literature available at the time of its publication and sets forth some of the factors that parents should consider before selecting and using a car safety seat.

Please note: Listing of resources does not imply an endorsement by the American Academy of Pediatrics (AAP). The AAP is not responsible for the content of the resources mentioned in this brochure. Phone numbers and Web site addresses are as current as possible, but may change at any time.

The information contained in this publication should not be used as a substitute for the medical care and advice of your pediatrician. There may be variations in treatment that your pediatrician may recommend based on individual facts and circumstances.

American Academy
of Pediatrics

DEDICATED TO THE HEALTH OF ALL CHILDREN™

The American Academy of Pediatrics is an organization of 60,000 primary care pediatricians, pediatric medical subspecialists, and pediatric surgical specialists dedicated to the health, safety, and well-being of infants, children, adolescents, and young adults.

American Academy of Pediatrics
Web site—www.aap.org

Copyright © 2002
American Academy of Pediatrics, Updated 1/04

Safe Transportation of Children With Special Needs:

A Guide for Families Part I Safety Information

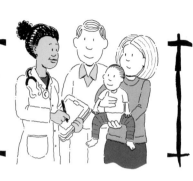

All children must ride in cars and other vehicles as safely as possible. Some children with certain medical conditions can ride in the standard types of car safety seats that are commonly found in stores. Children with breathing or muscle control conditions, casts, or other health care needs may need to use special medical car safety seats or restraints. If your child has special needs, a variety of child restraint options are available.

General guidelines for transporting a child with special needs

- Talk to your pediatrician or surgeon about your child's positioning and transportation needs.
- Remember that some children with special needs are able to use standard child restraints such as infant-only seats, convertible seats, forward-facing seats/restraints, or belt-positioning booster seats. (See "Standard car safety seats.")
- Check the label on the car safety seat and make sure it states that the seat meets or exceeds Federal Motor Vehicle Safety Standards.
- Never try to alter a car safety seat to fit a child with special needs. Never use a car safety seat that has been altered to fit a child with special needs unless it has been crash tested with the change.
- Stay up-to-date on what might be available for your child. New child restraints offer more options every year.
- Keep your child in the type of car safety seat that gives the most protection until your child reaches the top weight or height recommended by the manufacturer.
(See Part II Product Information.)

Getting help with costs

Car safety seats for children with special needs are often expensive. However, you may be able to get help with the cost. Insurance, including Medicaid, may cover the cost of a specialized restraint in some cases. For special needs car safety seat programs in your area, contact

- Your pediatrician.
- A local children's hospital.
- Your rehabilitation therapist.
- A Child Passenger Safety Technician in your area. To find one check the National Highway Traffic Safety Administration (NHTSA) Technician Contact Locator at www.nhtsa.dot.gov or 888/DASH-2-DOT (888/327-4236).
- Easter Seals at 800/221-6827.

Positioning guidelines

- Read the instructions for the car safety seat/restraint **and** your vehicle. Both sets of instructions will be necessary to make sure that your child is secure in the safety seat/restraint and the safety seat/restraint is correctly installed in your vehicle.

Standard car safety seats

Infant-only seats are for babies who weigh up to 20 to 35 pounds, depending on the seat's manufacturer. They must be rear-facing (the baby faces the back of the vehicle) and keep the baby in a semi-reclined position.

Convertible seats are for babies and toddlers. They are used rear-facing for babies who weigh up to 20 to 35 pounds, depending on the manufacturer. When a child is at least 1 year of age **and** weighs at least 20 pounds, the seat can be used forward-facing for toddlers up to 40 pounds.

Combination seats are only used forward-facing. They are used as car safety seats with a harness for children who are at least 1 year of age **and** who weigh at least 20 to 30 pounds, depending on the manufacturer. When your child reaches 40 pounds, you may remove the harness and the seat may be used as a belt-positioning booster seat with a lap and shoulder belt.

Forward-facing seats/restraints allow children who are at least 1 year of age **and** who weigh at least 20 pounds to stay in a harness system until they weigh 40 to 80 pounds, depending on the manufacturer.

Belt-positioning booster seats are designed for children who have outgrown car safety seats but are too small for seat belts. They raise the child up to position the lap belt low on the child's thighs and the shoulder belt across the child's shoulder and chest.

A new anchor system, Lower Anchors and Tethers for Children (LATCH) will be available in most new cars and on all new car safety seats in 2002. This system allows you to install standard car safety seats without using seat belts.

For more information on standard car safety seats, ask your pediatrician about the American Academy of Pediatrics (AAP) brochure *Car Safety Seats: A Guide for Families.*

- Make sure that all harness adjustments are made according to instructions.
- Be sure that all harness straps are snug and flat against your child's body.
- Position plastic chest or harness retainer clips at armpit level to keep the harness straps over the shoulders.
- Never place anything under or behind your child in a car safety seat/restraint.
- You may place rolled blankets, foam, or towels along each side of your child to keep him centered in the car safety seat.
- To help keep your child from sliding down in the seat, you may place a rolled cloth such as a washcloth or diaper between the crotch strap and your child's diaper area.

Travel guidelines

- The **back seat** is the safest place for all children to ride.
- **Never** put a rear-facing baby in front of a passenger air bag. In a crash, the air bag inflates very quickly and with great force. The child safety seat could be hit by the air bag and cause serious injuries or even death to the baby (see picture).

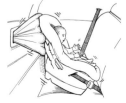

Car beds

Car beds that meet Federal Motor Vehicle Safety Standards allow babies to travel while lying down. There are many reasons why a baby may need to travel in a car bed, including the following:

- Problems breathing when sitting upright or semi-reclined
- Decreased muscle control
- Bones that break very easily
- Recent surgery on the spine
- Wearing a cast

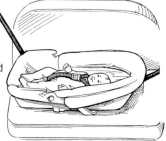

At this time there are a number of car beds available. They are designed for babies, not larger children. Although the beds vary in design, all of them must be installed lengthwise with the baby's head toward the center of the car.

- If you have no other option than to transport a child who is medically fragile in the front seat and your car has a passenger air bag, you will need to have your air bag switched off. Contact the NHTSA for a permission form and details (888/DASH-2-DOT [888/327-4236] or www.nhtsa.dot.gov).
- Depending on your child's condition, it may be wise to limit the amount of car travel.
- Stop often if your trip is long.
- When possible, an adult should ride in the back seat next to your child to watch her closely.
- Develop a medical care plan in case your child has a medical emergency during travel. Some parents attach a copy of the plan to the child's car safety seat/restraint.
- Carry with you an emergency kit that includes any special medications or supplies that your child may need. A checklist will help you ensure that the right medications and supplies are always with you. Do not leave this kit in the vehicle.
- Keep a cellular phone with you to contact help, if needed. Some cellular phones can dial 911 even if you do not purchase a service contract.
- Never use a reclined vehicle seat to transport a child. In a crash, the child can slip out of position and not be protected by the seat belt.
- In some instances, such as very tall children in casts, professional transport may be needed.
- Apply for a handicap parking permit on behalf of your child if it is hard to get her in and out of the car safety restraint. Handicap parking often allows more space to maneuver.
- **Never** leave your child alone in a vehicle, even to do an errand that should only take a minute. Your child's safety is worth the effort to remove her from the car safety seat/restraint, take her with you, and then secure her again when you return.

Premature and small babies

If your baby was born prematurely (early) or is small, the following information will help you transport your child safely:

- Select a car safety seat that fits your baby. Seats that have the shortest distance from the seat back to the crotch strap will help keep your baby from slouching. Seats that have the shortest distance from the harness slots to the seat bottom will fit better by keeping the harness over your baby's shoulders and holding your baby in the seat.

- Do not use a car safety seat with a shield or tray. In a crash or sudden stop, your small baby's neck or head could hit the shield or tray.
- Place rolled receiving blankets on both sides of your baby to center him in the car safety seat. Place a rolled diaper or washcloth between your child's diaper area and the crotch strap to keep your baby from slipping down (see picture). Do not place these behind or under the baby.

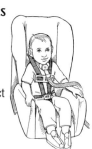

Some babies who were born prematurely have breathing problems when they sit semi-reclined in a car safety seat. Make sure that the hospital staff observes and monitors your baby in a car safety seat before going home. Your baby may need to use a car bed if he has any of the following while in a car safety seat:

- A decrease in oxygen levels
- Slow heart rate
- Apnea (breathing stops for a moment or two)

Babies and toddlers with tracheostomies

Most babies and toddlers with tracheostomies (a breathing tube placed into the windpipe) are able to use standard car safety seats. However, avoid using child restraints with tray or shield harness systems. In a crash or sudden stop, these could come in contact with the tracheostomy, and injure your child or block her airway.

Babies and toddlers in hip spica casts

Hip spica casts and other devices, such as splints, can make it impossible for a baby or toddler to sit in a standard car safety seat. The Spelcast convertible car seat is designed for babies and toddlers in casts. It is used rear-facing for babies 10 to 20 pounds and forward-facing for toddlers up to 40 pounds and 40 inches. A tether strap is available for use forward-facing. (See "Tether straps.") Other options for young children in hip spica casts may be car beds for babies or combination car seat/booster seats with low sides for toddlers.

Tether straps

Many child restraints that are designed for children with special needs must be installed with a tether strap and a seat belt. A tether strap limits forward movement of the child safety restraint in the vehicle. It attaches to the restraint and is bolted into your car at a vehicle anchor point (see picture). The tether strap and hardware come from the car safety seat or restraint manufacturer. If your car safety seat requires a tether, be sure to take your vehicle to a dealer who can help you find the hole or drill one for you in your vehicle if necessary. Never drill a hole yourself. You could puncture the gas line or damage your vehicle. If you have a newer car, you may already have tether anchors. However, **these anchors are for use with standard car safety seats and may not be strong enough to tether heavier, specialized medical restraints.** Follow the child restraint manufacturer's instructions and vehicle owner's manual regarding tether installation.

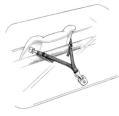

Should you keep your child rear-facing?

Babies are safest riding rear-facing until they are at least 1 year of age **and** weigh at least 20 pounds. In a rear-facing car safety seat, a baby sits back at an angle to help prevent his head from falling forward and affecting his breathing. This position helps to support his head and back and spreads the forces of a crash over these areas instead of his neck.

The rear-facing position also can help children who
- Have trouble holding up their heads because of a nerve or muscle disorder
- Break their bones easily
- Have trouble breathing
- Are small for their age

Many car safety seats allow babies and small children to ride rear-facing until they reach about 30 to 35 pounds or the top of the head is near the top of the seat. If a car safety seat holds children rear-facing to higher weights, the child should remain rear-facing until reaching the top weight or height allowed for the car safety seat for best protection. Check the labels on your car safety seat and the instruction manual for the seat for rear-facing weight and height limits.

Older children in hip spica casts

The modified E-Z-On Vest is designed for children 2 to 12 years of age who weigh 20 to 100 pounds. It allows a child to lie down in the back seat of the vehicle (see picture). The vest must be installed with 2 seat belts. One seat belt is secured under the chest strap of the vest, and the other seat belt is secured under the hip strap of the vest. Older children in hip spica casts may also fit in a combination car seat/booster with low sides.

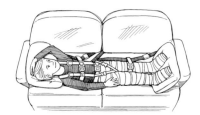

Remember, never use a reclined vehicle seat to transport a child. In some instances, professional transport may be needed.

Babies and children who can bend at their hips or sit up in their casts

Most babies and children who can bend at their hips or sit up in their casts can use standard car safety seats. Make sure the cast does not get in the way of the buckle and fits inside the restraint. A Spelcast car safety seat, forward-facing car seat/restraint, or combination car seat/booster seat with low sides can be useful for children in broomstick casts whose legs are spread widely apart. A convertible car seat with a 5-point harness is an option for children who have a thick, long leg cast that prevents buckling of a tray or T-shield harness.

If an older child is in a cast and can sit up, she may be able to use a belt-positioning booster seat or a seat belt if she is big enough. Make sure she is using the booster seat or seat belt properly and has enough legroom. The lap belt should be worn low and snug across the thighs. The shoulder belt should be across the chest, never behind the back or under the arm. Put padding or blankets on the floor so that the child's legs will be better supported during travel.

Larger children and forward-facing medical seats

Some children still need the support of a child restraint even after they have outgrown a standard car safety seat. This might include children with cerebral palsy; decreased head, neck, and trunk control; skeletal disorders; and various nerve and muscle disorders. There are forward-facing medical seats that fit children who weigh up to 105 pounds (see picture). These seats come with extra pads and devices to help position the child in the seat. Work with an occupational or physical therapist to position your child in these types of seats. These child restraints also come with an extra strap called a tether. (See "Tether straps.") The tether, along with the vehicle seat belt, must be used to install the restraint correctly.

Children and upright vests

If your older child does not need the added support and positioning features of a medical seat but has difficulty sitting still in a vehicle or gets out of his seat belt, an upright vest may be used. It is installed in the car with the vehicle seat belt and a tether. In some cases, a vest can be used on a school bus. Check with your pediatrician and your school transportation director for current information.

Older children and belt-positioning booster seats

If your child is able to sit up without help and is too large for a standard car safety seat with a harness or a forward-facing seat/restraint, he should use a belt-positioning booster seat until he is large enough to use a seat belt. Belt positioning booster seats raise a child up so that the lap and shoulder belts fit properly (see picture). This helps protect the upper body and head. These seats must be used with a lap/shoulder belt.

Older children and seat belts

Typically, a child is ready to use a seat belt when all 3 of the following conditions occur:
- The child is tall enough so that when she sits against the vehicle seat back her legs bend at the knee and her feet hang down.
- The shoulder belt lies across the chest, not the neck or throat.
- The lap belt lies low and snug across the thighs, not the stomach.

Children usually do not fit seat belts until they are between 8 to 12 years of age and are about 4 feet 9 inches tall. When your child is ready to wear a seat belt, make sure it fits properly. Shoulder belts should be worn across the chest. Never place a shoulder belt behind a child's back or under a child's arms. This could cause injury to the child.

Children and wheelchairs

Most wheelchairs are not crash tested. When possible, buckle your child in a car safety seat or restraint that fits her size and positioning needs. If you must transport your child in a wheelchair, install it in a forward-facing position with 4-point tie-down devices attached to the main frame of the wheelchair (see picture). Then restrain your child separately with a shoulder/lap belt. Positioning belts used with wheelchairs are not safety restraints. Lap trays attached to the wheelchair should be removed and secured separately during transport.

Several wheelchair manufacturers now offer certified transit models of their chairs. The tie-down attachment points on these chairs have been crash tested. Check with your child's therapist to determine if a certified transit model will meet your child's positioning, mobility, and safety needs. You can find more information on wheelchairs on the Internet at www.wheelchairnet.org.

When a child goes to school

When a child with special needs is ready to enter school, federal laws ensure her right to have equal services, including transportation. Any special transportation needs should be noted in the child's Individual Education Plan. The child's parents or caregivers, school representatives, and medical or rehabilitation personnel develop this plan.

Adapted vehicles

In some instances, families need an adapted vehicle to meet the transportation needs of their children. In general, families should work with a qualified rehabilitation specialist to decide the changes needed to protect everyone in the vehicle. For names of qualified driver rehabilitation specialists, contact a local rehabilitation center or the Association for Driver Rehabilitation Specialists at 800/290-2344 or www.driver-ed.org. When choosing a vehicle, families should work with a reputable dealer of adaptive vehicles. *Adapting Motor Vehicles for People With Disabilities* is a brochure published by the NHTSA to help families learn more about adapting vehicles. To get a free copy, call 888/DASH-2-DOT (888/327-4236) or view it on the Internet at www.nhtsa.dot.gov.

Medical home

For children with special needs, it is very important to have a medical home. A medical home is the group of people who work together to provide your child's health care. The medical home doctor (often a pediatrician or other primary care doctor) works as a partner with your family and others who care for your child. The same caring people meet all of your child's needs in your community from birth until she grows up. In addition to providing medical care, the people involved can help your family get special equipment and services for your child. Experts can help you find ways to pay the costs.

More information is available at www.aap.org/medhome or by sending an e-mail to medical_home@aap.org.

Resources

The *Emergency Information Form for Children With Special Needs* is available from the AAP and the American College of Emergency Physicians. This form is on the Internet at www.aap.org/advocacy/emergprep.htm.

The American Academy of Pediatrics
www.aap.org

Medem, an e-health network
www.medem.com

Medical equipment
Some children must travel with devices such as apnea monitors, oxygen tanks, ventilators, walkers, and crutches. Secure these in the vehicle so that they do not become flying objects in the event of a crash or sudden stop. At this time, there is no single product available to secure medical devices. Try wedging the equipment on the vehicle floor with pillows or securing it with seat belts not being used by a passenger. Make sure that any devices that use batteries have enough power for at least double the length of your trip.

Automotive Safety for Children Program
Riley Hospital for Children
575 West Dr, Room 004
Indianapolis, IN 46202
317/274-2977
www.preventinjury.org

Easter Seals
230 W Monroe, Suite 1800
Chicago, IL 60606
800/221-6827
www.easter-seals.org

National Highway Traffic Safety Administration (NHTSA)
Office of Occupant Protection-NTS-13
400 7th St, NW
Washington, DC 20590
888/DASH-2-DOT (888/327-4236)
www.nhtsa.dot.gov

Web site devoted to issues related to wheelchairs.
www.wheelchairnet.org

There may be car safety seats/restraints available that are not listed in this brochure. The products listed here are current only as of the date of publication. Some of the products noted may accommodate children with medical conditions not listed here. Addresses, phone numbers and Web site addresses are as current as possible, but may change at any time.

Suggested retail prices may vary.

American Academy of Pediatrics
DEDICATED TO THE HEALTH OF ALL CHILDREN™

The American Academy of Pediatrics is an organization of 60,000 primary care pediatricians, pediatric medical subspecialists, and pediatric surgical specialists dedicated to the health, safety, and well-being of infants, children, adolescents, and young adults.
American Academy of Pediatrics
Web site — www.aap.org
Copyright © 2002
American Academy of Pediatrics

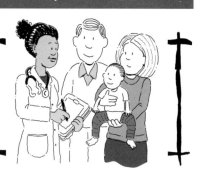

Safe Transportation of Children With Special Needs:

A Guide for Families   Part II   Product Information

Special Needs Car Safety Seats/Restraints Product Information

Model Name	Manufacturer	Price	Weight Limits	Height Limits	Conditions	Comments
Standard infant-only seats						
Varies	Varies For more information about standard car seats, ask your pediatrician about the American Academy of Pediatrics brochure, *Car Safety Seats: A Guide for Families.*	Varies	Upper limit varies from 20–35 pounds.	Up to 35"	Premature or small babies	Choose seats with smaller harness size. Use seats without shield or tray for best fit. Use rolled receiving blankets along both sides of baby for side support and a rolled cloth under the crotch strap to prevent slouching. At least 1 infant-only seat rear-faces to higher weights. Check instructions for weight and height limits.
Standard convertible seats						
Varies	Varies	Varies	Rear-facing varies from 20–35 pounds; forward-facing up to 40 pounds.	Up to 40"	Decreased head and neck control, trache-ostomies, long leg casts, eyeglasses	Use rear-facing for all children until they are at least 1 year of age AND at least 20 pounds. Use seats that rear-face to higher weights for larger babies or children with decreased head, neck, and trunk control. In forward-facing position, use a seat that can be semi-reclined for children with decreased head and neck control. Use 5-point harness for children with tracheostomies, eye-glasses, and thick, long leg casts.
Standard combination seats						
Varies	Varies	Varies	Up to 40 pounds with harness; up to 80 pounds used as booster seat without harness	Up to 40" with harness; up to 54" used as booster seat without harness	Some casts, behav-ioral conditions, decreased muscle tone	Forward-facing car seat with harness. After 40 pounds, harness is removed and seat becomes a high-back belt-positioning booster seat. Must have a lap and shoulder belt when used as a booster seat.
Standard forward facing seats/restraints						
Varies -	Varies	Varies	Upper limit varies from 40–80 pounds.	Upper limit varies from 40"–53".	Some casts, behav-ioral conditions, decreased muscle tone	Forward-facing only. Some require use of a tether.
Standard booster seats						
Varies	Varies	Varies	Varies from 80–100 pounds.	Varies from 50"–56".	For children who can sit up unassisted	Must be used with a lap and shoulder belt. Low-back and high-back models are available.
Car beds						
Angel Ride Infant Car Bed	Mercury Distributing 800/815-6330 www.mercurydistributing.com Angel Guard Products, Inc www.angel-guard.com	$45	Up to 9 pounds	20" or less	Small and premature babies	Harness with dual- tongue buckle. Install lengthwise with baby's head toward the center of the vehicle.
Ultra Dream Ride Car Bed	Cosco, Inc 2525 State St Columbus, IN 47201 800/544-1108 www.djgusa.com	$70	Up to 20 pounds	Up to 26"	Useful for babies who must travel flat because of breathing problems, fragile bones, Pierre Robin Sequence, spina bifida, and orthopedic conditions.	Install lengthwise with baby's head toward the center of the vehicle. If it is medically necessary for the baby to travel on his stomach, he will outgrow the bed before weighing 20 pounds.

Special Needs Car Safety Seats/Restraints Product Information, continued

Model Name	Manufacturer	Price	Weight Limits	Height Limits	Conditions	Comments
Car beds, continued						
Snug Seat Car Bed	Snug Seat, Inc PO Box 1739 Matthews, NC 28106 800/336-SNUG (7684) www.snugseat.com	$500	4–21 pounds	Up to 29"	Useful for babies who must travel lying down because of conditions such as breathing problems, osteogenisis imperfecta, Pierre Robin Sequence, spina bifida, and ortho-pedic conditions.	Baby is secured in a sturdy cloth bunting (sleeping bag) inside the bed. Snug Seat may modify sleeping bag for special applications. Install lengthwise with baby's head toward the center of the vehicle.
Specialized convertible car seat						
Spelcast	Snug Seat, Inc PO Box 1739 Matthews, NC 28106 800/336-SNUG (7684) www.snugseat.com	$295	10–20 pounds rear-facing; 20–40 pounds forward-facing	Up to 40"; child's head should not go above seat.	Designed for babies and toddlers who cannot use a standard car seat because of hip spica casts or other orthopedic devices.	Designed specifically for children in casts. Tether recommended for forward-facing position. Check with manufacturer to see how the weight of the cast affects how you use the seat.
Forward facing medical seats						
Columbia Orthopedic Positioning Seat	Columbia Medical PO Box 633 Pacific Palisades, CA 90272 800/454-6612 www.columbiamedical.com	$745	20–102 pounds	Up to 60"	Lack of upper body strength	Comes with adjustable head support pads, 4 positioning pads, crotch strap pad, and tether. Optional seat depth extender and abductor pad. Fits in many stroller bases including Columbia Stroller Base. Tether required for installation for children more than 65 pounds.
Carrie Car Seat	Tumble Forms Bergeron Health Care 15 S Second St Dolgeville, NY 13329 800/371-2778 www.tumbleforms.com	$745–$885 (depend-ing on size)	Four sizes • 20–40 pounds (preschool) • 30–60 pounds (elementary) • 50–100 pounds (junior) • 60–130 pounds (small adult)	Four sizes • 30"–38" (preschool) • 38"–48" (elementary) • 48"–58" (junior) • 56"–68" (small adult)	Decreased head, neck, and trunk control	Lateral head support and molded seat shape. Adjustable seat-to-back angle. Tether required. Optional footrest adjusts to maintain hip, knee, and ankle flexion. Optional stroller base and Cozee cover. Seat designed to stabilize the pelvis to assist with positioning problems.
Traveller Plus	Britax Child Safety, Inc 13501 S Ridge Dr Charlotte, NC 28273 704/409-1700 www.britaxusa.com	$450	20–105 pounds and minimum 1 year of age	19"–56"	Decreased head, neck, and trunk control	Forward-facing only. Comes with seat extender, recline bar, and crotch pommel. Must use top tether. Tether anchored to 2 points for children 80–105 pounds. Interchangeable foam padding allows for customizing seat.
Gorilla Postural Seat	Snug Seat, Inc PO Box 1739 Matthews, NC 28106 800/336-SNUG (7684) www.snugseat.com	$595	20–105 pounds and minimum 1 year of age.	Child's head not to extend above car seat back height	Cerebral palsy, spina bifida, muscular dystrophy, and similar conditions	Forward-facing only. Tether required. Comes with adjustable head support pads. Optional seat extension kit and seat recline wedge. Optional stroller base.
Snug Seat I Postural Seat	Snug Seat, Inc PO Box 1739 Matthews, NC 28106 800/336-SNUG (7684) www.snugseat.com	$750	20–45 pounds	Child's head not to extend above car seat back height	Decreased head, neck, and trunk control and skeletal deformities	Forward-facing only. Tether required. Foam pad positioning system for customized fit. Crash tested in conjunction with the Transport Stroller Base for tie-down in school buses.
Snug Seat 1000 Car Seat	Snug Seat, Inc PO Box 1739 Matthews, NC 28106 800/336-SNUG (7684) www.snugseat.com	$295	30–60 pounds	Child's head not to extend above car seat back height.	Decreased trunk control and weak neck muscles	Forward-facing only. Uses shoulder/lap belt. Has 5-point positioning harness. Comes with adjustable head support pads, built-in abduction, support tray, and seat wedge. Optional trunk and hip pads available. Lightweight.
Travel vests						
BESI Restraining Harness	Besi Manufacturing 9445 Sutton Pl Hamilton, OH 45011 800/543-8222 www.besi-inc.com	$85	Up to 164 pounds	None; for waists 22"–43"	Behavioral con-ditions; decreased trunk control	For school bus use only. Need hip measurement. Adjustable sizes. Cam wrap required for school bus installation, along with lap belt.

Special Needs Car Safety Seats/Restraints Product Information, continued

Model Name	Manufacturer	Price	Weight Limits	Height Limits	Conditions	Comments
Travel vests, continued						
E-Z-On Vest	E-Z-On Products, Inc of Florida 605 Commerce Way W Jupiter, FL 33458 800/323-6598 www.ezonpro.com	$77–$102 (varies with size and model)	Manufacturer recommends for ages 2 years and older and 40–164 pounds.	None; for waists 22"–43"	Behavioral conditions; decreased trunk control	Standard and fully adjustable sizes. Optional crotch strap. Tether required for vehicle installation; cam wrap required for school bus installation. Styles include "adjustable" zippers and shoulder straps.
E-Z-On 86-Y Universal Harness	E-Z-On Products, Inc of Florida 605 Commerce Way W Jupiter, FL 33458 800/323-6598 www.ezonpro.com	$60–$80	Manufacturer recommends for ages 4 years and older and 40–164 pounds.	None	Behavioral conditions	Harness supplements vehicle lap belt with 2 straps to hold upper body. Attaches to car with single bolt.
Q'Vest	Q'Straint 5553 Ravenswood Rd Bldg 110 Fort Lauderdale, FL 33312 800/987-9987 www.qstraint.com	$84	Two sizes • 20–60 pounds • 60 pounds or more	None	Behavioral conditions; decreased trunk control	Manufacturer recommends for school bus use only.
Travel vests (reclined)						
Modified E-Z-On Vest	E-Z-On Products, Inc of Florida 605 Commerce Way West Jupiter, FL 33458 800/323-6598 www.ezonpro.com	$111–$132	Manufacturer recommends for ages 2–12; 20–100 pounds.	Child must fit lengthwise on a bench seat. Sizes are for hips 22"–32".	For older children who must lie down because of conditions such as spinal injuries, body casts, long leg casts, or hip spica casts	Need hip measurement to determine size. Standard and adjustable models. Optional crotch strap. Requires 2 seat belts for installation.
Mobility base systems						
Kid Kart Xpress	Sunrise Medical 7477 E Dry Creek Pkwy Longmont, CO 80503 800/388-5278 www.sunrisemedical.com	$2,195 (standard package)	Seat is built on basis of child's measurements; maximum user weight of 55 pounds.	Based on specific measurements of child.	Decreased head, neck, and trunk control and other conditions requiring use of wheelchair	For use in school bus or van. Tie-down locations on mobility base tested and approved for transit. Manufacturer recommends use of Q'Straint tie-down system. Center mount joystick. Seating system options and accessories, including vent base frame, IV pole, and spica cast support.
Kid Kart TLC	Sunrise Medical 7477 E Dry Creek Pkwy Longmont, CO 80503 800/388-5278 www.sunrisemedical.com	$2,750 (standard package)	Seat is built on basis of child's measurements; maximum user weight of 75 pounds.	Based on specific measurements of child	Decreased head, neck, and trunk control and other conditions requiring use of wheelchair	For use in school bus or van. Tie-down locations on mobility base tested and approved for transit. Manufacturer recommends use of Q'Straint tie-down system. Seating system options and accessories, including vent and battery tray, and IV pole.
Mulholland Growth Guidance System	Mulholland Positioning Systems, Inc 215 N 12th St PO Box 391 Santa Paula, CA 93061 800/543-4769 www.mulhollandinc.com	$2,500–$4,500	Up to 50 pounds	None	Decreased head, neck, and trunk control	Postural support system with stroller base. Remove from stroller for installation in vehicle. Requires a tether. Install in bus or van only with Positioning Systems, Inc tie-down system.
Pixie Positioning Chair	Sammons Preston PO Box 5071 Bollingbrook, IL 60440-5071 800/323-5547 www.sammonspreston.com	$1,435–$1,625	Children ages 3–12; small and large sizes up to 110 pounds	None	Cerebral palsy and conditions that require positioning	Height-adjustable footrest and multiple harness settings. Folds for storage and travel.

The appearance of the name American Academy of Pediatrics (AAP) does not constitute a guarantee or endorsement of the products listed or claims made.

The information contained in this publication should not be used as a substitute for the medical care and advice of your pediatrician. There may be variations in treatment that your pediatrician may recommend based on individual facts and circumstances.

Although the American Academy of Pediatrics (AAP) is not a testing or standard-setting organization, this guide sets forth the Academy's recommendations based on the peer-reviewed literature available at the time of its publication and sets forth some of the factors that parents should consider before selecting and using a car safety seat or safety restraint.

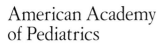

American Academy of Pediatrics

DEDICATED TO THE HEALTH OF ALL CHILDREN™

The American Academy of Pediatrics is an organization of 60,000 primary care pediatricians, pediatric medical subspecialists, and pediatric surgical specialists dedicated to the health, safety, and well-being of infants, children, adolescents, and young adults.

American Academy of Pediatrics
Web site — www.aap.org

Copyright © 2002
American Academy of Pediatrics

Choosing Child Care: What's Best for Your Family?

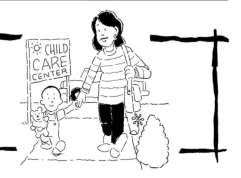

The child care that you choose for your family will play a key role in your child's health and development. Finding high-quality child care is very important, but not always easy. You will need to consider many questions. But you are not alone—an increasing number of parents rely on quality child care so that they can work or attend school. The following information may help you in your search for the child care option that is best for your family.

Types of child care

You can choose from the following 3 types of care:

- **In-home care**—the caregiver comes into your home.
- **Family child care**—you take your child to the home of the caregiver.
- **Center-based care**—you take your child to a place that is organized and staffed specifically to care for a group or groups of children.

    Consider the pros and cons of each type of care with your child's and your family's needs in mind.

In-home care

Having the caregiver come to or live in your home can be very convenient. In-home caregivers often can arrange their schedules to match your needs. Your child stays at home and does not have to adjust to a new setting. Your child will not be exposed to many seasonal illnesses because he will not be with groups of children. Your child may receive more individual attention, especially if the caregiver does not pursue other interests while caring for your child. If your caregiver also does housekeeping for your family, stress that your child's needs come first.

    Your in-home caregiver needs to know exactly what you expect. Discuss the following issues specifically with prospective caregivers:

- Activities and interactions that you want for your child, such as reading and playtime.
- How to use positive, effective discipline with your child, and what rules and limits you have set for your child.
- What the caregiver will and will not do in your home.
- Outings that are acceptable for your child and how to use the proper car safety seat, booster seat, or seat belt for your child in motor vehicles.
- **Limits for television,** video games, or other media. The American Academy of Pediatrics (AAP) does not recommend television for children younger than 2 years. For older children, the AAP recommends no more than 1 to 2 hours per day of educational, nonviolent programs.
- How and when the caregiver can contact you with questions or if there is an emergency.

    The caregiver should provide you with a daily schedule of what is planned and a daily report of what occurred. However, it is hard to know for sure what the caregiver does when you are not there. You will want to arrange for frequent, unannounced visits by a friend or family member who can observe how the caregiver interacts with your child and tell you about it. Keep in mind that relationships with in-home caregivers tend to be very personal.

Your caregiver

Selecting the right person to care for your child is one of the most important decisions you will make. Caregivers can be family members, people you knew before considering them as caregivers, or people with whom you will develop new relationships. Whatever type of care you choose, the relationship between you and your child's caregiver will be an important aspect of your life. Plan to spend some time together with your caregiver and your child so that you can learn about each other.

    It is important to check your caregiver's background, training, and references. The **training of caregivers** should include the following:

- Child development and early education (ie, the types of behavior that are typical for children your child's age and the types of activities that will help your child learn and grow)
- Using positive, effective discipline (including how to handle challenging behavior)
- Recognizing signs of illness
- Cleanliness and safety standards to prevent illness and injury (including how to use the proper car seats, booster seats, and seat belts for children in motor vehicles)
- First aid and proper response to choking and other emergencies
- How to evacuate the home or child care center safely in an emergency

At times you may function as both employer and friend or extended family for the caregiver.

    Skilled in-home caregivers are difficult to find. You will need a backup plan for the times when the caregiver is sick, has a personal need for time off, or goes on vacation. In some areas, agencies may provide training, placement, and supervision for in-home caregivers.

Family child care

This type of care takes place in the caregiver's home. Many family child care providers have young children of their own. They may care for children who are the same age as their own children or for children of different ages. Carefully review the program, policies, caregiver's qualifications, and condition of the home. Ask about children, teenagers, or other adults who live in the home. Who are they, what are their backgrounds, and how may they interact with your child?

    The AAP recommends that a child care home should not have more than 6 children per adult caregiver, including the caregiver's own children. (Some states allow more children when at least 2 adults are available at all times in larger family child care homes.) The total number of children should be fewer when infants and toddlers are included. No caregiver working alone should handle more than 2 children younger than 2 years.

    Because there usually is only 1 adult, backup care in an emergency situation must be nearby. In some areas, caregivers belong to a network of family child care providers who may provide training, shared toys, and backup help.

Family child care providers usually work alone. This makes it hard to judge their work. Look for caregivers who are licensed or registered with the state and, as a result, have unannounced visits by an inspector. Some family child care providers have earned accreditation as well. (See "Accreditation", right.)

Center-based care

Center-based care has many names—child care center, preschool, nursery school, or learning center. Center-based care also may have different sponsors, including churches, schools, colleges, universities, social service agencies, Head Start, independent owners and chains, and employers.

Regardless of what type of center-based care you choose, there are some basic things to consider. Centers should be licensed and inspected regularly for health, safety, cleanliness, staffing, and program content. (Some programs are exempt from state licensing.) Just because a center is licensed, do not assume it is regularly inspected. Check to see how often the center had announced and unannounced inspections in the past year and what was checked.

Keep in mind that state licensing regulations set the lowest legal limit for staying in business. High-quality care requires more than complying with regulations. To find out about what is covered by the regulations in your area, contact your city, county, or state department of social services. State licensing regulations can also be reviewed at the local licensing agency. Most are listed at the National Resource Center for Health and Safety in Child Care Web site at nrc.uchsc.edu.

High-quality centers should be accredited or in the process of obtaining accreditation. (See "Accreditation", above right.)

Parents should be welcome to make unannounced visits to the center to see their child, and they should be notified quickly if their child needs medical attention. Policies should be written and should explain how the center's staff promotes positive, effective discipline and responds to sick children. There should be a daily schedule that is used and posted for review by parents. Toys and activities should be suited to the children's ages and abilities. The facility should follow safety guidelines. Caregivers and center directors should be trained (see "Your caregiver" on page 1). Look for centers that have at least 2 caregivers per group and 1 group per room, a window or glass door for supervisors to view activities, and a plan for ongoing staff training.

Where to begin

When you start to look for child care, you may wish to contact a group such as Child Care Aware by phone at 800/424-2246 or online at www.childcareaware.org. This group can provide resources on high-quality child care and tell you if there is a local Child Care Resource and Referral agency in your community. All types of child care may be listed through this agency.

Once you receive a list of caregivers in your area, review written material that these caregivers make available, then call them. Ask questions on the phone to help you select those that you want to visit. Whatever type of child care you choose—in-home, family, or center-based—consider the following factors as you begin your search:

- **Location**—How far is the child care from home? From your work? Is this convenient for both parents? Can either parent get there quickly in an emergency?

Accreditation

Accreditation means that an outside observer has determined that the facility generally meets the criteria for high-quality child care. Family child care providers can be accredited through the National Association for Family Child Care (NAFCC).

Several independent groups of early childhood care and education professionals offer accreditation for centers. These include the National Association for the Education of Young Children (NAEYC) and the National Child Care Association (NCCA). If a seemingly good center is not accredited by either of these organizations, ask why. Encourage the staff to consider seeking accreditation.

- **Hours**—What hours of care are available? What happens if you are late in picking up your child? How are vacations and holidays scheduled?
- **Licensing/accreditation**—Is the facility or home licensed or registered with the appropriate local government agencies? Are there any outstanding violations? Is the program currently accredited; if so, by what organization?
- **Inspections/consultations**—Is there a qualified health professional, such as a doctor or nurse, who serves as a consultant for the child care program? (The national standard is that center-based infant-toddler programs should be visited by a health professional at least monthly, and all other child care programs should be visited at least quarterly.)
- **Visiting policy**—Are you welcome to visit during normal operating hours before and after enrolling your child? Can you see all the areas that your child will use?
- **Caregiver experience and training**—What education, training, and experience do the caregiver or center director and staff have? (See "Your caregiver" on page 1.) What type of training has the staff had during the past year? Do outside experts provide training?
- **Adequate staffing**—Are there enough trained adults available to children on a regular basis? Are there enough caregivers to fill in if one is ill or on vacation?

Do the child–staff ratios and the size of the groups of children fall within nationally recognized standards? (See chart below. For the recommended child–caregiver ratio for family child care homes, see "Family Child Care" on page 1.)

Age	Child–staff ratio*	Maximum group size*
Birth–12 months	3:1	6
13–30 months	4:1	8
31–35 months	5:1	10
3-year-olds	7:1	14
4–5-year-olds	8:1	16
6–8-year-olds	10:1	20
9–12-year-olds	12:1	24

*As recommended by the AAP. For more information, see *Caring for Our Children: National Health and Safety Performance Standards: Guidelines for Out-of-Home Child Care Programs*, listed in "Resources" on page 13.

- **Health standards**—What is the policy regarding sick children? Is a health assessment required before children enroll? Have caregivers and others who may spend time with your child been checked by a doctor to be sure that they are healthy?

- **Quality of program**—Are children cared for in small groups? Are activities proper for the children's level of development? Is there a daily schedule? Are there daily opportunities for indoor and outdoor play? Is television viewing permitted and, if so, what is watched and for how long? (See "In-home care" on page 1 for recommended limits for television.)

- **Policies**—Check the center's policies. Are the policies in writing? What is the discipline policy? Do the children go on any outings? If they travel by car, van, or bus, are the proper child safety seats, booster seats, and seat belts used?

- **Consistency**—Are the program's policies on meals, discipline, and issues such as toilet training the same as yours? How long have the caregivers who will take care of your child worked at the facility with children of your child's age? Will your child be able to have a stable relationship with 1 caring adult for at least 1 year?

- **Backup plans**—What happens if your child is sick or when the caregiver is not available or the child care program is closed?

- **Fees and services**—What is the cost for child care and/or optional services? How are payments collected? Are there other services available in addition to child care? Is safe transportation available daily and/or for trips?

- **References**—Ask for references and contact information from several parents who are currently using the program, as well as at least 1 parent whose child was in the program during the past year but is now too old to receive care at the facility.

- **Communication**—Can you talk with the caregiver on a regular basis? You will need to spend time with your child and the caregiver every day, both before you leave and when you return.

It is ultimately your responsibility to ensure that your child receives the best care. When problems occur, your caregiver should be able and willing to work through the situation with you. If at any time problems persist and you suspect your child's health or safety is in question, you will need to find other child care for your child right away.

What to observe

Visit the child care settings that you are seriously considering for your child. As you observe, consider the following questions:

1. Are there enough adults to meet the children's needs?
2. Do the caregivers seem to enjoy caring for the children? Are there joyful interactions between the children and caregivers?
3. Do the adults and the children often talk with each other? Are children encouraged to talk with each other?
4. Do the children in the program seem happy? When a child cries or acts out, how does the caregiver respond?
5. Is the noise level in the child care areas comfortable?
6. Is the center or home bright, cheerful, clean, safe, and well ventilated? Is all equipment clean, safe, and in good working order?
7. Is there a posted plan of activities being followed that includes large muscle play (ie, running, climbing), quiet play with toys the child chooses, time for reading and talking, rest, and snacks and meals?
8. Is the indoor space large enough? Look for 50 square feet, measured wall-to-wall, per child.

9. Is there a sleeping or quiet area large enough for all the children to rest during nap time? (There should be at least 3 feet of space between children unless each has a separate partitioned sleeping compartment.) Are there individual cribs, beds, cots, or mats to sleep on? Do sleeping children stay within view of caregivers? Do caregivers place infants to sleep on their backs? Are cribs free of blankets, toys, or other objects that could pose a hazard?
10. Does each child have a place for her own belongings?
11. Is there a clean diaper-changing area for infants and toddlers? Is a sink within the caregiver's reach near the diaper-changing area?
12. Are infants always fed in an upright position and, until they can sit by themselves for feeding, held by an adult? (No bottles should be allowed in bed or propped.)
13. Is the food nutritious, well prepared, suitable for the age group, and served in an appetizing way? Do you see posted menus, or are menus given to parents in advance? Do the menus match the food that is served?
14. Are there enough safe toys easily within reach of children? Are the toys suited to the age group?
15. Are dangerous toys and equipment such as baby walkers not used?
16. Are toys that are mouthed by infants or toddlers sanitized before other children are allowed to play with them?
17. Is there protective surfacing under all indoor and outdoor climbing equipment? Indoor climbing equipment requires the same types of impact-absorbing materials and fall zones as equipment installed outdoors.
18. Are the outside play area and equipment free of sharp edges, pinch points, rocks, uneven surfaces, and ditches? Is the area free of hazards such as high climbing equipment, tall slides, merry-go-rounds, trampolines, unprotected seesaws, and swings with wooden or plastic swing seats?
19. Is equipment sized and planned for use by the age group using it and inaccessible to those who are too young or too little to use it safely? Is the equipment properly installed, well maintained, and in good working order?
20. Is there well-maintained impact-absorbing material such as soft sand, wood chips, smooth gravel, or specially manufactured rubber mats under and extending at least 6 feet out from equipment?
21. Is the outside play area completely surrounded by the building and fencing?
22. Are the toilets and sinks clean and easy to reach? Can children reach clean towels, liquid soap, and toilet paper?
23. Do caregivers and children wash their hands at the following times:
    - Upon arrival for the day
    - When moving from one child care group to another
    - Before and after eating, handling food, or feeding a child
    - Before giving medication to a child
    - Before playing in water that is used by more than 1 person
    - After playing in sandboxes
    - After changing a diaper, using the toilet, or helping a child use the toilet
    - After handling any sort of bodily fluids, such as those from noses, mouths, cuts, or sores
    - After handling pets or other animals
    - After cleaning or handling garbage
24. Does the facility use disposable paper towels to ensure that each child uses only his own towel?

25. Are there sinks in each room (in centers), with separate sinks for food preparation and hand washing?
26. Is the center or home free of secondhand tobacco smoke?

Different children, different care

One key to good child care is whether the caregiver can adapt to the needs of each child and family. Not all children of the same age are at the same level of development; each child has unique character traits. A good caregiver understands these personal and developmental differences and creates a program to meet each child's needs. The type of child care that is best for your child may change as she grows older.

Finding programs and caregivers to meet the needs of children with disabilities or other special needs may be challenging. Inclusive programs usually work closely with parents and the child's pediatrician to find the best ways to provide a safe and supportive environment for every child. Discuss your child's needs with your pediatrician and caregiver to help your child function well in a positive environment.

Ask your pediatrician for advice about child care for your child. Your pediatrician can help you and your child's caregiver plan for your child's special needs, development, activities suitable for his age, health, safety, and any problems that come up while you are using child care.

Preparing your child

Most young infants, up to 7 months, adapt to caring adults and seldom have problems adjusting to good child care. Older infants may be upset when left with strangers. They may feel separation anxiety, which is a normal part of development for some children. They will need extra time and your support to "get to know" the caregiver.

Some children show changes in behavior when they start child care. Toddlers may cry, pout, refuse to go to child care, or act angry in other ways. Preschoolers may regress and behave like a younger child. They may be more wakeful at night. This behavior usually goes away after a few days or weeks in high-quality child care.

You can help your child adjust to a new child care arrangement. Arrange a visit with in-home caregivers while you are at home or when you need child care for a short time. Visit the center or family child care home that you have chosen with your child before beginning care. Show your child that you like and trust the caregiver.

Some children like to carry a reminder of home when they go to child care. A family photograph or small toy can be helpful. Talking to your child about child care and the care-giver is helpful. Being prepared makes any new experience easier for children. There also are storybooks about child care that you and your child can read together. (Check with your local library.)

After a child has been in child care, a sudden change in caregivers may be upsetting. This can happen even if the new caregiver is kind and competent. If you are concerned about your child's feelings, you may want to arrange a meeting with the caregiver or ask your pediatrician for advice. Parents need to help the caregivers and the child deal with any changes in the child's routine at home or child care.

High-quality child care helps children grow in every way and promotes their physical, social, and mental development. It offers support to working parents. Your pediatrician wants your child to grow and develop with enjoyment in a setting that supports you as a parent.

Planning for child care costs

Child care can be expensive, so families must budget ahead of time. Although the cost may seem high, consider how little the caregiver is actually earning per hour for the responsibility of ensuring your child's healthy growth and development during the hours when you use child care. Ask your employer for assistance from
- Direct payment through cafeteria plans
- Dependent-care spending accounts (tax savings)
- Voucher programs
- Employer discounts
  High-quality child care is an important investment for your child.

Resources

The following is a list of child care and early education resources. Check with your pediatrician for resources in your community.

American Academy of Pediatrics
Web site: www.aap.org

American Academy of Pediatrics
Healthy Child Care America
141 Northwest Point Blvd
Elk Grove Village, IL 60007
Phone: 888/227-5409
Fax: 847/228-6432
Web site: www.aap.org/advocacy/hcca.htm

Publications from the American Academy of Pediatrics
- *Caring for Your Baby and Young Child: Birth to Age 5*
- *Caring for Your School-Age Child: Ages 5–12*
- *Caring for Our Children: National Health and Safety Performance Standards: Guidelines for Out-of-Home Child Care Programs*
- *Preparing for Illness: A Joint Responsibility for Parents and Caregivers*

Medem (an e-health network)
Web site: www.medem.com

National Association for the Education of Young Children
1509 16th St, NW
Washington, DC 20036-1426
Phone: 800/424-2460
Web site: www.naeyc.org

National Association of Child Care Resource and Referral Agencies
1319 F St, NW, Suite 500
Washington, DC 20004-1106
Phone: 202/393-5501
Web site: www.naccrra.org

Child Care Aware (a program of the National Association of Child Care Resource and Referral Agencies)
Phone: 800/424-2246
Web site: www.childcareaware.org

National Child Care Information Center

243 Church St, NW, 2nd Floor

Vienna, VA 22180

Phone: 800/616-2242

TTY: 800/516-2242

Web site: www.nccic.org

National Resource Center for Health and Safety in Child Care

Campus Mail Stop F541

PO Box 6508

Aurora, CO 80045-0508

Phone: 800/598-KIDS (800/598-5437)

Web site: nrc.uchsc.edu

Please note: Inclusion on this list does not imply endorsement by the AAP. The AAP is not responsible for the content of the resources mentioned above. Addresses, phone numbers, and Web site addresses are as current as possible, but may change at any time.

The information contained in this publication should not be used as a substitute for the medical care and advice of your pediatrician. There may be variations in treatment that your pediatrician may recommend based on individual facts and circumstances.

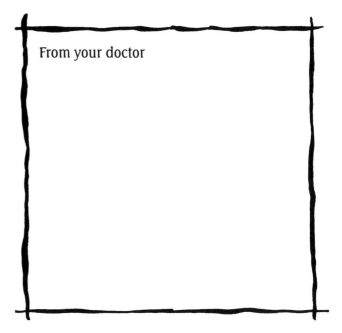

From your doctor

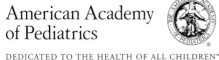

American Academy
of Pediatrics

DEDICATED TO THE HEALTH OF ALL CHILDREN™

The American Academy of Pediatrics is an organization of 60,000 primary care pediatricians, pediatric medical subspecialists, and pediatric surgical specialists dedicated to the health, safety, and well-being of infants, children, adolescents, and young adults.

American Academy of Pediatrics

Web site — www.aap.org

Copyright © 2002

American Academy of Pediatrics

Circumcision:
Information for Parents

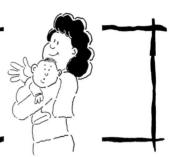

Circumcision is a surgical procedure in which the skin covering the end of the penis is removed. Scientific studies show some medical benefits of circumcision. However, these benefits are not sufficient for the American Academy of Pediatrics to recommend that all infant boys be circumcised. Parents may want their sons circumcised for religious, social, and cultural reasons. Since circumcision is not essential to a child's health, parents should choose what is best for their child by looking at the benefits and risks. This brochure answers common questions you may have about circumcision. Use this as a guide to help you decide what is best for your baby boy.

What is circumcision?

At birth, boys have skin that covers the end of the penis, called the foreskin. Circumcision surgically removes the foreskin, exposing the tip of the penis. Circumcision is usually performed by a doctor in the first few days of life. An infant must be stable and healthy to safely be circumcised.

Many parents choose to have their sons circumcised because "all the other men in the family were circumcised" or because they do not want their sons to feel "different." Others feel that circumcision is unnecessary and choose not to have it done. Some groups such as followers of the Jewish and Islamic faiths, practice circumcision for religious and cultural reasons. Since circumcision may be more risky if done later in life, parents may want to decide before or soon after their son is born if they want their son circumcised.

Common questions about circumcision

Is circumcision painful?

When done without pain medicine, circumcision is painful. There are pain medicines available that are safe and effective. The American Academy of Pediatrics recommends that they be used to reduce pain from circumcision. Local anesthetics can be injected into the penis to lower pain and stress in infants. There are also topical creams that can help. Talk to your pediatrician about which pain medicine is best for your son. Problems with using pain medicine are rare and usually not serious.

What should I expect for my son after circumcision?

After the circumcision, the tip of the penis may seem raw or yellowish. If there is a bandage, it should be changed with each diapering to reduce the risk of the penis becoming infected. Petroleum jelly should be used to keep the bandage from sticking. Sometimes a plastic ring is used instead of a bandage. The plastic ring that is left on the tip of the penis usually drops off within 5 to 8 days. It takes about 1 week to 10 days for the penis to fully heal after circumcision.

Reasons parents may choose circumcision

Research studies suggest that there may be some medical benefits to circumcision. These include the following:

- A slightly lower risk of urinary tract infections (UTIs). A circumcised infant boy has about a 1 in 1,000 chance of developing a UTI in the first year of life; an uncircumcised infant boy has about a 1 in 100 chance of developing a UTI in the first year of life.
- A lower risk of getting cancer of the penis. However, this type of cancer is very rare in both circumcised and uncircumcised males.
- A slightly lower risk of getting sexually transmitted diseases (STDs), including HIV, the AIDS virus.
- Prevention of foreskin infections.
- Prevention of phimosis, a condition in uncircumcised males that makes foreskin retraction impossible.
- Easier genital hygiene.

Reasons parents may choose not to circumcise

The following are reasons why parents may choose NOT to have their son circumcised:

- Possible risks. As with any surgery, circumcision has some risks. Complications from circumcision are rare and usually minor. They may include bleeding, infection, cutting the foreskin too short or too long, and improper healing.
- The belief that the foreskin is necessary to protect the tip of the penis. When removed, the tip of the penis may become irritated and cause the opening of the penis to become too small. This can cause urination problems that may need to be surgically corrected.
- The belief that circumcision makes the tip of the penis less sensitive, causing a decrease in sexual pleasure later in life.
- Almost all uncircumcised boys can be taught proper hygiene that can lower their chances of getting infections, cancer of the penis, and sexually transmitted diseases.

Are there any problems that can happen after circumcision?

Problems after a circumcision are very rare. However, call your pediatrician right away if

- Your baby does not urinate normally within 6 to 8 hours after the circumcision.
- There is persistent bleeding.
- There is redness around the tip of the penis that gets worse after 3 to 5 days.

It is normal to have a little yellow discharge or coating around the head of the penis, but this should not last longer than a week.

What if I choose not to have my son circumcised?

If you choose not to have your son circumcised, talk to your pediatrician about how to keep your son's penis clean. When your son is old enough, he can learn how to keep his penis clean just as he will learn to keep other parts of his body clean.

The foreskin usually does not fully retract for several years and should *never* be forced. The uncircumcised penis is easy to keep clean by gently washing the genital area while bathing. You do not need to do any special cleansing, such as with cotton swabs or antiseptics.

Later, when the foreskin fully retracts, boys should be taught how to wash underneath the foreskin every day. Teach your son to clean his foreskin by

- Gently pulling it back away from the head of the penis
- Rinsing the head of the penis and inside fold of the foreskin with soap and warm water
- Pulling the foreskin back over the head of the penis

See the AAP brochure *Newborns: Care of the Uncircumcised Penis* for more details. See your pediatrician if you notice any signs of infection such as redness, swelling, or foul-smelling drainage.

Female "circumcision"

Female genital mutilation, sometimes called female circumcision, is common in many cultures. It involves removing part or all of a female's clitoris. It may also involve sewing up the opening of the vagina. It is often done without any pain medicine. The purpose of this practice is to prove that a female is a virgin before she gets married, reduce her ability to experience sexual pleasure after marriage, and promote marital fidelity. There are many serious side effects, including the following:

- Pelvic and urinary tract infections
- Negative effects on self-esteem and sexuality
- Inability to deliver a baby vaginally

The Academy is absolutely opposed to this practice in all forms as it is disfiguring and has no medical benefits.

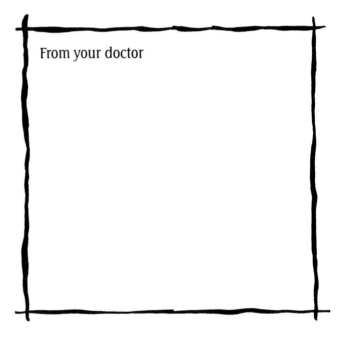

From your doctor

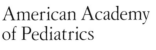

American Academy of Pediatrics

DEDICATED TO THE HEALTH OF ALL CHILDREN™

The American Academy of Pediatrics is an organization of 60,000 primary care pediatricians, pediatric medical subspecialists, and pediatric surgical specialists dedicated to the health, safety, and well-being of infants, children, adolescents, and young adults.

American Academy of Pediatrics
Web site — www.aap.org

Copyright © 1995
American Academy of Pediatrics, Updated 3/00

Diaper Rash

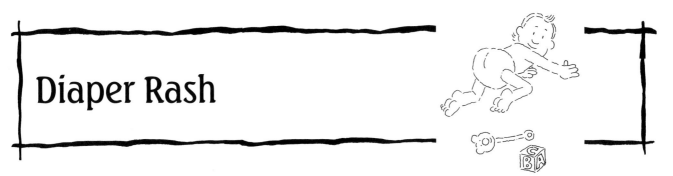

Diaper rash affects most babies, but it is usually not serious. Below we explain the causes of diaper rash, steps you can take to help prevent it, and how to treat it if it develops.

What is diaper rash?

Diaper rash can be any rash that develops inside the diaper area. In mild cases, the skin might be red. In more severe cases, there may be painful open sores. You will usually see a rash around the abdomen, genitalia, and inside the skin folds of the thighs and buttocks. Mild cases clear up within 3 to 4 days without any treatment. If a rash persists or develops again after treatment, consult your pediatrician.

What causes diaper rash?

Over the years diaper rash has been blamed on various causes, such as teething, diet, and ammonia in the urine. However, medical experts now believe it is caused by any of the following:

- Too much moisture
- Chafing or rubbing
- Prolonged contact of the skin with urine, feces, or both
- Yeast infection
- Bacterial infection
- Allergic reaction to diaper material

When skin stays wet for too long, the layers that protect it start to break down. When wet skin is rubbed, it also damages more easily. Moisture from a soiled diaper can harm your baby's skin and make it more prone to chafing. When this happens, a diaper rash may develop.

Further rubbing between the moist folds of the skin only makes the rash worse. This is why diaper rash often forms in the skin folds of the groin and upper thighs.

More than half of babies between 4 months and 15 months of age develop diaper rash at least once in a 2-month period. Diaper rash occurs more often in the following instances:

- As infants get older—mostly between 8 to 10 months of age
- If babies are not kept clean and dry
- In babies who have frequent stools, especially when the stools stay in their diapers overnight
- When babies begin to eat solid foods
- When babies are taking antibiotics, or in nursing babies whose mothers are taking antibiotics

Infants taking antibiotics are more likely to get diaper rashes caused by yeast infections. Yeast infects the weakened skin and causes a bright red rash with red spots at its edges. You can treat this with over-the-counter antifungal medications. If you see these symptoms, you may wish to consult with your pediatrician.

What can I do to prevent diaper rash?

To help prevent diaper rash from developing, you should:

- Change the diaper promptly after your child wets or has a bowel movement. This limits moisture on the skin.
- Do not put the diaper on airtight, especially overnight. Keep the diaper loose so that the wet and soiled parts do not rub against the skin as much.
- Gently clean the diaper area with water. You do not need to use soap with every diaper change or after every bowel movement. (Breastfed infants may stool as many as 8 times a day.) Use soap only when the stool does not come off easily.
- Do not use talcum or baby powder because they could cause breathing problems in your infant.
- Avoid over-cleansing with wipes that can dry out the skin. The alcohol or perfume in these products may irritate some babies' skin.

What can I do if my baby gets diaper rash?

If diaper rash develops despite your best efforts to prevent it, try the following:

- Change wet or soiled diapers often.
- Use clear water to cleanse the diaper area with each diaper change.
- Using water in a squirt bottle lets you clean and rinse without rubbing.
- Pat dry; do not rub. Allow the area to air dry fully.
- Apply a thick layer of protective ointment or cream (such as one that contains zinc oxide or petrolatum) to form a protective coating on the skin. These ointments are usually thick and pasty and do not have to be completely removed at the next diaper change. Remember, heavy scrubbing or rubbing will only damage the skin more.
- Check with your pediatrician if the rash:
  - Has blisters or pus-filled sores
  - Does not so away within 48 to 72 hours
  - Gets worse
- Use creams with steroids only if your pediatrician recommends them. They are rarely needed and may be harmful.

Which type of diaper should I use?

There are many different brands of diapers. Diapers are made of cloth or disposable materials. After they get soiled, you can wash cloth diapers and use them again and you throw away disposable diapers.

Research suggests that diaper rash is less common with the use of disposable diapers. In child care settings, children who wear super-absorbent disposable diapers tend to have lower rates of diaper rash. Regardless of which type of diaper you use, diaper rash occurs less often and is less severe when you change diapers often. If you use a cloth diaper, you can use a stay-dry liner inside it to keep your baby drier.

If you choose not to wash cloth diapers yourself, you can have a diaper service clean them. If you do your own washing, you will need to presoak heavily soiled diapers. Keep and wash soiled diapers separate from other clothes. Use hot water and double-rinse each wash. Do not use fabric softeners or antistatic products on the diapers because they may cause rashes in young, sensitive skin.

Whether you use cloth diapers, disposables, or both, always change diapers as needed to keep your baby clean, dry, and healthy.

> Remember—never leave your baby alone on the changing table or on any other surface above the floor. Even a newborn can make a sudden turn and fall to the floor.

Diaper rash is usually not serious, but it can cause your child discomfort. Follow the steps listed above to help prevent and treat diaper rash. Discuss any questions you have about these steps with your pediatrician.

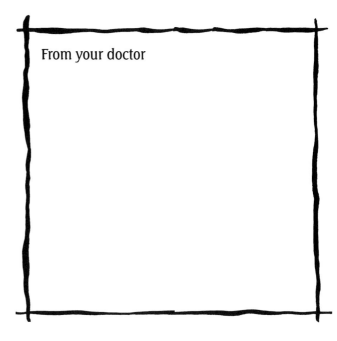

From your doctor

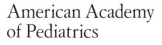

American Academy of Pediatrics

DEDICATED TO THE HEALTH OF ALL CHILDREN™

The American Academy of Pediatrics is an organization of 60,000 primary care pediatricians, pediatric medical subspecialists, and pediatric surgical specialists dedicated to the health, safety, and well-being of infants, children, adolescents, and young adults.

American Academy of Pediatrics
Web site—www.aap.org

Copyright © 1996
American Academy of Pediatrics, Reaffirmed 3/99

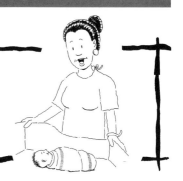

Newborn Hearing Screening and Your Baby

Before you bring your newborn home from the hospital, your baby needs to have a hearing screening. Although most babies can hear normally, 2 to 3 of every 1,000 babies are born with some degree of hearing loss. Without newborn hearing screening, it can be difficult to detect hearing loss in the important first months and years of your baby's life. About half of the children with hearing loss have no risk factors for it.

Newborn hearing screening can detect possible hearing loss in the first days of a baby's life. If a possible hearing loss is found, further tests will be done to confirm the results. If a hearing loss is confirmed, treatment and early intervention can start promptly. Early intervention helps babies with hearing loss and their families learn important communication skills.

That is why the American Academy of Pediatrics (AAP) recommends that all babies receive newborn hearing screening before they go home from the hospital.

What is hearing loss?

Hearing loss is the decreased ability to hear sounds. It may be mild to profound (severe), temporary or permanent, and can make it difficult to hear different kinds of sounds (especially consonants), which are essential in learning to talk.

It can affect one or both ears, and can occur anywhere along the hearing channel, including the following:

- **Outer ear** (eg, because of too much wax or a block in the outside ear canal)
- **Middle ear** (eg, because of an infection or fluid in the middle ear)
- **Cochlea** (inner ear), where sound waves are detected and passed on to the hearing nerve
- **Hearing nerve,** which connects to the brain
- **The hearing center in the brain**

Why do newborns need hearing screening?

Babies learn from the time they are born. One of the ways they learn is through hearing. If they have problems with hearing and do not receive the right treatment and early intervention services, babies will have trouble with language development. For some babies early intervention services may include the use of sign language and/or hearing aids. Studies show that children with hearing loss who receive appropriate early intervention services by age 6 months usually develop good language and learning skills.

Some parents think they would be able to tell if their baby could not hear. This is not always the case. Babies may respond to noise by startling or turning their heads toward the sound. This does not mean they have normal hearing. Most babies with hearing loss can hear some sounds but still not hear enough to develop full speaking ability.

Timing is everything. Your baby will have the best chance for normal language development if any hearing loss is discovered and treated by the age of 6 months—and the earlier, the better.

How is newborn hearing screening done?

There are 2 screening tests that may be used.

Auditory brainstem response (ABR)—This test measures how the brain responds to sound. Clicks or tones are played through soft earphones into the baby's ears. Three electrodes placed on the baby's head measure the brain's response.

Otoacoustic emissions (OAE)—This test measures sound waves produced in the inner ear. A tiny probe is placed just inside the baby's ear canal. It measures the response (echo) when clicks or tones are played into the baby's ears.

Both tests are quick (about 5 to 10 minutes), painless, and may be done while your baby is sleeping or lying still. Either or both tests may be used.

Can I assume that my hospital will screen my newborn's hearing?

It is best to ask. Most hospitals do hearing screening for all newborns. Some only screen newborns who are considered high risk, such as those with a family history of hearing loss.

Most states now have Early Hearing Detection and Intervention (EHDI) programs. Such programs try to ensure that all newborns in the state are screened for hearing loss and that those who need help get it.

What if my baby passes the hearing screening?

If your baby does not have any risk factors for hearing loss and has passed the newborn screening test, then your baby's pediatrician still will look at your baby's hearing and speech/language development along with other milestones at each of your baby's regular visits. Keep in mind that some forms of hearing loss develop as a child gets older.

If your baby has certain risk factors (eg, family history of hearing loss, premature birth, face/skull deformities), your baby's pediatrician should arrange for regular hearing tests to make sure that your baby continues to hear well.

What if my baby does not pass the hearing screening?

If your baby does not pass the hearing screening at birth, it does not mean that your baby has hearing loss. In fact, most babies who do not pass the screening test have normal hearing. But to be sure, it is extremely important to have further testing. This should include a more thorough hearing evaluation and a medical evaluation. These tests should be done as soon as possible, but definitely before your baby is 3 months old. These tests can confirm whether hearing is normal or not.

If hearing loss is found, what can be done?

This depends on the type of hearing loss that your baby has. Every baby with hearing loss should be seen by a hearing specialist (audiologist) experienced in testing babies and a pediatric ear/nose/throat doctor (otolaryngologist).

Special hearing tests can be performed by the audiologist who, together with the otolaryngologist, can tell you the degree of hearing loss and what can be done to help.

If the hearing loss is permanent, hearing aids and speech and language services may be recommended for your baby. The Individuals with Disabilities Education Act (IDEA) requires that free early intervention programs be offered to children with hearing loss, beginning at the time the child's hearing loss is identified.

The outlook is good for children with hearing loss who begin an early intervention program before the age of 6 months. Research shows these children usually develop language skills on par with those of their peers.

What if I do not receive my baby's hearing screening results?

Usually parents receive the results of their babies' hearing screening before mother and baby leave the hospital. If you did not get the results of your baby's hearing screening, call your baby's pediatrician to confirm the results.

How will I pay for newborn hearing screening and early intervention services?

Hearing screening tests usually cost between $25 and $40. Check with your health insurance company to see if it will cover the cost of newborn hearing screening and follow-up services. In some cases, your local school system, state programs, or local service clubs may cover the cost.

What if my baby did not receive hearing screening as a newborn?

If your baby did not receive hearing screening as a newborn in the hospital, call your baby's pediatrician and ask to have your baby screened (with ABR and/or OAE) as soon as possible. It is important to know that hearing can be tested at any age. Talk to your baby's pediatrician if you are concerned at any time about your baby's hearing or speech development.

Resources

Alexander Graham Bell Association for the Deaf and Hard of Hearing
202/337-5220
www.agbell.org

American Society for Deaf Children
Voice/TTY: 800/942-2732
www.deafchildren.org

American Speech-Language-Hearing Association
Voice/TTY: 800/638-8255
www.asha.org

Family Voices
888/835-5669
www.familyvoices.org

Medem (an e-health network)
www.medem.com

National Association of the Deaf
Voice: 301/587-1788
TTY: 301/587-1789
www.nad.org

National Center for Hearing Assessment and Management
Voice/TTY: 435/797-3584
www.infanthearing.org

National Institute on Deafness and Other Communication Disorders
Voice: 800/241-1044
TTY: 800/241-1055
www.nidcd.nih.gov

Please note: Inclusion on this list does not imply an endorsement by the American Academy of Pediatrics. The AAP is not responsible for the content of the resources mentioned above. Addresses, phone numbers, and Web site addresses are as current as possible, but may change at any time.

The information contained in this publication should not be used as a substitute for the medical care and advice of your pediatrician. There may be variations in treatment that your pediatrician may recommend based on individual facts and circumstances.

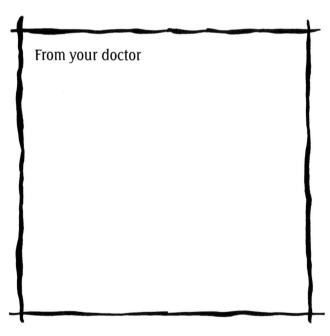

From your doctor

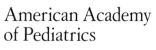

American Academy of Pediatrics

DEDICATED TO THE HEALTH OF ALL CHILDREN™

The American Academy of Pediatrics is an organization of 60,000 primary care pediatricians, pediatric medical subspecialists, and pediatric surgical specialists dedicated to the health, safety, and well-being of infants, children, adolescents, and young adults.

American Academy of Pediatrics
Web site—www.aap.org

Copyright © 2002
American Academy of Pediatrics

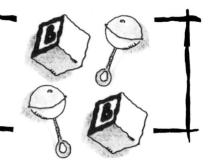

Early Arrival:
Information for Parents of Premature Infants

Your Very Special Delivery

Congratulations! You have welcomed a new baby to your family! While every child brings his own joys and challenges, you may be worried because your baby was born earlier than expected. But as you will see, while premature infants may need extra care at first, they have bright futures.

Premature Birth Is Common

Every year, about 11% of babies are born prematurely. But, thanks to medical advances, children born after 28 weeks and weighing more than 2 lb 3 oz, have a 95% or better chance of survival. They usually catch up in height and weight with their peers by age 2. In fact, 80% of babies born after the 30th week of pregnancy have no long-term health or developmental problems.

Premature Babies Need Special Care

At the Hospital
Because premature babies are born before they are physically ready to leave the womb, they require extra medical attention immediately after delivery. Your child may need special tests as well as medical help that is different from that needed by full-term babies. It may be a few days or weeks before his lungs fully develop, before he begins to breathe and feed on his own, and before he is able to maintain his own body temperature.

Your baby will probably be admitted to a *neonatal intensive care unit* or a *neonatal intermediate care unit*. There, a specially educated team of doctors and nurses can give your child the care he needs.

At Home
Like any child, your premature baby needs your love and attention in order to thrive. There are many things you can do at home to make sure your baby has a healthy start. This booklet will help you care for your child so that you can help him stay healthy and grow strong.

Answers to Parents' Common Questions

Q: Why was my baby premature? Is it my fault?

A: Many mothers of premature infants worry that they might have done something during pregnancy that caused their babies to be born early. Smoking, drinking alcohol, and using drugs during pregnancy can contribute to prematurity; however, no one knows for sure why most premature babies are born early. If you smoke, have a drinking problem, or use drugs, get help right away. These behaviors can harm your baby after she is born, too. Your new baby needs you to be as healthy as possible.

Q: Will I be able to hold my baby?

A: All babies need to be touched, held, snuggled, and talked to. This can reduce stress and help their brains develop. Although your baby may look fragile, you should gently touch, hold, and cradle her if your doctor says it is OK.

Q: Why does my baby look different?

A: Babies who are born early do not look like full-term infants. Your baby's head may seem larger compared to the rest of her body. Her body will have less fat and her skin may look thin. Her blood vessels may show underneath. Also, your baby's facial features may appear sharper. But don't worry, she will begin to look like a typical newborn as she grows.

Q: What will happen to my baby when I leave the hospital without her?

A: Leaving your baby, even for a short time, can be difficult, but your baby is in good hands. You can visit often to spend time with your child. Use the time away from the hospital to rest and get ready for your baby's homecoming.

Q: Will my child always have problems because she was born early?

A: Though premature babies are at higher risk for some problems, most of them grow into healthy children. Early diagnosis, treatment, and ongoing care can give your child a brighter future.

Some Helpful Definitions

- **Apgar Score:** This exam measures your baby's heart rate, breathing, muscle tone, reflex response, and color at birth. The Apgar score helps the hospital staff know how your baby is doing as he gets used to life outside the womb. Because of their early birth, premature babies are more likely to have lower scores.
- **Cardiorespiratory Monitor:** Because your baby's lungs are still immature, he may have trouble breathing. His breathing and heart rate can be watched using special equipment called a cardiorespiratory monitor. If he needs help breathing, the doctors may give him extra oxygen or use other equipment to help him breathe.
- **Warmer/Incubator:** Because your baby has less body fat, he can get cold in normal room temperatures. For that reason, he will be placed in a warmer bed or an incubator. These special beds have built-in heaters to help keep your baby warm.

Your Baby's Nutrition Needs

Because premature infants are small, they have a great need for food to gain strength and build resistance to disease. At first they may need to receive fluids intravenously (through an IV) or through a feeding tube.

Breast milk is the best nutrition for your baby. However, if your baby is not able to nurse at first, you can pump your milk and it can be given to her. Express your milk at the times when your baby would usually feed, so that your body becomes used to the schedule (usually about 8 times per day at the start). Most hospitals have breastfeeding experts to help you get started. Once you start to breastfeed, let your baby nurse often to build up your milk supply.

Breastfeeding is best for most infants, however, for medical or personal reasons, your baby may need infant formula. You and your pediatrician should discuss this decision.

Special Health Issues

Premature infants are not as fully developed as full-term babies. That is why they have a somewhat higher risk for certain health problems.

- **Respiratory Distress Syndrome (RDS)**
  What It Is: RDS is a breathing problem caused by immature lungs. Premature infants' lungs may lack a liquid substance called surfactant that gives fully developed lungs the elastic qualities required for easy breathing. Without surfactant, the lungs tend to collapse, forcing a tiny baby to work harder to breathe.
  Treatment: Many infants will require a ventilator, or respirator, to breathe for them. Artificial surfactants are now available and are very effective in treating RDS. Many babies respond very well to this treatment. Lung problems in premature infants usually improve within several days to several weeks.

- **Chronic Lung Disease/Bronchopulmonary Dysplasia (BPD)**
  What It Is: Babies who need oxygen for more than a month are described as having bronchopulmonary dysplasia (BPD) or chronic lung disease. They may need oxygen and other treatments for several weeks or months.
  Treatment: Babies often outgrow BPD as their lungs mature and grow, although some premature infants continue to require oxygen when they go home.

- **Respiratory Syncytial Virus (RSV)**
  What It Is: RSV is the leading cause of lower respiratory tract illness in infants and children. In the United States, RSV outbreaks usually occur between October and May. Infants who get RSV may develop apnea (pauses in a baby's breathing that last more than 15 seconds); bronchiolitis (an infection of the small breathing tubes of the lungs); or long-term lung problems. Premature infants and babies with BPD are at highest risk for complications from RSV infection.
  Prevention and Treatment: RSV is very contagious. It can be spread in the hospital or after babies are sent home. Make sure that family and friends who visit your new baby do not have colds or other infections. Ask them to wash their hands before touching your baby. There is no proven effective treatment for RSV infection. As a result, your pediatrician may recommend medication to prevent RSV infection if your baby is at very high risk for serious complications.

- **Retinopathy of Prematurity (ROP)**
  What It Is: ROP is an eye disease that occurs when part of the eye, called the retina, has not fully developed.
  Treatment: Most cases of ROP are mild and will resolve without treatment. However, in some cases ROP can result in serious vision problems. Severe cases of ROP are often treated with surgery. Your pediatrician will talk to you about this treatment if it is needed.

- **Apnea and Bradycardia**
  What It Is: Apnea refers to pauses in your baby's breathing that last more than 15 seconds. This is common in preterm babies. When apnea occurs, the heart rate will often decrease as well. This is called bradycardia.
  Treatment: If your baby has apnea spells, your pediatrician may prescribe a medicine to help regulate breathing. Your baby's heart and breathing will also be watched by monitors. Most premature babies outgrow this before they go home. If your baby does not, he may need a home apnea monitor.

- **Jaundice**
  What It Is: Jaundice happens because a baby's liver has not matured enough to completely filter a yellowish substance called bilirubin from the blood. Newborns often produce more bilirubin than their livers can handle.
  Treatment: Most cases can be treated effectively by placing the baby under special lights. During the treatment, most of the baby's skin is exposed and his eyes are covered to protect them from the light.

- **Other Health Problems**
  Premature infants may also develop other conditions such as anemia of prematurity (low blood cell count) and heart murmurs. Heart murmurs are sounds that the flow of blood makes as it goes through the heart. Your pediatrician and the other health care professionals caring for your baby will keep you informed about your baby's condition and progress.

Choosing a Pediatrician

Because your baby arrived early, you may not have had time to choose a pediatrician for your child. Your baby's doctor or nurse at the hospital may be able to recommend a pediatrician. You can also write the American Academy of Pediatrics for the names of pediatricians in your area. See the "Helpful Organizations" section at the end of this booklet for the address.

A Happy Homecoming

The OK to Go
You finally get to bring your baby home! Your pediatrician will approve the discharge of your baby from the hospital, based on the following guidelines. Your baby should be:
- breathing on her own,
- able to maintain body temperature,
- able to be fed by breast or bottle, and
- gaining weight steadily at time of discharge.

Other medical problems should also be resolved, or home care should be set up before your baby leaves the hospital.

Questions to Ask Before You Leave the Hospital
Your pediatrician will talk with you before your baby leaves the hospital. Be sure that he or she explains the following:
- How to care for your baby at home
- When to call his or her office or go to the hospital
- How to know if your baby is eating properly, getting enough sleep and gaining enough weight
- What medicines to give, if any are needed
- How often you will need to bring your baby in for an exam. Regular contact with your pediatrician is very important to your child's health. Be sure to discuss any worries that you have about your baby.

Safe Traveling With Your Baby
It is not only unsafe, but also illegal for any baby to ride in a car without being secured in a car safety seat. Premature infants should be observed in a car seat before discharge from the hospital to see if the semireclined position adds to or causes breathing problems. If your pediatrician recommends that your baby lie flat during travel, a crash-tested car bed may be used for a short period.

The back seat is the only safe place for babies. Whenever possible, an adult should ride in the back seat next to your baby to watch her closely. Depending on your baby's condition, you may want to limit her amount of car travel for the first month or two at home. You can check this with your pediatrician.

If You Must Bring the Hospital Home With You
Some premature babies need monitors and other equipment at home. For example, if apnea is a problem, monitoring may be done at home. Some babies may also need to go home with oxygen or other treatments. You and other caregivers will be trained on how to take care of your child's special needs before you take her home. You will also be taught how to perform *infant cardiopulmonary resuscitation* (CPR).

Settling in at Home
Premature babies need to be fed more often, and it will take a little while for them to adjust to being at home. Accept any offers of help around the house during the first few weeks, so you can take time to get used to having a new baby in the house.

A Good Night's Rest for Both of You
Your baby needs plenty of sleep in order to grow and develop. He will rest easier—and you will, too—if you follow a few simple rules when you put your baby down for a nap or for the night.

Sleeping Position: Back to Sleep
The American Academy of Pediatrics recommends that healthy infants be placed on their backs to sleep. Babies who are placed on their stomachs to sleep are at higher risk for sudden infant death syndrome (SIDS).

Placing babies on their backs to sleep does not increase the risk of other problems (for example, choking, flat head, or poor sleep). However, premature infants with certain medical problems (such as lung problems) may need to sleep on their side. Whether your baby sleeps on his back or side, a certain amount of "tummy time" is needed when he is awake. Ask your pediatrician about the best sleeping position for your baby.

In addition to proper sleeping position, you can reduce the risk of SIDS by:
- keeping blankets, pillows, soft bedding, and large stuffed toys out of your baby's crib;
- making sure your baby's room is not too hot or too cold;
- not smoking in your home;
- getting regular health care for your child; and
- breastfeeding.

Your Child's Growth and Development
Your baby's first year is a time of great change, just as it would be if she had been born on or near her due date. A child's development is complex, ongoing process. No two children mature at the same rate or in the same way. Development even varies from day to day and week to week. Over time, you will get to know your baby as an individual.

Timing Is Everything
Because your child was born early, you should think of her progress in terms of "adjusted age." For example, if your baby was 8 weeks early, adjust your expectations by 2 months. Therefore, a 4-month-old premature baby may act like a full-term 2 month old. Try not to compare your child with full-term babies or focus too much on developmental charts. Your pediatrician will follow your child's developmental progress.

Early Intervention Can Help
If there are any developmental problems, the important thing is to catch them early, so that your child can be helped to adapt.

Some problems can show up right away; others do not show up for some time. You are in the best position to monitor your child's development. Become familiar with your child's general pattern of development, and if you think your child is showing signs of a hearing, vision, speech, muscle, or learning delay, see your pediatrician as soon as possible. Early intervention programs that work with children from birth to 3 years may do a lot to lessen any long-term effect on your child's learning.

Keeping Your Child Healthy
One of the most important things you can do to keep your child healthy is to make sure he receives all recommended check-ups and immunizations. Check-ups will help make sure your baby's growth is on track, give your pediatrician a chance to catch any health problems early, and help you get your questions answered. If your baby has trouble gaining weight, has breathing problems, or any other problems that are of concern, your pediatrician may wish to see your child more often.

Immunizations can make sure your child's health is not put at risk by serious childhood diseases, such as whooping cough, hepatitis, and meningitis. These diseases can cause death or leave your child with long-term health problems.

When to Begin Immunizations
Some parents think their children do not need immunizations until they enter school. Actually, they should start when they are infants. Children should receive most of their immunizations during their first 2 years.

Most premature infants need to receive their immunizations at the same age as full-term infants, unless your pediatrician feels that this is not appropriate. Your pediatrician can help you make sure your child's immunizations are given on time and are up-to-date.

Immunizations Your Child Needs

Your child needs all of these immunizations to stay healthy:

- Hepatitis B
- Diphtheria, Tetanus, Pertussis (DTaP/DTP)
- *Haemophilus influenzae* type b (Hib)
- Polio
- Measles, Mumps, Rubella (MMR)
- Varicella (Chicken Pox)

Talk to your pediatrician about when your baby should have these immunizations.

If You Need Support

Sometimes parents need help taking care of a premature baby. Or they may need a shoulder to lean on when facing the stresses of being a new parent. If this is the case:

- Talk to your pediatrician, he or she can be a great source of support.
- Take a parenting class or join a parent support group. Your local hospital may offer these or can refer you to counselors or other professionals who can help.
- If you need more information or support, contact the other organizations listed below.

Helpful Organizations

For parents of PREMATURE BABIES:

Association for the Care of Children's Health
7910 Woodmont Ave, Suite 300
Bethesda, MD 20814
609/224-1742

The National Perinatal Association
3500 E Fletcher Ave, Suite 209
Tampa, FL 33613
813/971-1008

La Leche League
1400 N Meacham
PO Box 4079
Schaumburg, IL 60168-4079
847/519-7730 or
800/LaLeche

Healthy Mothers/Healthy Babies Coalition
409 12th St, SW
Washington, DC 20024-8811
202/863-2458

March of Dimes
1275 Mamaroneck Ave
White Plains, NY 10605
888/663-4637

For a referral to a pediatrician in your area, send the name of the area where you live and a self-addressed, stamped envelope to:

American Academy of Pediatrics
Pediatrician Referral Source
PO Box 927
Elk Grove Village, IL 60009-0927

Look Forward to the Future

Because your child was born early and may have some health problems, you may be afraid to plan too far ahead. But it is never too early to start bonding with your child. Today, premature babies have a good chance of doing well, thanks to medical advancements and early intervention.

Pediatrician's Name: _____
_____
Address: _____
_____
Phone Number: _____

Immunization Record
Record month/day/year below

DTaP/DTP	Hepatitis B	Td
_____	_____	_____
_____	_____	_____
_____	_____	**Other**
_____	**Polio**	_____
_____	_____	_____
Hib	_____	_____
_____	_____	_____
_____	**Varicella**	_____
_____	_____	
_____	_____	
MMR		
_____		
_____		

The information contained in this publication should not be used as a substitute for the medical care and advice of your pediatrician. There may be variations in treatment that your pediatrician may recommend based on individual facts and circumstances.

American Academy of Pediatrics

DEDICATED TO THE HEALTH OF ALL CHILDREN™

The American Academy of Pediatrics is an organization of 60,000 primary care pediatricians, pediatric medical subspecialists, and pediatric surgical specialists dedicated to the health, safety, and well-being of infants, children, adolescents, and young adults.

American Academy of Pediatrics
Web site—www.aap.org

Copyright © 1998
American Academy of Pediatrics

Prevent Shaken Baby Syndrome

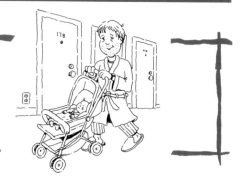

Taking care of a baby can be a most rewarding and exciting experience. However, it also can be frustrating when the baby gets fussy, especially when an end to the crying seems to be nowhere in sight. Too often, parents or other caregivers lose control and shake, jerk, or jolt a baby in an effort to stop the crying.

Most people know the dangers of hitting an infant or child. But did you know that shaking your baby also is very dangerous? Your pediatrician and the American Academy of Pediatrics want you to be aware of the dangers of shaking a baby. If you ever have felt frustrated when taking care of a fussy baby, read on to find out why shaking a baby can be deadly.

What is shaken baby syndrome?

Shaken baby syndrome is a serious type of head injury that happens when an infant or toddler is severely or violently shaken. Babies are not able to fully support their heavy heads. As a result, violent and forceful shaking causes a baby's brain to be injured. Too often, this leads to the death of a baby. It also can lead to

- Bleeding around the brain
- Blindness
- Hearing loss
- Speech or learning disabilities
- Chronic seizure disorder
- Brain damage
- Mental retardation
- Cerebral palsy

Shaken baby syndrome usually occurs when a parent or other caregiver shakes a baby out of anger or frustration, often because the baby will not stop crying. Shaken baby syndrome is a serious form of child abuse. Remember, it is *never* okay to shake a baby.

What are the signs and symptoms of shaken baby syndrome?

When a baby is violently shaken, brain cells are destroyed and the brain cannot get enough oxygen. As a result, a victim of shaken baby syndrome may show one or all of the following signs and symptoms:

- Irritability
- Lethargy (difficulty staying awake)
- Difficulty breathing
- Tremors (shakiness)
- Vomiting
- Seizures
- Coma
- Death

Spread the word!

Parents, if other people help take care of your baby, make sure they know about the dangers of shaken baby syndrome. This includes child care providers, older siblings, grandparents, and neighbors — *anyone* who cares for your baby. Make sure they know it is *never* okay to shake a baby.

What do I do if my baby is shaken?

If you think your baby might have been injured from violent shaking, the most important step is to get medical care right away. Call your pediatrician or take your baby to the nearest emergency department. If your baby's brain is damaged or bleeding inside from severe shaking, it will only get worse without treatment. Getting medical care right away may save your baby's life and prevent serious health problems from developing.

Be sure to tell your pediatrician or the doctor in the emergency room if your baby was shaken. Do not let embarrassment, guilt, or fear get in the way of your baby's health or life. Without the correct information, your pediatrician or the doctor may assume your baby has an illness. Mild symptoms of shaken baby syndrome are very similar to colic, feeding problems, and fussiness. Your baby may not get the right treatment if the doctor does not have all the facts.

When babies cry

It is not always easy to figure out why babies cry. They may be hungry or overtired. They may be cold or need their diapers changed. Sometimes it seems like they cry for no reason. The following are a few ideas to try when your baby does not stop crying:

- Check to see if your baby's diaper needs changing.
- Wrap your baby in a warm, soft blanket.
- Feed your baby slowly, stopping to burp often.
- Offer your baby a pacifier.
- Hold your baby against bare skin, like on your chest, or cheek-to-cheek.
- Rock your baby using slow, rhythmic movements.
- Sing to your baby or play soft, soothing music.
- Take your baby for a walk in a stroller.
- Go for a ride with your baby in the car (remember to always use a car seat).

If you have tried all of these and your baby continues to cry, go back and try them again. Most babies get tired after crying for a long time and eventually will fall asleep.

When your baby cries, take a break – don't shake!

If you have tried to calm your crying baby but nothing seems to work, it is important to stay in control of your temper. Remember, it is never okay to shake, throw, or hit your baby — and it never solves the problem! If you feel like you are getting angry and might lose control, try the following:

- Take a deep breath and count to 10.
- Place your baby in a safe place, leave the room, and let your baby cry alone.
- Call someone close to you for emotional support.
- Call your pediatrician. There may be a medical reason why your baby is crying.

Be patient. Colicky and fussy babies eventually grow out of their crying phase. Keeping your baby safe is the most important thing you can do. Even if you feel frustrated, stay in control and never shake your baby.

The information contained in this publication should not be used as a substitute for the medical care and advice of your pediatrician. There may be variations in treatment that your pediatrician may recommend based on individual facts and circumstances.

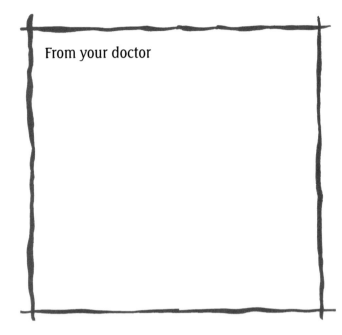

From your doctor

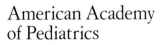

American Academy of Pediatrics

DEDICATED TO THE HEALTH OF ALL CHILDREN™

TThe American Academy of Pediatrics is an organization of 60,000 primary care pediatricians, pediatric medical subspecialists, and pediatric surgical specialists dedicated to the health, safety, and well-being of infants, children, adolescents, and young adults.

American Academy of Pediatrics
Web site — www.aap.org

Copyright © 2003
American Academy of Pediatrics

SIDS: Important Information for Parents

Sudden infant death syndrome (SIDS) is the sudden, unexplained death of a baby younger than 1 year. To lower the risk of SIDS, all healthy infants should sleep on their backs—at nap time and at night. Here's how you can lower your baby's risk.

The safest position to sleep

- Place your baby on his back to sleep; it's the safest position.
- Babies who sleep on their stomachs are at a higher risk for SIDS.
- Side sleeping is not as safe as back sleeping and is not advised.

The safest place to sleep

- Place your baby in a safety-approved crib with a firm mattress and a fitted sheet.
- Never put your baby to sleep on a chair, sofa, water bed, cushion, or sheepskin.
- The safest place for your baby to sleep is in the room where you sleep, but not in your bed.
- Place your baby's crib or bassinet near your bed (within an arm's reach) to make breastfeeding easier and help you watch over your baby.
- If bumper pads are used, they should be thin, firm, well secured, and not "pillow-like."
- Blankets, if used, should be tucked in around the crib mattress. They should not reach any higher than your baby's chest. Try using sleep sacks or sleep clothing instead of a blanket to avoid the risk of overheating.
- Keep pillows, quilts, comforters, sheepskins, and stuffed toys out of your baby's crib. They can cover your infant's face—even if she is lying on her back.

Other ways to reduce the risk

- Do not let your baby get too warm during sleep. Use light sleep clothing. Keep the room at a temperature that feels comfortable for an adult.
- Do not smoke during pregnancy. Also, do not allow smoking around your baby. Infants have a higher risk of SIDS if they are exposed to secondhand smoke. One of the most important things parents and caregivers who smoke can do for their own health and the health of their children is to stop smoking.
- Pacifiers may help reduce the risk of SIDS. However, if your baby doesn't want it or if it falls out of his mouth, don't force it. If you are breastfeeding, wait until your baby is 1 month old before using a pacifier.

- Avoid products that claim to prevent SIDS. Most have not been tested for safety. None have been shown to reduce the risk of SIDS.
- Home monitors should also be avoided. While they can be helpful for babies with breathing or heart problems, they have not been found to reduce the risk of SIDS.
- Give your baby plenty of "tummy time" when he is awake. This will help strengthen neck muscles and avoid flat spots on his head.
- Share this information with anyone who cares for your baby, including babysitters, grandparents, and other caregivers.

These recommendations are for healthy infants. A very small number of infants with certain medical conditions may need to be placed to sleep on their stomachs. Your pediatrician can advise you if a position other than the back is needed.

The information contained in this publication should not be used as a substitute for the medical care and advice of your pediatrician. There may be variations in treatment that your pediatrician may recommend based on individual facts and circumstances.

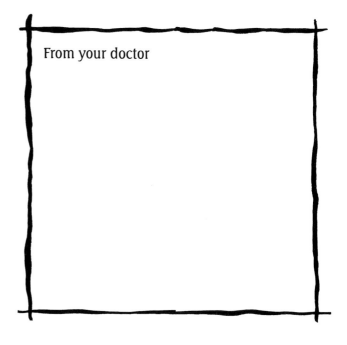

From your doctor

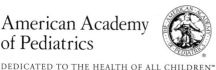

American Academy of Pediatrics

DEDICATED TO THE HEALTH OF ALL CHILDREN™

The American Academy of Pediatrics is an organization of 60,000 primary care pediatricians, pediatric medical subspecialists, and pediatric surgical specialists dedicated to the health, safety, and well-being of infants, children, adolescents, and young adults.

American Academy of Pediatrics
Web site—www.aap.org

Copyright © 2006
American Academy of Pediatrics, Updated 11/05

Fun in the Sun: Keep Your Baby Safe

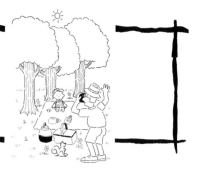

Warm, sunny days are wonderful. The sun feels good on your skin. But what feels good can be very bad for you, your family, and especially your baby. Before you take your baby to the park, beach, or even out into the backyard, please read this. It will help you learn how to protect your entire family and develop safe sun habits that can last a lifetime.

Skin cancer and the sun

The sun provides energy to all living things on earth. But it can also harm us. Its ultraviolet (UV) rays can cause sunburn and skin cancer.

The sun is the main cause of skin cancer, the most common form of cancer in the United States. There will be a million new cases of skin cancer this year. Skin cancer can and does occur in children and young adults, but most of the people who get skin cancer are older. Older people get skin cancer because they have already received too much of the sun's damaging rays. Your skin remembers each sunburn and each suntan year after year.

All skin cancers are harmful and some, especially malignant melanoma, can be deadly if left untreated. Malignant melanoma is the second most common form of cancer in women 25 to 34 years of age. Sun exposure in early childhood and adolescence contributes to skin cancer.

The sun and your baby's skin

Your baby's skin is very delicate and it's up to you to protect it. Sunburns hurt. Sunburns can also cause dehydration and fever. Too many sunburns and too much sun exposure over the years can cause not only skin cancer, but also wrinkles and cataracts of the eye.

Most of our sun exposure—between 60% and 80%—happens before we turn 18 years of age. That's because children spend more time outdoors than most adults, especially in the summer.

The dangers of sunburns

Research has shown that two or more blistering sunburns as a child or teen increase the risk of developing skin cancer later in life. It is very important, therefore, to protect babies and children from sunburn.

- A baby's sensitive skin is thinner than adult skin and a baby will sunburn more easily than an adult. Even babies with naturally darker skin need protection.
- It's up to you to protect your baby. A baby can't tell you when he is too hot or beginning to sunburn. Your baby can't move out of the sun and into the shade without your help.

Protecting your baby

Follow these simple rules to protect your baby from sunburns now and from skin cancer later in life:

- Babies under 6 months of age should be kept out of direct sunlight. Move your baby to the shade or under a tree, umbrella, or the stroller canopy.
- Dress your baby in clothing that covers the body, such as comfortable lightweight long pants, long-sleeved shirts, and hats with brims that shade the face and cover the ears.
- Select clothes made of tightly woven fabrics. Clothes that have a tighter weave—the way a fabric is constructed—generally protect better than clothes with a broader weave. If you're not sure about how tight a fabric's weave is, hold the clothing up to a lamp or window and see how much light shines through. The less light, the better. Clothing made of cotton is both cool and protective.
- When using a cap with a bill, make sure the bill is facing forward to shield the baby's face. Child-sized sunglasses with UV protection are also a good idea for protecting your child's eyes.

Remember...

- The sun's rays are the strongest between 10:00 am and 4:00 pm. Try to keep your baby out of the sun during these hours.
- The sun's damaging UV rays can bounce back from sand, snow, or concrete; so be particularly careful in these areas.
- Most of the sun's rays can come through the clouds on an overcast day; so use sun protection *even on cloudy days.*

Sunscreen for your baby

Choose a sunscreen made for children. For babies *under* 6 months of age, sunscreen may be used on small areas of the body such as the face and the backs of the hands if adequate clothing and shade are not available. For babies over 6 months of age, test the sunscreen on your baby's back for a reaction before applying it all over. Apply carefully around the eyes, avoiding the eyelids. If your baby rubs sunscreen into her eyes, wipe the eyes and hands clean with a damp cloth. If the sunscreen irritates her eyes, try a different brand or try a sunscreen stick or sunblock with titanium dioxide or zinc oxide. If a rash develops, talk to your pediatrician.

When choosing a sunscreen, look for the words "broad-spectrum" on the label—it means that the sunscreen will screen out both ultraviolet B (UVB) and ultraviolet A (UVA) rays. A sunscreen with a sun protection factor (SPF) of 15 should be adequate in most cases.

Use enough sunscreen and rub it in well, making sure to cover all exposed areas, especially your baby's face, nose, ears, feet, and hands and even the backs of the knees. Put it on 30 minutes before going outdoors. The sunscreen needs time to work on the skin. Reapply the sunscreen frequently, especially if your baby is playing in the water. Zinc oxide, a very effective sunblock, can be used as extra protection on the nose, cheeks, tops of the ears, and the shoulders.

Remember...

- Sunscreens should be used for sun protection and not as a reason to stay in the sun longer.

Sunburn can be dangerous

If your baby gets a sunburn and is under 1 year of age, contact your pediatrician at once—a severe sunburn is an emergency. For babies over the age of 1 year, tell your pediatrician if there is blistering, pain, or fever.

Remember...

- Avoid sunburns—they can be very dangerous to a baby.
- If your baby gets a sunburn, give juice or water to your baby to replace lost fluids.
- Cool water soaks may help your baby's skin feel better.
- *Do not use* any medicated lotions on your baby's skin unless your pediatrician recommends it.
- Keep your baby completely out of the sun until the sunburn is totally healed.

Set a good example

Make sun protection a regular family event. Your baby needs you for protection from the sun and from sunburns. Since babies learn by imitation, you can be the best teacher by practicing sun protection yourself. Teach all members of your family how to protect their skin.

Sun myths

Myth: A suntan is good for your baby.
Fact: A tan is a sign of skin damage.

Myth: Babies can't get sunburned on a cloudy day.
Fact: Most of the sun's rays can come through clouds and cause sunburns.

Myth: Baby oil is good sun lotion.
Fact: Baby oil causes the skin to burn faster and offers no protection at all.

Myth: Your baby needs the vitamins that the sun provides.
Fact: A proper well-balanced diet and minimum sunlight will give your baby all the necessary vitamins.

The information contained in this publication should not be used as a substitute for the medical care and advice of your pediatrician. There may be variations in treatment that your pediatrician may recommend based on individual facts and circumstances.

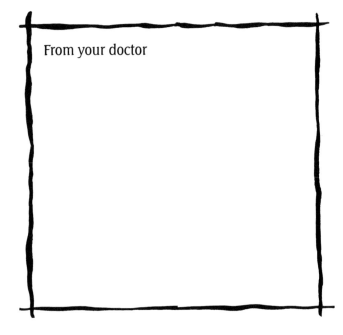

From your doctor

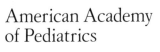

American Academy
of Pediatrics

DEDICATED TO THE HEALTH OF ALL CHILDREN™

The American Academy of Pediatrics is an organization of 60,000 primary care pediatricians, pediatric medical subspecialists, and pediatric surgical specialists dedicated to the health, safety, and well-being of infants, children, adolescents, and young adults.

American Academy of Pediatrics
Web site — www.aap.org

Copyright © 1995
American Academy of Pediatrics, Updated 1/00

Thumbs, Fingers, and Pacifiers

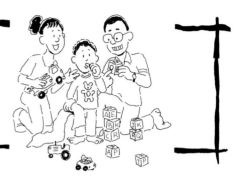

Does your baby suck his thumb or use a pacifier? Don't worry, these habits are very common and have a soothing and calming effect. The need to suck is present in all infants. Some infants suck their thumbs even before they are born, and some will do it right after being born. This brochure has been developed by the American Academy of Pediatrics to inform parents about thumb and finger sucking, and the use of pacifiers. The information in this brochure is based on the Academy's parenting manual, *Caring for Your Baby and Young Child: Birth to Age 5.*

Thumb and finger sucking

Thumb and finger sucking is normal for young children. Most children suck their thumbs or fingers at some time in their early life. Many thumb or finger suckers stop by age 6 or 7 months. The only time it might cause you concern is if it goes on beyond 6 to 8 years of age or affects the shape of your child's mouth or teeth. If you see changes in the roof of your child's mouth (palate) or in the way the teeth are lining up, talk to your pediatrician or pediatric dentist.

Children who suck their thumbs past 6 to 8 years often get teased by friends, brothers, sisters, and relatives. Sometimes these comments are enough to get the child to stop. If not, talk to your pediatrician about other ways to help your child stop.

Pacifiers

Many parents have strong feelings about pacifiers. Some oppose their use because of the way they look. Some resent the idea of "pacifying" a baby with an object. Others believe that using a pacifier can harm a baby. This is not true. Pacifiers do not cause any medical or psychological problems. If your baby wants to suck beyond what nursing or bottle-feeding provides, a pacifier will satisfy that need.

A pacifier should not be used to replace or delay meals. Offer a pacifier only after or between feedings, when you are sure your baby is not hungry. If your child is hungry, and you offer a pacifier as a substitute, he may become so upset that it interferes with feeding. It may be tempting to offer your child the pacifier when it is easy for you. However, it is best to let your child decide whether and when to use it.

Some babies use a pacifier to fall asleep. The trouble is, they often wake up when it falls out of their mouths. Once your baby is older and has the skill to find and replace it, there is no problem. Until then, your child may cry for you to find the pacifier. **Do not attempt to solve this problem by tying a pacifier to your child's crib, or around your child's neck or hand. This is very dangerous and could cause serious injury or even death.** Babies who suck their fingers or hands have a real advantage here, because their hands are always readily available.

Shopping for a pacifier

When buying a pacifier, keep the following points in mind:
- Look for a one-piece model that has a soft nipple (some models can break into two pieces).
- The shield should be at least 1½ inches across, so a baby cannot put the entire pacifier into her mouth. Also, the shield should be made of firm plastic with air holes.
- Make sure the pacifier is dishwasher-safe. Follow the instructions on the pacifier and either boil it or run it through the dishwasher before your baby uses it. Clean it this way frequently until your baby is 6 months old so that your child is not exposed to germs. After that, your baby is less likely to get an infection in that way, so you can just wash it with soap and rinse it in clear water.
- Pacifiers come in two sizes, one for the first 6 months and another for children after that age. For your baby's comfort, make sure the pacifier is the right size.
- You will also find a variety of nipple shapes, from squarish "orthodontic" versions to the standard bottle type. Try different shapes until you find the one your baby prefers.
- Buy some extras. Pacifiers have a way of getting lost or falling on the floor or street when you need them most.
- *Never* tie a pacifier around your baby's neck or hand, or to your child's crib. The danger of serious injury or even death is too great.
- Do not use the nipple from a baby bottle as a pacifier. If the baby sucks hard, the nipple may pop out of the ring and choke her.
- Pacifiers fall apart over time. Inspect them every once in a while to see whether the rubber has changed color or torn. If so, replace them.

How to help your child stop

As children grow and develop, their need to suck usually goes away, most often by the time they are 6 to 8 years old. Also, with increases in peer pressure, children are more able to control their behavior.

As a first step in dealing with your child's sucking habits, ignore them! Most often, they will disappear with time. Harsh words, teasing, or punishment may upset your child, and the habit will get worse. Punishment is not an effective way to get rid of habits.

Older children (more than 3 years of age) may use sucking to relieve boredom. Try getting your child's attention with an activity that she finds fun. Rewarding good behavior is the best way to produce a change. Praise and reward your child when she does not suck her thumb or use the pacifier. Star charts, daily rewards, and gentle reminders, especially during the daytime hours, are also very helpful.

If these measures do not work and your child wants to stop, your pediatrician might recommend trying a reminder such as covering the thumb with a plastic strip or "thumb guard" (an adjustable plastic cap that is taped to the thumb).

Your child should be directly involved with the treatment chosen. Before using these methods, be sure to explain them to your child. If they make your child afraid or tense, stop them at once. If your child's teeth are affected by the behavior and you have tried all the methods described above, talk to a pediatric dentist. Some dentists will install a device in the mouth that prevents the fingers or thumb from putting pressure on the palate or teeth. In fact, this device usually makes it so unpleasant to place the thumb or finger into the mouth that your child removes his thumb or finger.

Severe emotional upsets or stress-related problems might cause your child to suck his thumb or use a pacifier for a long time. It is also possible that your child may be one of the very few who cannot seem to stop. However, most children stop daytime sucking habits before they get very far in school. This is because of peer pressure. These same children might still use sucking as a way of going to sleep or calming themselves when they are upset. This is usually done in private and causes no harm either emotionally or physically. Putting too much pressure on your child to stop this type of behavior may cause more harm than good. Even these children eventually stop the habit on their own.

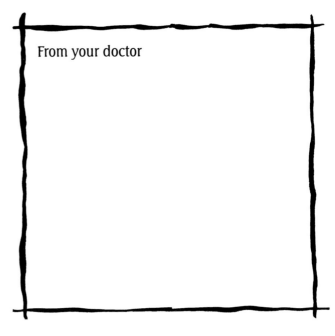

From your doctor

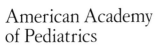

American Academy of Pediatrics

DEDICATED TO THE HEALTH OF ALL CHILDREN™

The American Academy of Pediatrics is an organization of 60,000 primary care pediatricians, pediatric medical subspecialists, and pediatric surgical specialists dedicated to the health, safety, and well-being of infants, children, adolescents, and young adults.

American Academy of Pediatrics
Web site—www.aap.org

Copyright © 1997
American Academy of Pediatrics

Toilet Training

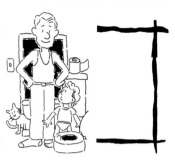

Bowel and bladder control is a necessary social skill. Teaching your child to use the toilet takes time, understanding, and patience. The important thing to remember is that you cannot rush your child into using the toilet. The American Academy of Pediatrics has developed this brochure to help you guide your child through this important stage of social development.

When is a child ready for toilet training?

There is no set age at which toilet training should begin. The right time depends on your child's physical and psychological development. Children younger than 12 months have no control over bladder or bowel movements and little control for 6 months or so after that. Between 18 and 24 months, children often start to show signs of being ready, but some children may not be ready until 30 months or older.

Your child must also be emotionally ready. He needs to be willing, not fighting you or showing signs of fear. If your child resists strongly, it is best to wait for a while.

It is best to be relaxed about toilet training and avoid becoming upset. Remember that no one can control when and where a child urinates or has a bowel movement except the child. Try to avoid a power struggle. Children at the toilet-training age are becoming aware of their individuality. They look for ways to test their limits. Some children may do this by holding back bowel movements.

Look for any of the following signs that your child is ready:

- Your child stays dry at least 2 hours at a time during the day or is dry after naps.
- Bowel movements become regular and predictable.
- Facial expressions, posture, or words reveal that your child is about to urinate or have a bowel movement.
- Your child can follow simple instructions.
- Your child can walk to and from the bathroom and help undress.
- Your child seems uncomfortable with soiled diapers and wants to be changed.
- Your child asks to use the toilet or potty chair.
- Your child asks to wear grown-up underwear.

How to teach your child to use the toilet

Decide what words to use

You should decide carefully what words you use to describe body parts, urine, and bowel movements. Remember that friends, neighbors, teachers, and other caregivers also will hear these words. It is best to use proper terms that will not offend, confuse, or embarrass your child or others.

Avoid using words like "dirty," "naughty," or "stinky" to describe waste products. These negative terms can make your child feel ashamed

Stress in the home may make learning this important new skill more difficult. Sometimes it is a good idea to delay toilet training in the following situations:

- Your family has just moved or will move in the near future.
- You are expecting a baby or you have recently had a new baby.
- There is a major illness, a recent death, or some other family crisis.

However, if your child is learning how to use the toilet without problems, there is no need to stop because of these situations.

and self-conscious. Treat bowel movements and urination in a simple, matter-of-fact manner.

Your child may be curious and try to play with the feces. You can prevent this without making her feel upset by simply saying, "This is not something to be played with."

Pick a potty chair

Once your child is ready, you should choose a potty chair. A potty chair is easier for a small child to use, because there is no problem getting on to it and a child's feet can reach the floor.

Children are often interested in their family's bathroom activities. It is sometimes helpful to let children watch parents when they go to the bathroom. Seeing grown-ups use the toilet makes children want to do the same. If possible, mothers should show the correct skills to their daughters, and fathers to their sons. Children can also learn these skills from older brothers and sisters, friends, and relatives.

Help your child recognize signs of needing to use the potty

Encourage your child to tell you when he is about to urinate or have a bowel movement. Your child will often tell you about a wet diaper or a bowel movement *after* the fact. This is a sign that your child is beginning to recognize these bodily functions. Praise your child for telling you, and suggest that "next time" he let you know in advance.

Before having a bowel movement, your child may grunt or make other straining noises, squat, or stop playing for a moment. When pushing, his face may turn red. Explain to your child that these signs mean that a bowel movement is about to come.

It often takes longer for a child to recognize the need to urinate than the need to move bowels. Some children do not gain complete bladder control for many months after they have learned to control bowel movements. Some children achieve bladder control first. It is better for boys to learn to urinate sitting down first, and then change to standing up after they use the potty for stools. Remember that all children are different!

Make trips to the potty routine

When your child seems to need to urinate or have a bowel movement, go to the potty. Keep your child seated on the potty for only a few minutes at a time. Explain what you want to happen. Be cheerful and casual. If she protests strongly, do not insist. Such resistance may mean that it is not the right time to start training.

It may be helpful to make trips to the potty a regular part of your child's daily routine, such as first thing in the morning when your child wakes up, after meals, or before naps. Remember that you cannot control when your child urinates or has a bowel movement.

Success at toilet training depends on teaching at a pace that suits your child. You must support your child's efforts. Do not try to force quick results. Encourage your child with lots of hugs and praise when success occurs. When a mistake happens, treat it lightly and try not to get upset. Punishment and scolding will often make children feel bad and may make toilet training take longer.

Teach your child proper hygiene habits. Show your child how to wipe carefully. (Girls should wipe thoroughly from front to back to prevent bringing germs from the rectum to the vagina or bladder.) Make sure both boys and girls learn to wash their hands well after urinating or a bowel movement.

Some children believe that their wastes are part of their bodies; seeing their stools flushed away may be frightening and hard for them to understand. Some also fear they will be sucked into the toilet if it is flushed while they are sitting on it. Parents should explain the purpose of body wastes. To give your child a feeling of control, let her flush pieces of toilet paper. This will lessen the fear of the sound of rushing water and the sight of things disappearing.

Encourage the use of training pants

Once your child has repeated successes, encourage the use of training pants. This moment will be special. Your child will feel proud of this sign of trust and growing up. However, be prepared for "accidents." It may take weeks, even months, before toilet training is completed. Continue to have your child sit on the potty at specified times during the day. If your child uses the potty successfully, it is an opportunity for praise. If not, it is still good practice.

In the beginning, many children will have a bowel movement or will urinate right after being taken off the toilet. It may take time for your child to learn how to relax the muscles that control the bowel and bladder. If these "accidents" happen a lot, it may mean your child is not really ready for training.

Sometimes your child will ask for a diaper when a bowel movement is expected and stand in a special place to defecate. Instead of considering this a failure, praise your child for recognizing the bowel signals. Suggest that he have the bowel movement in the bathroom while wearing a diaper. Encourage improvements and work toward sitting on the potty without the diaper. If this behavior continues for more than a few weeks, consult your pediatrician. It may represent a power struggle or fear.

Stooling patterns vary. Some children move their bowels 2 or 3 times a day. Others may go 2 or 3 days between movements. Soft, comfortable stools brought about by a well-balanced diet make training easier for both child and parent. Trying too hard to toilet train your child before he is ready can result in long-term problems with bowel movements.

Talk with your pediatrician if there is a change in the nature of the bowel movements or if your child becomes uncomfortable. Do not use laxatives, suppositories, or enemas unless your pediatrician advises these for your child.

Most children achieve bowel control and daytime urine control by 3 to 4 years of age. Even after your child is able to stay dry during the day, it may take months or years before he achieves the same success at night. Most girls and more than 75% of boys will be able to stay dry at night after 5 years of age.

Most of the time, your child will let you know when he is ready to move from the potty chair to the "big toilet." Make sure your child is tall enough, and practice the actual steps with him. Provide a stool to brace his feet.

Your pediatrician can help

If any concerns come up before, during, or after toilet training, talk with your pediatrician. Often the problem is minor and can be resolved quickly, but sometimes physical or emotional causes will require treatment. Your pediatrician's help, advice, and encouragement can help make toilet training easier. Also, your pediatrician is trained to identify and manage problems that are more serious.

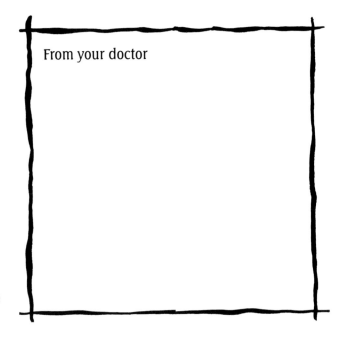

From your doctor

American Academy of Pediatrics

DEDICATED TO THE HEALTH OF ALL CHILDREN™

The American Academy of Pediatrics is an organization of 60,000 primary care pediatricians, pediatric medical subspecialists, and pediatric surgical specialists dedicated to the health, safety, and well-being of infants, children, adolescents, and young adults.

American Academy of Pediatrics
Web site—www.aap.org

Copyright © 1993
American Academy of Pediatrics, Updated 4/03

Care of the Uncircumcised Penis

One of the first decisions you will make for your new baby boy is whether or not to have him circumcised. If you have chosen not to have your son circumcised, there are some things you should be aware of and teach your son as he gets older.

What is foreskin retraction?

Sometime during the first several years of your son's life, his foreskin, which covers the head of the penis, will separate from the glans. Some foreskins separate soon after birth or even before birth, but this is rare. When it happens is different for every child. It may take a few weeks, months, or years.

After the foreskin separates from the glans, it can be pulled back away from the glans toward the abdomen. This is called *foreskin retraction.*

Most boys will be able to retract their foreskins by the time they are 5 years old, yet others will not be able to until the teenage years. As a boy becomes more aware of his body, he will most likely discover how to retract his own foreskin. But *foreskin retraction should never be forced.* Until separation occurs, do not try to pull the foreskin back — especially an infant's. Forcing the foreskin to retract before it is ready may severely harm the penis and cause pain, bleeding, and tears in the skin.

What is smegma?

When the foreskin separates from the glans, skin cells are shed. These skin cells may look like whitish lumps, resembling pearls, under the foreskin. These are called *smegma.* Smegma is normal and nothing to worry about.

Does my son's foreskin need special cleaning?

Your son's intact or uncircumcised penis requires no special care and is easy to keep clean. When your son is an infant, bathe or sponge him regularly and wash all body parts, including the genitals. Simply wash the penis with soap and warm water. Remember, do not try to forcibly retract the foreskin.

If your son's foreskin is separated and retractable before he reaches puberty, an occasional retraction with cleansing beneath will do. Once your son starts puberty, he should retract the foreskin and clean beneath it on a regular basis. It should become a part of your son's total body hygiene, just like shampooing his hair and brushing his teeth. Teach your son to clean his foreskin in the following way:

- Gently pull the foreskin back away from the glans.
- Rinse the glans and inside fold of the foreskin with soap and warm water.
- Pull the foreskin back over the head of the penis.

Is there anything else I should watch for?

While your son is still a baby, you should make sure the hole in the foreskin is large enough to allow a normal stream when he urinates. Talk to your pediatrician if any of the following occurs:

- The stream of urine is never heavier than a trickle.
- Your baby seems to have some discomfort while urinating.
- The foreskin becomes considerably red or swollen.

The information contained in this publication should not be used as a substitute for the medical care and advice of your pediatrician. There may be variations in treatment that your pediatrician may recommend based on individual facts and circumstances.

From your doctor

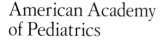
American Academy
of Pediatrics

DEDICATED TO THE HEALTH OF ALL CHILDREN™

The American Academy of Pediatrics is an organization of 60,000 primary care pediatricians, pediatric medical subspecialists, and pediatric surgical specialists dedicated to the health, safety, and well-being of infants, children, adolescents, and young adults.

American Academy of Pediatrics
Web site—www.aap.org

Copyright © 2000
American Academy of Pediatrics

Developmental Issues

Understanding Autism Spectrum Disorders (ASDs):
An introduction

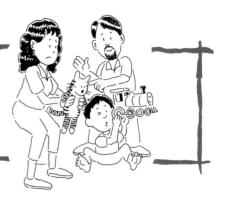

Autism spectrum disorders (ASDs) are a group of related brain-based disorders that affect a child's behavior, social, and communication skills. They include 3 of 5 disorders known as pervasive developmental disorders (PDDs). These are autistic disorder, Asperger syndrome, and PDD-not otherwise specified (PDD-NOS).

Because most children with ASD will master the early motor skills such as sitting, crawling, and walking on time, delays in social and communication skills may not be as obvious to parents. Looking back, many parents of children with ASD can think of specific examples that suggest something was different, but nothing indicating a serious problem.

Autism spectrum disorders are lifelong conditions with no known cure. However, children with ASD can progress developmentally and learn new skills. Some children may improve so much that they no longer meet the criteria for ASD, although milder symptoms may often persist.

It is important to start an intervention program as soon as possible. The sooner autism is identified, the sooner an intervention program can start. Each child with autism has different needs. What works for one child may not work for another.

The following are excerpts from the American Academy of Pediatrics' (AAP) booklet *Understanding Autism Spectrum Disorders (ASDs)*.

How common are autism spectrum disorders?
Autism spectrum disorders affect an estimated 4 to 6 out of every 1,000 children. The reported number of children with ASD has increased since the early 1990s. The reason for the increase is unclear. It may be because of many factors, including an increased awareness of what ASDs are, more screening tools and services, and/or changes in how ASD has been defined and diagnosed. In the past, only children with the most severe autism were diagnosed (the tip of the iceberg). Now children with milder symptoms are being identified and referred to intervention and educational programs.

What are the symptoms of autism spectrum disorders?
No 2 children with ASD have the exact same symptoms, but the criteria are somewhat standardized. The number of symptoms and how severe they are can vary greatly. The following are examples of how a child with ASD may act:

Social differences
- Doesn't snuggle when picked up, but arches back instead
- Doesn't keep eye contact or makes very little eye contact
- Doesn't respond to parent's smile or other facial expressions
- Doesn't look at objects or events parents are looking at or pointing to
- Doesn't point to objects or events to get parents to look at them
- Doesn't bring objects to show to parents just to share his interest
- Doesn't often have appropriate facial expressions

- Unable to perceive what others might be thinking or feeling by looking at their facial expressions
- Doesn't show concern (empathy) for others
- Unable to make friends

Communication differences
- Doesn't say single words by 15 months or 2-word phrases by 24 months
- Repeats exactly what others say without understanding its meaning (parroting or echolalia)
- Doesn't respond to name being called, but does respond to other sounds (like a car horn or a cat's meow)
- Refers to self as "you" and others as "I" (pronominal reversal)
- Often doesn't seem to want to communicate
- Doesn't start or can't continue a conversation
- Doesn't use toys or other objects to represent people or real life in pretend play
- May have a good rote memory, especially for numbers, songs, TV jingles, or a specific topic
- Loses language milestones, usually between the ages of 15 to 24 months in a few children (regression)

Behavioral differences (stereotypic, repetitive, and restrictive patterns)
- Rocks, spins, sways, twirls fingers, or flaps hands (stereotypic behavior)
- Likes routines, order, and rituals
- Obsessed with a few activities, doing them repeatedly during the day
- Plays with parts of toys instead of the whole toy (for example, spinning the wheels of a toy truck)
- May have splinter skills, such as the ability to read at an early age, but often without understanding what it means
- Doesn't cry if in pain or seem to have any fear
- May be very sensitive or not sensitive at all to smells, sounds, lights, textures, and touch
- Unusual use of vision or gaze—looks at objects from unusual angles
- May have unusual or intense but narrow interests

What are the different types of autism spectrum disorders?
As mentioned earlier, ASD includes 3 of 5 disorders known as PDDs. Pervasive developmental disorders are defined in the fourth edition of the *Diagnostic and Statistical Manual of Mental Disorders (DSM-IV)* and the revised *Diagnostic and Statistical Manual of Mental Disorders, Fourth Edition, Text Revision (DSM-IV-TR)*. These manuals are published by the American Psychiatric Association and describe behavioral and mental health conditions. Pediatricians may use the *Diagnostic and Statistical Manual of Mental*

Disorders, Primary Care (DSM-PC) version published by the AAP. Although many doctors use the term PDD as published in the *DSM,* most experts in the field now use the term ASD.

The following are descriptions of autistic disorder, Asperger syndrome, and PDD-NOS:

Autistic disorder

Autistic disorder is the term used when a child meets all the necessary criteria listed in the *DSM-IV.* Children with autistic disorder have problems with language skills that are absent, delayed, or abnormal; problems relating to others socially; and unusual or repetitive behaviors. While social symptoms are usually present in the first year of life, language problems show up in the second year and stereotypic behaviors show up later. Many of these children will have intellectual deficits; others might *appear* to have deficits when, in fact, scores on intelligence tests are low because of lack of cooperation. Others may have normal scores on intelligence tests, yet they may have trouble with abstract and real-life reasoning. Children with autism are often labeled as *high functioning* when intelligence is in the normal range.

Asperger syndrome

Asperger syndrome is usually not diagnosed until preschool age or later. This is because early speech development, especially language and sentence structure, is relatively normal. Sometimes children with Asperger syndrome speak in an odd way. Some children may speak in the same tone of voice without raising or decreasing the pitch of their voice. Other children may speak in language above what you would expect for their age like "little professors." They may make little eye contact while talking and may have trouble maintaining a back-and-forth conversation. They usually obsess over 1 or 2 topics and will talk about these topics whether the listener is interested. Children with Asperger syndrome often interpret language literally and may have particular trouble with humor, teasing, and figures of speech. Many may also have problems with motor coordination. Intelligence is normal. Some experts do not consider this a separate disorder from high-functioning autism.

Pervasive developmental disorder-not otherwise specified

Children with PDD-NOS or atypical autism show some signs of autism or other PDD, but don't meet the criteria to be diagnosed with one specific disorder.

What causes autism spectrum disorders?

No one knows exactly what causes ASD. Years ago "poor, non-nurturing" parenting was thought to be a possible cause of ASD, but this is not the case. Today scientists know from twin and other family studies that genetics play a major role. Although many chromosomal and gene abnormalities have been identified, none of these are present in all children with ASD. If a family already has a child diagnosed with ASD, the chances that siblings might also have some form of ASD are 10 times higher than in the general population. Environmental factors may also play a secondary role, but this has not been proven yet.

Studies have shown that in families with autism, there are often other developmental problems. These problems may include language delays, learning disabilities, anxiety, or mood disorders among family members.

Autism spectrum disorders, particularly autistic disorder, also tend to occur more often in people with certain medical conditions, such as fragile X syndrome, tuberous sclerosis, congenital rubella syndrome, and untreated phenylketonuria (PKU).

Two prescription medicines that have potentially been linked to ASD are thalidomide and valproate.

Current scientific proof does not support a link between the measles-mumps-rubella (MMR) vaccine or any combination of vaccines and ASD. There also is no scientific proof to support a link between thimerosal (a mercury-containing preservative) and ASD. In any event, vaccines no longer contain mercury.

What are the early signs of autism spectrum disorders?

Many children with ASD may show developmental differences throughout their infancy, especially in social and language skills. Because they usually sit, crawl, and walk on time, these more subtle differences often go unnoticed.

Social skills

In looking back on their child's development, parents will often say that something seemed different from the beginning. For example, a child with ASD may have

- Not smiled back to you or smiled less often or less enthusiastically than you expected.
- Not cuddled like other children.
- Not made as much eye contact with others.
- Not responded to her name being called.
- Seemed to tune others out. At other times, she may have seemed to hear environmental sounds, even very faint ones, perfectly well. This was probably confusing and may have caused you to worry about a hearing problem.

One of the most important developmental differences between children with ASD and other children is a delay or lack of *joint attention.* Looking back and forth between the same object or event and another person and connecting with that person is called joint attention. It is a building block for later social and communication skills. Engaging in many back-and-forth social interactions, such as exchanging lots of emotional expressions, sounds, and other gestures, is called *reciprocal social interaction.* Delays in joint attention skills are found in most children with ASD and rarely seen in children with other types of developmental problems. Thus, joint attention deficits are thought to be among the most characteristic deficits of ASD. There are several stages of joint attention. Children with ASD usually show delays or absent skills at every stage.

Other differences in children with autism spectrum disorders

- **May use fewer gestures or none at all.** For example, they may not wave goodbye, reach up to parents to be held, or play patty-cake.
- **May be attached to hard objects.** Many typically developing children become attached to a comfort item that helps to soothe and console them in times of stress. Usually this is a soft object such as a favorite blanket, stuffed animal, or pillow. However, children with ASD often insist on carrying a hard object with them at all times. The object could be a pen, a piece of string, an action figure from a favorite TV show or video, or sometimes an unusual object like a toilet plunger or soft soap dispenser. The children may have severe temper tantrums if the object is taken away. These unusual attachments often change from one object to another over time.
- **May demonstrate repetitive actions** such as hand flapping, rocking, head banging, twirling, or pacing back and forth across the room.

- **May not engage in pretend or make-believe play** with dolls or stuffed animals as if they were having a tea or birthday party.

  On the other hand, some children with ASD may be especially talented in putting complex puzzles together or playing computer games.

Language delays

All children with autism show significant language delays. Those children later diagnosed with Asperger syndrome will seem to have met language milestones during the toddler years, but use of language may be abnormal.

Regression in developmental milestones

About 25% of children will seem to have normal development until about 18 months, after which they will gradually or suddenly

- Stop talking (if they had begun to say a few words).
- Stop waving goodbye.
- Stop turning their heads when their names are called.
- Withdraw into a shell and seem more distant and less interested in their surroundings.

  However, a careful review of home videos of these children taken at their 1-year-old birthday parties (*before* they actually regress) often shows subtle signs of ASD that were missed at the time. One of the most common signs in these videos is children not consistently turning their heads when their names were called.

How is the diagnosis made?

Diagnosis of ASD involves many factors. There are no specific lab tests for ASD, so pediatricians must rely on information from parents and what can be observed during well-child checkups. The condition is complex and symptoms are different for each child.

When an ASD is suspected as a cause of language and social delays, a full evaluation should follow. This may be done by a doctor or psychologist who has expertise in the diagnosis of ASD or, preferably, by a team of specialists that may include developmental pediatricians, child neurologists, child psychiatrists, psychologists, speech or language pathologists, occupational or physical therapists, educators, and social workers. Typically, an evaluation will include the following:

- **Careful observation of play and child-caregiver interactions.**
- **Detailed history and physical exam.**
- **Developmental assessment of all skills** (motor, language, social, self-help, cognitive). Autism spectrum disorders are suspected when the child's social and language functioning is significantly more impaired than the overall level of motor, adaptive, and cognitive skills.
- **Standardized autism-specific tool.** Special training is usually needed to administer a standardized behavioral or developmental tool that has been specifically developed to help diagnose ASD. There may be few clinicians in a given community with these qualifications. However, every school district should have at least one professional (usually a child psychologist) that can administer an autism-specific tool. Tools may include the Childhood Autism Rating Scale, Gilliam Autism Rating Scale, Autism Diagnostic Interview-Revised, and Autism Diagnostic Observation Schedule.
- **Hearing test.** All children with any speech delays or those suspected of having ASD should have their hearing evaluated by a pediatric audiologist.
- **Language evaluation** that provides standardized scores of expressive language (including speech) and receptive language, as well as an evaluation of pragmatic language (social use of language) and articulation (pronunciation).

Medical tests

In fewer than 10% of children diagnosed, ASD may be associated with a known syndrome or medical condition. Lab tests may be needed to rule out other possible medical causes with similar symptoms. Your pediatrician will recommend what's best based on your child's history and physical exam. Tests should be ordered only if the results will provide useful information. Your child may be referred to other specialists, such as a geneticist or a pediatric neurologist, to help with this search for an underlying cause.

Living with autism spectrum disorders

There are many different strategies and techniques to help children with ASD interact with others and learn new skills that will help them talk, interact, play, learn, and care for their needs. So far, no one technique has been proven significantly better than others. However, effective programs should be intense, address behavior management as well as communication and social skills development, and encourage parents to get involved. The ultimate goal of all programs should be the successful integration of the child with ASD into inclusive environments with typically developing peers as early as possible.

According to an expert panel writing for the National Academy of Sciences, effective educational programs designed for children with ASD from birth to 8 years of age should

- **Offer choices.** The program should offer a variety of behavioral, language, social, play, and cognitive strategies that are individualized to the child. If possible, the child should also receive direct speech, occupational, and physical therapies.
- **Have clear goals.** An individualized plan should include specific, observable, and measurable goals and objectives in each developmental and behavioral area of intervention.
- **Be intense.** The program should be intense, with 20 to 25 hours of planned intervention or instruction per week. It should be given year-round. The majority of children benefit from a staffing ratio of 1:1 or 1:2 with an adult. For each child there should be 1 teacher, and there should be no more than 2 children per teacher.
- **Encourage parents to be fully involved.** Siblings and peers should also be part of the program. Children often learn best by modeling typically developing children in inclusive settings.
- **Take place in everyday settings.** To promote generalization of newly acquired skills, interventions should take place in everyday settings. Natural reinforcers should also be used.
- **Address behavior problems.** A functional analysis of behavior should be done when there are behavior problems. Information gained should be used to design a behavior management plan.
- **Monitor progress often.** If goals and objectives are not being met in a reasonable amount of time, the program should be evaluated and revised as needed.

The types and quality of services may vary depending on where you live. Unfortunately, few communities have programs with all, or even most, of these recommendations. Usually this is because there isn't enough public funding and/or experienced staff. Efforts are being made nationally to increase funding and training, but such changes will take time. However, many children will still benefit from a limited program versus no program at all. Often this is possible because of a team effort from staff and parents.

In general, whichever techniques are used, the more and sooner, the better. Children should be referred to an appropriate program as soon as a delay is suspected. Parents should not wait for a definitive diagnosis of autism because this may take quite some time. When ASD or another developmental disability is diagnosed, the program can be changed to best meet the needs of the child and family. Keep in mind that this can be an ongoing process as additional signs and symptoms become noticeable or others improve.

Although *all* children with ASD will need developmental and educational services and most will need therapy and behavioral interventions, only certain children may need medicine. Medicine may be needed to control behaviors that could interfere with ASD interventions. Aggressive or disruptive behaviors can become a problem when they cause physical harm to others (or to the child himself) or when they prevent him from cooperating with therapists or teachers.

Parents are encouraged to learn as much as they can about all the different treatments available. Treatment should focus on supporting the child to succeed in the real world.

The future

Children with ASD are affected by many factors that will shape their future. Overall, the long-term outcomes of children with ASD have been improving. In general, the sooner ASD is identified, the sooner appropriate intervention programs can begin and the better the outcomes. However, children may be limited in what they can do depending on their intelligence, the severity of autistic symptoms, and whether they have associated medical problems such as seizures.

Children with intelligence in the normal range and milder autistic symptoms generally have better outcomes. Those with Asperger syndrome are thought to have somewhat better outcomes than children with other types of ASD if they don't have additional medical or emotional problems.

The goal of all parents, whether their child has a disability, is to try their very best to help their child reach his full potential with the help of all available resources.

Resources

Books

Gabriels RL, Hill DE. *Autism: From Research to Individualized Practice.* London, England: Jessica Kinglsey Publishers; 2002

Gray C, McAndrew S. *My Social Stories Book.* London, England: Jessica Kinglsey Publishers; 2002

Howlin P, Baron-Cohen S, Hadwin J. *Teaching Children with Autism to Mind-Read: A Practical Guide for Teachers and Parents.* Chichester, England: John Wiley and Sons; 1999

Naseef RA. *Special Children, Challenged Parents: The Struggles and Rewards of Raising a Child with a Disability.* Rev ed. Baltimore, MD: Paul H. Brookes Co; 2001

Ozonoff S, Dawson G, McPartland J. *A Parent's Guide to Asperger Syndrome and High Functioning Autism: How to Meet the Challenges and Help Your Child Thrive.* New York, NY: Guilford Press; 2002

Schopler E. *Parent Survival Manual: A Guide to Crisis Resolution in Autism and Related Developmental Disorders.* New York, NY: Plenum Press; 1995

Siegel B. *The World of the Autistic Child: Understanding and Treating Autistic Spectrum Disorders.* New York, NY: Oxford University Press; 1996

Szatmari P. *A Mind Apart: Understanding Children With Autism and Asperger Syndrome.* New York, NY: Guilford Press; 2004

Volkmar FR, Wiesner LA. *Healthcare for Children on the Autism Spectrum: A Guide to Medical, Nutritional and Behavioral Issues.* Bethesda, MD: Woodbine House; 2004

Wetherby AM, Prizant BM. *Autism Spectrum Disorders: A Transactional Developmental Perspective.* Baltimore, MD: Paul Brookes; 2000

Wheeler M. *Toilet Training for Individuals With Autism and Related Disorders: A Comprehensive Guide for Parents and Teachers.* Arlington, TX: Future Horizons; 1998

Wrobel M, Rielly P. *Taking Care of Myself: A Hygiene, Puberty and Personal Curriculum for Young People With Autism.* Arlington, TX: Future Horizons; 2003

Web sites

American Academy of Pediatrics National Center of Medical Home Initiatives for Children With Special Needs
www.medicalhomeinfo.org/health/autism.html

Autism Society of America
www.autism-society.org

Centers for Disease Control and Prevention Autism Information Center
www.cdc.gov/ncbddd/dd/ddautism.htm

Cure Autism Now
www.cureautismnow.org

National Alliance for Autism Research
www.naar.org

Please note: Listing of resources does not imply an endorsement by the American Academy of Pediatrics (AAP). The AAP is not responsible for the content of the resources mentioned in this brochure. Web site addresses are as current as possible, but may change at any time.

The information contained in this publication should not be used as a substitute for the medical care and advice of your pediatrician. There may be variations in treatment that your pediatrician may recommend based on individual facts and circumstances.

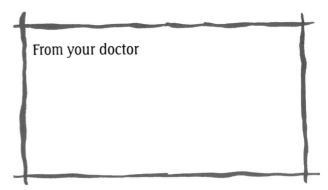

From your doctor

American Academy of Pediatrics

DEDICATED TO THE HEALTH OF ALL CHILDREN™

The American Academy of Pediatrics is an organization of 60,000 primary care pediatricians, pediatric medical subspecialists, and pediatric surgical specialists dedicated to the health, safety, and well-being of infants, children, adolescents, and young adults.

American Academy of Pediatrics
Web site—www.aap.org

Copyright © 2006
American Academy of Pediatrics

Is Your One-Year-Old Communicating With You?

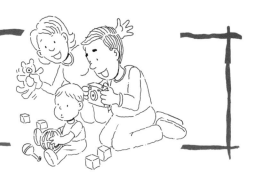

"Da-da." "Ma-ma." "Ba-ba." What will your baby's first word be?

Whatever the word is, when you hear it, it's an exciting moment in your child's language development.

However, language skills begin long before the first spoken words. Your child starts to communicate with you during the first year of life. She may respond to you and the world around her with eye gazes, smiles, gestures, or sounds. Later on, you'll notice more obvious "speech" skills or milestones.

Read more to learn about early language and social milestones and possible signs of language delay.

> If you have *any* concerns about your baby's development, share them with your pediatrician—the sooner the better.

Milestones

Remember, children develop at different rates, but they usually are able to do certain things at certain ages. The following developmental milestones are only guidelines:

By 12 months your baby should

- ☐ Look for and be able to find the source of sounds.
- ☐ Respond to his name most of the time when you call it.
- ☐ Wave goodbye.
- ☐ Look where you point when you say, "Look at the _____."
- ☐ Change from monotone babble to babble with inflection as if telling a story in a foreign language.
- ☐ Take turns "talking" with you—listens to you when you speak and then resumes babbling when you stop.
- ☐ Say "da-da" to dad and "ma-ma" to mom.
- ☐ Say at least 1 or more words.
- ☐ Point to items he wants that are out of reach or make sounds while pointing.

Between 12 and 24 months your baby should

- ☐ Follow simple commands with, and then later without, gestures.
- ☐ Get objects from another room when asked.
- ☐ Point to a few body parts when asked.
- ☐ Point to interesting objects or events to get you to look at them too.
- ☐ Bring things to you to "show you."
- ☐ Point to objects so you will name them.
- ☐ Name a few common objects and pictures when asked.
- ☐ Enjoy pretending (for example, has a tea party). She will use gestures and words with you or a favorite stuffed animal.
- ☐ Learn about 1 new word per week as she approaches her 2nd birthday.

About developmental language delay

Delays in language are the most common types of developmental delay. One in 5 children will show a developmental delay in the speech or language area. Some children will also show behavioral challenges because they are frustrated when they can't express everyday needs, desires, or interests.

Simple speech delays are sometimes temporary. They may resolve on their own or with a little extra help from family. Sometimes formal speech therapy is needed.

It's important to encourage your baby to "talk" to you with gestures and/or sounds before filling a need. In some cases, your baby will need more help from a trained professional.

Sometimes delays may be a warning sign of a more serious disorder that could include a hearing loss, global developmental delays, or autism. Delays also could be a sign of a possible learning problem you may not notice until the school years. It's important to have your child evaluated if you are concerned about your child's language development.

By 24 months your toddler should

- ☐ Point to many body parts and common objects.
- ☐ Point to some pictures in books.
- ☐ Follow 2-step commands.
- ☐ Say about 50 to 100 words.
- ☐ Say several 2-word phrases like "daddy go," "doll mine," and "all gone."
- ☐ May say a few 3-word sentences like "I want juice" or "Me go bye-bye."
- ☐ Be understood about 50% of the time.

Not typical behaviors

Sometimes language delays are associated with behaviors that may concern you, like if your baby

- ☐ Doesn't cuddle like other babies
- ☐ Doesn't return a happy smile back to you
- ☐ Doesn't seem to notice if you are in the room
- ☐ Doesn't seem to notice certain noises (for example, seems to hear a car horn or a cat's meow but not when you call his name)
- ☐ Acts as if he is in his own world
- ☐ Prefers to play alone; seems to "tune others out"
- ☐ Doesn't seem interested in or play with toys but likes to play with objects in the house
- ☐ Shows a strange attachment to hard objects (would rather carry around a flashlight or ballpoint pen than a stuffed animal or favorite blanket)
- ☐ Can say the ABCs, numbers, or words to TV jingles but can't ask for things he wants
- ☐ Doesn't seem to have any fear

☐ Doesn't seem to feel pain
☐ Laughs for no clear reason
☐ Uses words or phrases that are inappropriate for the situation

---

If your child seems delayed or shows any of the above behaviors, tell your pediatrician. Also, tell your pediatrician if your baby stops talking or doing things that he used to do.

What your pediatrician might do

After you share your concerns with your pediatrician, he or she may

- Ask you some questions, or ask you to fill out a questionnaire.
- Evaluate certain aspects of your child's development by interacting with your child in various ways.
- Order a hearing test and refer you to a speech and language therapist for testing. The therapist will evaluate your child's speech (expressive language) and ability to understand speech and gestures (receptive language).

If your pediatrician doesn't seem to be concerned and instead tries to reassure you that children develop at different rates and that your child will "catch up in time," it's OK to say you are still concerned. You might also ask your pediatrician if a referral to a developmental specialist might be appropriate.

If any of the steps above lead to the conclusion that *expressive language ONLY* is delayed, you may be given suggestions to help your child at home. Formal speech therapy may also be recommended.

If *BOTH receptive and expressive* language are delayed and the hearing test is normal, your child will need further evaluation. This will determine whether the delays are due to a true communication disorder, global developmental delays, autism, or some other developmental problem.

When autism is the reason for language delays, the child will also show some or all of the above-listed behaviors. Most likely, your child will then be referred to a specialist or a team of specialists knowledgeable about autism and its many related disorders. The specialist(s) may then recommend speech therapy but also specific interventions to improve social skills, behavior, and the "desire" to communicate.

Programs

Regardless of the cause of your child's delays, your pediatrician may refer you to a local developmental or school program that provides intervention services to children with various delays. The staff there might do an independent evaluation. You may be reassured that your child's development is, indeed, within normal limits, or the staff might feel that he would benefit from some type of intervention.

If your child is younger than 3 years, the referral may be to an *Early Intervention Program (EIP)* in your area. This is a federal- and state-funded program that helps children with delays or behavioral challenges. You may also contact the EIP directly.

If your child is eligible for services, a team of specialists will, with your input, develop an *Individualized Family Service Plan (IFSP)*. This plan becomes a guide for the services that will be provided until your child turns 3 years of age. It may include parent training and support, direct therapy, respite, and special equipment. Other services may be offered if they benefit your child and/or your family. If your child needs help after 3 years of age, the EIP staff will refer your child to the local school district.

If your child is 3 years of age or older at the time of a concern, the referral may be to your local public school. You may also contact the local public school directly. If your child is eligible, the school district staff will, with your input, develop an *Individualized Education Plan (IEP)*. This plan provides many of the same services as the EIP but the focus is different; school services are mainly for the child. The level of services also may be different. If your child continues to need special education and services, the IEP will be reviewed and revised from time to time. The EIP should be revised to meet your child's changing needs as she grows older and develops new skills.

Resources

American Academy of Pediatrics
National Center of Medical Home Initiatives
for Children with Special Needs
www.medicalhomeinfo.org

Family Voices
www.familyvoices.org

Remember

Your instincts as a parent should be followed. If you continue to have concerns about your child's development, ask for a reevaluation or referral for more formal testing.

Please note: Listing of resources does not imply an endorsement by the American Academy of Pediatrics (AAP). The AAP is not responsible for the content of the resources mentioned in this brochure. Web site addresses are as current as possible, but may change at any time.

The information contained in this publication should not be used as a substitute for the medical care and advice of your pediatrician. There may be variations in treatment that your pediatrician may recommend based on individual facts and circumstances.

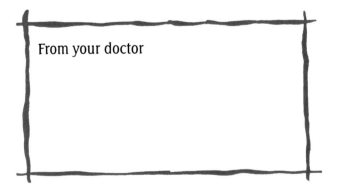

From your doctor

American Academy of Pediatrics

DEDICATED TO THE HEALTH OF ALL CHILDREN™

The American Academy of Pediatrics is an organization of 60,000 primary care pediatricians, pediatric medical subspecialists, and pediatric surgical specialists dedicated to the health, safety, and well-being of infants, children, adolescents, and young adults.
American Academy of Pediatrics
Web site—www.aap.org

Copyright © 2005
American Academy of Pediatrics

Your Child's Growth:
Developmental Milestones

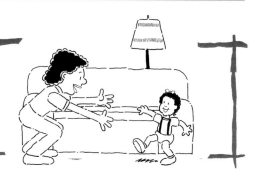

Watching a young child grow is a wonderful and unique experience for a parent. Learning to sit up, walk, and talk are some of the major developmental milestones your child will achieve.

Although no two children develop at the same rate, they should be able to do certain things at certain ages. This list of milestones by age is a good way to see how your child is doing. Keep in mind that a "No" answer to any of these questions does not mean that there is a problem. However, if you see large differences between your child and what is listed here, talk with your pediatrician.

3 Months

- When your baby is lying on his back, does he move both arms equally well? Check "No" if your baby uses only one arm all the time.
  ☐ Yes   ☐ No
- Does your baby make sounds such as gurgling, cooing, babbling, or other noises besides crying?
  ☐ Yes   ☐ No
- Does your baby respond to your voice?
  ☐ Yes   ☐ No
- Are your baby's hands frequently open?
  ☐ Yes   ☐ No
- Can your baby hold his head up for a few seconds when held upright?
  ☐ Yes   ☐ No

6 Months

- Does your baby play with her hands by touching them together?
  ☐ Yes   ☐ No
- Does your baby turn her head to sounds coming from a different room?
  ☐ Yes   ☐ No
- Can your baby roll over from stomach to back or from back to stomach?
  ☐ Yes   ☐ No
- When you hold your baby under her arms, does she seem like she's trying to stand?
  ☐ Yes   ☐ No
- When your baby is on her stomach, does she try to push up with her hands?
  ☐ Yes   ☐ No
- Does your baby see small objects, like crumbs?
  ☐ Yes   ☐ No
- Does your baby produce a string of sounds?
  ☐ Yes   ☐ No
- Does she react to the emotions of others?
  ☐ Yes   ☐ No

- Does your baby relax when you read her a story?
  ☐ Yes   ☐ No
- Does your baby like looking at herself in a mirror?
  ☐ Yes   ☐ No
- Does your baby reach for you?
  ☐ Yes   ☐ No

9 Months

- When you come up quietly behind your baby, does he sometimes turn his head as though he hears you? (Only check "Yes" if you have seen him respond to quiet sounds or whispers.)
  ☐ Yes   ☐ No
- Can your baby sit without support and without holding up his body with his hands?
  ☐ Yes   ☐ No
- Does your baby crawl or creep on his hands and knees?
  ☐ Yes   ☐ No
- Does your baby hold his bottle?
  ☐ Yes   ☐ No
- Does your baby drop or throw toys on purpose?
  ☐ Yes   ☐ No
- Does he bang and shake his toys?
  ☐ Yes   ☐ No
- When you show your baby a book, does he get excited and try to grab and taste it?
  ☐ Yes   ☐ No
- Is your baby wary of people he doesn't know?
  ☐ Yes   ☐ No
- Does your baby make sounds that use vowels and consonants?
  ☐ Yes   ☐ No

12 Months

- Does your baby like to play peekaboo?
  ☐ Yes   ☐ No
- Does your baby pull up to stand?
  ☐ Yes   ☐ No
- Does your baby walk holding on to furniture?
  ☐ Yes   ☐ No
- Does your baby say at least one word other than "ma-ma" or "da-da"?
  ☐ Yes   ☐ No

- Does your baby turn her head in the direction of where a sound is made?
  ☐ Yes ☐ No
- Does your baby copy familiar behaviors, like using a cup or telephone?
  ☐ Yes ☐ No
- Does your baby turn her books face up, but turn several pages at once?
  ☐ Yes ☐ No
- Does your baby look for and find toys?
  ☐ Yes ☐ No
- Does your baby like to explore objects and spaces?
  ☐ Yes ☐ No

18 Months

- Can your child use a cup without spilling?
  ☐ Yes ☐ No
- Can your child walk across a large room without falling or wobbling from side to side?
  ☐ Yes ☐ No
- Can your child take off his own shoes?
  ☐ Yes ☐ No
- Can your child feed himself?
  ☐ Yes ☐ No
- Does your child clearly look to you in stressful situations?
  ☐ Yes ☐ No
- Does your child have temper tantrums?
  ☐ Yes ☐ No
- Does your child say at least 4 to 10 words?
  ☐ Yes ☐ No
- Can your child point to pictures that you name in a book?
  ☐ Yes ☐ No
- Does your child pretend to talk?
  ☐ Yes ☐ No

2 Years

- Can your child say things like "all gone," "go bye-bye," or other 2-word sentences?
  ☐ Yes ☐ No
- Does your child say about 50 words?
  ☐ Yes ☐ No
- Can your child take off her own clothes? (Diapers, hats, and socks do not count.)
  ☐ Yes ☐ No
- Can your child run without falling? (Occasional falls do not count.)
  ☐ Yes ☐ No
- Does your child look at pictures in a book?
  ☐ Yes ☐ No
- Does your child pretend to read to you?
  ☐ Yes ☐ No
- Does your child tell you what she wants?
  ☐ Yes ☐ No
- Does your child repeat words others say?
  ☐ Yes ☐ No

- Can your child point to at least one named body part?
  ☐ Yes ☐ No
- Does your child like to play with or around other children?
  ☐ Yes ☐ No
- Does your child show increasing independence, wanting to do things her way?
  ☐ Yes ☐ No
- Does your child like to collect or hoard things?
  ☐ Yes ☐ No

3 Years

- Can your child name at least one picture when you look at animal books together?
  ☐ Yes ☐ No
- Does your child enjoy sitting together for at least 5 minutes for story time?
  ☐ Yes ☐ No
- Can your child answer "what" questions about the story that you have just read together?
  ☐ Yes ☐ No
- Can your child throw a ball overhand from a distance of 5 feet?
  ☐ Yes ☐ No
- Is your child easily understood by most adults?
  ☐ Yes ☐ No
- Does your child help put things away?
  ☐ Yes ☐ No
- Can your child answer the question, "Are you a boy or girl?"
  ☐ Yes ☐ No
- Can your child name at least one color?
  ☐ Yes ☐ No
- Does your child talk in 3-word sentences most of the time?
  ☐ Yes ☐ No

4 Years

- Can your child pedal a tricycle at least 10 feet forward?
  ☐ Yes ☐ No
- Does your child play hide-and-seek, cops-and-robbers, or other games where he takes turns and follows rules?
  ☐ Yes ☐ No
- Does your child turn paper pages in a book one at a time?
  ☐ Yes ☐ No
- Does your child retell stories that are familiar?
  ☐ Yes ☐ No
- Can your child tell you what action is taking place in a picture?
  ☐ Yes ☐ No
- Does your child use action words (verbs)?
  ☐ Yes ☐ No
- Does your child play pretend games, such as with toys, dolls, animals, or even an imaginary friend?
  ☐ Yes ☐ No
- Can your child copy a circle?
  ☐ Yes ☐ No

- Does your child pretend to write, making marks on a page that only he can read?
  ☐ Yes   ☐ No
- Does your child use 4- or 5-word sentences?
  ☐ Yes   ☐ No

5 Years

- Can your child button her clothing or her doll's clothes?
  ☐ Yes   ☐ No
- Does your child react well when you leave her with a friend or sitter?
  ☐ Yes   ☐ No
- Can your child name at least 3 colors?
  ☐ Yes   ☐ No
- Can your child walk down stairs alternating her feet?
  ☐ Yes   ☐ No
- Can your child jump with her feet apart?
  ☐ Yes   ☐ No
- Can your child point while counting at least 3 different objects?
  ☐ Yes   ☐ No
- Can your child name a coin correctly?
  ☐ Yes   ☐ No
- Can your child sit and listen to a 10- to 20-minute story?
  ☐ Yes   ☐ No
- Can your child copy a square?
  ☐ Yes   ☐ No
- Can your child name at least some letters of the alphabet when she sees them?
  ☐ Yes   ☐ No
- Can your child identify and print the first letter in her name?
  ☐ Yes   ☐ No
- Can your child recognize and name several single numbers?
  ☐ Yes   ☐ No
- Does your child recognize common street and store signs (eg, "Stop," "Open")?
  ☐ Yes   ☐ No

6 Years

- Can your child tie his shoes?
  ☐ Yes   ☐ No
- Can your child dress himself without help?
  ☐ Yes   ☐ No
- Can your child catch a small bouncing ball? (Large balls do not count.)
  ☐ Yes   ☐ No

- Can your child skip?
  ☐ Yes   ☐ No
- Can your child tell his age?
  ☐ Yes   ☐ No
- Can your child repeat at least 4 numbers in the proper sequence?
  ☐ Yes   ☐ No
- Can your child recognize and name at least 10 letters in the alphabet?
  ☐ Yes   ☐ No
- Does your child know the sounds of most letters of the alphabet?
  ☐ Yes   ☐ No
- Can your child recognize and read 15 or more common words?
  ☐ Yes   ☐ No
- Can your child copy a few simple words from a book?
  ☐ Yes   ☐ No

Remember, these milestones are an aid, not a test. If you have any questions or concerns about your child, talk with your pediatrician. If there is a problem, early treatment is important.

Copyrighted information used in this brochure was granted courtesy of William Frankenburg, MD, and Josiah Dodds, MD.

The information contained in this publication should not be used as a substitute for the medical care and advice of your pediatrician. There may be variations in treatment that your pediatrician may recommend based on individual facts and circumstances.

From your doctor

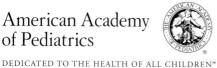

American Academy of Pediatrics

DEDICATED TO THE HEALTH OF ALL CHILDREN™

The American Academy of Pediatrics is an organization of 60,000 primary care pediatricians, pediatric medical subspecialists, and pediatric surgical specialists dedicated to the health, safety, and well-being of infants, children, adolescents, and young adults.

American Academy of Pediatrics
Web site—www.aap.org

Copyright © 2006
American Academy of Pediatrics, Updated 12/05

Learning Disabilities:
WHAT PARENTS NEED TO KNOW

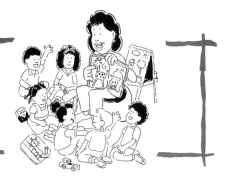

Your child will learn many things in life—how to listen, speak, read, write, and do math. Some skills may be harder to learn than others. If your child is trying his best to learn certain skills but is not able to keep up with his peers, it's important to find out why. There can be many reasons. If your child has a learning disability (LD), the sooner you know, the sooner you can get your child help. Though there's no cure, your child can learn how to succeed in school, work, and relationships.

What is an LD?

Learning disability is a term used to describe a range of learning problems. These problems have to do with the way the brain gets, uses, stores, and sends out information. Children with LD may have trouble with one or more of the following skills: reading, writing, listening, speaking, reasoning, and math. This isn't the same as learning problems that are mainly caused by visual, hearing, or motor handicaps.

What causes LD?

The causes of LD aren't always known. There could be many possible causes. Often children with LD have a parent or relative with the same or similar learning difficulties. In some cases, children with LD were born with a low birth weight or prematurely. In other cases, an injury or illness during childhood may have caused LD (for example, severe head injury, lead poisoning, or a childhood illness like meningitis).

How do I know if my child has an LD?

Learning disabilities aren't always obvious. However, there are some signs that could mean your child needs help. Keep in mind that children develop and learn at different rates. Let your pediatrician know if your child shows any of the following signs:

Preschool children may have

- **Delays in language development.** By 2½ years of age, your child should be able to talk in short sentences.
- **Trouble with speech.** By 3 years of age, your child should speak well enough so that adults can understand most of what she says.
- **Trouble with coordination.** By 5 years of age, your child should be able to button, cut, and hop. She should be able to copy a circle, square, or triangle.
- **Short attention spans.** Between 3 to 5 years of age, your child should be able to sit still and listen to a short story. As your child gets older, she should be able to pay attention for a longer time.

Is there a cure?

There is no single cure for LD. Be cautious of people and groups who claim to have simple answers or solutions. You may hear about eye exercises, body movements, special diets, vitamins, and nutritional supplements. There's no good evidence that these work. If in doubt, talk with your pediatrician. Also, you can contact trusted resources like the ones listed at the end of this brochure for more information.

School-aged children and teens may find it difficult to

- Follow directions.
- Get and stay organized at home and school.
- Understand verbal directions.
- Learn facts and remember information.
- Learn subjects taught in school (for example, math, reading, or spelling) but seem smart in other things.
- Fit in with their peers or communicate with others.
- Sound words out and read or spell.
- Write clearly (may have poor handwriting).
- Concentrate and finish schoolwork (may daydream a lot).

What are common LD?

The following are brief descriptions of some common LD. Keep in mind, not every child with an LD fits neatly within one of these types. Careful evaluation is important.

Children with a **reading disorder**

- May not remember the names of letters and the sounds they make.
- May not understand words that are read to them.
- May not understand that words are made up of sounds and that letters stand for those sounds.
- May not be able to sound out words at the right speed and correctly.
- May have trouble spelling.
- May take longer to read words they know.

Children with a **writing (graphomotor) disorder**

- May have trouble using a pen or pencil.
- May not remember how letters are formed.
- May have trouble copying shapes or drawing lines and spacing things out correctly.
- May have trouble writing words to express themselves.
- May have trouble organizing and writing their thoughts on paper.

Children with a **math disorder**

- May have trouble with math concepts such as number values, quantity, and order.
- May have trouble with fractions, percentages, geometry, and algebra.

- May have trouble with things like time, money, and measuring.
- May have other problems, including problems with shapes and drawing.

Children with **nonverbal LD**
- May have problems with nonverbal cues, like body language.
- May have poor coordination.

Children with **speech and language disabilities**
- May have problems understanding and using language (this may affect how well they can read and write).
- May struggle to understand instructions or new information.

Children with **central auditory processing disorders**
- May have no problem hearing but they may not interpret and store what is heard.
- May have a specific weakness in learning from sounds. These children may have even more difficulty when there's a lot of background noise.

Who can help?

Schools are required by law to help *all* children with language or learning difficulties at no cost to parents. If you're concerned about your child's problems with learning or think your child may have an LD, talk with your child's teacher and your pediatrician. Informal screening and formal evaluation are ways that teachers and other education specialists can help determine if there's a problem.

Your pediatrician may want to test your child's vision and hearing to rule out other possible problems. You may also want to see a pediatrician who specializes in neurodevelopmental disabilities, developmental and behavioral pediatrics, or child neurology. Other professionals that can help are psychologists and private educational specialists.

Children with LD may be eligible to receive special services to help them do well in school. These may include tutoring, non-timed tests, or sometimes changes in the classroom that are geared toward the child's specific learning style. One way to ensure that your child is being helped is for teachers and parents (and sometimes your pediatrician) to meet and develop a written plan that clearly describes the services your child needs. This plan is called an Individualized Education Program (IEP). Once this plan is in place, it should be reviewed regularly to make sure your child's needs are being met.

How can I help my child?

Most children who have problems learning can reach their goals by developing different ways of learning. Love and support from parents, friends, and teachers as well as the right medical care are important, too.

Here are 3 ways you can encourage your child.

- **Focus on strengths.** All children have special talents as well as weaknesses. Find your child's strengths and help him learn to use them. Your child might be good at math, music, or sports. He could be skilled at art, working with tools, or caring for animals.
- **Develop social skills.** Disabilities combined with the challenges of growing up can make your child sad, angry, or withdrawn. Help your child by pointing out that an LD is not tied to how smart he is. Try to find clubs, teams, and other activities that stress friendship and fun.

These activities should also build confidence. And remember, competition isn't just about winning.
- **Plan for the future.** Many parents of children with LD worry about their child's future. Remind your child that an LD isn't tied to how smart he is. In fact, many people with LD are very bright and grow up to be very successful in life. You can help your child plan for adulthood by encouraging him to make career and education choices during high school. There are special career and vocational programs that help build confidence by teaching decision making and job skills.

Where can I find more information?

If you have any questions about LD, contact your pediatrician or any of the following resources:

American Academy of Pediatrics National Center of Medical Home Initiatives for Children With Special Needs
847/434-4917
www.medicalhomeinfo.org

Children and Adults With Attention-Deficit/Hyperactivity Disorder (CHADD)
800/233-4050 (National Resource Center on AD/HD)
www.chadd.org

Council for Exceptional Children
888/CEC-SPED (888/232-7733)
www.cec.sped.org

Healthy & Ready to Work National Center
352/207-6808
www.hrtw.org

Learning Disabilities Association of America
888/300-6710
www.ldanatl.org

National Center for Learning Disabilities
888/575-7373
www.ncld.org

Office of Special Education and Rehabilitative Services (OSERS)
202/245-7468
www.ed.gov/about/offices/list/osers/index.html?src=oc

Remember
Children with LD can learn and succeed, if they get the right help and support. Early identification is important—if you have any concerns about your child's learning, talk with your pediatrician.

American Academy of Pediatrics
DEDICATED TO THE HEALTH OF ALL CHILDREN™

The American Academy of Pediatrics is an organization of 60,000 primary care pediatricians, pediatric medical subspecialists, and pediatric surgical specialists dedicated to the health, safety, and well-being of infants, children, adolescents, and young adults.
American Academy of Pediatrics
Web site—www.aap.org
Copyright © 2005
American Academy of Pediatrics

Helping Your Child Learn to Read

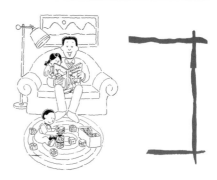

Does your child listen closely during story time? Does your child like to look through books and magazines? Does your child like learning the names of letters? If the answer is "yes" to any of these questions, your child may have already learned some important early reading skills and may be ready to learn some of the basics of reading. This brochure gives tips on how to make reading a family tradition and how to help your child develop a love of learning.

Reading tips

The following are a few tips to keep in mind as your child learns to read:

- Set aside time every day to read together. Many children like to have stories read to them at bedtime. This is a great way to wind down after a busy day and get ready for sleep.
- Leave books in your child's room for her to enjoy on her own. Make sure her room is reading-friendly with a comfortable bed or chair, bookshelf, and reading lamp.
- Read books that your child enjoys. After a while, your child may learn the words to her favorite book. When this happens, let your child complete the sentences or take turns reciting the words.
- Do not drill your child on letters, numbers, colors, shapes, or words. Instead, make a game out of it and find ways to encourage your child's curiosity and interests.

Start the process early

A child as young as 6 months of age can begin to enjoy books. The following are some age-by-age activities to help your young child learn language and begin to make the connection between words and meaning:

Birth to 1 year of age

- Play frequently with your baby. Talk, sing, recite rhymes, and do finger plays. This helps your baby learn spoken language and builds a strong foundation for reading.
- Talk with your baby, making eye contact. Allow time for your baby to respond before moving on to the next idea.
- Give your baby board books or soft books to look at, chew on, or bang on the table.
- Look at picture books with your baby and name the objects that he sees. Say things like "See the baby!" or "Look at the puppy!"
- Snuggle with your baby on your lap and read aloud to him. He may not understand the story, but he will love to hear the sound of your voice and the rhythm of the language.

1 to 3 years of age

- Read to your child every day. Allow your child to pick which books he wants, even if he picks the same one time and time again!
- Let your child "read" to you by naming objects in the book or making up a story.

- Make regular trips to the library with your child. Most children find it very exciting to get a library card. Make this moment something to celebrate.
- Continue to talk, sing, recite rhymes, and play with your child.

3 to 5 years of age

- By 3 to 5 years of age, most children are just beginning to learn the alphabet—singing their ABCs, knowing the letters of their names. Read alphabet books with your child and point out letters as you read.
- Help your child recognize whole words as well as letters. Learning and remembering what words look like are the first steps to learning to read. Point out common, everyday things like the letters on a stop sign or the logo on a favorite restaurant.
- As you read together, ask your child to make up his own story about what is happening in the book. Keep reading a part of your child's bedtime routine.
- Some educational television shows, videos, and computer programs can help your child learn to read. They can also make learning fun. But you need to be involved, too. If your child is watching *Mr. Rogers' Neighborhood* or *Sesame Street*, for example, sit and talk about what the program is trying to teach. Limit screen time to no more than 1 or 2 hours per day of educational, nonviolent programs.
- If possible, give your child a subscription to a children's magazine. Children love getting mail, and it is something they can read as well!
- Provide opportunities for your child to use written language for many purposes. Write shopping lists together. Compose letters to send to friends or relatives.

Reading aloud with your child

Reading books aloud is one of the best ways you can help your child learn to read. This can be fun for you, too. The more excitement you show when you read a book, the more your child will enjoy it. The most important thing to remember is to let your child set her own pace and have fun at whatever she is doing. Do the following when reading to your child:

- Run your finger under the words as you read to show your child that the print carries the story.
- Use funny voices and animal noises. Do not be afraid to ham it up! This will help your child get excited about the story.
- Stop to look at the pictures; ask your child to name things she sees in the pictures. Talk about how the pictures relate to the story.
- Invite your child to join in whenever there is a repeated phrase in the text.
- Show your child how events in the book are similar to events in your child's life.
- If your child asks a question, stop and answer it. The book may help your child express her thoughts and solve her own problems.
- Keep reading to your child even after she learns to read. A child can listen and understand more difficult stories than she can read on her own.

Listening to your child read aloud

Once your child begins to read, have him read out loud. This can help build your child's confidence in his ability to read and help him enjoy learning new skills. Take turns reading with your child to model more advanced reading skills.

If your child asks for help with a word, give it right away so that he does not lose the meaning of the story. Do not force your child to sound out the word. On the other hand, if your child wants to sound out a word, do not stop him.

If your child substitutes one word for another while reading, see if it makes sense. If your child uses the word "dog" instead of "pup," for example, the meaning is the same. Do not stop the reading to correct him. If your child uses a word that makes no sense (such as "road" for "read"), ask him to read the sentence again because you are not sure you understand what has just been read. Recognize your child's energy limits. Stop each session at or before the earliest signs of fatigue or frustration.

Most of all, make sure you give your child lots of praise! You are your child's first, and most important, teacher. The praise and support you give your child as he learns to read will help him enjoy reading and learning even more.

Learning to read in school

Most children learn to read by 6 or 7 years of age. Some children learn at 4 or 5 years of age. Even if a child has a head start, she may not stay ahead once school starts. The other students most likely will catch up during the second or third grade. Pushing your child to read before she is ready can get in the way of your child's interest in learning. Children who really enjoy learning are more likely to do well in school. This love of learning cannot be forced.

As your child begins elementary school, she will begin her formal reading education. There are many ways to teach children to read. One way emphasizes word recognition and teaches children to understand a whole word's meaning by how it is used. Learning which sounds the letters represent—phonics—is another way children learn to read. Phonics is used to help "decode" or sound out words. Focusing on the connections between the spoken and written word is another technique. Most teachers use a combination of methods to teach children how to read.

Reading is an important skill for children to learn. Most children learn to read without any major problems. Pushing a child to learn before she is ready can make learning to read frustrating. But reading together and playing games with books make reading fun. Parents need to be involved in their child's learning. Encouraging a child's love of learning will go a long way to ensuring success in school.

The American Academy of Pediatrics gratefully acknowledges the assistance of the Reach Out and Read program in the development of this brochure. Reach Out and Read is a pediatric early literacy program that makes literacy promotion and giving out books part of pediatric primary care. This program is endorsed by the American Academy of Pediatrics. For more information about Reach Out and Read, please contact the program at

Reach Out and Read
National Center
29 Mystic Ave
Somerville, MA 02145
617/629-8042
www.reachoutandread.org

Dyslexia

Does your child reverse letters or numbers or see them upside down? Does he read very slowly, really struggle to decode words, or continually misspell fairly simple words?

Most children have these problems when they are first learning to read. However, if no improvements are made over several years, these problems may be a sign of *dyslexia*, a reading disorder. Today, dyslexia is easier to identify than other learning problems. Talk to your pediatrician if, by 7 years of age, your child often does the following:

- Confuses the order of letters in words
- Does not look carefully at all the letters in a word, guessing what the word is from the first letter
- Loses his place on a page while reading, sometimes in the middle of a line
- Reads word by word, struggling with almost every one of them
- Reads very slowly and tires easily from reading

The information contained in this publication should not be used as a substitute for the medical care and advice of your pediatrician. There may be variations in treatment that your pediatrician may recommend based on individual facts and circumstances.

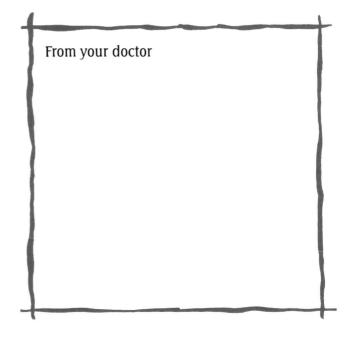

From your doctor

 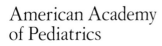

Nutrition and Fitness

calcium and you

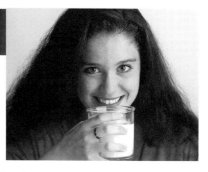

As you grow, you need calcium **to build strong bones and a healthy body.** Getting plenty of calcium while you are young also makes your bones strong and **keeps them strong for your entire lifetime.**

In fact, your body's ***need for calcium is at its highest point between the ages of 9 and 18 years.*** However, most young people in the United States don't get enough calcium in their diets.

What is calcium?

Calcium is a mineral that many parts of your body need. **Its main job is to build strong bones and teeth,** which contain 99% of your body's calcium. Your bones are a ***bank for calcium.*** A very small amount of calcium is in body fluids such as blood. But this small amount of calcium does important things. It has a role in helping your muscles move and in controlling your blood pressure.

If you make the right choices, the foods you eat or the things you drink can provide the calcium you need. If you don't get enough calcium, your bones will weaken. This is because your body will take calcium from your bones to meet its needs.

Why should I bank calcium?

When you are young, your body can deposit calcium in your "bone bank" by increasing your **bone density.** Density is a measure of how thick your bones are. Higher density bones are stronger and less likely to break.

As you get older, you lose the ability to bank calcium. By the time you reach young adulthood, your bones reach their *peak bone density.* That means your bones are as dense (or packed with calcium) as they will get—for life. Then your body mainly withdraws calcium from your bone bank.

People who do not have enough calcium in their bone bank can get osteoporosis when they get older. ***Osteoporosis is a disease that can make bones so fragile that they can break from the stress of just bending over.*** People with osteoporosis may not know they have the disease until 1 or more bones fracture. By this time, it is usually too late to undo the damage to their bones.

Is calcium all I need for strong bones?

Calcium does not work alone. A healthy diet, weight-bearing physical activity, and vitamin D are also important for developing strong bones.

- **Healthy diet**—Proper nutrition is very important to keep bones healthy.

- **Physical activity**—Studies show that regular, weight-bearing activities (such as walking, running, and jumping and playing tennis, basketball, or soccer) help you build strong bones.
- **Vitamin D**—Sources of vitamin D include the following:
  ~ Sunlight (Your body makes vitamin D when your skin is exposed to sunlight.)
  ~ Milk and other dairy products fortified with vitamin D
  ~ Vitamin D–fortified drinks and other foods, such as cereals (check the label)
  ~ Multivitamins

How much calcium do I need?

How much calcium your body needs varies according to age. You need the most calcium between 9 and 18 years of age.

The American Academy of Pediatrics recommends the following daily intake of calcium:

Daily calcium needs		
Age	Calcium Need (mg per day)	Servings of Milk to Meet Need
4–8 years	800	3 servings
9–18 years	1,300	4 servings
19–50 years	1,000	3–4 servings

How can I get calcium?

The best way to get the calcium that you need is by **eating and drinking foods that naturally contain calcium.** Many foods contain calcium.

Low-fat milk and other dairy products are very good sources of calcium. They naturally offer the most calcium per serving. For example, 1 cup of milk has about the same amount of calcium as 4 cups of broccoli.

Many foods contain some calcium, but the best sources include the following:

- Low-fat milk, yogurt, and other milk products are generally super sources of calcium.
- Flavored milks, such as chocolate or strawberry, have as much calcium as plain milk but may have more calories.
- Dark green, leafy vegetables such as kale and turnip greens are low in calories and high in calcium. However, spinach is not a good source of calcium.
- Broccoli, tofu, chickpeas, lentils, split peas, and canned salmon and sardines (and other fish with bones) also are good sources of calcium.
- Calcium-fortified juices and cereals can help boost the calcium in your diet, but limit yourself to 8 to 12 ounces (1½ cups) of juice a day.

(See "Counting Calcium" at the end of this handout.)

Calcium supplements

Certain medical conditions, diets, or lifestyle choices can make it hard for you to get enough calcium by eating the right foods. In some cases, your pediatrician may recommend a calcium supplement, such as a daily dose of a calcium-containing antacid or another type of calcium supplement. If you take calcium supplements, don't take more than a total of 1,000 mg of them a day.

Lactose intolerance

Some young people have significant lactose intolerance, which means they have **trouble digesting lactose** (the sugar in milk). In most people, lactose intolerance is of a mild form. These people can digest dairy products in small amounts with a meal. Cheeses and yogurts in which the lactose is partially broken down can provide good sources of calcium for them. There are preparations of the enzyme lactase that make lactose easier to digest. Also available is milk with reduced lactose. Nondairy foods that are rich in calcium, as well as calcium-fortified foods, also can be **good choices for people who have lactose intolerance.** In some cases, your pediatrician may recommend a calcium supplement.

What decreases my calcium intake?

The following can hurt your bone health:

- **Drinking a lot of soda (pop or soft drinks)**—Studies show that this may make you more prone to bone fractures. This may be because sodas often take the place of milk or other calcium-rich drinks. Cola-type sodas also contain phosphorus, which may interfere with how your body handles calcium.
- **Certain diets**—Some diets may not provide enough calcium, such as a vegetarian diet that excludes dairy products. Before you start any diet, check with your pediatrician to make sure it includes enough calcium.
- **Caffeine, alcohol, and tobacco**—All of these can cause you to lose calcium from your bones.
- **Certain medicines and diseases**—Some medicines and kidney and intestinal diseases can cause you to lose calcium from your bones. Ask your pediatrician if any of the medicine you are taking affects your bones and what you can do to protect them.

What can I do to get more calcium?

There are many ways to get more calcium, such as

- Choose milk or smoothies instead of soda at restaurants or school cafeterias.
- Boost the calcium in salads with beans (such as garbanzo or kidney), cheese, broccoli, almonds, or tofu.
- Choose yogurt as a light meal or snack.
- Create special drinks with milk. Add flavorings. Make shakes or smoothies.
- Use low-fat yogurt on its own or with fresh fruit. Add it to pancakes or waffles, shakes, salad dressings, dips, and sauces.
- Try calcium-rich foods that may be new to you and your family.
- Try calcium-fortified juice and calcium-fortified waffles or cereal for breakfast.

How to read food labels

Food labels list the amount of calcium in a serving as "% Daily Value," not as milligrams (mg).

100% of the Daily Value = 1,000 mg of calcium per day

To find out how many milligrams of calcium are in a serving, place a "0" at the end of the number listed for the daily value. For example, a serving of calcium-fortified orange juice might list the amount of calcium as 30% of the daily value.

30% Daily Value = 300 mg calcium

In general, a food that lists a daily value of 20% or more for calcium is high in calcium. Any food that contains less than 5% of the daily value is low in calcium.

When possible, **choose sources of calcium that are either low in fat or have no fat at all.** Or **make trade-offs** in your food choices. For example, if you go for a thick, chocolate milk shake, skip the French fries. (Removing fat from a food does not take away calcium.)

Counting calcium

If you are between the ages of 9 years and 18 years, you need about **1,300 mg of calcium each day.** Keep track of what you eat for a few days to see if you are getting enough calcium.

If a medical condition or restricted diet is keeping you from getting the calcium you need, talk with your pediatrician.

The following tables show the amount of calcium in a variety of foods. **Calcium amounts may vary. Check nutrition labels on products for exact amounts.**

Milk Group	Calcium (mg)
Milk*, regular or low fat, 1 cup	245–265
Yogurt, nonfat, fruit, 1 cup	260
Cheese, 1-oz slice	200
Cheese, pasteurized, ¾-oz slice	145
Ice cream, ½ cup	90
Ice cream, soft-serve, ½ cup	115
Frozen yogurt, ½ cup	105
Pudding, instant, ½ cup	150
Soy milk, calcium-fortified, 1 cup	200–500
Protein Group	**Calcium (mg)**
Almonds, chopped, 1 oz	65
White beans, cooked, boiled, 1 cup	160
Salmon, canned with bones, 3 oz	205
Tofu, firm, calcium-fortified, ½ cup	205

Vegetables/Fruits	Calcium (mg)
Broccoli, cooked, 1 cup	60
Collards, cooked, 1 cup	265
Tomatoes, canned, stewed, 1 cup	85
Orange juice, calcium-fortified, 1 cup	300
Orange, 1 medium	50
Grains	**Calcium (mg)**
English muffin, plain, enriched, 1	95
Pancakes (made with milk), 1	80
Corn tortilla, 1	45
Selected breakfast cereals, calcium-fortified, ¾–1 cup	100
Instant oatmeal (made with water), calcium-fortified, ½ cup	65
Prepared Foods	**Calcium (mg)**
Bean and cheese burrito	110
Cheese pizza, 1 slice	120
Cheeseburger	140
Taco, 1 small	220

*Low-fat milk has as much or more calcium than whole milk.
Source: US Department of Agriculture

The information contained in this publication should not be used as a substitute for the medical care and advice of your pediatrician. There may be variations in treatment that your pediatrician may recommend based on individual facts and circumstances.

The persons whose photographs are depicted in this publication are professional models. They have no relation to the issues discussed. Any characters they are portraying are fictional.

From your doctor

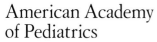
American Academy of Pediatrics
DEDICATED TO THE HEALTH OF ALL CHILDREN™

The American Academy of Pediatrics is an organization of 60,000 primary care pediatricians, pediatric medical subspecialists, and pediatric surgical specialists dedicated to the health, safety, and well-being of infants, children, adolescents, and young adults.
American Academy of Pediatrics
Web site—www.aap.org
Copyright © 2006
American Academy of Pediatrics, Updated 2/06

Encourage Your Child to Be Physically Active

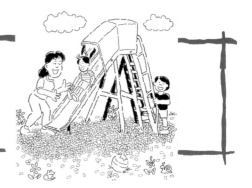

Today's youth are less active and more overweight than any previous generation.

Did you know?

- Children on average spend nearly 3 hours a day watching TV.
- Only half of children and teens, aged 12 to 21, regularly exercise.
- Illinois is the only state that still mandates that physical education be offered in public schools.
- More than 15% of all school children are considered obese or overweight.
- Overweight teens have a 70% chance of becoming overweight or obese adults.
- Eighty-five percent of children diagnosed with type 2 diabetes are either overweight or obese.
- Sleep apnea occurs in approximately 7% of children who are obese.

Get the entire family moving

With participation in all types of physical activity declining dramatically as a child's age and grade in school increases, it is important that physical activity be a regular part of family life. Studies have shown that lifestyles learned as children are much more likely to stay with a person into adulthood. If sports and physical activities are a family priority, they will provide children and parents with a strong foundation for a lifetime of health.

The benefits of physical activity

While exercise is vital to the health and well-being of children, many of them either do not appreciate or fully understand the many emotional and physical health benefits of physical activity.

The benefits of physical activity include

Benefits to the body

- Builds and maintains healthy bones, muscles, and joints.
- Controls weight and body fat.
- Improves appearance.
- Increases muscle strength, endurance, and flexibility.
- Improves ability to fall asleep quickly and sleep well.
- Reduces the risk of diabetes, high blood pressure, and heart disease later in life.
- Builds and improves athletic skills.

Mental benefits

- Increases enthusiasm and optimism.
- Organized sports foster teamwork and friendship.
- Boosts self-esteem.
- Reduces anxiety, tension, and depression.

Getting started

Parents can play a key role in helping their child become more physically active.

Following are 11 ways to get started:

1. **Talk to your pediatrician.** Your pediatrician can help your child understand why physical activity is important. Your pediatrician also can suggest a sport or activity that is best for your child.

2. **Find a fun activity.** Help your child find a sport that she enjoys. The more she enjoys the activity, the more likely it is that she will continue. Get the entire family involved. It is a great way to spend time together.

3. **Choose an activity that is developmentally appropriate.** For example, a 7- or 8- year-old child is not ready for weight lifting or a 3-mile run, but soccer, bicycle riding, and swimming are all appropriate activities.

4. **Plan ahead.** Make sure your child has a convenient time and place to exercise.

5. **Provide a safe environment.** Make sure your child's equipment and chosen site for the sport or activity are safe. Make sure your child's clothing is comfortable and appropriate.

6. **Provide active toys.** Young children especially need easy access to balls, jump ropes, and other active toys.

7. **Be a model for your child.** Children who regularly see their parents enjoying sports and physical activity are more likely to do so themselves.

8. **Play with your child.** Help her learn a new sport.

9. **Turn off the TV.** Limit television watching and computer use. The American Academy of Pediatrics recommends no more than 1 to 2 hours of total screen time, including TV, videos, and computers and video games, each day. Use the free time for more physical activities.

10. **Make time for exercise.** Some children are so overscheduled with homework, music lessons, and other planned activities that they do not have time for exercise.

11. **Do not overdo it.** When your child is ready to start, remember to tell her to listen to her body. Exercise and physical activity should not hurt. If this occurs, your child should slow down or try a less vigorous activity. As with any activity, it is important not to overdo it. If your child's weight drops below an average, acceptable level, or if exercise starts to interfere with school or other activities, talk with your pediatrician.

Remember

There is a powerful relationship between childhood obesity and lifelong weight and related medical problems.

Exercise along with a balanced diet provides the foundation for a healthy, active life. One of the most important things parents can do is encourage healthy habits in their children early on in life. It is not too late to start. Ask your pediatrician about tools for healthy living today.

The information contained in this publication should not be used as a substitute for the medical care and advice of your pediatrician. There may be variations in treatment that your pediatrician may recommend based on individual facts and circumstances.

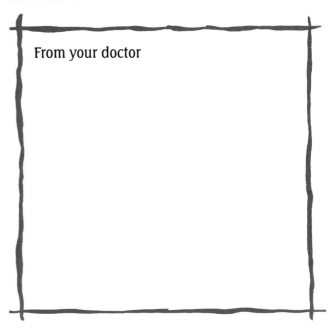

From your doctor

American Academy of Pediatrics

DEDICATED TO THE HEALTH OF ALL CHILDREN™

The American Academy of Pediatrics is an organization of 60,000 primary care pediatricians, pediatric medical subspecialists, and pediatric surgical specialists dedicated to the health, safety, and well-being of infants, children, adolescents, and young adults.

American Academy of Pediatrics
Web site—www.aap.org

Copyright © 2003
American Academy of Pediatrics

© 2007 American Academy of Pediatrics

Feeding Kids Right Isn't Always Easy

Tips for Preventing Food Hassles

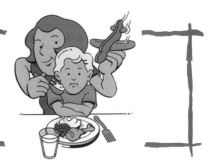

Feeding Kids — What's Your Role?

While parents are the best judges of **what** children should eat and **when,** children are the best judges of **how much** they should eat.

*Here are **five** important feeding jobs for parents and caregivers:*

1. Offer a variety of healthful and tasty foods. Be adventurous!
2. Serve meals and snacks on a regular schedule.
3. Make mealtime pleasant.
4. Teach good manners at the table.
5. Set a good example.

Happy encounters with food at any age help set the stage for sensible eating habits throughout life. Handling food and eating situations positively encourages healthful food choices.

This brochure gives helping hints for food and nutrition for young children. For specific advice, talk to your child's pediatrician or a registered dietitian.

Mealtime: Not a Battleground

"Clean your plate."

"No dessert until you eat your vegetables."

"If you behave, you can have a piece of candy."

To parents and caregivers, these phrases probably sound familiar. However, food should be used as nourishment, not as a reward or punishment. In the long run, food bribery usually creates more problems than it solves.

Did You Know That...

...encouraging your child to wash his or her hands thoroughly before meals may help prevent foodborne illness?

Mealtime Is More Than Food

Youngsters are too smart to heed the old saying "Do as I say, not as I do." Children learn by imitating what they see. Adults who eat poorly can't expect their children to eat well. Set a good example by eating meals at regular times and by making healthful and tasty food choices.

Parents and caregivers are "gatekeepers," who control what foods come into the house. Having lots of healthful foods around helps children understand that these food choices are a way of life.

Mealtime is family time. Children learn many things as you eat together. And pleasant social encounters with food help develop good food habits.

Three, Two, One ... Let's Eat!

Prepare children for meals. A five-minute warning before mealtime lets them calm down, wash their hands and get ready to eat. A child who is anxious, excited or tired may have trouble settling down to eat.

Consistent food messages encourage children to eat and help prevent arguments over food.

Here are six common childhood eating situations. Try these simple tips to make mealtime a more pleasant experience.

Feeding Challenges...	Feeding Strategies...
Food Jags: Eats one and only one food, meal after meal	Allow the child to eat what he or she wants if the "jag" food is wholesome. Offer other foods at each meal. After a few days, the child likely will try other foods. Don't remove the "jag" food, but offer it as long as the child wants it. Food jags rarely last long enough to cause any harm.
Food Strikes: Refuses to eat what's served, which can lead to "short-order cook syndrome"	Have bread, rolls or fruit available at each meal, so there are usually choices that the child likes. Be supportive, set limits and don't be afraid to let the child go hungry if he or she won't eat what is served. Which is worse, an occasional missed meal or a parent who is a perpetual short-order cook?
"The TV Habit": Wants to watch TV at mealtime	Turn off the television. Mealtime TV is a distraction that prevents family interaction and interferes with a child's eating. Value the time spent together while eating. Often it is the only time during the day that families can be together. An occasional meal with TV that the whole family can enjoy is fine.
The Complainer: Whines or complains about the food served	First ask the child to eat other foods offered at the meal. If the child cannot behave properly, have the child go to his or her room or sit quietly away from the table until the meal is finished. Don't let him or her take food along, return for dessert or eat until the next planned meal or snack time.
"The Great American White Food Diet": Eats only white bread, potatoes, macaroni and milk	Avoid pressuring the child to eat other foods. Giving more attention to finicky eating habits only reinforces a child's demands to limit foods. Continue to offer a variety of food-group foods. Encourage a taste of red, orange or green foods. Eventually the child will move on to other foods.
Fear of New Foods: Refuses to try new foods	Continue to introduce and reinforce new foods over time. It may take many tries before a child is ready to taste a new food... and a lot of tastes before a child likes it. Don't force children to try new foods.

Try these simple steps:
- Be a smart gatekeeper. Buy a variety of foods you want the child to eat. Be adventurous with food!
- Be flexible. Don't worry if the child skips a meal.

- Be sensible. Set an example by eating a variety of healthful foods yourself.
- Let children make their own food choices from the healthful choices you provide.

Occasional Meal Skipping and Finicky Food Habits Are Okay

Well-meaning adults often view a child's odd food and eating behaviors as a problem. However, childhood food jags, a fear of new foods and other feeding challenges are usually part of normal development.

There's no need to worry if a child skips a meal or won't eat the vegetables on his or her plate. Keep the big picture in mind. Offer a variety of healthful, tasty and nourishing foods. Over time, a child will get everything needed to grow and develop normally. Plenty of food variety and a relaxed, happy atmosphere at mealtime are the "ingredients" for a well-fed child.

Children often use the table as a stage for showing their independence. Sometimes, food is not the issue at all. The eating process is just one more way children learn about the world.

Work Up an Appetite!

Active play, along with eating right, promotes good health ... and a healthy appetite! And it is the best exercise for toddlers and young children.

Making a snowman, playing tag, throwing balls, riding a bike and taking a nature walk are healthful and fun for the whole family. Don't just watch. Join in and be active, too. When you're physically active, you set a good example.

The New Food Guide Pyramid

For the latest information from the US Department of Agriculture about making healthy food choices and keeping physically active, visit their Web site at www.mypyramid.gov to learn about **MyPyramid.**

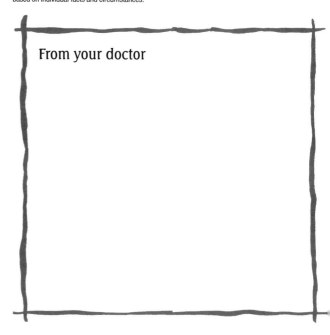

From your doctor

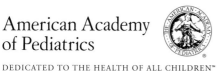

American Academy of Pediatrics

DEDICATED TO THE HEALTH OF ALL CHILDREN™

The American Academy of Pediatrics is an organization of 60,000 primary care pediatricians, pediatric medical subspecialists, and pediatric surgical specialists dedicated to the health, safety, and well-being of infants, children, adolescents, and young adults.

American Academy of Pediatrics
Web site—www.aap.org

Copyright © 1991
American Academy of Pediatrics, Updated 1/02

Growing Up Healthy

Fat, Cholesterol and More

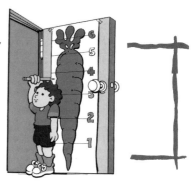

Children and Heart Disease: A Generation at Risk

Many Americans consume too many calories and too much fat, especially saturated fat, and cholesterol. These eating patterns are one cause of America's high rates of obesity and heart disease. As a parent or caregiver, you can help your child develop eating and physical activity habits to stay healthy now — and throughout life.

What's a Parent to Do?

Food and physical activity habits begin at home. Although many things influence children, adults are still the most important role models for developing healthful eating and lifestyle habits.

The information in this brochure provides eating and physical activity guidelines for healthy children ages two years and over. For specific food and nutrition advice, talk to your child's pediatrician or a registered dietitian.

The New Food Guide Pyramid

For the latest information from the US Department of Agriculture about making healthy food choices and keeping physically active, visit their Web site at www.mypyramid.gov to learn about **MyPyramid.**

Fat in Food: How Much for Children?

If heart disease runs in your family, your child is at greater risk for heart disease in adulthood. To help protect your child from heart disease later in life, help him or her learn healthful eating and lifestyle habits during childhood.

Most nutrition experts agree that childhood is the best time to *start* cutting back on total fat, saturated fat and cholesterol. But adult goals aren't meant for young children under the age of two years. Fat is an essential nutrient that supplies energy, or calories, they need for growth and active play.

Between the ages of two and five, as children eat with their family, encourage them to gradually choose foods with less fat and saturated fat. By age five, their overall food choices, like yours, should be low in fat.

You might wonder: how is saturated fat different than other fat? It's more solid at room temperature. Saturated fats come mostly from animal sources, such as butter, cheese, bacon and meat, as well as stick margarine.

Caution: A low-fat eating plan is not advised for children under two years of age because of special needs for rapid growth and development during these years.

Healthful Eating

For healthful eating, offer foods from the five major food groups. Encourage nutrient-rich foods with less fat: grain products; fruits; vegetables; low-fat dairy foods; and lean meats, poultry, fish, and cooked dry beans.

Most young children — age two and over — need the minimum number of servings from each food group. Although children will decide how much

they can eat, a child-size serving is one-fourth to one-third the size of an adult portion. That's about one measuring tablespoon per year of the young child's age.

Good Nutrition: It's a Juggling Act

Chances are that some of your child's favorite foods are higher in fat and energy (or calories) compared to the amount of nutrients they provide. Any food that supplies energy and nutrients can fit into a nutritious eating plan for your child.

Follow this nutrition advice: Offer your child many different food-group foods. Be flexible; what children eat over several days, not one day or one meal, is what counts. Help your child eat sensibly. Here are ways to be sensible about fat, saturated fat and cholesterol in food choices:

Food Group...	Most Days...	Some Days...
Bread, Cereal, Rice and Pasta	bagel or English muffin	doughnut or danish
	pretzels, baked chips	regular corn chips
	graham crackers, crackers, fig bars, vanilla wafers	chocolate chip cookies, cupcakes
Vegetable	baked potato	french fries
	raw vegetables	creamy cole slaw
Fruit	fresh fruit and juice	—
Milk, Yogurt and Cheese	reduced-fat cheese	cheese
	low-fat frozen yogurt or ice cream	ice cream
Meat, Poultry, Fish, Dry Beans, Eggs and Nuts	baked and grilled chicken	fried chicken
	baked fish	fried fish sticks

Smart Ideas for the Whole Family

Try these simple tips to limit extra fat, saturated fat and cholesterol:

- Have plenty of fresh fruits and vegetables available and ready to eat.
- Offer skim or l % milk* and low-fat yogurt. Choose cheeses that are lower in fat.
- Include starchy foods, such as potatoes, rice, pasta, and whole-grain breads and cereals often.
- Choose lower fat or fat-free toppings like grated parmesan cheese, herbed cottage cheese and nonfat/low-fat gravy, sour cream, or yogurt.
- Select lean meats, such as skinless chicken and turkey, fish, lean beef cuts (round, loin, lean ground beef) and lean pork cuts (tenderloin, chops, ham). Trim off all visible fat, and remove skin from poultry before eating.
- Choose margarine and vegetable oils made from canola, corn, sunflower, soybean and olive oils. Choose tub and liquid margarine, rather than regular margarine in sticks, too.
- Try angel food cake, frozen fruit bars, and low-fat/fat-free frozen desserts such as fudge bars, yogurt or ice cream.
- Use nonstick vegetable sprays when cooking.

* Children *under* two years old should only drink whole milk.

- Use fat-free cooking methods, such as baking, broiling, grilling, poaching or steaming, when preparing meat, poultry or fish.
- Serve vegetable- and broth-based soups. Or use skim or 1% milk* or evaporated skim milk when making cream soups.
- Use the Nutrition Facts label on food packages to find foods with less fat per serving. Be sure to check serving size as you make choices. Remember that the % Daily Values on food labels are based on calorie levels for adults.

* Children *under* two years old should only drink whole milk.

Parent Tip: Forget "Forbidden" Foods

Forcing children to eat food doesn't work. Neither does forbidding foods. Foods that are "forbidden" just may become more desirable for children.

It's important for both children and adults to be sensible and enjoy all foods, but not to overdo on any one type of food. Sweets and higher-fat snack foods in appropriate portions are okay. Just make sure your child is offered wise food choices from all the food groups.

Caution:

- Restricting a child's eating pattern too much may harm growth and development, or encourage undesirable eating behaviors.
- Before making any drastic changes in a child's eating plan or physical activity habits, talk to your child's pediatrician or a registered dietitian.
- Don't restrict fat or calories for children under two years of age, except on the advice of your child's pediatrician.

Teach Good Habits by Example

Children learn more from ACTIONS than from WORDS. Practice what you preach. Your actions will make you healthier, too!

Get Up and Move...Turn Off That Tube!

Too much television usually results in not enough physical activity or creative play. Pediatricians recommend limiting TV time to no more than one or two hours each day.

Be active. Join your children in doing other activities. These activities will please almost any young child:

- Playing tag
- Jumping rope
- Throwing balls
- Riding a tricycle or bicycle
- Pulling a wagon
- Flying a kite
- Digging in the sand
- Making a snowman

- Ice skating or sledding
- Jumping in leaves
- Playing on swings
- "Driving" a toy truck
- Swimming
- Walking with the family
- Dancing
- Pushing a toy shopping cart

The information contained in this publication should not be used as a substitute for the medical care and advice of your pediatrician. There may be variations in treatment that your pediatrician may recommend based on individual facts and circumstances.

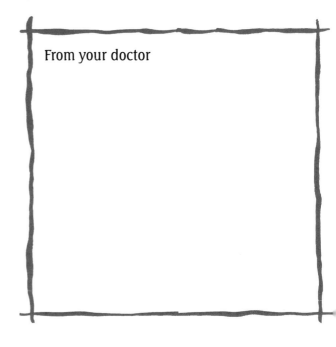

From your doctor

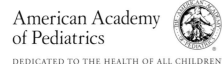

American Academy
of Pediatrics

DEDICATED TO THE HEALTH OF ALL CHILDREN™

The American Academy of Pediatrics is an organization of 60,000 primary care pediatricians, pediatric medical subspecialists, and pediatric surgical specialists dedicated to the health, safety, and well-being of infants, children, adolescents, and young adults.

American Academy of Pediatrics
Web site—www.aap.org

Copyright © 1991
American Academy of Pediatrics, Updated 10/05

Right From the Start

ABC's of Good Nutrition for Young Children

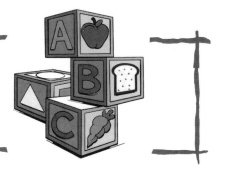

Good Nutrition: The Results Are Worth It

Proper nutrition begins at the supermarket with the foods you buy and continues at home as you prepare and serve meals. Giving your child a healthy start with good eating habits promotes his or her lifelong health.

This brochure focuses on feeding young children. It is meant to help you set the stage for healthful eating habits and food choices. The ABCs of good family nutrition start with love and common sense.

For specific advice about food and nutrition for young children, talk to your child's pediatrician or a registered dietitian.

Active Play Is Important to Health

Along with proper nutrition, your child needs physical activity for lifelong health. In the form of active play, physical activity not only promotes your child's appetite. It also helps develop a sense of well-being and confidence in his or her physical activities. From the early childhood years, encourage your child to live an active life.

Actions Speak Louder Than Words

As children grow and develop, they watch for clues about food choices. Youngsters often copy food habits, likes and dislikes. When you make wise food choices, your actions speak louder than words.

The ABCs of Good Nutrition

A variety of foods provides the nutrients that young children need to build strong bodies and stay healthy. Food also supplies the energy that children need to grow normally, play, learn and explore the world around them.

Offering a variety of tasty foods is the best way to supply the nutrition that a growing child needs.

A wide variety of foods are part of the five different food groups. Each food group makes special nutrient contributions. And each nutrient has certain jobs in the body.

Foods from all the groups work together to supply energy and nutrients necessary for health and growth. No one food group is more important than another. For good health, you and your child need them all.

Foods to Choose

- *From the Bread, Cereal, Rice and Pasta Group:* a whole-grain bread, crackers, cereal, grits, pasta, rice, bagel, tortilla, cornbread, pita bread, muffin, English muffin, matzo crackers, rice cake, pancakes, breadsticks, pretzels
- *From the Vegetable Group:* asparagus, beets, bok choy, broccoli, carrot, cauliflower, collard greens, corn, cucumber, green and red peppers, green beans, jicama, kale, okra, peas, potato, pumpkin, snow peas, squash, spinach, sweet potato, tomato, vegetable juices, zucchini

- *From the Fruit Group:* apple, applesauce, apricot, banana, berries, cantaloupe, fruit cocktail, figs, fruit juices, grapefruit, kiwifruit, mango, nectarine, orange, papaya, peach, pear, plum, pineapple, raisins, prunes, starfruit, strawberries, tangerine, watermelon
- *From the Milk, Yogurt and Cheese Group:* skim, l %, 2 % and whole* milk, yogurt, cheese, string cheese, cottage cheese, pudding, custard, frozen yogurt, ice milk, calcium-fortified soybean milk
- *From the Meat, Poultry, Fish, Dry Beans, Eggs and Nuts** Group:* lean cuts of beef, veal, pork, ham and lamb; skinless chicken and turkey; fish; shellfish; cooked beans (kidney beans, black-eyed peas, pinto beans, lentils, black beans); refried beans (made without lard); peanut butter; eggs; reduced-fat deli meats; tofu; nuts**; peanuts**

*   Children under two years of age should *only* drink whole milk.
** Nuts, peanuts and seeds are not recommended for children under four years of age because they are a choking hazard. Small pieces of hard, uncooked fruits and vegetables also pose a choking hazard to children under age four.

The New Food Guide Pyramid

For the latest information from the US Department of Agriculture about making healthy food choices and keeping physically active, visit their Web site at www.mypyramid.gov to learn about **MyPyramid.**

How Do I Know If My Child Is Eating Enough?

Children eat when they are hungry and usually stop when they are full. Some parents worry because young children appear to eat very small amounts of food, especially when compared to adult portions. A child who is growing well is getting enough to eat.

To check your child's eating pattern, pay attention to his or her food choices.

- Make sure no one food group is completely left out. If this happens for a few days, don't worry. But prolonged neglect of a food group could keep your child from getting enough nutrients.
- Encourage your child to be adventurous and eat a variety of foods within the food groups, too. Even within a food group, different foods provide different nutrients.

Child-Size Servings: Be Realistic

For youngsters, adult-size servings can be overwhelming. Offering child-size servings encourages food acceptance.

Here's an easy guide to child-size servings:

- Serve one-fourth to one-third of the adult portion size, or one measuring tablespoon for each year of the young child's age.
- Give less than you think the child will eat. Let the child ask for more if he or she is still hungry.

Snacks Count, Too

Snacks make up an important part of childhood nutrition. Children must eat frequently. With their small stomachs, they cannot eat enough at meals alone for their high energy needs. Three meals and two or three healthful snacks a day help youngsters meet their daily nutrition needs.

To make the most of snacks, parents and caregivers should control the type of snack and time it is served.

Type. Offer a variety of food-group snacks. Choose mostly snack foods that supply enough nutrients to justify their energy, or calories.

Timing. Plan snacks. Schedule snacks around normal daily events, and space them at least two hours before meals. Children should learn to get and feel hungry, instead of feeling full all the time.

Quick and Smart Snack Food Ideas

For more nutrition, mix and match snacks from more than one food group:

- Fresh, frozen or canned fruit (banana, strawberries, cantaloupe pieces, orange sections, apple slices) or fruit juice
- Raw vegetables (baby carrots, cucumber slices, zucchini sticks, broccoli florets*)
- Vegetable soup
- Graham, animal crackers or fig bars
- Soft pretzels or breadsticks
- English muffin or bagel
- Low-fat yogurt or string cheese
- Skim or 1 % milk ** (flavored or unflavored)
- Turkey or meat cubes
- Hard-cooked egg

* Small pieces of hard, uncooked fruits and vegetables pose a choking hazard to children under age four.

** Children under two years of age should *only* drink whole milk.

The information contained in this publication should not be used as a substitute for the medical care and advice of your pediatrician. There may be variations in treatment that your pediatrician may recommend based on individual facts and circumstances.

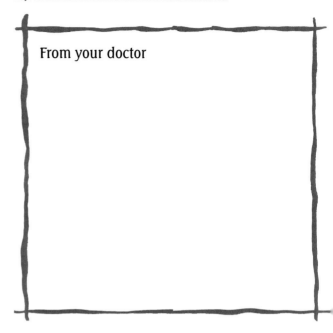

From your doctor

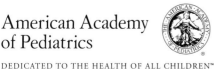

American Academy of Pediatrics

DEDICATED TO THE HEALTH OF ALL CHILDREN™

The American Academy of Pediatrics is an organization of 60,000 primary care pediatricians, pediatric medical subspecialists, and pediatric surgical specialists dedicated to the health, safety, and well-being of infants, children, adolescents, and young adults.

American Academy of Pediatrics
Web site—www.aap.org

Copyright © 1991
American Academy of Pediatrics, Updated 5/05

© 2007 American Academy of Pediatrics

Starting Solid Foods

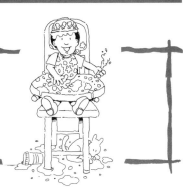

Until now, your baby's diet has been made up of breast milk and/or formula. But once your child reaches 4 to 6 months of age, you can begin adding solid foods. This brochure has been developed by the American Academy of Pediatrics to give parents information on how to introduce solid foods to their infants.

When can my baby eat solid foods?

Most babies are ready to eat solid foods at 4 to 6 months of age. Before this age, most babies do not have enough control over their tongues and mouth muscles. Instead of swallowing the food, they push their tongues against the spoon or the food. This tongue-pushing reflex helps babies when they are nursing or drinking from a bottle. Most babies lose this reflex at about 4 months of age. Energy needs of babies increase around this age as well, making this an ideal time to introduce solids.

You may start solid foods at any feeding. At first you may want to pick a time when you do not have many distractions. However, keep in mind that as your child gets older, she will want to eat with the rest of the family.

Feeding your baby solid foods

To prevent choking, make sure your baby is sitting up when you introduce solid foods. If your baby cries or turns away when you give him the food, do not force the issue. It is more important that you both enjoy mealtimes than for your baby to start solids by a specific date. Go back to nursing or bottle-feeding exclusively for a week or two, then try again.

It is important for your baby to get used to the process of eating — sitting up, taking bites from a spoon, resting between bites, and stopping when full. Always use a spoon to feed your baby solid foods. Some parents try putting solid foods in a bottle or infant feeder with a nipple. This is not a good idea. Feeding your baby this way can cause choking. It also greatly increases the amount of food your baby eats and can cause your baby to gain too much weight. These early experiences will help your child learn good eating habits throughout life.

How to start

Start with half a spoonful or less and talk to your baby through the process ("Mmm, see how good this is!"). Your baby may not know what to do at first. She may look confused or insulted, wrinkle her nose, roll the food around her mouth, or reject it altogether. This is a normal reaction, because her feedings have been so different up to this point.

One way to make eating solids for the first time easier is to give your baby a little milk first, then switch to very small half-spoonfuls of food, and finish with more milk. This will prevent your baby from getting frustrated when she is very hungry.

Do not be surprised if most of the first few solid-food feedings wind up on your baby's face, hands, and bib. Increase the amount of food gradually, with just a teaspoonful or two to start. This allows your baby time to learn how to swallow solids.

What kinds of foods should my baby eat?

For most babies it does not matter what the first solid foods are. Many pediatricians recommend cereals first. The first cereals usually are offered in this order:

- Rice cereal
- Oatmeal cereal
- Barley cereal

It is a good idea to give your baby wheat and mixed cereals last, because they may cause allergic reactions in very young babies.

You can use premixed baby cereals in a jar or dry cereals to which you add breast milk, formula, or water. The premixed foods may be easier to use, but the dry ones are richer in iron and allow you to control the thickness of the cereal. Whichever type of cereal you choose, make sure that it is made for babies. Only baby foods contain the extra nutrients your child needs at this age.

Once your baby learns to eat one food, gradually give him other foods such as

- Infant cereals
- Fruit
- Strained vegetables
- Meat

Give your baby eggs last, because they occasionally cause allergic reactions. Babies are born with a preference for sweets. The order of introducing foods does not change this.

Warning: do not home-prepare beets, turnips, carrots, spinach, or collard greens

In some parts of the country, these vegetables have large amounts of nitrates, chemicals that can cause an unusual type of anemia (low blood count) in young infants. Baby food companies are aware of this problem and screen the produce they buy for nitrates. They also avoid buying these vegetables in parts of the country where nitrates have been found. Because you cannot test for this chemical yourself, it is safer to use commercially prepared forms of these foods, especially while your child is an infant. If you choose to prepare them at home anyway, serve them fresh and do not store them. Storage of these foods may actually increase the amount of nitrates in them.

Give your baby one new food at a time, and wait at least 2 to 3 days before starting another. After each new food, watch for any allergic reactions such as diarrhea, rash, or vomiting. If any of these occur, stop using the new food and talk with your pediatrician.

Within 2 or 3 months of starting solid foods, your baby's daily diet should include the following foods each day:
- Breast milk or formula
- Cereal
- Vegetables
- Meats
- Fruits

Finger foods

Once your baby can sit up and bring her hands or other objects to her mouth, you can give her finger foods to help her learn to feed herself. To avoid choking, make sure anything you give your child is soft, easy to swallow, and cut into small pieces. Some examples include small pieces of banana, wafer-type cookies, or crackers; and well-cooked and cut-up yellow squash, peas, and potatoes. Do not give your baby any food that requires chewing at this age.

At each of your child's daily meals, she should be eating about 4 ounces, or the amount in one small jar of strained baby food. (Do not give your child foods that are made for adults. These foods often have added salt and preservatives.)

If you want to give your baby fresh food, use a blender or food processor, or just mash softer foods with a fork. All fresh foods should be cooked with no added salt or seasoning. Though you can feed your baby raw bananas (mashed), most other fruits and vegetables should be cooked until they are soft. Refrigerate any food you do not use and look for any signs of spoilage before giving it to your baby. Fresh foods are not bacteria-free, so they will spoil more quickly than food from a can or jar.

What can I expect after my baby starts solids?

When your child starts eating solid foods, his stools will become more solid and variable in color. Due to the added sugars and fats, they will have a much stronger odor too. Peas and other green vegetables may turn the stool a deep-green color; beets may make it red. (Beets sometimes make urine red as well.) If your baby's meals are not strained, his stools may contain undigested pieces of food, especially hulls of peas or corn, and the skin of tomatoes or other vegetables. All of this is normal. Your child's digestive system is still immature and needs time before it can fully process these new foods. If the stools are extremely loose, watery, or full of mucus, however, it may mean the digestive tract is irritated. In this case, reduce the amount of solids and let him build a tolerance for them a little more slowly. If the stools continue to be loose, watery, or full of mucus, consult your pediatrician to see if your child has a digestive problem.

Should I give my baby juice?

Babies do not need juice. Babies less than 6 months of age should not be given juice. However, if you choose to give your baby juice, do so only after she is 6 months of age and offer it only in a cup, not in a bottle. Limit juice intake to no more than 4 ounces a day and offer it only with a meal or snack. Any more than this can fill up your baby, giving her less of an appetite for other, more nutritious foods, including breast milk or formula. Too much juice also can cause diaper rash, diarrhea, or excessive weight gain. To help prevent tooth decay, avoid putting your child to bed with a bottle.

Give your child extra water if she seems to be thirsty between feedings. During the hot months when your child is losing fluid through sweat, offer water two or more times a day. If you live in an area where the water is fluoridated, these feedings also will help prevent future tooth decay.

Junior foods

When your child reaches about 8 months of age, you may want to introduce "junior" foods. These are slightly coarser than strained foods and are packaged in larger jars — usually 6 to 8 ounces. They require more chewing than baby foods. You also can expand your baby's diet to include soft foods such as puddings, mashed potatoes, yogurt, and gelatin. As always, introduce one food at a time, then wait 2 or 3 days before trying something else to be sure your child does not develop an allergic reaction.

As your baby's ability to use his hands improves, give him his own spoon and let him play with it at mealtimes. Once he has figured out how to hold the spoon, dip it in his food and let him try to feed himself. But do not expect much in the beginning, when more food is bound to go on the floor and high chair than into his mouth. A plastic cloth under his chair will help minimize some of the cleanup.

Be patient, and resist the temptation to take the spoon away from him. For a while you may want to alternate bites from his spoon with bites from a spoon that you hold. Your child may not be able to use a spoon on his own until after his first birthday. Until then, you may want to fill the spoon for your child but leave the actual feeding to him. This can help decrease the mess and waste.

Good finger foods for babies include the following:
- Crunchy toast
- Well-cooked pasta
- Small pieces of chicken
- Scrambled egg
- Ready-to-eat cereals
- Small pieces of banana

Offer a variety of flavors, shapes, colors, and textures, but always watch your child for choking in case he bites off a piece that is too big to swallow.

Choosing a high chair

Select a chair with a wide base, so it cannot be tipped over if someone bumps against it.

If the chair folds, be sure it is locked each time you set it up.

Whenever your child sits in the chair, use the safety straps. This will prevent your child from slipping down and causing serious injury or even death. Never allow your child to stand in the high chair.

Do not place the high chair near a counter or table. Your child may be able to push hard enough against these surfaces to tip the chair over.

Never leave a young child alone in a high chair and do not allow older children to climb or play on it, as this could tip it over.

A high chair that hooks on to a table is not a good substitute for a more solid one. If you plan to use this type of chair when you eat out or when you travel, look for one that locks on to the table. Be sure the table is heavy enough to support your child's weight without tipping. Also, check to see whether your child's feet can touch a table support. If your child pushes against the table, it may dislodge the seat.

Because children often swallow without chewing, do not offer children younger than 4 years of age the following foods:

- Chunks of peanut butter
- Nuts and seeds
- Popcorn
- Raw vegetables
- Hard, gooey, or sticky candy
- Chewing Gum

Other firm, round foods like grapes, cooked carrots, hot dogs, meat sticks (baby food "hot dogs"), or chunks of cheese or meat always should be cut into **very small** pieces. Before cutting a hot dog, remove the slippery peel.

Good eating habits start early

Babies and small children do not know what foods they need to eat. Your job as a parent is to offer a good variety of healthy foods. Watch your child for cues that she has had enough to eat. Do not overfeed!

Begin to build good eating habits. Usually eating five to six times a day (three meals and two to three snacks) is a good way to meet toddlers' energy needs. Children who "graze," or eat constantly, may never really feel hungry. They can have problems from eating too much or too little.

If you are concerned that your baby is *already* overweight, talk with your pediatrician before making any changes to her diet. During these months of rapid growth, your baby needs a balanced diet that includes fat, carbohydrates, and protein. It is not wise to switch a baby under 2 years of age to skim milk, for example, or to other low-fat substitutes for breast milk or formula. A better solution might be to slightly reduce the amount of food your child eats at each meal. This way, your child will continue to get the balanced diet she needs.

Your pediatrician will help you determine if your child is overfed, not eating enough, or eating too many of the wrong kinds of foods. Because prepared baby foods have no added salt, you do not have to worry about salt at this age. However, be aware of the eating habits of others in your family. As your baby eats more and more "table foods," she will imitate the way you eat, including using salt and nibbling on snacks. For your child's sake as well as your own, cut your salt use and watch how much fat you consume. Provide a good role model by eating a variety of healthy foods.

The information contained in this publication should not be used as a substitute for the medical care and advice of your pediatrician. There may be variations in treatment that your pediatrician may recommend based on individual facts and circumstances.

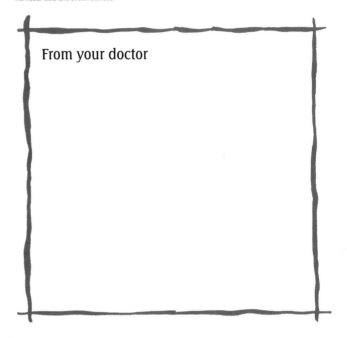

From your doctor

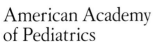

What's to Eat?

Healthy Foods for Hungry Children

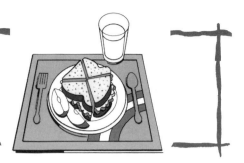

A Menu for Good Health

Ask anyone who cares for children — feeding kids can be challenging! This brochure gives meal suggestions that are tasty, convenient and nutritious*. From breakfast through dinner, these ideas will please even the fussiest eater. For specific food and nutrition advice, talk to your child's pediatrician or a registered dietitian.

* The amount of food and number of servings children need daily from each food group depends on their age and how active they are.

The New Food Guide Pyramid

For the latest information from the US Department of Agriculture about making healthy food choices and keeping physically active, visit their Web site at www.mypyramid.gov to learn about **MyPyramid.**

Off to a Good Start…The Breakfast Bonus

Breakfast provides energy to carry a child through an active morning. Children who skip breakfast may not concentrate well at school or may lack energy to play. Not everyone enjoys traditional breakfast foods, such as cereal and toast. These breakfast ideas are a little different:
- Breakfast shake: combine skim or I % milk*, fruit and ice in a blender.
- Frozen banana: dip a banana in yogurt, then roll it in crushed cereal. Freeze.
- Peanut butter spread on crackers, a tortilla, apple slices or jicama slices.
- Leftover spaghetti, chicken or pizza: serve hot or cold!

* Skim and I % milk are recommended for children over two years old. Children under two years of age should only drink whole milk.

Cereal Choices

Cereal with milk is the number-one breakfast favorite. Check the Nutrition Facts label — found on most packaged foods — for the amount of iron, other nutrients and fiber. Look at the % Daily Values to find how much.

If your child prefers a sweet taste, you might jazz up unsweetened cereal with sliced peaches or bananas, strawberries, or blueberries.

Active Play Is Important, Too!

Physical activity, along with proper nutrition, promotes lifelong health. Active play is the best exercise for kids! Parents can join their children and have fun while being active, too. Some fun activities for parents and kids to do together include playing on swings, riding tricycles or bicycles, jumping rope, flying a kite, making a snowman, swimming or dancing.

Lunches Worth Munchin'

Children who help make their own lunches are more likely to eat them. Include these brown bag perks to make lunches fun!
- Use cookie cutters to cut sandwiches in fun, interesting shapes.
- Decorate lunch bags with colorful stickers.

- Put a new twist on a sandwich favorite. Top peanut butter with raisins, bananas or apple slices.
- For color and crunch, use a variety of veggies as "sandwich toppers": cucumber slices, sprouts, grated carrots or zucchini.

Brown Bag Food Safety

Remember the golden rule for food safety:

Keep Hot Foods Hot and Cold Foods Cold.

When there's no refrigerator to store a bag lunch, keep food safe by:
- Tucking an ice- or freezer-pack into the lunch bag. Or use an insulated container to keep hot foods hot.
- Adding a box of frozen fruit juice.
- Freezing the sandwich bread and filling — or other freezable foods — the night before.

You may also help prevent food-borne illness by:
- Encouraging your child to wash his or her hands thoroughly before meals.

Did You Know That…

Most regular deli meats, such as salami and bologna, are very high in fat. Try reduced-fat deli meats. Turkey breast, ham and roast beef are usually lower-fat choices. Check the Nutrition Facts label on packaged meats to learn the fat content.

Pretzels, baked tortilla chips and baked potato chips are virtually fat-free and make a good alternative for potato chips and other high-fat snacks.

The Meal Dilemma… Dealing with Picky Eaters

Even the most nutritious meal won't do any good if a child refuses to eat it. Some youngsters are naturally finicky eaters. Others eat only certain foods — or refuse food — as a way to assert themselves. If your child refuses one food from a group, try offering a substitute from the same food group. Try these ideas to make your family meals happy ones:

If Your Child Refuses…	Instead Try…
Green vegetables	Deep-yellow or orange vegetables
Milk	Chocolate milk, cheese, yogurt
Beef	Chicken, turkey, fish, pork

- Boost the nutritional value of prepared dishes with extra ingredients. Perhaps add nonfat dry milk to cream soups, milkshakes and puddings. Or mix grated zucchini and carrots into quick breads, muffins, meatloaf, lasagna and soups.
- Serve a food your child enjoys along with a food that he or she has refused to eat in the past.
- Try serving a food again if it was refused before. It may take many tries before a child likes it.

- Let children help with food preparation. It can make eating a food more fun.
- Add eye appeal. Cut foods into interesting shapes. Or create a smiling face on top of a casserole with cheese, vegetables or fruit strips.
- Set a good example by eating well yourself. Whenever possible, eat meals as a family.

How Much Food Is Enough?

Some parents worry because young children seem to eat small amounts of food, especially when compared with adult portions. Don't worry about how little a child eats. A child who is growing well is getting enough to eat.

Hungry And In a Hurry? Food for Fast Times

When it comes to food, families want convenience. It's no surprise that fast-food restaurants are so popular. However, some fast foods supply a lot of fat and calories. These tips help you get the most from foods that are fast:

- Most fast foods can fit within a healthful eating plan. Children and adults can afford to eat these foods every once in a while if other food choices are sensible. Try these ways to enjoy them:

  Share: split an order of fries with other family members.

  Choose food-group foods: in combination meals, substitute fruit juice or skim or 1 % milk* for soft drinks.

  Balance high-fat choices with low-fat choices: order a small hamburger and the salad bar for your child. Kids like the fresh fruit, carrot sticks and broccoli florets.

- Most fast-food spots offer lower-fat choices: salad bar (low-fat dressing), plain baked potatoes (topped with salad bar veggies), chili, skim or 1 % milk*, low-fat frozen yogurt, English muffins, fruit juice and grilled (non-fried) chicken sandwiches.
- Supermarkets offer a variety of nutritious foods that are fast. Ready-made deli sandwiches (made with reduced-fat deli meats), fresh fruits and the salad bar are some "fast foods" from the grocery store.

* Children under two years of age should *only* drink whole milk.

Microwave Magic — Safely!

A microwave oven can help you cook in a healthful way. Vegetables cooked in a microwave oven stay nutrient-rich. For one reason, nutrients don't dissolve in any cooking water; short cooking time is another factor. Meat, fish and poultry dishes can be cooked or reheated with little or no added fat.

Microwaving also can help you cook faster and easier. But it can pose potential hazards — especially when children cook with the microwave oven. BURNS are the most common microwave injury. Children can be burned by:

- Removing dishes from the microwave oven — *make sure they use a pot holder.*
- Spilling hot foods — *keep the oven out of a young child's reach.*
- Opening microwave popcorn packages and other containers — *show older children how to open the container so steam escapes away from their hands and face.*
- Eating food that is cooked unevenly or has "hot spots" — *show older children how to stir food well before tasting it, or let food "rest" so that heat distributes evenly.*

Here's a common sense rule for microwave ovens: *If children are too young to read or follow written directions, they are too young to use a microwave oven without supervision.*

The information contained in this publication should not be used as a substitute for the medical care and advice of your pediatrician. There may be variations in treatment that your pediatrician may recommend based on individual facts and circumstances.

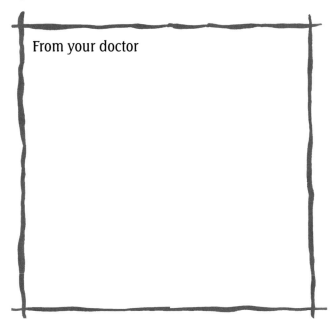

From your doctor

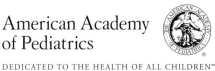

American Academy of Pediatrics

DEDICATED TO THE HEALTH OF ALL CHILDREN™

The American Academy of Pediatrics is an organization of 60,000 primary care pediatricians, pediatric medical subspecialists, and pediatric surgical specialists dedicated to the health, safety, and well-being of infants, children, adolescents, and young adults.

American Academy of Pediatrics
Web site—www.aap.org

Copyright © 1991
American Academy of Pediatrics, Updated 8/05

Sports and Your Child

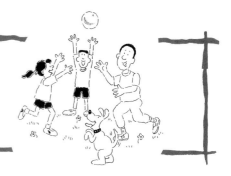

Whether on a court, in a pool, on a field, or in a gym, more American children than ever are competing in sports. Sports help boys and girls keep their bodies fit and feel good about themselves. However, there are some important issues that parents need to be aware of if their children participate in organized sports.

The following are answers to common questions parents have about sports and children. Talk with your pediatrician if you have other questions or concerns.

Q: At what age should my child get started in sports?

A: Before school age, children should stay physically active and healthy through unstructured "free play." For preschool-aged children, "sports" classes that emphasize fun are a great way to introduce athletics without competition. Most older children are ready for organized team sports when they are about 6 years of age. This is when they can follow directions and understand the concept of teamwork. Beginning around age 8, contact sports may be acceptable.

Keep in mind that all children are unique individuals. They grow and mature at different rates. Age, weight, and size shouldn't be the only measures used to decide if your child is ready to play a sport. Emotional development is also important. Children shouldn't be pushed into a sport or be placed in a competition they are not physically or emotionally ready to handle. Consider allowing your child to participate only if his interest is strong and you feel he can handle it. Remember, most children play sports to have fun.

Q: Should boys and girls play in sports together?

A: Until puberty, boys and girls can play sports together because they are usually about the same size and weight. After puberty, most boys are stronger and bigger than most girls. At that point, boys and girls should no longer compete against each other in most sports. However, if there is no team for girls in a certain sport, girls should be allowed to try out for a spot on the boys' team (in fact, it's the law in some states).

Q: What are the risks of injury?

A: All sports have a risk of injury; some more than others. In general, the more contact in a sport, the greater the risk of injury.

Most sports injuries involve the soft tissues of the body, not the bones. Only about 5% of sports injuries involve broken bones. However, the areas where bones grow in children are at more risk of injury during the rapid growth phase of puberty.

The main types of sports injuries are sprains (injuries to ligaments) and strains (injuries to muscles). Many injuries are caused by overuse. Overuse is when a child overdoes it (by pitching too many innings, for example). This places stress on the tendons, joints, bones, and muscles and can cause damage.

Q: How can the risk of injury be reduced?

A: The following are ways to help reduce the risk of injury:

- **Wear the right gear.** Players should wear the appropriate protective equipment such as pads (neck, shoulder, elbow, chest, knee, shin), helmets, mouthpieces, face guards, protective cups, and/or eyewear.
- **Increase flexibility.** Stretching exercises before and after games can help increase flexibility of muscles and ligaments used in play.
- **Strengthen muscles.** Conditioning exercises during practice and before games can help strengthen muscles used in play.
- **Use the proper technique.** Proper technique should be reinforced throughout the season of play.
- **Take breaks.** Rest periods are important during practice and games to reduce the risk of overuse injuries.
- **Play safe.** There should be strict rules against headfirst sliding (in baseball and softball), spearing (in football), and body checking (in ice hockey) to prevent serious head and spine injuries.
- **Stop the workout** if there is pain.
- **Avoid heat injury.** Heat injury or illness results from excessive exercise in high temperature and humidity. Rules for safe exercise in the heat include the following:
  —Drink plenty of proper fluids before, during, and after exercise or play.
  —Decrease or stop practices or competitions during periods when the combination of excessive heat and humidity approaches dangerous levels.
  —Wear lightweight clothing.

It's also important to make sure your child has a complete physical exam by your pediatrician before participating in any sport. Most organized sports teams require an exam before a child can play. These exams are not designed to stop children from participating, but to make sure they are in good health and can safely play the game.

Q: What if my child wants to quit?

A: Sometimes a child will lose interest in playing a sport, find another sport more interesting, or follow their friends to a new activity. If your child wants to quit, get as many facts as you can. Talk with your child to find out the reasons for quitting. There may be a simple reason, such as not getting along with a coach, or the frustration of being "benched" and never playing in any games. If this is the case, talk with your child's coach to try to solve the problem.

Base your decision on what your child says and what you see. While it may not be wise for your child to make a habit of quitting when things get tough, "sticking it out" may not be the answer.

Q: How can sports-related stress be prevented?

A: The main source of stress in sports is the pressure to win. Sadly, many coaches and parents place winning above everything else. Young athletes should be judged on effort and not just winning. They should be rewarded for trying hard and for improving their skills rather than punished or criticized for losing. Remember, children would rather play on a losing team than sit on the bench with a winning team.

Reduce stress in your child's sport with the following tips:

- **Look for positive programs.** Avoid placing your child in a "win at all costs" program or intensive programs for elite players that play 4 to 5 times each week.
- **Get to know the coaches.** Stay away from coaches who are abusive toward or overly demanding of any child.
- **Find a good fit.** Make sure your child plays with and against other children in the same age range and ability.
- **Get help.** Help your child improve her skills with extra practices, sports camps, or outside help.

    If your child is under too much stress, either from the sport or from other sources like school or home, withdrawing from the sport may be necessary. Signs of stress include loss of appetite, headache, or vomiting. Depression is also a sign of stress. The signs of depression include sleeping more often than usual and acting tired or withdrawn.

    Learning to cope with stress is an important part of growing up. In many ways, sports can help children cope with stress. This is one reason why pediatricians encourage children to play sports.

Q: Should bad grades keep a child from playing sports?

A: In most cases, the answer is no. A child having trouble in school still needs all the benefits of exercise, competition, and a sense of accomplishment. Sports may be the only place a child feels successful, and it could be harmful to take away a source of achievement.

    If your child is not doing well in school, make sure other things are not the cause, such as conflicts with a job, other duties, or too much TV. If you feel that your child is simply not studying enough, you may want to tell him he can only play if his grades improve. Ask your child what you can do to help him do better in school.

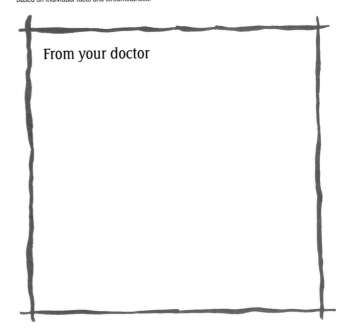

The information contained in this publication should not be used as a substitute for the medical care and advice of your pediatrician. There may be variations in treatment that your pediatrician may recommend based on individual facts and circumstances.

From your doctor

American Academy of Pediatrics

DEDICATED TO THE HEALTH OF ALL CHILDREN™

The American Academy of Pediatrics is an organization of 60,000 primary care pediatricians, pediatric medical subspecialists, and pediatric surgical specialists dedicated to the health, safety, and well-being of infants, children, adolescents, and young adults.

American Academy of Pediatrics
Web site—www.aap.org

Copyright © 2005
American Academy of Pediatrics, Updated 10/05

get fit, stay healthy

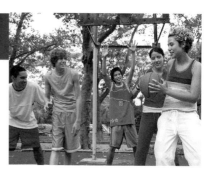

Being fit means you're in **good shape,** you have *energy,* you're active, and you don't get tired easily during the day. Most people who are fit also **feel pretty good** about themselves.

Any type of regular, physical activity can **improve your fitness and your health**—even walking, climbing up a flight of stairs, or mowing the lawn. The most important thing is that you keep moving!

Feel better, look better

There are a lot of **benefits** to being physically active. It can help

- **Keep you at a healthy weight.** This doesn't necessarily mean being thin. Everybody's ideal weight is different—it depends on your **height and body size.** Ask your pediatrician what the right weight is for you.
- **Prevent heart disease.** Heart disease is the leading cause of death in the United States. Research has shown that the risk factors for heart disease start during childhood. A lack of physical activity is one of the major risk factors of heart disease.
- **Strengthen your bones. Regular exercise keeps bones healthy** and can help prevent a bone disease called osteoporosis. This disease is common in older people and causes bones to break easily.
- **Reduce stress.** We all have stress, but learning to *cope* with it is an important way to stay healthy. Many things can cause stress like problems with parents or friends or the pressures of school. Major things like moving to a new home or breaking up with someone can also cause stress. Exercise can help you relax and helps your body handle stress.

Total fitness

To **be fit,** you might find it helpful to work on all aspects of fitness, including the following:

Aerobic endurance—This is how well your heart, lungs, and blood vessels provide oxygen and nutrients throughout your body. When you exercise, you **breathe harder** and your **heart beats faster.** This helps your body get the oxygen it needs. If you are not fit, your heart and lungs have to work extra hard, even to do everyday things like walking up the stairs.

Body fat—How much you weigh is not the only way to tell if you are overweight. It's actually determined by your body mass index (BMI), which includes your weight and height and gives an idea of *how much of your body weight comes from fat.* People who are overweight have more body fat in relation to the amount of bone and muscle in their bodies. Eating too much and not exercising enough can cause you to have too much body fat. Your risk of health problems like diabetes, cancer, high blood pressure, knee and back pain, and heart attacks is increased when you're overweight.

Muscle strength and endurance—This is the amount of work and the amount of time that your muscles are able to do a certain activity before they get tired. *The more fit you are, the longer you are able to play a sport,* work out, or do other activities before you have to stop.

Flexibility—This is how well you can move and stretch your joints, ligaments, and muscles through a full range of motion. For example, people with good flexibility can bend over and touch the floor easily. Poor flexibility may increase the risk of getting hurt during athletic and everyday activities.

What can I do to become more fit?

Just do it! Make the commitment and **stick to it.** Exercise should be a regular part of your day, like brushing your teeth, eating, and sleeping. It can be in gym class, joining a sports team, or working out on your own.

Stay positive and have fun. A **good mental attitude** is important. Find an activity that you think is fun. You are more likely to keep with it if you choose something you like. A lot of people find it's more fun to exercise with someone else, so see if you can find a friend or family member to be active with you.

Take it one step at a time. *Small changes can add up to better fitness.* For example, walk or *ride your bike to school* or to a friend's house instead of getting a ride. Get on or off the bus several blocks away and walk the rest of the way. Use the stairs instead of taking the elevator or escalator.

Get your heart pumping. Whatever you choose, make sure it includes aerobic activity that makes you breathe harder and increases your heart rate. This is the best type of exercise because **it increases your fitness level** and makes your heart and lungs work better. It also **burns off body fat.** Examples of aerobic activities are basketball, running, or swimming. (See the Fitness Activity Chart at the end of this brochure for more ideas.)

Don't forget to warm up with some easy exercises or mild stretching before you do any physical activity. This warms your muscles up and may help protect against injury. Stretching makes your muscles and joints *more flexible* too. It is also important to stretch out *after* you exercise to cool down your muscles.

How often should I exercise?

Your goal should be to do some type of exercise **every day.** It is best to do some kind of aerobic activity without stopping for at least **20 to 30 minutes** each time. Do the activity as often as possible, but don't exercise to the point of pain.

Like all things, *exercise can be overdone.* You may be exercising too much if

Is it safe to train with weights?

Strength training, also called "weight training" or "resistance training," is an activity in which you use free weights, weight machines, resistance bands, or even your own weight to increase **muscle strength** and muscle endurance. The goal is **not to bulk up,** but to build strength and coordination. Do not focus on how much weight you are lifting, but rather on doing the exercises slowly and safely. When done correctly, this can be a great way to increase your strength and fitness.

Start with light weights and use smooth, controlled motions. Increase the number of times you lift the weight (repetitions) gradually. Avoid strength training more than 3 times per week and make sure you have *a day of rest in between* each workout. Too much weight training can be harmful and there are no extra benefits to strength training more often.

Safety measures should be taken during strength training. Most strength training injuries happen when exercises are not done correctly, when too much weight is lifted, or when there is no adult supervision.

Weight training isn't the same as weight lifting, power lifting, and body building. Avoid these activities until your body has reached full adult development (usually after the age of 18) because these sports can result in serious injury. Ask your pediatrician when it is a good time for you to start.

- Your **weight falls** below what is normal for your age, height, and build.
- It starts to get in the way of school and your other activities.
- You start to have bone, joint, or muscle *pain* that affects your daily activities.
- You are a **girl** and your periods become irregular, sporadic, or stop completely.

If you notice any of these signs, **talk with your parents or pediatrician** before health problems occur.

A healthy lifestyle

In addition to exercise, making **just a few other changes** in your life can help keep you healthy, such as

- Watch less TV or spend less time playing computer or video games. (Use this time to exercise instead!) Or exercise while watching TV (for example, sit on the floor and do sit-ups and stretches; use hand weights; or use a stationary bike, treadmill, or stair climber).

- Eat 3 **healthy meals** a day, including at least 4 servings of *fruits,* 5 servings of *vegetables,* and 4 servings of *dairy products.*
- Make sure you **drink plenty of fluids** before, during, and after any exercise (water is best but flavored sports drinks can be used if they do not contain a lot of sugar). This will help replace what you lose when you sweat.
- Stop drinking or drink fewer regular soft drinks.
- Eat less junk food and fast food. (They're often full of fat, cholesterol, salt, and sugar.)
- Get 9 to 10 hours of **sleep** every night.
- **Don't** *smoke* cigarettes, *drink* alcohol, or *do* drugs.

Fitness Activity Chart

Activity	Calories Burned During 10 Minutes of Continuous Activity	
	77-lb Person	132-lb Person
Basketball (game)	60	102
Cross Country Skiing	23	72
Biking (9.3 mph)	36	60
Judo	69	118
Running (5 mph)	60	90
Sitting (complete rest)	9	12
Soccer (game)	63	108
Swimming (33 yd)		
Breaststroke	34	58
Freestyle	43	74
Tennis	39	66
Volleyball (game)	35	60
Walking		
2.5 mph	23	34
3.7 mph	30	43

Modified from Bar-Or O. *Pediatric Sports Medicine for the Practitioner.* New York, NY: Springer-Verlag; 1983: 349–350

Ferguson JM. *Habits, Not Diets.* Palo Alto, CA: Bull Publishing Co; 1988

From your doctor

American Academy of Pediatrics

DEDICATED TO THE HEALTH OF ALL CHILDREN™

The American Academy of Pediatrics is an organization of 60,000 primary care pediatricians, pediatric medical subspecialists, and pediatric surgical specialists dedicated to the health, safety, and well-being of infants, children, adolescents, and young adults.

American Academy of Pediatrics
Web site—www.aap.org

Copyright © 2006
American Academy of Pediatrics, Updated 3/06

SECTION FIVE

Safety and Prevention

Air Bag Safety

An air bag can save your life. However, air bags and young children do not mix. The following information will help keep you and your children safe:

- The safest place for *all* infants and children younger than 13 years to ride is in the back seat.
- *Never* put an infant in the front seat of a car, truck, SUV, or van with a passenger air bag.

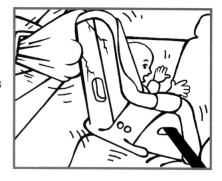

- Infants must always ride in rear-facing car safety seats in the back seat until they are at least 20 pounds AND at least 1 year of age. The American Academy of Pediatrics recommends that infants ride rear-facing until they reach the maximum weight and height allowed by the manufacturer for use of the car safety seat.
- All children should be properly secured in car safety seats, belt positioning booster seats, or the shoulder/lap belts correct for their size.
- Seat belts must be worn correctly at all times by all passengers who have outgrown booster seats and fit shoulder/lap belts properly to provide the best protection.
- Side air bags improve safety for adults in side impact crashes, but children who are not properly restrained and are seated near a side air bag may be at risk for serious injury. Check your vehicle owner's manual to see what it says about children and side air bags.
- You may have heard recently about new "advanced" air bags. These make travel safer for adults, but it is not yet known how they will affect the safety of children. Even though these new air bags may be safer, the back seat is still the safest place for children younger than 13 years to ride.

What Parents Can Do

- Eliminate potential risks of air bags to children by buckling them in the *back* seat for every ride.
- Plan ahead so that you do not have to drive with more children than can be safely restrained in the back seat.

- For most families, installation of air bag on/off switches is not necessary. Air bags that are turned off provide no protection to older children, teens, parents, or other adults riding in the front seat.
- Air bag on/off switches should only be used if your child has special health care needs for which, your pediatrician recommends constant observation during travel and no other adult is available to ride in the back seat with your child.
- If no other arrangement is possible and an older child *must* ride in the front seat, move the vehicle seat back as far as it can go, away from the air bag. Be sure the child is restrained properly for his size. Keep in mind that your child may still be at risk for

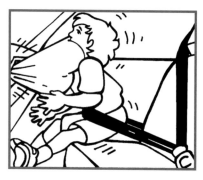

injuries from the air bag. The back seat is the safest place for children to ride.

The information contained in this publication should not be used as a substitute for the medical care and advice of your pediatrician. There may be variations in treatment that your pediatrician may recommend based on individual facts and circumstances.

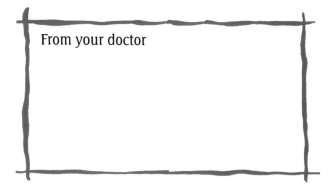

From your doctor

American Academy of Pediatrics

DEDICATED TO THE HEALTH OF ALL CHILDREN™

The American Academy of Pediatrics is an organization of 60,000 primary care pediatricians, pediatric medical subspecialists, and pediatric surgical specialists dedicated to the health, safety, and well-being of infants, children, adolescents, and young adults.

American Academy of Pediatrics
Web site — www.aap.org

Copyright © 1996
American Academy of Pediatrics, Updated 12/03

Anesthesia and Your Child

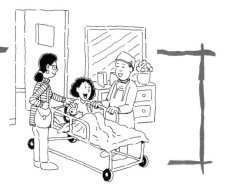

Any time a child requires a hospital visit, it can cause anxiety—for both parent and child. This especially may be the case when the visit involves any type of procedure that might require anesthesia. Examples of such procedures are surgery, some types of x-rays, and certain tests to examine the stomach or intestines.

The purpose of anesthesia is to enable your child's surgery, medical test, or treatment to occur without pain, memory, or movement.

Your child's comfort and safety are very important. The person(s) providing your child's anesthesia will monitor heart rate, blood pressure, breathing, temperature, and the oxygen level in the blood before, during, and after anesthesia. Your child's unique needs, the procedure involved, and your child's health will help determine the type of anesthesia.

Most anesthesia providers work as a team. Anesthesiologists (doctors), residents (doctors-in-training), certified registered nurse anesthetists (CRNAs), physician's assistants, and nurses may all be part of this team.

Preparing for anesthesia

Before having anesthesia, your child will need a physical examination. At this time, either your pediatrician or a member of the anesthesia care team will review your child's current health and medical history. You will answer questions about your child's health. This may take place on the day of the surgery, test, or treatment, or in the days just before it occurs.

It is important to tell the doctor about any of the following that apply to your child:

- Allergies, including allergies to food, drugs, or latex (rubber).
- All medications that your child is taking, including herbal or natural types and inhaled (breathed in) medications.
- Breathing problems, including asthma, croup or wheezing, snoring, and apnea (periods when breath is held during sleep).
- Any recent illnesses, especially bad colds.
- Any problems that your child had as a newborn, such as premature birth, breathing problems such as croup or asthma, or birth defects.
- Heart problems, including holes between the heart chambers, valve problems, heart murmurs, or irregular heartbeats.
- Any other medical problems that your child has or has had, especially if they required visits to a doctor or a stay in the hospital.
- Any previous surgery or procedure using anesthesia.
- Previous problems with anesthesia or surgery, such as airway problems, problems going to sleep or waking up from anesthesia, or problems with nausea and vomiting after surgery.
- Any family history (both sides of the family) of problems with anesthesia.
- Family history of bleeding problems.
- Whether your child or anyone in the household smokes.
- If your child has any loose teeth. (Sometimes loose teeth must be removed for your child's safety.)
- Whether your child may be pregnant.

Your child may need blood tests prior to anesthesia. Other tests, such as x-rays, are needed sometimes. Most of the time few, if any, tests are required.

What is a pediatric anesthesiologist?

A *Pediatric Anesthesiologist* has the experience and training to help ensure a successful surgery, test, or treatment for your child.

A pediatric anesthesiologist is a fully trained anesthesiologist who has completed at least 1 year of specialized training in anesthesia care of infants and children. Most pediatric surgeons deliver care to children in the operating room along with a pediatric anesthesiologist. Many children who need surgery have complex medical problems that affect many parts of the body. The pediatric anesthesiologist has special training and experience to evaluate these complex problems and to plan a safe anesthetic for each child.

What are the risks of anesthesia for my child?

Minor side effects of anesthesia, such as a sore throat, nausea, and vomiting, are common. Major problems are rare. Ask the anesthesiologist to explain the specific risks for your child.

What do I tell my child about anesthesia?

Begin talking about the hospital visit 5 to 6 days in advance for older children, and 2 or 3 days ahead for toddlers. Be honest with your child. Depending on your child's age, use familiar words such as "sore" for pain or "taking a nap" for being put under anesthesia.

Explain that the sleep from anesthesia is different from sleep at home. During anesthesia a person does not feel pain. Your child will not wake up in the middle of the procedure. At the end of the surgery, test, or treatment, the anesthesiologist will take away the medicine that provides this type of "sleep" and your child will awaken and return to his family.

Children between the ages of 3 and 12 may not be ready to hear about the risks of surgery or anesthesia. Often, they understand enough to be scared, but not enough to be reassured. Your anesthesiologist may want to tell you about the risks when your child is not present.

If your child becomes worried when you talk about what anesthesia will be like, explain that it is OK to be scared. Point out that the anesthesia care team will work hard to make your child feel safe and comfortable. You can help keep your child's fears to a minimum by being calm and reassuring.

Some hospitals offer special programs that explain the anesthesia and surgery process to children and families. Ask for books and videotapes that can help you prepare your child and yourself.

What if my child gets sick just before the scheduled time?

Call your anesthesia care team and your doctor if your child becomes ill near the time scheduled for the procedure. If your child develops a cold or other illness, the surgery, test, or treatment may have to be rescheduled because the risk of added problems may increase. If your child is exposed to chickenpox within 3 weeks of the procedure, it may be rescheduled because of the risk to other patients. Your child may be able to spread chickenpox before skin spots develop.

The day of the procedure

Can my child eat, drink, or take medicine on the day of anesthesia?

Except for emergencies, your child's stomach should be empty when anesthesia is started. This helps to prevent vomiting, which may cause food or stomach acid to get into the lungs. It is important to check with your surgeon or anesthesiologist prior to your child's anesthesia for specific guidelines for your child. The following are general recommendations:

Infants younger than 1 year of age may have
- Solid food until 8 hours before anesthesia (NOTE: baby food and cereal are solid foods)
- Infant formula until 6 hours before anesthesia
- Breast milk until 4 hours before anesthesia
- Clear liquids until 2 to 4 hours before anesthesia

Children of all ages may have
- Solid food until 8 hours before anesthesia (NOTE: baby food and cereal are solid foods). In general, no solid foods are allowed after a certain time the evening before anesthesia.
- Clear liquids (eg, apple juice, clear soda, Popsicles, or a prepared electrolyte solution) until 2 hours before anesthesia (NOTE: orange juice with pulp, milk, and baby formula **are not** clear liquids).

Remember, each health care facility has its own guidelines for eating and drinking prior to anesthesia. Check with your anesthesia care team to learn the instructions for your child. Failing to follow your health care facility's guidelines may result in the delay of your child's procedure.

In addition, ask your anesthesiologist which, if any, of your child's routine medications may be taken on the day of anesthesia. Some medications may be given on the morning of anesthesia with small sips of water, but not mixed with solids such as applesauce. However, other medications, including herbal and natural types, may interact with drugs used for anesthesia and must be stopped prior to anesthesia.

On the morning that your child is to receive anesthesia

- Be sure to follow the fasting (not eating) instructions.
- Dress your child in loose-fitting, comfortable clothes.
- Give any medications (that your anesthesiologist has approved) with a sip of water.
- Bring a favorite comfort object such as a blanket, stuffed animal, or toy.
- Be a calm and reassuring parent for your child.

What will my child do while waiting for anesthesia?

Most large hospitals have a special waiting area with space and toys for play. If you have not done so already, you will meet the anesthesia care team at this time. They will review your child's records, briefly examine your child, tell you how they will keep your child safe, discuss the risks, and answer any remaining questions or concerns.

Will my child be worried?

A calm and supportive family can provide the most help in ensuring that your child will not be overly worried or upset. As mentioned, a special blanket, stuffed animal, or toy also may provide comfort.

Often, sedatives (medications to help your child relax) are given before the start of anesthesia to help reduce fear and worry. The choice of whether to provide a sedative will depend on your child's age, level of anxiety, medical condition, and your hospital's practices. Sedatives may be given through the mouth, nose, or rectum (the anal opening), or as an injection.

How will anesthesia be given to my child?

Most children get to choose one of the following ways for anesthesia to be started:
- By breathing anesthetic gases through a mask
- Through a needle that is put into a vein (IV)
- Through a needle that is put into a muscle (an injection)

When a mask is used, there is no need for shots and no pain is involved. However, some children do not like having masks placed on their faces. An injection can be briefly painful and frightening to a child. However, it is quick and does not require your child to remain still. If an IV is used, the use of local anesthetic (numbing medicine) at the IV site will make this less painful.

If a mask will be used to start anesthesia, talk to your child about this before the day of the surgery, test, or treatment. Explain that the mask contains special air that helps children feel sleepy. The mask may be treated with a special smell to make the process more comfortable. This method may not be used in certain cases, such as for some emergencies, in the case of stomach or bowel problems, or if your child has eaten recently.

Once a child reaches about 10 years of age, anesthesia usually is started by IV. No matter how anesthesia is started, your child will be kept comfortable and asleep with a combination of gas and IV anesthetics. Your child will not awaken during the surgery, test, or treatment. She will awaken once the procedure is completed, unless there is a need for intensive care at that time. If your child needs this type of care, your anesthesiologist will explain this to you.

Can I be with my child when anesthesia is started?

Some hospitals allow 1 support person (usually a parent) to go with the child into the operating room or other area where your child is to receive anesthesia. Check on the policy at your hospital ahead of time. Your child's anesthesiologist will make the final decision.

Many anesthesiologists feel that giving children sedatives makes separation much easier and that parents do not need to be present. Whatever the decision, remember that the anesthesia care team has a lot of experience with helping children stay calm during these moments.

If you are able to be present for the start of anesthesia, ask the anesthesiologist beforehand what you should expect to see and how your child might react. Understanding what is to happen will make you feel more comfortable.

It is important to realize that even if you are allowed to be with your child for the start of anesthesia, it is no guarantee that your child will not get upset before going to sleep. This depends on your child's age, temperament, and past experiences.

After the procedure

Where will my child go after the procedure?

Your child will go to a recovery room or an intensive care unit, depending on the type of surgery, test, or treatment, and your child's medical condition. Usually, parents are allowed to be present once their child is admitted to these areas and the child's condition is stable. After a routine procedure, the recovery stay is usually 30 minutes to 2 hours. Then your child may go to a regular hospital bed or a short-stay unit, or be discharged and able to go home.

How will my child behave after the procedure?

Children come out of anesthesia in different ways. Some are alert and calm right away. Others may remain groggy for a longer period of time. Infants and toddlers may be irritable until the effects of the anesthesia have worn off. If this is the case, your child may need more sedative medication while "sleeping off" the remaining effects of anesthesia.

Will my child feel pain?

One of the main goals of anesthesia is to prevent pain during and after the procedure. If your child is in pain in the recovery room, he may get more pain medicine. Pain medication comes in many different forms and can be given in many different ways. Your child's doctors will discuss the options with you and your child ahead of time.

Will nausea and vomiting be a problem?

Nausea and vomiting are very common after anesthesia and may be due to your child's condition, the procedure, or the side effects of anesthesia. If your child is vomiting a lot, she may need to stay in the hospital longer. Sometimes an unplanned overnight stay in the hospital is needed. There are medications that can be given to your child during or after anesthesia to reduce the chance that this will be a problem.

Discuss your questions or concerns with your anesthesia care team and your pediatrician or other doctor(s) who are involved. These health care professionals are trained to ensure your child's comfort and safety throughout the process.

You can reach someone from your anesthesia care team at

_____ .

Be sure to keep your anesthesia care team informed about your child's health just before the procedure. Call this number and/or the doctor who is performing the procedure if your child develops a cold or other illness or has been exposed to chickenpox within 3 weeks of the procedure.

The information contained in this publication should not be used as a substitute for the medical care and advice of your pediatrician. There may be variations in treatment that your pediatrician may recommend based on individual facts and circumstances.

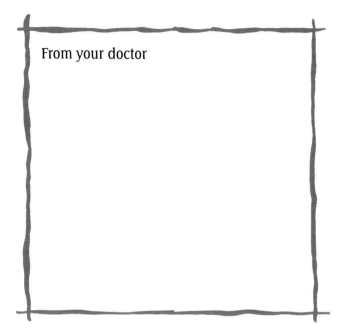

From your doctor

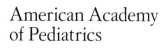

American Academy
of Pediatrics

DEDICATED TO THE HEALTH OF ALL CHILDREN™

The American Academy of Pediatrics is an organization of 60,000 primary care pediatricians, pediatric medical subspecialists, and pediatric surgical specialists dedicated to the health, safety, and well-being of infants, children, adolescents, and young adults.

American Academy of Pediatrics
Web site — www.aap.org

Antibiotics and Your Child

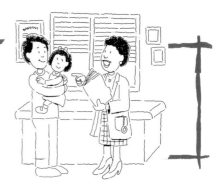

Is an antibiotic the right treatment for your child? That depends. Antibiotics are powerful medicines, but they don't always work. First, your pediatrician will need to find out what's making your child sick. It's important that antibiotics are taken only if needed and just as your pediatrician tells you. When antibiotics aren't used the right way, they can do more harm than good.

The following are answers to common questions about the use of antibiotics. Talk with your pediatrician if you have other questions or concerns.

Q: When do antibiotics work?

A: Antibiotics only work for infections caused by certain bacteria. They don't work on viruses.

Bacteria cause many ear infections, some sinus infections, and pneumonia. They also cause strep throat and urinary tract and skin infections. Keep in mind that all prescribed doses of an antibiotic should be finished. If your child stops taking the medicine too soon, the infection could start again.

Viruses cause all colds and flu, most coughs, and most sore throats. There's no medicine to cure infections caused by viruses. However, you can help your child feel better while the illness runs its course. Your pediatrician may suggest ways you can ease the symptoms.

Q: When are antibiotics harmful?

A: Antibiotics can kill or slow down certain bacteria from growing, but each time they're used there's a chance that resistant bacteria will develop. These resistant bacteria are more likely to cause your child's next infection and may make it harder to treat your child the next time. A few bacterial infections have already become resistant to many antibiotics and are untreatable. There's a growing concern that more bacterial infections will become untreatable by commonly prescribed antibiotics.

Q: What are resistant bacteria?

A: Resistant bacteria are bacteria that are no longer killed by most antibiotics. Repeated use and misuse of antibiotics are some of the main causes of the increase in resistant bacteria. These resistant bacteria can also be spread to other children and adults.

Q: Can resistant bacteria be treated?

A: Some resistant bacteria can be treated with stronger medicines. These medicines may need to be given by vein (IV) in the hospital. To lower your child's risk of infection caused by resistant bacteria, use antibiotics only when they are needed.

Using antibiotics safely

Keep the following in mind if your child gets sick:

- **Antibiotics aren't always the answer when your child is sick.** Ask your pediatrician what the best treatment is for your child.
- **Antibiotics only treat bacterial infections.** They don't work on colds and flu.
- **Finish all prescribed doses of an antibiotic.** If your child feels better and stops the medicine too soon, the infection could return.
- **Throw away unused antibiotics.** Never save antibiotics for later use.

Q. What are the side effects?

A: Side effects may include nausea, diarrhea, and stomach pain. Some people may have an allergic reaction that causes a rash, itching, or hives. In severe cases, some people may have trouble breathing. Some antibiotics kill "good" bacteria that help our bodies. When this happens the helpful bacteria are replaced by bacteria and yeast that can cause diarrhea or skin or mouth infections. Always let your pediatrician know if your child has any side effects.

Q: What if my child has an ear infection and is in pain?

A: Despite what you may think, antibiotics may not help your child's ear infection. One reason is that bacteria don't cause all ear infections. Your pediatrician will decide what the best treatment is for your child. Some children with a low fever and mild symptoms may be observed without antibiotics; some children with bacterial infections may not be given antibiotics right away. Because pain is often the first and most uncomfortable symptom of ear infection, it's important to help comfort your child by giving her pain medicine. In most cases, your child will feel better after the first 1 to 2 days.

Acetaminophen and ibuprofen are over-the-counter pain medicines that may help lessen much of the pain. Be sure to use the right dose for your child's age and size. There are also eardrops that may help ear pain for a short time. Ask your pediatrician whether these drops should be used. Over-the-counter cold medicines (decongestants and antihistamines) don't help clear up ear infections.

Q: If some viral infections lead to bacterial infections, why doesn't my pediatrician prescribe antibiotics?

A: **Most viral infections in children don't develop into bacterial infections.** Treating viral infections with antibiotics may occasionally lead to an infection caused by resistant bacteria instead of stopping an infection. Let your pediatrician know if the illness gets worse or lasts a long time so that the right treatment can be given as needed.

Q: Doesn't yellow or green mucus mean that my child has a bacterial infection?

A: **No, it's normal for the mucus to change from clear to yellow or green.** Mucus gets thick and changes color during a viral cold as part of the normal healing process.

The information contained in this publication should not be used as a substitute for the medical care and advice of your pediatrician. There may be variations in treatment that your pediatrician may recommend based on individual facts and circumstances.

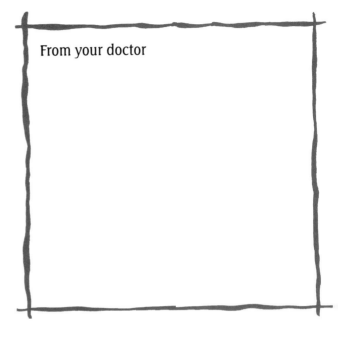

From your doctor

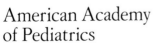

Safety of Blood Transfusions

Part I: About Blood and Blood Transfusions

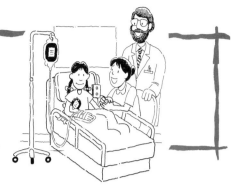

Because of illness or injury, some children need to receive transfusions of blood and blood products. This procedure can be frightening for parents and their children. Many parents also are concerned about the safety of transfusions. While the blood supply in the United States is considered very safe, parents should know a few things about blood transfusions and the safety of blood products for children.

A quick lesson about blood

The blood in our bodies does many important things. It carries oxygen and nutrients to all of our body's tissues. It helps remove carbon dioxide and other wastes from our body. It helps fight against infections and heal wounds and provides all the substances that are necessary for blood to clot.

Human blood is made up of several parts often called components. Each component has a specific job.

- **Red blood cells** carry oxygen from the lungs to all the tissues of the body and carry carbon dioxide from tissues back to the lungs.
- **White blood cells** attack bacteria and other germs and help the body prevent infections.
- **Platelets** control bleeding by starting the process by which blood clots.
- **Plasma** carries the red and white blood cells and platelets throughout the body. Plasma is made up of water, nutrients, and proteins, including those that interact and combine to form clots.

Techniques now exist in blood banks to separate these components and transfuse them separately.

Blood types

There are many different types of blood. The four major blood types (A, B, AB, and O) are classified by the presence of certain sugars ("A" or "B" substance) on the surface of the red blood cells.

Blood Type	Description
A	"A" substance is present.
B	"B" substance is present.
AB	Both "A" and "B" substances are present.
O	Neither "A" or "B" substance is present.

Anyone can receive type O blood with the plasma removed. That is why people with type O blood are called "universal donors." People who have AB blood can receive blood that is type A, B, or O. That is why they are called "universal recipients." When the transfusion is not an emergency, transfusion services try to provide people with blood matched to their type.

The blood type as usually reported by a laboratory also contains information about the Rh factor. This has to do with another substance on the surface of red blood cells called "Rh" substance. The presence or absence of "Rh" substance classifies the blood as positive or negative. For example, "O positive" blood is blood type O with Rh factor; "O negative" blood is blood type O without Rh factor.

It is important to know what type of blood a patient has because mixing different blood types can lead to serious medical problems. That is why blood is tested for its type and presence of Rh factor before a blood transfusion can take place.

Who needs blood transfusions?

One out of every 10 people admitted to a hospital needs a blood transfusion. A blood transfusion occurs when a patient receives whole blood components from another person (a donor). Patients with certain medical problems may require blood transfusions, such as

- Victims of car crashes or other severe injuries
- Victims of burns
- Patients with cancer
- Patients with transplants
- Patients who have had heart surgery
- Patients with hemoglobin disorders (eg, sickle cell disease)
- Patients with bleeding disorders (eg, hemophilia)
- Patients with severe anemia
- Patients with life-threatening infections and few white blood cells

Are blood transfusions safe?

Stories in the news of people becoming infected with various diseases from contaminated blood may lead parents to fear and question the safety of blood transfusions. While there have been cases of patients receiving contaminated blood, the risk of this actually is very low. In the United States, all blood donors are screened (eg, health history, sexual practice, travel, drug use) and the blood products they donate are carefully checked for a wide variety of infectious agents (germs) that could be spread through transfusions. These include

- Human immunodeficiency virus (HIV), the virus that causes acquired immunodeficiency syndrome (AIDS)
- Human T-lymphotropic virus (HTLV), a virus associated with a rare form of leukemia

- Syphilis
- Hepatitis B
- Hepatitis C

If a donor is considered to be at significant risk for having a transmissible infection, the donor is not accepted. If a unit of blood is found to be unsafe, it is destroyed. The donor is then contacted and advised not to donate blood in the future.

The information contained in this publication should not be used as a substitute for the medical care and advice of your pediatrician. There may be variations in treatment that your pediatrician may recommend based on individual facts and circumstances.

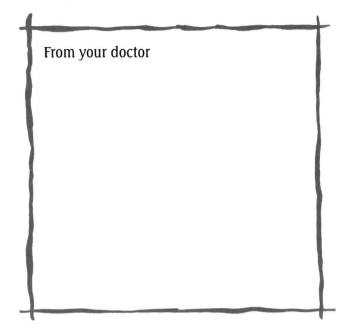

From your doctor

American Academy of Pediatrics

DEDICATED TO THE HEALTH OF ALL CHILDREN™

The American Academy of Pediatrics is an organization of 60,000 primary care pediatricians, pediatric medical subspecialists, and pediatric surgical specialists dedicated to the health, safety, and well-being of infants, children, adolescents, and young adults.

American Academy of Pediatrics
Web site — www.aap.org

Copyright © 2003
American Academy of Pediatrics

Safety of Blood Transfusions

Part II: Blood Transfusion Options and Procedures

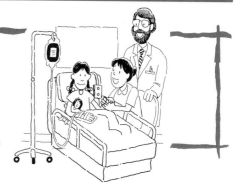

Where can the blood come from?

If your child needs a blood transfusion, you may be able to choose where the blood comes from. See "Blood Transfusion Options" below.

What you should know before giving consent

All medical procedures have risks. As mentioned, the risks of receiving blood or blood products may include disease transmission and allergic reactions. Before your child receives a transfusion of blood or blood products, you will be asked to give your permission or consent. To do this, you need to have as much information as possible. Ask as many questions as you need and make sure you understand the following:

- Your child's condition and why he needs a transfusion
- Other treatments besides a transfusion and their risks and benefits
- What will happen if you choose not to permit the transfusion

In an emergency, it may be difficult for you to understand everything the doctor is telling you. Ask questions until you understand what is happening to your child. Keep in mind that the doctor who is treating your child may not be able to predict all possible risks and cannot give you any guarantees. In an emergency, there may not be time to discuss why your child needs a transfusion. However, the reasons for the transfusion should be fully explained to you when your child is recovering.

How are transfusions done?

If your child is old enough to understand, try to prepare her for the procedure by going over what will happen.

- Before the transfusion begins, a small amount of your child's blood will be tested to identify its type and to make sure it matches the donor. This is done by inserting a needle into a vein in your child's arm (this should only sting for a few seconds) and withdrawing the blood into a test tube to be used by the laboratory.
- Next, a sterile, single-use plastic tube (catheter) or steel needle (butterfly) will be placed into a vein in your child's arm and taped in place.
- The nurse will make sure the blood is the correct blood for your child. You may be asked to identify your child.
- A plastic bag holding the blood or blood product will then be hung on a pole next to your child's hospital bed.
- Finally, a plastic tube will be attached from the bag to the tube or needle in your child's arm. The transfusion begins when the contents of the bag start to flow.

Blood Transfusion Options

Option	Description	Advantages	Disadvantages
Autologous transfusion	A patient donates his or her own blood before surgery to be used if needed.	No risk of disease transmission or allergic reactions.	Not suitable for children younger than 9 or 10 years. Cannot be used for emergency surgery because the donation must be planned in advance. May not be possible for patients with certain medical conditions.
Blood recycling	Blood lost during surgery is collected, cleaned, and returned to the patient.	No risk of disease transmission or allergic reactions.	Cannot be used for emergency surgery because the recycling process must be planned in advance. May not be possible for patients with certain medical conditions.
Directed donation	Patients choose their own blood donors. For example, parents can donate blood to their children.	Patients feel safer by selecting their own donors.	Blood types must be the same or compatible. Still has a risk of disease transmission and allergic reactions. Must be planned in advance. Some hospitals do not allow this type of donation.
Random donor blood	Volunteer blood donors.	Readily available; screened for diseases.	Blood types must be the same or compatible. Small risk of disease transmission and allergic reactions.

Blood alternatives

Some alternatives to human blood and blood products have been developed. For example, children with hemophilia now can be given highly purified clotting factors or factors made without human protein in the laboratory by what are called "recombinant DNA techniques." The recombinant factors are virtually 100% free of germs that can be transferred from a donor to a transfusion recipient. There also are hormones or growth factors available that cause the body to increase blood cell production. When time permits, treatment with one of these may eliminate the need for a transfusion.

Research is being carried out in a number of laboratories on several red blood cell substitutes. Such substitutes would eliminate the need for donors of red blood cells and make transfusions simpler and safer.

Investigators are making progress in this area and hope that someday an effective, safe alternative to human blood for transfusions will be available.

Once the transfusion begins, your child should not feel any pain. If she complains of pain or a burning sensation, becomes itchy, or feels anxious, let the nurse know. Because the blood has been refrigerated, your child may feel cold after a few minutes. Ask the nurse for a blanket if your child gets uncomfortably cold.

Most transfusions take 1 to 4 hours. However, if your child requires more than 1 unit of blood or requires another blood product, the transfusion could last longer. When the transfusion is over, the nurse will remove the tube or needle from your child's arm and cover the opening in the vein with a bandage.

Remember

If your child needs to receive blood or blood products, talk with your pediatrician about any concerns or fears you have about the procedure. If necessary, seek out a specialist in transfusion medicine (usually a clinical pathologist affiliated with a hospital blood bank). Learn all you can about your child's condition and make sure you understand the benefits and risks of receiving blood or blood products.

The information contained in this publication should not be used as a substitute for the medical care and advice of your pediatrician. There may be variations in treatment that your pediatrician may recommend based on individual facts and circumstances.

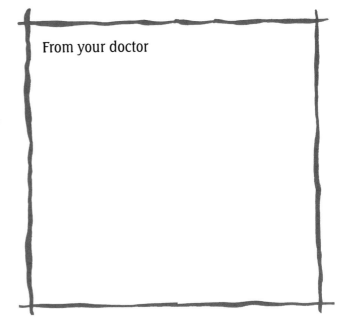

From your doctor

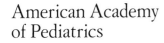

American Academy
of Pediatrics

DEDICATED TO THE HEALTH OF ALL CHILDREN™

The American Academy of Pediatrics is an organization of 60,000 primary care pediatricians, pediatric medical subspecialists, and pediatric surgical specialists dedicated to the health, safety, and well-being of infants, children, adolescents, and young adults.

American Academy of Pediatrics
Web site — www.aap.org

Copyright © 2003
American Academy of Pediatrics

Choking Prevention and First Aid for Infants and Children

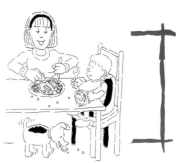

When children begin crawling, or eating table foods, parents must be aware of the dangers and risks of choking. Children younger than 5 years can easily choke on food and small objects.

Choking occurs when food or small objects get caught in the throat and block the airway. This can prevent oxygen from getting to the lungs and the brain. When the brain goes without oxygen for more than 4 minutes, brain damage or even death may occur. Many children die from choking each year. Most children who choke to death are younger than 5 years. Two thirds of choking victims are infants younger than 1 year.

Balloons, balls, marbles, pieces of toys, and foods cause the most choking deaths.

Read more about choking prevention and first aid.

Dangerous foods

Do not feed children younger than 4 years round, firm food unless it is chopped completely. Round, firm foods are common choking dangers. When infants and young children do not grind or chew their food well, they may try to swallow it whole. The following foods can be choking hazards:

- Hot dogs
- Nuts and seeds
- Chunks of meat or cheese
- Whole grapes
- Hard, gooey, or sticky candy
- Popcorn
- Chunks of peanut butter
- Raw vegetables
- Fruit chunks, such as apple chunks
- Chewing gum

Dangerous household items

Keep the following household items away from infants and children:

- Balloons
- Coins
- Marbles
- Toys with small parts
- Toys that can be squeezed to fit entirely into a child's mouth
- Small balls
- Pen or marker caps
- Small button-type batteries
- Medicine syringes

What you can do to prevent choking

- *Learn CPR (cardiopulmonary resuscitation)* (basic life support).
- *Be aware that balloons pose a choking risk* to children up to 8 years of age.
- *Keep the above foods from children* until 4 years of age.
- *Insist that children eat at the table,* or at least while sitting down. They should never run, walk, play, or lie down with food in their mouths.
- *Cut food for infants and young children* into pieces no larger than one-half inch, and teach them to chew their food well.
- *Supervise mealtime* for infants and young children.
- *Be aware of older children's actions.* Many choking incidents occur when older brothers or sisters give dangerous foods, toys, or small objects to a younger child.
- *Avoid toys with small parts,* and keep other small household items out of the reach of infants and young children.
- *Follow the age recommendations on toy packages.* Age guidelines reflect the safety of a toy based on any possible choking hazard as well as the child's physical and mental abilities at various ages.
- *Check under furniture and between cushions* for small items that children could find and put in their mouths.
- *Do not let infants and young children play with coins.*

First aid for the child who is choking

Make a point to learn the instructions on the reverse side of this brochure. Post the chart in your home. However, these instructions should *not* take the place of an approved class in basic first aid, CPR, or emergency prevention. Contact your local American Red Cross office or the American Heart Association to find out about classes offered in your area. Most of the classes teach basic first aid, CPR, and emergency prevention along with what to do for a choking infant or child. Your pediatrician also can help you understand these steps and talk to you about the importance of supervising mealtime and identifying dangerous foods and objects.

From your doctor

American Academy of Pediatrics

DEDICATED TO THE HEALTH OF ALL CHILDREN™

The American Academy of Pediatrics is an organization of 60,000 primary care pediatricians, pediatric medical subspecialists, and pediatric surgical specialists dedicated to the health, safety, and well-being of infants, children, adolescents, and young adults.
American Academy of Pediatrics
Web site — www.aap.org

Copyright ©2006
American Academy of Pediatrics, Updated 4/06

CHOKING/CPR

LEARN AND PRACTICE CPR (CARDIOPULMONARY RESUSCITATION)

IF ALONE WITH A CHILD WHO IS CHOKING...

1. SHOUT FOR HELP.   2. START RESCUE EFFORTS.   3. CALL 911 OR YOUR LOCAL EMERGENCY NUMBER.

YOU SHOULD START FIRST AID FOR CHOKING IF...	DO NOT START FIRST AID FOR CHOKING IF...
• The child cannot breathe at all (the chest is not moving up and down). • The child cannot cough or talk, or looks blue. • The child is found unconscious. (Go to CPR.)	• The child can breathe, cry, or talk. • The child can cough, sputter, or move air at all. The child's normal reflexes are working to clear the airway.

FOR INFANTS YOUNGER THAN 1 YEAR

INFANT CHOKING

If the infant is choking and is unable to breathe, cough, cry, or speak, follow these steps. Have someone call 911, or if you are alone call 911 as soon as possible.

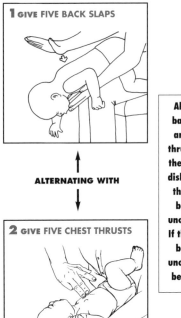

1 GIVE FIVE BACK SLAPS

ALTERNATING WITH

2 GIVE FIVE CHEST THRUSTS

Alternate back slaps and chest thrusts until the object is dislodged or the infant becomes unconscious. If the infant becomes unconscious, begin CPR.

INFANT CPR

To be used when the infant is unconscious or when breathing stops.

1 OPEN AIRWAY
- Open airway (tilt head, lift chin).
- Take 5 to 10 seconds to check if the child is breathing after the airway is opened. **Look** for up and down movement of the chest and abdomen. **Listen** for breath sounds at the nose and mouth. **Feel** for breath on your cheek. If opening the airway results in breathing, other than an occasional gasp, do not give breaths.
- If there is no breathing **look** for a foreign object in the mouth. **If you can see** an object in the infant's mouth, sweep it out carefully with your finger. Then attempt rescue breathing. **Do NOT** try a blind finger sweep if the object is not seen, because it could be pushed farther into the throat.

2 RESCUE BREATHING
- **Position** head and chin with both hands as shown—head gently tilted back, chin lifted.
- Take a normal breath (not a deep breath).
- **Seal** your mouth over the infant's mouth and nose.
- Give 2 breaths, each rescue breath over 1 second with a pause between breaths. Each breath should make the chest rise.

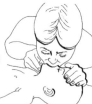

If no rise or fall after the first breath, repeat steps 1 and 2. If still no rise or fall, continue with step 3 (below).

3 CHEST COMPRESSIONS
- **Place** 2 fingers of 1 hand on the breastbone just below the nipple line.
- **Compress** chest $\frac{1}{3}$ to $\frac{1}{2}$ the depth of the chest.
- **Alternate** 30 compressions with 2 breaths.
- **Compress** chest at rate of 100 times per minute.

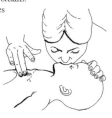

Be sure someone calls 911 as soon as possible. If you are alone, call 911 or your local emergency number after 5 cycles of breaths and chest compressions (about 2 minutes).

If at any time an object is coughed up or the infant/child starts to breathe, call 911 or your local emergency number.

Ask your pediatrician for information on choking/CPR instructions for children older than 8 years and for information on an approved first aid or CPR course in your community.

CHOKING/CPR

LEARN AND PRACTICE CPR (CARDIOPULMONARY RESUSCITATION)

IF ALONE WITH A CHILD WHO IS CHOKING...

1. SHOUT FOR HELP.   2. START RESCUE EFFORTS.   3. CALL 911 OR YOUR LOCAL EMERGENCY NUMBER.

YOU SHOULD START FIRST AID FOR CHOKING IF...	DO NOT START FIRST AID FOR CHOKING IF...
• The child cannot breathe at all (the chest is not moving up and down). • The child cannot cough or talk, or looks blue. • The child is found unconscious. (Go to CPR.)	• The child can breathe, cry, or talk. • The child can cough, sputter, or move air at all. The child's normal reflexes are working to clear the airway.

FOR CHILDREN 1 TO 8 YEARS OF AGE*

CHILD CHOKING

If the child is choking and is unable to breathe, cough, cry, or speak, follow these steps.
Have someone call 911, or if you are alone call 911 as soon as possible.

CONSCIOUS

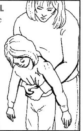

FIVE ABDOMINAL THRUSTS just above the navel and well below the bottom tip of the breastbone and rib cage. Give each thrust with enough force to produce an artificial cough designed to relieve airway obstruction.

> If the child becomes unconscious, begin CPR.

CHILD CPR

To be used when the child is **UNCONSCIOUS** or when breathing stops.

1 OPEN AIRWAY

- Open airway (tilt head, lift chin).
- Take 5 to 10 seconds to check if the child is breathing after the airway is opened. **Look** for up and down movement of the chest and abdomen. **Listen** for breath sounds at the nose and mouth. **Feel** for breath on your cheek. If opening the airway results in breathing, other than an occasional gasp, do not give breaths.
- If there is no breathing **look** for a foreign object in the mouth. **If you can see** an object in the child's mouth, sweep it out carefully with your finger. Then attempt rescue breathing. **Do NOT** try a blind finger sweep if the object is not seen, because it could be pushed farther into the throat.

2 RESCUE BREATHING

- **Position** head and chin with both hands as shown—head gently tilted back, chin lifted.
- Take a normal breath (not a deep breath).
- **Seal** your mouth over the child's mouth.
- **Pinch** the child's nose.
- Give 2 breaths, each rescue breath over 1 second with a pause between breaths. Each breath should make the chest rise and fall.

If no rise or fall after the first breath, repeat steps 1 and 2. If still no rise or fall, continue with step 3 (below).

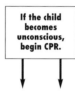

3 CHEST COMPRESSIONS

Place heel of 1 hand over the lower half of the breastbone OR use 2 hands: place heel of 1 hand over the lower half of the breastbone, then place other hand over first hand (to keep them off of the chest).

- **Compress** chest ⅓ to ½ depth of chest.
- **Alternate** 30 compressions with 2 breaths.
- **Compress** chest at rate of 100 times per minute.

Check for signs of normal breathing, coughing, or movement after every 5 cycles (about 2 minutes).

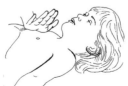
1-hand technique

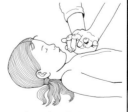
2-hand technique

> Be sure someone calls 911 as soon as possible. If you are alone, call 911 or your local emergency number after 5 cycles of breaths and chest compressions (about 2 minutes).
>
> *For children 8 years and older, adult recommendations for choking/CPR apply.

If at any time an object is coughed up or the infant/child starts to breathe, call 911 or your local emergency number.

Ask your pediatrician for information on choking/CPR instructions for children older than 8 years and for information on an approved first aid or CPR course in your community.

A Guide to Children's Dental Health

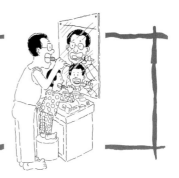

The road to a bright smile begins long before the first tooth breaks through the gum. Parents play a big part in helping their children develop healthy teeth. Early monitoring by a pediatrician or dentist is important.

Steps to good dental health include

- Regular care by a dental professional
- Getting enough fluoride
- Regular brushing and flossing
- Eating right

It's important for parents to care for their teeth too because cavity-causing bacteria can be easily transferred when sharing food or drinks. By following these steps and teaching them to your children, your entire family can benefit from good dental health.

Read more to learn why fluoride is important, when to start cleaning your child's teeth, if pacifier use or thumb sucking hurt teeth, about foods that can lead to tooth decay, about pediatric dentists, and good dental habits.

Why is fluoride important?

Fluoride is a natural chemical that can be added to drinking water and toothpaste. It strengthens *tooth enamel* (the hard outer coating on teeth). Fluoride also helps repair early damage to teeth.

The fluoride content of local water supplies varies. Check with your local water department to find out the exact water fluoride level in your area. Then talk with your child's pediatrician or dentist to see if she needs additional fluoride, such as fluoride drops or tablets. The need for fluoride is based on your child's *caries* (tooth decay) risk.

When should I start cleaning my child's teeth?

Daily dental cleaning should start as soon as your infant's first tooth appears. Wipe the teeth with a piece of gauze or a damp cloth. Switch to a toothbrush with a fluoride toothpaste as your child gets older. Because children tend to swallow toothpaste, put only a small (pea-sized) amount of fluoride toothpaste on your child's toothbrush and press the toothpaste into the bristles. Taking in too much fluoride while brushing can result in *fluorosis* (spotting of the teeth).

Also, check the teeth for early signs of tooth decay. Cavities appear as white, yellow, or brown spots or lines on the teeth. Any 2 teeth that are touching each other should be flossed to prevent a cavity from forming between the teeth. An ideal baby bite should have spaces between the front teeth. If your child's teeth are touching early, this is a sign that dental crowding may occur in the adult teeth that may require future orthodontic care.

Does pacifier use or thumb sucking hurt teeth?

If a child sucks strongly on a pacifier, his thumb, or his fingers, this habit may affect the shape of his mouth or how his teeth are lining up. If a child stops using a pacifier by 3 years of age, his bite will most likely correct itself. If a child stops sucking on a pacifier, his thumb, or his fingers before his permanent front teeth come in, there's a chance his bite will correct itself. If your child continues his sucking habit after his adult teeth have come in, then orthodontic care may be needed to realign his teeth.

Food that can lead to tooth decay

Sweets like candy or cookies can lead to tooth decay. Sugar from fruits and fruit juices left on the teeth for a long time is not healthy for teeth. Frequent sipping on drinks such as fruit juices and sodas can also cause tooth decay. Starchy foods, such as crackers, and sticky foods and candies, such as raisins, fruit roll-ups, and gummy bears, tend to stay on the teeth longer. These foods also are more likely to lead to tooth decay.

Starches and fruits, however, are a necessary part of any child's diet. To avoid tooth decay, give your child these foods only at mealtime (before the teeth have been brushed). For healthy teeth, offer your child a well-balanced diet with a variety of foods. Drinking water with fluoride is an excellent way to keep teeth healthy.

Pediatric dentists

During regular well-child visits, your child's pediatrician will check her teeth and gums to make sure they are healthy. If your child has dental problems, your child's pediatrician may refer her to a dental professional.

A pediatric dentist specializes in the care of children's teeth, but some general dentists also treat children. Pediatricians may refer children younger than 1 year to a dental professional if the child

- Chips or injures a tooth or has an injury to the face or mouth.
- Has teeth that show any signs of discoloration. This could be a sign of tooth decay.
- Complains of tooth pain or is sensitive to hot or cold foods or liquids. This could also be a sign of decay.
- Has any abnormal lesion (growth) inside the mouth.
- Has an unusual bite—the teeth do not fit together right.

Good dental habits

Regular dental checkups, a balanced diet, fluoride, injury prevention, habit control, and brushing and flossing are all important for healthy teeth. Starting children off with good dental habits now will help them grow up with healthy smiles.

The American Academy of Pediatrics (AAP) recommends that all infants receive oral health risk assessments by 6 months of age. Infants at higher risk of early dental caries should be referred to a dentist as early as 6 months of age and no later than 6 months after the first tooth erupts or 12 months of age (whichever comes first).

All children should have a comprehensive dental exam by a dentist in the early toddler years.

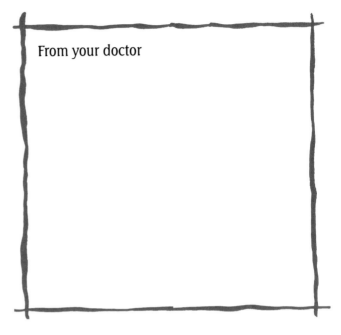

From your doctor

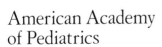

American Academy of Pediatrics

DEDICATED TO THE HEALTH OF ALL CHILDREN™

The American Academy of Pediatrics is an organization of 60,000 primary care pediatricians, pediatric medical subspecialists, and pediatric surgical specialists dedicated to the health, safety, and well-being of infants, children, adolescents, and young adults.

American Academy of Pediatrics
Web site — www.aap.org

Copyright © 2004
American Academy of Pediatrics

The Teen Driver
Guidelines for Parents

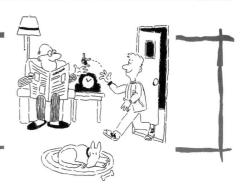

Traffic crashes are the leading cause of death for teens and young adults. More than 5,000 young people die every year in car crashes and thousands more are injured. Drivers who are 16 years old are more than 20 times as likely to have a crash as are other drivers. State and local laws, safe driving programs, and driver's education classes all help keep teens safe on the roads. Parents can also play an important role in keeping young drivers safe. This information has been developed by the American Academy of Pediatrics to inform parents about the risks that teen drivers face and how parents can help keep them safe on the roads.

Why teens are at risk

There are two main reasons why teens are at a higher risk for being in a car crash: lack of driving experience and their tendency to take risks while driving.

- **Lack of experience.** Teens drive faster and do not control the car as well as more experienced drivers. Their judgment in traffic is often insufficient to avoid a crash. In addition, teens do most of their driving at night, which can be even more difficult. Standard driver's education classes include 30 hours of classroom teaching and 6 hours of behind-the-wheel training. This is not enough time to fully train a new driver.
- **Risk taking.** Teen drivers are more likely to be influenced by peers and other stresses and distractions. This can lead to reckless driving behaviors such as speeding, driving while under the influence of drugs or alcohol, and not wearing safety belts.

Programs that help

Graduated licensing laws. Most teens get their driver's licenses in two stages: a learner's permit followed a few months later by a regular driver's license. The US Department of Transportation recommends "graduated licensing" so that learning to drive is spread over three stages. Each stage gives teens more driving privileges. Teen drivers have to meet certain restrictions for at least 6 months in each stage in order to move to the next stage. Driver's education classes would cover more and more complex decision-making and skills training during each stage. Twelve states have some form of graduated licensing laws.

Minimum drinking age and zero tolerance laws. Drunk and drugged driving are major problems for American teens. In one study, an estimated 6% to 14% of drivers younger than 21 years who were stopped at roadside sobriety checkpoints had been drinking. The misuse of alcohol and other drugs can severely hurt teenagers in many ways—especially on the road. A teen driver with a blood alcohol level (BAC) above 0.05% is more likely to be involved in a crash than is a sober teen driver.

Two types of laws exist to help lower the number of teens who drive after drinking alcohol. These are *minimum drinking* age laws and zero tolerance laws. Minimum drinking age laws prohibit the sale of alcohol to anyone under 21 years of age. These laws have helped reduce the number of alcohol-related crashes by 40%. But in some states, these laws have many loopholes and are hard to enforce. Many states have or will soon adopt zero tolerance laws that lower the allowable BAC limits for minors. Some states also require that licenses be suspended, sometimes for up to 1 year, after drivers younger than 21 years of age are arrested for driving drunk. These laws work. In Maryland, alcohol-related crashes decreased by at least 11% as a result of zero tolerance laws.

Safety belt laws. Even though all states have laws that require the use of safety belts, these laws may not apply to all passengers or all seats in a vehicle. In addition, studies show that teens do not use safety belts as often as older drivers do. Young people between 10 and 20 years old use safety belts only about 35% of the time—the lowest usage rate of any group. Strictly enforced safety belt laws, along with air bags, could greatly reduce the number of teens who are injured and killed in car crashes. In addition, teen drivers need to learn to take the responsibility of making sure all passengers are buckled up.

Curfew laws. Curfew laws ban teen driving during certain hours at night, such as midnight to 5 am. States with nighttime driving curfews for young drivers have lower crash rates than other states. The more strict the law, the fewer fatal crashes occur.

Educational efforts. Various state and national groups have programs to educate teens about unsafe driving practices, such as not wearing a safety belt and drunk driving. Pediatricians also play a role in such efforts.

There are several groups that encourage alternatives to drinking and driving by hosting social events for teens such as alcohol-free proms and parties. They also help teens and parents communicate. For example, SADD (Students Against Driving Drunk) encourages parents and teens to sign a contract in which both parties agree to avoid using alcohol or other drugs before driving and avoid riding with those who have. The contract also states that if a teen has been drinking he or she will call home for a ride. The group also encourages young people to help other teens change drinking habits and save lives on the roadways.

Safe ride programs. In some areas, "safe ride" programs help parents get involved by volunteering to drive to proms and other parties. Other programs give rides to teens who might otherwise have to drive home after drinking or ride with someone who has been drinking. A California program, for example, combines an educational program about alcohol abuse and an escort service for "stranded" teens on weekend nights. Teens can use this service in confidence. Teens volunteer to be drivers, but adults are also on-call in case questions or problems come up. Volunteer drivers stay in the car when they drop teens at home. They watch the teens enter their homes but do not talk with parents. Adults on-call handle any questions from parents.

How parents can help

Establish and discuss "house rules" about driving even before your teen gets a license. Remind your teen that these rules are in place because you care about his or her safety. If your teen complains about the rules, stand firm. You might say something like, "I don't care what other parents are doing—I care about you and don't want you to get in a crash." Remember, you control the car keys. Don't hesitate to take away driving privileges if your teen breaks any rules. Resist the urge to break the house rules yourself and let your teen drive because it is too much trouble for you to drive. Instead, try to arrange a car pool of parents and take turns driving.

You do not need to wait for graduated licensing laws to be passed in your state to adopt your own graduated driving rules. By slowly increasing driving privileges, you can help your teen get the experience needed to drive safely and responsibly. Here are some suggestions on how you can create a graduated licensing program for your teen driver. It may not be necessary to use all of the following restrictions; choose the ones that make the most sense for you and your teen.

Stage one
- teen must be at least 15½ years old or have a legal learner's permit
- teen must drive with a licensed adult driver at all times, the parent if possible
- no driving between 10 pm and 5 am or no driving after sunset
- driver and all passengers must wear safety belts
- no use of tobacco, alcohol, or other drugs
- teen must remain ticket-free and crash-free for 6 months before moving up to the next stage

Stage two
- teen must be at least 16 years old or have driven with a learner's permit for at least 6 months
- teen must drive with a licensed adult driver during nighttime hours, the parent if possible
- teen allowed to drive unsupervised during daytime hours
- passengers restricted to one nonfamily member during daytime hours

- no use of tobacco, alcohol, or other drugs
- driver and all passengers must wear safety belts
- teen must remain ticket-free and crash-free for 12 months before moving up to the next stage

Stage three
- teen must be at least 18 years old or have driven at least 2 years at the previous stage
- no restrictions on driving as long as the teen driver remains ticket-free and crash-free for 6 months
- no use of tobacco, alcohol, or other drugs
- all passengers must wear safety belts
Other ways parents can help:
- Require that your teen maintain good grades in school before he or she can drive. Check with your auto insurance company to see if any "good student" discounts are available.
- Set a good driving example (no use of alcohol or other drugs, no speeding, always wear your safety belt, and require that safety belts be worn by all passengers).
- Remind your teen how important it is to stay focused on driving, not getting distracted by excessively loud music or talking on a cellular phone.
- Let your teen know that driving after drinking or using other drugs will not be tolerated. Tell your teen to always call you or someone else for a ride any time he or she or any other driver has been drinking or using drugs. Let your teen know that you will pick him or her up. However, if you find he or she was drinking, it may be better to wait until the next day before you discuss the incident.
- Be alert to any signs that your teen has a drinking or other substance abuse problem. If you suspect a problem, urge your teen to talk with his or her pediatrician or school counselor. Such trusted adults can refer your teen for other help, if needed.
- Support efforts to protect teens. These might include "safe ride" programs or Mothers Against Drunk Driving (MADD). Encourage alcohol-free community events.
- Encourage schools to teach about the dangers of driving after drinking or using drugs.
- Support showing safety films in schools. Also support efforts to promote safety belt use in all vehicles that take children and teens to and from school.

Driving is a privilege and a big responsibility. Teen drivers, because of their age and inexperience, are at a higher risk for car crashes. Licensing programs, rules of the road, and safe ride programs are designed to help teen drivers stay safe. Along with support and encouragement from parents, these programs are the best way to help teens learn to become responsible drivers.

American Academy of Pediatrics

DEDICATED TO THE HEALTH OF ALL CHILDREN™

The American Academy of Pediatrics is an organization of 60,000 primary care pediatricians, pediatric medical subspecialists, and pediatric surgical specialists dedicated to the health, safety, and well-being of infants, children, adolescents, and young adults.

American Academy of Pediatrics
Web site — www.aap.org

Copyright © 1996
American Academy of Pediatrics

Your Child and the Environment

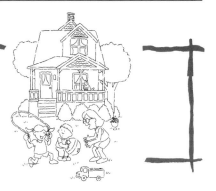

Environmental dangers are everywhere. Most of these dangers are more harmful to children than adults. However, there are things you can do to reduce your child's contact with them. Read more to learn about how to protect your family from environmental dangers.

Where children live

Air pollution is not just a problem outside. There can be things in the air inside your home that can harm your child. There can also be hazards found in the dust and dirt in or around your home and yard. The following are examples of hazards found where children live:

Asbestos

Asbestos is a natural fiber that was often used for fireproofing, insulating, and soundproofing between the 1940s and 1970s. Asbestos is only dangerous when it becomes crumbly. If that happens, asbestos fibers get into the air and are breathed into the lungs. Breathing in these fibers can cause chronic health problems, including a rare form of lung cancer. Asbestos can still be found in some older homes, often as insulation around pipes. Schools are required by law to remove asbestos or make sure that children are not exposed to it.

WHAT YOU CAN DO

- ✓ Don't allow children to play near exposed or crumbling materials that may contain asbestos.
- ✓ If you think there is asbestos in your home, have an expert look at it.
- ✓ If your home has asbestos, use a certified contractor to help solve the problem. You could have more problems if the asbestos isn't contained or removed safely.

Carbon monoxide

Carbon monoxide (CO) is a toxic gas that has no taste, no color, and no odor. It comes from appliances or heaters that burn gas, oil, wood, propane, or kerosene. Carbon monoxide poisoning is very dangerous. If left unchecked, exposure to CO can lead to memory loss, personality changes, brain damage, and death.

WHAT YOU CAN DO

- ✓ See your doctor right away if everyone in your house has flu-like symptoms (headache, fatigue, nausea) at the same time, especially if the symptoms go away when you leave the house.
- ✓ Put CO detectors on each floor in your home.
- ✓ Never leave a car running in an attached garage, even if the garage door is open.
- ✓ Never use a charcoal grill inside the home or in a closed space.
- ✓ Have furnaces; woodstoves; fireplaces; and gas-fired water heaters, ovens, ranges, and clothes dryers checked and serviced each year.
- ✓ Never use a gas oven to heat your home.

Household products

Many cleaning products give off dangerous fumes or leave residues. These products can be harmful if they are not thrown out properly (for example, if they are left in the garage).

WHAT YOU CAN DO

- ✓ Only use these products when needed.
- ✓ Always have enough ventilation when using these products.
- ✓ Store them in a safe place.
- ✓ Bring empty containers to your local hazardous waste disposal center.

Lead

Lead is one of the most serious environmental problems to children. Your child can get lead in her body if she swallows lead dust, breathes lead vapors, or eats soil or paint chips that have lead in them. Lead poisoning can cause learning disabilities, behavioral problems, anemia, or damage to the brain and kidneys.

Lead is most often found in
- Paint that is on the inside and outside of homes built before 1978
- Dust and paint chips from old paint
- Soil that has lead in it (particularly around older homes or by businesses that used lead)
- Hobby materials such as paints, solders, fishing weights, and buckshot
- Food stored in certain ceramic dishes (especially if dishes were made in another country)
- Older painted toys and furniture such as cribs
- Tap water, especially in homes that have lead solder on pipes
- Mini-blinds manufactured outside the United States before July 1997

A child who has high lead levels may not look or act sick. The only way to know if your child has lead in her body is with a blood test.

WHAT YOU CAN DO

If your home was built before 1978, test the paint for lead. If lead paint is found, get expert advice on how to repair it safely. (Remember, unsafe repairs can increase your child's risk for exposure to lead.)
- ✓ Don't scrape or sand paint that may have lead in it.
- ✓ Clean painted areas with soap and water and cover peeling, flaking, or chipping paint with new paint, duct tape, or contact paper.
- ✓ Make sure painted areas are repaired before putting cribs, playpens, beds, or highchairs next to them.
- ✓ Check with your health department to see if the water in your area contains lead.
- ✓ Always use cold water for mixing formula, cooking, and drinking. Run the water for 1 to 2 minutes before each use.
- ✓ Ask your pediatrician if your child needs a lead test. A blood test is the only accurate way to test for lead poisoning.

✓ Encourage your child to wash his hands often, especially before eating.
✓ Give your child a healthy diet with the right amounts of iron and calcium.
✓ Before moving into a home or apartment, check for possible lead problems.
✓ Never live in an old house while it's being renovated.

Molds

Molds grow almost anywhere and can be found in any part of a home. Common places where molds grow include the following:
- Damp basements
- Closets
- Showers and tubs
- Refrigerators
- Air conditioners and humidifiers
- Garbage pails
- Mattresses
- Carpets (especially if wet)

Children who live in moldy places are more likely to develop allergies, asthma, and other health problems.

WHAT YOU CAN DO
✓ Keep the surfaces in your home dry.
✓ Throw away wet carpets that can't be dried.
✓ Keep air conditioners and humidifiers clean and in good working order.
✓ Use exhaust fans in the kitchen and the bathroom to help keep the air dry.
✓ Avoid using items that are likely to get moldy, like foam rubber pillows and mattresses.

From-the-job hazards

From-the-job hazards brought into the home can be dangerous to children. This can happen when parents who work with harmful chemicals bring them into the home on their skin, hair, clothes, or shoes. People who work in the following places are most at risk:
- Painting and construction sites
- Car body or repair shops
- Car battery and radiator factories
- Shipyards

WHAT YOU CAN DO
✓ Find out if you or any adult in your home is exposed to lead, asbestos, mercury, or chemicals at work.
✓ If so, shower and change before coming home.
✓ Wash work clothes separately from other laundry.

Radon

Radon is a gas that can be found in water, building materials, and natural gas. It has no taste, no color, and no odor. Radon can seep into a home through cracks in the foundation, floors, and walls. High levels of radon have been found in homes in many parts of the United States. Breathing in radon doesn't cause health problems at first. However, over time it can increase your risk of lung cancer. Radon is believed to be the second most common cause of lung cancer (after smoking) in the United States.

WHAT YOU CAN DO
✓ Check with your health department to see if radon levels are high in your area.
✓ Test your home for radon. Home radon tests don't cost much and are easy to use. The results can be analyzed by a certified laboratory. You can't test yourself or your child for radon exposure.

Secondhand smoke

Secondhand smoke is also called environmental tobacco smoke (ETS). This is the smoke breathed out by a smoker or from the tip of a lit cigarette. Children are exposed to secondhand smoke any time they are around someone smoking a cigarette, pipe, or cigar. The chemicals in secondhand smoke can cause cancer. In fact, secondhand smoke has been linked to 3,000 lung cancer deaths each year in people who don't even smoke!

WHAT YOU CAN DO
✓ If you are a smoker, get help so you can quit! (Children whose parents smoke are more likely to try smoking than those whose parents give clear messages that smoking is not healthy.)
✓ Remove your children from places where there are smokers.
✓ If there are smokers in the house, have them smoke outside.
✓ Avoid smoking in your car.

What children eat and drink

Drinking water

Children drink 5 to 10 times more water for their size than adults. Most of this water is tap water. Tap water in most areas is protected by law. However, small water supplies, such as from private wells, are not.

Many people use bottled water because they think it's better than tap water. Some brands are better. However, other brands may only be tap water that's bottled and sold separately. Bottled water costs a lot more than tap water, but may be needed in some areas. Children need fluoride for good dental health. Only some brands of bottled water have fluoride, so read the labels.

Some of the things in drinking water that can make children sick include the following:
- Germs
- Nitrates
- Heavy metals
- Chlorine
- Radioactive particles
- By-products from cleaning products

The quality of water in the United States is among the best in the world, but problems do happen. County health departments and state environmental agencies are the best sources of information about the water where you live.

WHAT YOU CAN DO
✓ Find out where your water comes from. If you are on a municipal water supply, the water company must tell you what is in the water. If your water is not regulated or you have a well, have it tested each year.
✓ Always drink and cook with cold water. Contaminants can build up in water heaters.

✓ If you are not sure of your plumbing, run the water for 1 to 2 minutes each morning before you drink or cook with water. This flushes the pipes and reduces the chances of a contaminant getting into your water. In some areas more time is needed to flush water through the pipes. Ask your pediatrician or health department about recommendations specific to your area.

✓ If you have well water and a baby younger than 1 year, have your water tested for nitrates *before* giving it to your baby. Breastfeeding, using ready-to-feed formula, or using bottled water with powdered formula is wise until you know if your water is safe. If you have questions, call your local health department.

If you think your water may have germs, you can kill most of them by boiling the water and cooling it before use. Do not boil water for longer than 1 minute. This can cause a buildup of toxins and metals in the water. Water filters installed on faucets or pitchers that have built-in filters may also help remove harmful contaminants from tap water.

Mercury

Mercury that gets into oceans, lakes, rivers, and ponds can get into the fish we eat. Mercury can also be found in many other places. Because mercury can be toxic, especially in large doses, every effort should be made to reduce exposure to children and pregnant women.

WHAT YOU CAN DO

✓ Don't eat shark, swordfish, king mackerel, or tilefish because they contain high levels of mercury. Also, limit your child's intake of canned light tuna, shrimp, pollock, salmon, cod, catfish, clams, flatfish, crabs, and scallops to 2 meals per week. Albacore (white) tuna should be limited to 1 meal per week. Pregnant or nursing women should also limit the amount of these fish they eat.

✓ Check with local advisories about the safety of fish caught in your area. If no advice is available, only give your child up to 1 meal per week of fish from your local waters.

✓ Use a digital thermometer instead of one that contains mercury. If you have a mercury thermometer, keep it out of your child's reach. See if your community has a thermometer exchange program for the proper disposal of these thermometers.

✓ The material traditionally used to fill dental cavities contains small amounts of mercury. There is no scientific proof that this is dangerous to children. However, if this worries you, talk to your dentist about other treatment options.

✓ Talk with your pediatrician if your family uses mercury in folk remedies or in cultural traditions (such as Santeria [religion originating in Cuba]).

To do their part, drug companies have stopped using mercury as a preservative in vaccines (even though it was used only in very small amounts). All vaccines for children, except some influenza (flu) vaccine and Td (tetanus-diphtheria–containing) vaccines, are now free of mercury.

Pesticides

Pesticides are chemicals used to kill insects, weeds, and fungi. Many are toxic to the environment and to people. Too much exposure to pesticides can cause a wide range of health problems.

WHAT YOU CAN DO

✓ Wash all fruits and vegetables with water.

✓ Buy fruits and vegetables that are in season because they are less likely to be heavily sprayed.

✓ If possible, eat foods that are grown without the use of chemical pesticides.

✓ Use nonchemical pest control methods in your home and garden.

✓ Keep all pesticides out of children's reach to avoid accidental poisoning.

✓ Tell neighbors before you spray outdoors.

Where children play

Art supplies

Art supplies can cause health problems in children who use them. While older children can usually use these products safely, most younger children and some children with disabilities cannot. Harmful art supplies can include the following:

- Rubber cement
- Permanent felt-tip markers
- Pottery glazes
- Enamels
- Spray fixatives
- Prepackaged papier-mâché

WHAT YOU CAN DO

✓ Use only nontoxic art supplies.

✓ Read and follow all instructions carefully.

✓ Always use products in a well-ventilated room.

✓ Look for the ACMI (Art & Creative Materials Institute Inc.) nontoxic seal or other information on the label that says the product is safe for children.

✓ Talk with your school to make sure only safe art supplies are being used.

Insect repellent

Most insect repellents include a chemical called DEET (diethyltoluamide). This chemical is absorbed into the skin and can harm children.

WHAT YOU CAN DO

✓ Choose an insect repellent that is made for children. Make sure the brand you choose has no more than 30% DEET for infants older than 2 months and older children. Do not use DEET products on infants younger than 2 months.

Are electric and magnetic fields safe?

All electric appliances like microwaves, computers, and TVs produce electric and magnetic fields (EMFs) when they are used. There is some concern that exposure to these fields may cause health problems, including cancer. However, more research is needed and a definite link between cancer and EMFs has not been made. Until more is known about EMFs, reduce your child's exposure by

- Keeping your child away from microwaves while they are in use
- Having your child sit at least 3 feet from the TV screen
- Moving electric clocks, radios, and baby monitors away from your child's bed
- Not using electric bedding (blankets, mattress pads, heating pads, and waterbed heaters)

✓ Apply insect repellent to clothing when possible, rather than directly on the skin.

Lawn and garden fertilizers

Lawn and garden fertilizers can be harmful if children come in contact with them while playing in the yard. Many of these products are made with chemicals (pesticides) that are known to cause health problems, especially in children.

WHAT YOU CAN DO
✓ Use these chemicals only when needed.
✓ Read and follow the instructions carefully.
✓ Keep your child off a treated lawn until it has been watered twice and the odor of the chemicals is gone.

Ozone

Ozone is colorless gas found in the air and is harmful the closer it gets to the ground. Ozone levels are highest in summer, in the late afternoon. Ozone pollution can cause breathing problems in children with asthma.

WHAT YOU CAN DO
✓ Keep your child indoors as much as you can when there's a health advisory or smog alert.
✓ Take public transportation, carpool, walk, or ride a bike instead of driving when you can, or buy a fuel-economic car. This will help reduce the amount of air pollution caused by cars.

Sun

The sun is the main cause of skin cancer in the United States. Children's skin can burn easily. Sunburns can be very painful and can cause a child to become sick. The sun's rays can also damage the eyes.

WHAT YOU CAN DO
✓ Keep babies younger than 6 months out of direct sunlight.
✓ Choose a sunscreen made for children with a sun protection factor (SPF) of at least 15.
✓ Use hats and sunglasses to protect your child's head and eyes from the sun.
✓ Try to keep your child in the shade between 10 am and 4 pm. This is when the sun's rays are strongest.
✓ Dress your child in lightweight clothing that covers as much of the body as possible.

To learn more

Agency for Toxic Substances and Disease Registry
888/422-8737
www.atsdr.cdc.gov

American Lung Association
800/LUNGUSA (800/586-4872)
www.lungusa.org

Remember

Whether it is inside or outside, children love to explore their environment. This natural curiosity is an important way for children to learn. Be aware of the possible dangers that your child may face. Keep in mind that not all environmental dangers can be avoided completely, and do what you can to reduce your child's exposure.

Environmental Protection Agency
202/272-0167
www.epa.gov

Food and Drug Administration
888/INFO-FDA (888/463-6332)
www.fda.gov

National Coalition Against the Misuse of Pesticides
202/543-5450
www.beyondpesticides.org

National Pesticide Information Center
800/858-7378
www.npic.orst.edu

Hotlines
EMF InfoLine
800/363-2383

National Lead Information Center
800/424-LEAD (800/424-5323)

National Radon Hotline
800/767-7236

Safe Drinking Water Hotline
800/426-4791

Please note: Listing of resources does not imply an endorsement by the American Academy of Pediatrics (AAP). The AAP is not responsible for the content of the resources mentioned in this brochure. Phone numbers and Web site addresses are as current as possible, but may change at any time.

The information contained in this publication should not be used as a substitute for the medical care and advice of your pediatrician. There may be variations in treatment that your pediatrician may recommend based on individual facts and circumstances.

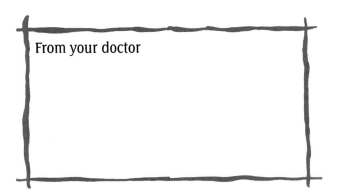

From your doctor

American Academy of Pediatrics

DEDICATED TO THE HEALTH OF ALL CHILDREN™

The American Academy of Pediatrics is an organization of 60,000 primary care pediatricians, pediatric medical subspecialists, and pediatric surgical specialists dedicated to the health, safety, and well-being of infants, children, adolescents, and young adults.

American Academy of Pediatrics
Web site — www.aap.org

Copyright © 2005
American Academy of Pediatrics, Updated 4/05

Keep Your Family Safe:
FIRE SAFETY AND BURN PREVENTION AT HOME

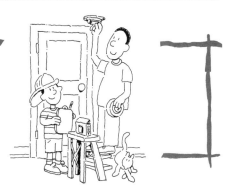

Fires and burns cause more than 4,000 deaths and more than 50,000 hospitalizations every year. Winter is an especially dangerous time, as space heaters, fireplaces, and candles get more use in the home. It is no surprise that most fires in the home occur between December and February. However, you might be surprised at how easy it is to reduce the risk of fire in your home. Follow these suggestions to keep your home and family safe from fire all year round.

Smoke alarms save lives

Most fatal fires in the home happen while people are sleeping. One of the most important steps you can take to protect your family against fire is to install smoke alarms and keep them in good working order. Smoke alarms are available at most home and hardware stores and often cost $10 or less. Check with your fire department to see if they give out and install free smoke alarms.

- Install smoke alarms outside every bedroom or any area where someone sleeps. Be sure there is at least one alarm on every level of your home or at each end of a mobile home.
- Place smoke alarms away from the kitchen and bathroom. False alarms can occur while cooking or even showering.
- Test smoke alarms every month by pushing the test button.
- Change the batteries when they get low, or at least once a year such as when you change your clocks back in the fall.
- Replace smoke alarms every 10 years.
- Never paint a smoke alarm.
- Clean smoke alarms monthly by dusting or vacuuming.
- Smoke alarms with a flashing light and an alarm should be used in homes with hard-of-hearing or deaf children or adults.

Prevention around the home

Take a careful look at each room of your home. Use the following checklists and safety tips to reduce the risk of fire:

- ☐ Make an escape plan. Practice it every 6 months. Every member of the family should know at least two exits from each room and where to meet outside.
- ☐ Inspect and replace any electrical cords that are worn, frayed, or damaged. Never overload outlets. Avoid running electrical cords under carpet or furniture as they can overheat and start a fire.
- ☐ Make sure doors and windows are easy to open.
- ☐ Automatic home fire sprinkler systems are affordable and practical for many homes.
- ☐ Wood stoves usually cannot be safely installed in mobile homes. If one is present, it should be inspected by the local fire department to be sure it is safely vented.

- ☐ Avoid using alternative heating sources such as kerosene heaters and electric space heaters. If they must be used, keep them away from clothing, bedding, and curtains, and unplug them at night. If kerosene heaters must be used, make sure there is adequate ventilation to prevent carbon monoxide poisoning.

Bedrooms

- ☐ Check the labels of your child's pajamas. Children should always wear flame-retardant and/or close-fitting sleepwear.
- ☐ If a bedroom is on an upper floor, make sure there is a safe way to reach the ground, such as a noncombustible escape ladder.
- ☐ In the event of a fire, test any closed doors with the back of your hand for heat. Do not open the door if you feel heat or see smoke. Close all doors as you leave each room to keep the fire from spreading.
- ❖ *Never smoke in bed or when you are drowsy or have been drinking. Tobacco and smoking products, matches, and lighters are the most common cause of fatal fires in the home.*

Living and family rooms

- ☐ Make sure all matches, lighters, and ashtrays are out of your child's sight and reach. Better yet, keep them in a locked cabinet.
- ☐ Use large, deep ashtrays that won't tip over, and empty them often. Fill ashtrays with water before dumping ashes in the wastebasket.
- ☐ Give space heaters plenty of space. Keep heaters *at least* 3 feet from anything that might burn, like clothes, curtains, and furniture. Always turn space heaters off and unplug them when you go to bed or leave the home.
- ☐ Have fireplaces and chimneys cleaned and inspected once a year.
- ☐ Use a metal screen or glass doors in front of the fireplace.
- ❖ *Never leave children alone in a room with candles, heaters, or with a burning fireplace.*

Kitchen

- ☐ Keep your stove and oven clean and free of anything that could catch fire. Do not place pot holders, curtains, or towels near the burners.
- ☐ Install a portable fire extinguisher in the kitchen, high on a wall, and near an exit. (Choose a multipurpose, dry chemical extinguisher). Adults should know how to use it properly when the fire is small and contained, such as in a trash can. Call your fire department for information on how to use fire extinguishers.
- ❖ *Never leave cooking food unattended.*
- ❖ *Never pour water on a grease fire.*
- ❖ *If a fire starts in your oven, keep the oven door closed and call the fire department.*

Garage, storage area, and basement

- ☐ Have your furnace inspected at least once a year.
- ☐ Do not store anything near a heater or furnace. Remove trash from the home.
- ☐ Clean your dryer vent after every use. Lint buildup can start a fire.
- ☐ Check to make sure paint and other flammable liquids are stored in their original containers, with tight-fitting lids. Store them in a locked cabinet if possible, out of your child's reach, and away from appliances, heaters, pilot lights, and other sources of heat or flame.
- ☐ Never use flammable liquids near a gas water heater.
- ☐ Store gasoline, propane, and kerosene outside the home in a shed or detached garage. Keep them tightly sealed and labeled in approved safety containers.
- ❖ *Gasoline should be used only as a motor fuel, never as a cleaning agent.*
- ❖ *Never smoke near flammable liquids.*

Outdoors

- ☐ Move barbecue grills away from trees, bushes, shrubs, or anything that could catch fire. *Never* use grills indoors, on a porch, or on a balcony.
- ☐ Place a barrier around open fires, fire pits, or campfires. *Never* leave a child alone around the fire. Always be sure to put the fire out completely before leaving or going to sleep.
- ❖ *Do not start lawnmowers, snowblowers, or motorcycles near gasoline fumes. Let small motors cool off before adding fuel.*
- ❖ *Be very careful with barbecue grills. Never use gasoline to start the fire. Do not add charcoal lighter fluid once the fire has started.*

Know what to do in a fire

- **If you get trapped by smoke or flames,** close all doors. Stuff towels or clothing under the doors to keep out smoke. Cover your nose and mouth with a damp cloth to protect your lungs. If there is no phone in the room, wait at a window and signal for help with a light-colored cloth or flashlight.
- **Crawl low under smoke.** Choose the safest exit. If you must escape through a smoky area, remember that cleaner air is always near the floor. Teach your child to crawl on her hands and knees, keeping her head less than 2 feet above the floor, as she makes her way to the nearest exit.
- **Don't stop. Don't go back.** In case of fire, do not try to rescue pets or possessions. Once you are out, do not go back in for any reason. Firefighters have the best chance of rescuing people who are trapped. Let firefighters know right away if anyone is missing.
- **Stop, drop, and roll! Cool and call.** Make sure your child knows what to do if his clothes catch fire.
  Stop! — Do not run.
  Drop! — Drop to the ground right where you are.
  Roll! — Roll over and over to put out the flames. Cover your face with your hands.
  Cool — Cool the burned area with water.
  Call — Call for help.

Fire and children

A child's curiosity about fire is natural and in most cases is no cause for concern. However, when a child begins to use fire as a weapon, it can be very dangerous. Almost half of all people arrested for arson are under the age of 18. Fire setting by children may be a call for help or a way to oppose authority. A child who sets fires may have depression, stress, anger, or a sense of failure or may be acting out against abuse. Use the following tips when talking to your child about preventing fires:

Fire drills — be prepared!

Even preschool-aged children (3 and older) can begin to learn what to do in case of a fire.

1. **Install at least one smoke alarm** on every level of your home.
2. **Have an escape plan** and practice it with your family. This will help you and your family reach safety when it counts. When a fire occurs, there will be no time for planning an escape.
3. **Draw a floor plan of your home.** Discuss with your family two ways to exit every room. Make sure everyone knows how to get out and that doors and windows can be easily opened. *If you live in an apartment building, never use an elevator during a fire. Use the stairs!*
4. **Agree on a meeting place.** Choose a spot outside your home near a tree, street corner, fence, or mailbox where everyone can gather after escaping. Teach your children that the sound of a smoke alarm means to go outside right away and meet at the designated place.
5. **Know how to call the fire department.** The fire department should be called from outside using a portable phone or from a neighbor's home. Whether the number is 911 or a regular phone number, everyone in the family should know it by heart. Make sure your children know your home address too. Teach your children that firefighters are friends and never to hide from them.
6. **Practice, practice, practice.** Practice your exit drill at least twice a year. Remember that fire drills are not a race. Get out quickly, but calmly and carefully. Try practicing realistic situations. Pretend that some exits or doorways are blocked or that the lights are out. The more prepared your family is, the better your chances of surviving a fire.

Note: Parents of children with special needs should consider a safety plan that fits their child's needs and abilities. For example, a child who is hard of hearing or deaf may need a smoke alarm with a flashing strobe-light feature.

- Teach your child that matches and lighters are tools for grown-ups only.
- Older children should be taught to use fire properly, and only in the presence of an adult.

If you suspect that your child is setting even very small fires, address the problem right away. Discuss any problems in the child's life that may be causing the behavior. Listen carefully to what your child says. Some children may have trouble talking openly with a parent. Consult your pediatrician, who can suggest ways to help. Many schools and fire departments offer programs to help children who play with fires or set fires.

For your sitters

When you are away from home and someone else cares for your children, take the following steps to ensure that your children and the sitter will be just as safe as when you are there.

- Let your sitter know where the safest exits are from your home. Discuss the family's escape plan.
- Tell the sitter where the outside meeting place is that the family has agreed upon in case of fire.
- Remind sitters *never* to leave the children alone.
- In case of fire, instruct the sitter to leave the house immediately with the children and call the fire department from a neighbor's house or an outside telephone.
- Remind sitters that you do not allow smoking in or around your home and children and not to bring matches or lighters into the home.
- Make sure to leave a list of emergency information near the phone. Include the following:v Local fire and police department phone numbers

- ❖ Poison control center phone number
- ❖ Your pediatrician's name and phone number
- ❖ Where you can be reached
- ❖ Children's full names
- ❖ Your full home address and phone number (and, if you live in a rural area, any fire identifiers)
- ❖ Neighbor's name and phone number
- ❖ Any special instructions
- • Provide your sitter with a copy of this brochure to read.

Burn prevention

Most burn injuries happen in the home. For a young child, there are many ordinary places in the home that can be dangerous. Hot bath water, radiators, and even food that is too hot can cause burns. The following tips and suggestions will help you avoid the possibility of burn injury to your child:

- • Keep matches, lighters, and ashtrays out of the reach of children.
- • Childproof all electrical outlets with plastic plugs.
- • Do not allow your child to play close to fireplaces, radiators, or space heaters.
- • Replace all frayed, broken, or worn electrical cords.
- • Never leave barbecue grills unattended.
- • Teach your children that irons, curling irons, grills, radiators, and ovens can get very hot and are dangerous to touch or play near. Never leave any of these items unattended with children near. Unplug all appliances after using them.

Kitchen concerns

- • *Never* leave a child alone in the kitchen when food is cooking.
- • Enforce a "kid-free" zone 3 feet around the oven or stove while you are cooking. Use a playpen, high chair, or other stationary device to keep your child from getting too close.
- • Never leave a hot oven door open.
- • Use back burners if possible. When using front burners, turn pot handles inward. Never let them stick out where a child could grab them.
- • Do not leave spoons or other utensils in pots while cooking.
- • Turn off burners and ovens when they are not being used.
- • Do not use wet pot holders, as they may cause steam burns.
- • Carefully place wet foods into a deep fryer or frying pan containing grease rather than tossing them in. The reaction between hot oil and water will splatter.
- • Remove pot lids carefully to avoid being burned by steam. Remember, steam is hotter than boiling water.
- • In case of a small pan fire, carefully slide a lid over the pan to smother the flames, turn off the burner, and wait for the pan to cool completely.
- • Never carry your child and hot liquids at the same time.
- • Never leave hot liquids, like a cup of coffee, where children can reach them. Don't forget that a child can get burned from hot liquids by pulling on hanging tablecloths.
- • Wear tight-fitting or rolled-up sleeves when cooking to reduce the risk of your clothes catching on fire.
- • In microwave ovens, use only containers that are made for microwaves. Test microwaved food for heat and steam before giving it to your child. (Never warm a bottle in the microwave. It can heat the liquid unevenly and burn your child.)
- • Avoid letting appliance cords hang over the side of countertops, where children could pull on them.

Different degrees of burns

Following are the four different levels of burns and the symptoms of each:

- • **1st degree burns are minor and heal quickly.** Symptoms are redness, tenderness, and soreness (like most sunburns).
- • **2nd degree burns are serious injuries.** First aid and medical treatment should be given as soon as possible. Symptoms are blistering (like a severe sunburn), pain, and swelling.
- • **3rd degree burns are severe injuries.** Medical treatment is needed right away. Symptoms are white, brown, or charred tissue often surrounded by blistered areas. There may be little or no pain at first.
  - ❖ Deep 2nd and 3rd degree burns are called *full-thickness burns* and are very serious.
- • **4th degree burns are severe injuries that involve both skin and underlying structures, such as muscle and bone.** These often occur with electrical burns and may be more severe than they appear. They may cause serious complications and should be seen by a doctor immediately.

Remember to call your pediatrician if your child suffers anything more than a minor burn. ALL electrical burns and any burn on the hand, foot, face, or genitals should receive medical attention right away.

Hot water

- • The temperature of your water heater should be set no higher than 120°F to prevent scalding.
- • When using tap water, always turn on the cold water first, then add hot. When finished, turn off the hot water first.
- • Test the temperature of bath water with your forearm or the back of your hand before placing your child in the water.
- • Use a cool-mist vaporizer to treat upper-respiratory illnesses, as hot water vaporizers can cause steam burns or can spill on your child.
- • Never leave children alone in the bathroom for any reason. They are at risk of burns and drowning.

First aid for burns

For severe burns, immediately call 911 or your local emergency number. Until help arrives, follow these steps

1. **Cool the burn.**
   For 1st and 2nd degree burns, cool the burned area with cool running water for 10 minutes. This helps stop the burning process, numbs the pain, and prevents or reduces swelling. *Do not use ice on a burn. It may delay healing. Also, do not rub a burn, it can increase blistering.*
   For 3rd degree burns, cool the burn with wet, sterile dressings until help arrives.

2. **Remove burned clothing.**
   Lay the person flat on her back and take off the burned clothing that isn't stuck to the skin. Remove any jewelry or tight-fitting clothing from around the burned area before swelling begins. If possible, elevate the injured area.

3. **Cover the burn.**
   After the burn has cooled, apply a clean, dry gauze pad to the burned area. Do not break any blisters. This could allow germs into the wound.
   Never put grease (including butter or medical ointments) on the burn. Grease holds in heat, which may make the burn worse.

4. Treat for shock.

Keep the person's body temperature normal. Cover unburned areas with a dry blanket.

Adapted from material provided by the National Fire Protection Association (NFPA). For more information, call 617/770-3000, or visit the NFPA Web site at www.nfpa.org or its family Web site at www.sparky.org.

The information contained in this publication should not be used as a substitute for the medical care and advice of your pediatrician. There may be variations in treatment that your pediatrician may recommend based on individual facts and circumstances.

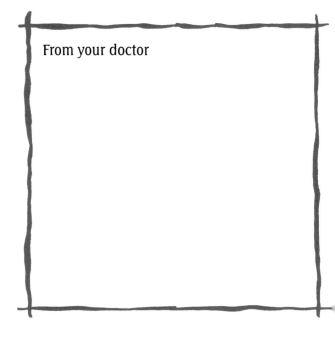

From your doctor

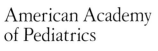

American Academy
of Pediatrics

DEDICATED TO THE HEALTH OF ALL CHILDREN™

The American Academy of Pediatrics is an organization of 60,000 primary care pediatricians, pediatric medical subspecialists, and pediatric surgical specialists dedicated to the health, safety, and well-being of infants, children, adolescents, and young adults.

American Academy of Pediatrics
Web site — www.aap.org

Copyright © 2000
American Academy of Pediatrics

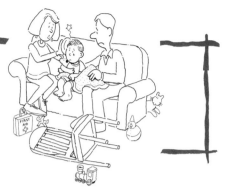

Minor Head Injuries in Children

Almost all children bump their heads every now and then. While these injuries can be upsetting, most head injuries are minor and do not cause serious problems. In very rare cases, problems can occur after a minor bump on the head. This brochure, developed by the American Academy of Pediatrics, will help parents understand the difference between a head injury that needs only a comforting hug and one that requires immediate medical attention.

The information in this brochure is intended for children who

- Were well before the injury
- Act normally *after* the injury
- Have no cuts on the head or face (this is called a closed head injury)
- Have no other injuries to the body

The information in this brochure is not intended for children who

- Are younger than 2 years of age
- Have possible neck injuries
- Already have nervous-system problems, such as seizures or movement disorders
- Have difficulties or delays in their development
- Have bleeding disorders or bruise easily
- Are victims of child abuse

Children with these conditions may have more serious problems after a mild head injury.

What should I do if my child has a head injury but does not lose consciousness?

For anything more than a light bump on the head, you should call your pediatrician. Your pediatrician will want to know when and how the injury happened and how your child is feeling.

If your child is alert and responds to you, the head injury is mild and usually no tests or X-rays are needed. Your child may cry from pain or fright, but this should last no longer than 10 minutes. You may need to apply a cold compress for 20 minutes to help the swelling go down and then watch your child closely for a period of time.

If there are any changes in your child's condition, call your pediatrician right away. You may need to bring your child to the pediatrician's office or directly to the hospital. The following are signs of a more serious injury:

- A constant headache that gets worse
- Slurred speech or confusion
- Dizziness that does not go away or happens repeatedly
- Extreme irritability or other abnormal behavior
- Vomiting more than 2 times
- Stumbling or difficulty walking
- Oozing blood or watery fluid from the nose or ears
- Difficulty waking up
- Unequal size of the pupils (the dark center part of the eyes)
- Unusual paleness that lasts for more than an hour

- Convulsions (seizures)
- Difficulty recognizing familiar people

What if my child loses consciousness?

If your child loses consciousness, call your pediatrician. Special tests may need to be done as soon as possible so that your pediatrician can find out how serious the injury is.

If the test results are normal, your pediatrician will want you to watch your child closely for a period of time. Your pediatrician will let you know if this can be done at home or in the hospital. If you take your child home and her condition changes, call your pediatrician right away since more care may be needed.

What kinds of tests may be needed? Where are they done?

A CAT scan is a special type of X-ray that gives a view of the brain and the skull. It is painless. A CAT scan is available at almost every hospital.

What is the difference between a head X-ray and CAT scan?

- *Head X-rays* can show fractures (bone breaks) of the skull, but do not show if there is a brain injury.
- *CAT scans* can show brain injury and may be helpful in deciding the seriousness of the injury. They can even show very minor injuries that may not need treatment.

What happens if the CAT scan or head X-ray shows a problem?

More tests will probably be needed and your pediatrician may want a head-injury specialist to examine your child.

What should I do if my child needs to be observed at home?

You or another responsible adult should stay with your child for the first 24 hours and be ready to take your child back to the pediatrician or hospital if there is a problem. Your child may need to be watched carefully for a few days because there could be a delay in signs of a more serious injury.

It is okay for your child to go to sleep. However, your pediatrician may recommend that you check your child every 2 to 3 hours to make sure he moves normally, wakes enough to recognize you, and responds to you.

If your pediatrician prescribes medicine, follow the directions carefully. Do not give pain medication, except for acetaminophen, unless your pediatrician says it is okay. Your pediatrician will let you know if your child can eat and drink as usual.

What if my child gets worse?

If your child gets worse, your pediatrician will need to examine her again. If a CAT scan has not been done, your pediatrician may order one. Your pediatrician also may talk with a specialist or admit your child to the hospital for closer observation.

Call your pediatrician or return to the hospital if your child experiences any of the following:

- Vomits more than twice
- Cannot stop crying
- Looks sicker
- Has a hard time walking, talking, or seeing
- Is confused or not acting normally
- Becomes more and more drowsy, or is hard to wake up
- Seems to have abnormal movements or seizures or any behaviors that worry you

Will my child have any permanent damage from a minor head injury?

If your child does well through the observation period, there should be no long-lasting problems. Remember, most head injuries are mild. However, be sure to talk with your pediatrician about any concerns or questions you might have.

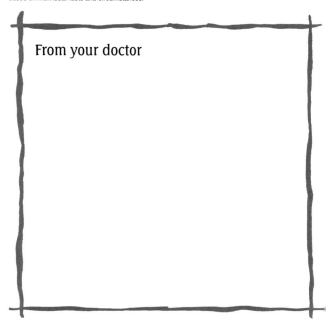

From your doctor

American Academy of Pediatrics

DEDICATED TO THE HEALTH OF ALL CHILDREN™

The American Academy of Pediatrics is an organization of 60,000 primary care pediatricians, pediatric medical subspecialists, and pediatric surgical specialists dedicated to the health, safety, and well-being of infants, children, adolescents, and young adults.

American Academy of Pediatrics
Web site—www.aap.org

Copyright © 1999
American Academy of Pediatrics, Updated 10/02

Home Safety Checklist

Use this checklist to help ensure that your home is safer for your child. A "full-house survey" is recommended at least every 6 months. Every home is different, and no checklist is complete and appropriate for every child and every household.

Your Child's Bedroom

☐ Is there a safety belt on the changing table to prevent falls?

☐ Is the baby powder out of baby's reach during diaper changing? Inhaled powder can injure a baby's lungs. Use cornstarch rather than talcum powder.

☐ Are changing supplies within your reach when baby is being changed?

☐ Never leave a child unattended on a changing table, even for a moment.

☐ Is there a carpet or a nonskid rug beneath the crib and changing table?

☐ Are drapery and blind cords out of the baby's reach from the crib and changing table? They can strangle children if they are left loose.

☐ Have bumper pads, toys, pillows, and stuffed animals been removed from the crib by the time the baby can pull up to stand? If large enough, these items can be used as a step for climbing out.

☐ Have all crib gyms, hanging toys, and decorations been removed from the crib by the time your baby can get up on his hands and knees? Children can get tangled in them and become strangled.

☐ Make sure the crib has no elevated corner posts or decorative cutouts in the end panels. Loose clothing can become snagged on these and strangle your baby.

☐ Does the mattress in the crib fit snugly, without any gaps, so your child cannot slip in between the crack and the crib side?

☐ The slots on the crib should be no more than 2⅜ inches apart. Widely spaced slots can trap an infant's head.

☐ Are all screws, bolts, and hardware, including mattress supports, in place to prevent the crib from collapsing?

☐ Make sure there are no plastic bags or other plastic material in or around the crib that might cause suffocation.

☐ Check the crib for small parts and pieces that your child could choke on.

☐ Make sure the night-light is not near or touching drapes or a bedspread where it could start a fire. Buy only "cool" night-lights that do not get hot.

☐ Is there a smoke detector in or near your child's bedroom?

☐ Make sure that window guards are securely in place to prevent a child from falling out the window. Never place a crib, playpen, or other children's furniture near a window.

☐ Are there plug protectors in the unused electrical outlets? These keep children from sticking their fingers or other objects into the holes.

☐ Make sure a toy box does not have a heavy, hinged lid that can trap your child. (It is safer with no lid at all.)

☐ To keep the air moist, use a cool mist humidifier (not a vaporizer) to avoid burns. Clean it frequently and empty it when not in use to avoid bacteria and mold from growing in the still water.

☐ To reduce the risk of SIDS (Sudden Infant Death Syndrome), put your baby to sleep on her back in a crib with a firm, flat mattress and no soft bedding underneath her.

Your Bedroom

☐ Do not keep a firearm anywhere in the house. If you must, lock up the gun and the bullets separately.

☐ Check that there are no prescription drugs, toiletries, or other poisonous substances accessible to young children.

☐ If your child has access to your bedroom, make sure drapery or blind cords are well out of reach. Children can get tangled in them and become strangled.

☐ Is there a working smoke detector in the hallway outside of the bedroom?

The Bathroom

☐ Is there a nonskid bath mat on the floor to prevent falls?

☐ Is there a nonskid mat or no-slip strips in the bathtub to prevent falls?

☐ Are the electrical outlets protected with Ground Fault Circuit Interrupters to decrease the risk of electrical injury?

☐ Are medications and cosmetics stored in a locked cabinet well out of your child's reach?

☐ Are hair dryers, curling irons, and other electrical appliances unplugged and stored well out of reach? They can cause burns or electrical injuries.

☐ Are there child-resistant safety latches on all cabinets containing potentially harmful substances (cosmetics, medications, mouthwash, cleaning supplies)?

☐ Are there child-resistant caps on all medications, and are all medications stored in their original containers?

☐ Is the temperature of your hot water heater 120°F or lower to prevent scalding?

☐ Do you need a doorknob cover to prevent your child from going into the bathroom when you are not there? Teach adults and older children to put the toilet seat cover down and to close the bathroom door when done—to prevent drowning.

☐ Remember, supervision of young children is essential in the bathroom, especially when they are in the tub—to prevent drowning.

The Kitchen

☐ Make sure that vitamins or other medications are kept out of your child's reach. Use child-resistant caps.

☐ Keep sharp knives or other sharp utensils well out of the child's reach (using safety latches or high cabinets).

☐ See that chairs and step stools are away from counters and the stove, where a child could climb up and get hurt.

☐ Use the back burners and make sure pot handles on the stove are pointing inward so your child cannot reach up and grab them.

☐ Make sure automatic dishwasher detergent and other toxic cleaning supplies are stored in their original containers, out of a child's reach, in cabinets with child safety latches.

☐ Keep the toaster out of your child's reach to prevent burns or electrical injuries.

☐ Keep electrical appliances unplugged from the wall when not in use, and use plug protectors for wall outlets.

☐ Are appliance cords tucked away so that they cannot be pulled on?

☐ Make sure that your child's high chair is sturdy and has a seat belt with a crotch strap.

☐ Is there a working fire extinguisher in the kitchen? Do all adults and older children know how to use it?

The Family Room

☐ Are edges and corners of tables padded to prevent injuries?

☐ Are houseplants out of your child's reach? Certain houseplants may be poisonous.

☐ Are televisions and other heavy items (such as lamps) secure so that they cannot tip over?

☐ Are there any unnecessary or frayed extension cords? Cords should run behind furniture and not hang down for children to pull on them.

☐ Is there a barrier around the fireplace or other heat source?

☐ Are the cords from drapes or blinds kept out of your child's reach to prevent strangulation?

☐ Are plug protectors in unused electrical outlets?

☐ Are matches and lighters out of reach?

Miscellaneous Items

☐ Are stairs carpeted and protected with non-accordion gates?

☐ Are the rooms in your house free from small parts, plastic bags, small toys, and balloons that could pose a choking hazard?

☐ Do you have a plan of escape from your home in the event of a fire? Have you reviewed and practiced the plan with your family?

☐ Does the door to the basement have a self-latching lock to prevent your child from falling down the stairs?

☐ Do not place your child in a baby walker with wheels. They are very dangerous, especially near stairs.

☐ Are dangerous products stored out of reach (in cabinets with safety latches or locks or on high shelves) and in their original containers in the utility room, basement, and garage?

☐ If your child has a playpen, does it have small-mesh sides (less than 3/4 inch mesh) or closely spaced vertical slats (less than 2⅜ inches)?

☐ Are the numbers of the Poison Control Center and your pediatrician posted on all phones?

☐ Do your children know how to call 911 in an emergency?

☐ Inspect your child's toys for sharp or detachable parts. Repair or throw away broken toys.

The Playground

☐ Are the swing seats made of something soft, not wood or metal?

☐ Is the surface under playground equipment energy absorbent, such as rubber, sand, sawdust (12 inches deep), wood chips, or bark? Is it well maintained?

☐ Is your home playground equipment put together correctly and does it sit on a level surface, anchored firmly to the ground?

☐ Do you check playground equipment for hot metal surfaces such as those on slides, which can cause burns? Does your slide face away from the sun?

☐ Are all screws and bolts on your playground equipment capped? Do you check for loose nuts and bolts periodically? Be sure there are no projecting bolts, nails, or s-links.

☐ Do you watch your children when they are using playground equipment— to prevent shoving, pushing, or fighting?

☐ Never let a child play on playground equipment with dangling drawstrings on a jacket or shirt.

The Pool

☐ Never leave your child alone in or near the pool, even for a moment.

☐ Do you have a 4-foot fence around all sides of the pool that cannot be climbed by children and that separates the pool from the house?

☐ Do fence gates self-close and self-latch, with latches higher than your child's reach?

☐ Does your pool cover completely cover the pool so that your child cannot slip under it?

☐ Do you keep rescue equipment (such as a shepherd's hook or life preserver) and a telephone by the pool?

☐ Does everyone who watches your child around a pool know basic lifesaving techniques and CPR?

☐ Does your child know the rules of water and diving safety?

The Yard

☐ Do you use a power mower with a control that stops the mower if the handle is let go?

☐ Never let a child younger than 12 years of age mow the lawn. Make sure your older child wears sturdy shoes (not sandals or sneakers) while mowing the lawn and that objects such as stones and toys are picked up from the lawn before it is mowed.

☐ Do not allow young children in the yard while you are mowing.

☐ Teach your child to never pick and eat anything from a plant.

☐ Be sure you know what is growing in your yard so, if your child accidentally ingests a plant, you can give the proper information to your local Poison Control Center.

The information contained in this publication should not be used as a substitute for the medical care and advice of your pediatrician. There may be variations in treatment that your pediatrician may recommend based on individual facts and circumstances.

American Academy
of Pediatrics

DEDICATED TO THE HEALTH OF ALL CHILDREN™

The American Academy of Pediatrics is an organization of 60,000 primary care pediatricians, pediatric medical subspecialists, and pediatric surgical specialists dedicated to the health, safety, and well-being of infants, children, adolescents, and young adults.

American Academy of Pediatrics
Web site—www.aap.org

Copyright © 1999
American Academy of Pediatrics

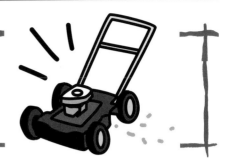

Lawn Mower Safety

Each year many children are injured severely by lawn mowers. Power mowers can be especially dangerous. However, most lawn mower-related injuries can be prevented by following these safety guidelines.

When is my child old enough to mow the lawn?

Before learning how to mow the lawn, your child should show the maturity, good judgment, strength and coordination that the job requires. In general, the American Academy of Pediatrics recommends that children should be at least

- 12 years of age to operate a walk-behind power mower or hand mower safely
- 16 years of age to operate a riding lawn mower safely

  It is important to teach your child how to use a lawn mower. Before you allow your child to mow the lawn alone, spend time showing him or her how to do the job safely. Supervise your child's work until you are sure that he or she can manage the task alone.

Before mowing the lawn:

1. Make sure that children are indoors or at a safe distance well away from the area that you plan to mow.
2. Read the lawn mower operator's manual and the instructions on the mower.
3. Check conditions
   - Do not mow during bad weather, such as during a thunderstorm.
   - Do not mow wet grass.
   - Do not mow without enough daylight.
4. Clear the mowing area of any objects such as twigs, stones, and toys, that could be picked up and thrown by the lawn mower blades.
5. Make sure that protective guards, shields, the grass catcher, and other types of safety equipment are placed properly on the lawn mower and that your mower is in good condition.
6. If your lawn mower is electric, use a ground fault circuit interrupter to prevent electric shock.
7. Never allow children to ride as passengers on ride-on lawn mowers or garden tractors.

While mowing:

1. Wear sturdy closed-toe shoes with slip-proof soles, close-fitting clothes, safety goggles or glasses with side shields, and hearing protection.
2. Watch for objects that could be picked up and thrown by the mower blades, as well as hidden dangers. Tall grass can hide objects, holes or bumps. Use caution when approaching corners, trees or anything that might block your view.
3. If the mower strikes an object, stop, turn the mower off, and inspect the mower. If it is damaged, do not use it until it has been repaired.
4. Do not pull the mower backwards or mow in reverse unless absolutely necessary, and carefully look for children behind you when you mow in reverse.
5. Use extra caution when mowing a slope.
   - When a walk-behind mower is used, mow across the face of slopes, not up and down, to avoid slipping under the mower and into the blades.
   - With a riding mower, mow up and down slopes, not across, to avoid tipping over.
6. Keep in mind that lawn trimmers also can throw objects at high speed.
7. Remain aware of where children are and do not allow them near the area where you are working. Children tend to be attracted to mowers in use.

Stop the engine and allow it to cool before refueling.

Always turn off the mower and wait for the blades to stop completely before

- Crossing gravel paths, roads or other areas
- Removing the grass catcher
- Unclogging the discharge chute
- Walking away from the mower

This information is based on the American Academy of Pediatrics' policy statement *Lawn Mower Injuries to Children*, published in June 2001. *Parent Pages* offers parents relevant facts that explain current policies about children's health.

The information contained in this publication should not be used as a substitute for the medical care and advice of your pediatrician. There may be variations in treatment that your pediatrician may recommend based on individual facts and circumstances.

American Academy of Pediatrics

DEDICATED TO THE HEALTH OF ALL CHILDREN™

The American Academy of Pediatrics is an organization of 60,000 primary care pediatricians, pediatric medical subspecialists, and pediatric surgical specialists dedicated to the health, safety, and well-being of infants, children, adolescents, and young adults.

American Academy of Pediatrics
Web site—www.aap.org

Copyright © 2001
American Academy of Pediatrics

Lead Screening for Children

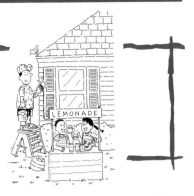

Of all the health problems caused by the environment, lead poisoning is the most preventable. Despite this, almost 1 million children in the United States have elevated levels of lead in their blood. Any child can be at risk for lead poisoning.

Read more to learn about the risks of lead poisoning and how to prevent it, and about lead screening and treatment for lead poisoning.

How can lead hurt my child?

Children, primarily those younger than 6 years, *can* be exposed to lead if they
- Get lead dust from old paint on their hands or toys and then put their hands in their mouths
- Breathe in lead dust from old paint
- Eat chips of old paint or dirt that contain lead
- Drink water from pipes lined or soldered with lead

Once lead enters the body, it travels through the bloodstream and is stored mainly in the bones where it can remain for a lifetime. Very high levels of lead in the body may cause many long-term problems, including
- Developmental delays
- Hearing loss
- Seizures and coma
- Kidney problems
- Anemia
- Growth problems

Most children with high lead levels in their blood show no obvious symptoms until they reach school age. At that point, some may show learning and behavioral problems. Others with high lead levels may experience symptoms such as stomach pain, headaches, vomiting, or muscle weakness.

Where can lead be found?

You may have heard that children can be harmed by the lead in pencils. This is not true. There is no actual lead in pencils and there is no lead in the paint on the outside of pencils. Lead is found in the following places:
- Dust and paint chips from old paint
- Homes built before 1950, particularly those that are in need of repair or are in deteriorating condition
- Homes built before 1978 that are being renovated
- Soil that has lead in it
- Hobby materials such as stained glass, paints, solders, fishing weights, and buckshot
- Folk remedies
- Workplace dust brought home on the clothing of people who have jobs that use lead, such as foundry workers, smelter workers, and radiator repair mechanics
- Food stored in some ceramic dishes (especially if made in another country)
- Older painted toys and antique furniture such as cribs

Should my child be screened for lead?

If you can answer "yes" to any of the following questions, especially numbers 1, 2, and 3, your child may need to be screened for lead. Talk to your pediatrician about lead screening for your child.

1. Does your child live in or regularly visit a house that was built before 1950, including a home child care center or the home of a relative?
2. Does your child live in or regularly visit a house built before 1978 that has been remodeled in the last 6 months? Are there any plans to remodel?
3. Does your child have a brother, sister, housemate, or playmate who is being treated for lead poisoning?
4. Does your child live with an adult whose job or hobby involves exposure to lead?
5. Does your child live near an active lead smelter, battery-recycling plant, or other industry likely to release lead into the environment?
6. Does your child live within 1 block of a major highway or busy street?
7. Has your child ever been given home remedies such as azarcon, greta, or pay looah?
8. Has your child ever lived outside the United States?
9. Does your family use pottery or ceramics for cooking, eating, or drinking?
10. Have you seen your child eat paint chips?
11. Have you seen your child eat soil or dirt?
12. Have you been told your child has low iron?

Adapted from the Centers for Disease Control and Prevention's *Screening Young Children for Lead Poisoning: Guidance for State and Local Public Health Officials.*

- Tap water in older homes that have lead pipes or lead solder in their pipes
- Automobile batteries

Prevention—what you can do

- If your home was built before 1950, ask your child's pediatrician to test your child for lead.
- If your home was built before 1978, talk with your child's pediatrician or your health department about safe ways to remodel *before* any work is done.
- When removing lead paint, be sure to use a certified contractor. Trying to remove the paint on your own can often make the condition worse. Know your state's laws regarding lead removal. Some states only allow certified contractors to remove lead. Be sure to seal off the room or area you are remodeling with heavy plastic until the job is done.

- Clean and cover any chalking, flaking, or chipping paint with a new coat of paint, duct tape, or contact paper. It is important to check for paint dust or flaking paint at window areas where children often play. Be aware that these are temporary measures only, and that lead must be completely removed for your child's best protection.
- Repair areas where paint is dusting, chipping, or peeling before placing cribs, playpens, beds, or highchairs next to them.
- Wet mop floors, damp sponge walls and horizontal surfaces, and vacuum with a high-efficiency particulate air vacuum (HEPA vac) if you are concerned about the possibility of lead dust in your home. Although good cleaning is a temporary solution, complete removal of the lead is the best protection.
- Encourage your children to wash their hands often, especially before eating.
- Have your home or apartment checked for possible lead contamination before moving in. Keep in mind that landlords are legally responsible for removing any lead found on their property.
- If you work around lead or have hobbies that involve lead, change clothes and shoes before entering your home. Keep clothes at work or wash work clothes as soon as possible.
- Check with your child's pediatrician or your health department to see if your area has a problem with lead in the water.
- If you have lead pipes, run the first morning tap water for 2 minutes before using it for drinking or cooking. Use cold tap water for mixing formula, drinking, or cooking because hot tap water can have higher amounts of lead in it.

You can also reduce the risks of lead by making sure your child eats a well-balanced diet. Give your child nutritious, low-fat foods that are high in calcium and iron, like meat, beans, spinach, and low-fat dairy products. Calcium and iron in particular reduce the amount of lead absorbed by the body.

Lead screening

The only way to know for sure if your child has been exposed to lead is to have your child's pediatrician test your child's blood. Lead screening tests use either a small amount of blood from a finger prick or a larger sample of blood from a vein in the arm. These tests measure the amount of lead in the blood.

Treatment

For children with *low* levels of lead in their blood, identify and eliminate the sources of lead to avoid future health problems. Children with *high* levels of lead in their blood usually need to take a drug that binds the lead in the blood and helps the body get rid of it. This treatment may be given as a series of shots or as oral medicine depending on the severity of the lead poisoning. Some children with lead poisoning need more than one type of treatment and several months of close follow-up. If the damage is severe, the child may need special schooling and therapy.

Remember

Most young children put things other than food into their mouths. They chew on toys, taste the sand at the park, and eat cat food if given the chance. This rarely causes any harm, as long as poisons, small items that children can choke on, and sharp objects are kept out of reach. Lead, however, can be very dangerous to children. Infants and toddlers can get lead poisoning by putting their fingers in their mouths after touching lead dust, eating lead paint chips, or breathing in lead dust. Lead poisoning can cause developmental delay, hearing loss, seizures and coma, kidney problems, anemia, and growth problems. Talk with your child's pediatrician about getting a blood test, especially if your child is younger than 3 years. Take the steps listed in this brochure to make sure your child is not exposed to lead.

The information contained in this publication should not be used as a substitute for the medical care and advice of your pediatrician. There may be variations in treatment that your pediatrician may recommend based on individual facts and circumstances.

From your doctor

American Academy of Pediatrics

DEDICATED TO THE HEALTH OF ALL CHILDREN™

The American Academy of Pediatrics is an organization of 60,000 primary care pediatricians, pediatric medical subspecialists, and pediatric surgical specialists dedicated to the health, safety, and well-being of infants, children, adolescents, and young adults.
American Academy of Pediatrics
Web site—www.aap.org

Copyright © 2005
American Academy of Pediatrics

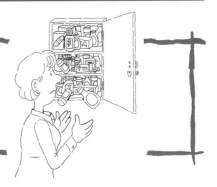

A Guide to Your Child's Medicines

If you are confused or have questions about your child's medicines, you are not alone. The instructions that come with medicines can be hard to read and understand. For your child's health and safety, it's important that you understand this information. Read on to find out more about your child's medicines.

Ask questions

Before you give your child any medicines, be sure you know how to use them. The following are questions you can ask your pediatrician or pharmacist:

- What is the name of the medicine?
- How will it help my child?
- Do I need to do anything *before* I give this medicine to my child?
- How much medicine do I give my child? When? For how long?
- Should my child avoid certain activities or not eat certain foods while using this medicine?
- Should my child not take other medicines, herbal products, or supplements?
- Are there any side effects?
- Is there anything special I need to know? (For example, is the dose larger than usual?)
- Is there any written information you can give me?
- What do I do if my child misses a dose?
- What do I do if I give my child too much?
- What if my child spits it out?
- Does it come in chewable tablets or liquid?
- Can you show me how to use this medicine?
- (If it's a prescription) Can this prescription be refilled? How many times?

Prescription medicines

Medicines that only a doctor (and some other health professionals) can order are called *prescription medicines*. They may be generic or brand name. Generic medicines cost less than brand-name medicines but aren't always available. Sometimes it's more important to use the brand name. Ask your pediatrician what's best for your child.

The following are common prescription medicines for children:

- **Antibiotics.** Used for some bacterial infections like strep throat. Also used for some types of infections of the ear, sinus, urinary tract, and skin. Antibiotics usually don't cause problems but can have some side effects. Side effects may include skin rash, loose stools, upset stomach, staining of urine, or allergic reactions. Antibiotics don't work on viral infections like colds and the flu. The overuse of antibiotics has caused some bacteria to become resistant to them. This is why your pediatrician may not always treat a bacterial infection with an antibiotic.

If your child goes to the hospital, do the following:

- Bring your child's health records.
- If your child is taking any medicines, including supplements, vitamins, herbal products, or home remedies, bring them to the hospital in their original containers. Write down when your child last took the medicines, and bring the note with you.
- Ask about any medicines your child is given while in the hospital. Keep a diary of what types of medicines are given to your child and when. Make sure to note any allergic reactions.

- **Ear drops.** Used for inflammation and infections of the ear canal. Side effects may include itching, feeling like the ears are clogged, or a "popping" sound in the ear.
- **Eyedrops or ointment.** Used for eye infections, allergies, or vision problems. Some children may get puffy eyes or say the drops hurt their eyes.
- **Inhalers.** Used to treat asthma and inflammation of the lungs. Your pediatrician will show you how to use an inhaler.
- **Nasal sprays.** Used to treat sinus problems or allergies. Certain types of sprays should only be used for a short time. Check with your pediatrician about how to use your nasal spray.
- **Skin products.** Used for skin infections, burns, parasites/mites, rashes, and acne. In general they are well tolerated, but your child's skin may get irritated. Also, special care is needed when using medicines that contain steroids or medicines for lice and scabies. They can have serious side effects if used too long.

All medicines have the potential to cause allergic reactions. Remember to let your pediatrician know if your child has any side effects to any medicine. Side effects may include vomiting or hives or other skin rashes.

Read the label

The following information is found on a prescription label:

a) **Prescription number.** Your pharmacy will ask for this number when you call in for a refill. You may also need this number when filling out insurance forms.
b) **Your child's name.** Never give your child's medicine to another child even if the other child has similar symptoms.
c) **Name of the medicine or the main ingredient.** Make sure this matches what your pediatrician told you. The strength of the medicine (for example, 10-mg tablets) may also be listed.

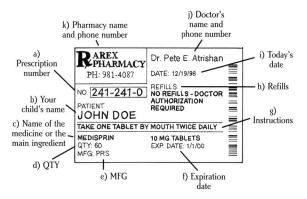

a) Prescription number

k) Pharmacy name and phone number

j) Doctor's name and phone number

i) Today's date

b) Your child's name

c) Name of the medicine or the main ingredient

d) QTY

e) MFG

f) Expiration date

g) Instructions

h) Refills

d) **QTY.** "Quantity" or how much is in the package.

e) **MFG.** "Manufacturer" or who makes the medicine.

f) **Expiration date.** Throw away or flush medicines past this date.

g) **Instructions.** The instructions tell you what condition or symptom is being treated and how your child needs to take the medicine. What your pediatrician tells you should match what is on the label. The following are some examples:

- **"Take full course."** Make sure your child takes the medicine for as long as directed, even if your child is feeling better.
- **"Take with food."** Give the medicine to your child after a meal. This is for medicines that work better when the stomach is full.
- **"Take 4 times a day."** Give the medicine to your child 4 times during the day—for example, at breakfast, lunch, dinner, and before bed. This is different than "take every 4 hours."
- **"Take every 4 hours."** Give the medicine to your child every 4 hours. This adds up to 6 times in a 24-hour period. For example, 6:00 am, 10:00 am, 2:00 pm, 6:00 pm, 10:00 pm, and 2:00 am. Most medicines don't have to be given at the exact time to work, but some do.
- **"Take as needed as symptoms persist."** Give the medicine to your child when needed.

h) **Refills.** The label will show the number of refills you can get. If "no refills—Dr authorization required" is on the label, you will need to call your pediatrician.

i) **Today's date.**

j) **Doctor's name and phone number.**

k) **Pharmacy name and phone number.**

The medicine may have an extra brightly colored safety label that says, for example, "Keep refrigerated," "Shake well before using," or "May cause drowsiness."

Over-the-counter medicines

You can get *over-the-counter (OTC) medicines* without a doctor's order. This doesn't mean that OTCs are harmless. Like prescription medicines, OTCs can be very dangerous to a child if not taken the right way. You need to read and understand the instructions before giving OTCs to your child.

The following are common OTCs for children. Talk with your pediatrician before you give your child any medicine.

- **Acetaminophen and ibuprofen (fever reducer or pain reliever).** Can help your child feel better if your child's head or body aches or he has a fever. They also can help relieve minor pain from bangs and bumps or soreness from a shot. You don't need to treat a mild fever if your child is playing, drinking fluids, and generally acting well.

A warning about aspirin

Never give aspirin or other salicylates (a type of medicine used to reduce pain or fever) to your child unless your pediatrician tells you it's safe. Aspirin has been linked to Reye syndrome, a serious and sometimes fatal liver disorder, especially when given to children with the flu or chickenpox. For more information on Reye syndrome or a list of medicines that contain aspirin, contact the National Reye's Syndrome Foundation at 800/233-7393 or www.reyessyndrome.org.

Acetaminophen and ibuprofen have few side effects and are quite safe if the right dose is given. They come in drops for infants, liquid (syrup or elixir) for toddlers, and chewable tablets for older children. Acetaminophen also comes in suppositories if your child is vomiting and can't keep down medicine taken by mouth. *Never* give a child aspirin (see "A warning about aspirin").

Keep in mind that infant drops are *stronger* (more concentrated) than syrup for toddlers. Some parents make the mistake of giving higher doses of infant drops to a toddler, thinking the drops are not as strong. Be sure the type you give your child is appropriate for his weight and age.

Ibuprofen tends to work better than acetaminophen in treating high fevers (103°F or higher). However, ibuprofen should only be given to children older than 6 months. Never give it to a child who is dehydrated or vomiting.

If your child has a kidney disease, asthma, an ulcer, or other chronic illness, ask your pediatrician if ibuprofen is safe for your child. Don't give your child ibuprofen or acetaminophen if he is taking any other pain reliever or fever reducer, unless your pediatrician says it's OK.

- **Antihistamines.** Can help your child feel better when he has a runny nose, itchy eyes, and sneezing due to allergies (but not colds). They also can help relieve itching from chickenpox or insect bites. They can even control hives or other allergic reactions. Antihistamines can make some children sleepy. Other children may become irritable, nervous, or restless. For that reason, don't give an antihistamine at bedtime unless you know your child will have no trouble sleeping.

- **Cough syrups.** Coughing helps clear the lungs of germs and mucus. A cough is "productive" if it sounds like mucus is coming up. This type of cough usually doesn't need to be treated. However, some coughs may be very dry and keep your child up at night. A humidifier may help loosen your child's cough. (Be sure to clean the humidifier often to prevent mold and bacteria buildup.) Some cough medicines, called *expectorants,* may also help loosen mucus. Cough *suppressants,* which help calm a cough, should be avoided as coughing helps clear the lungs. Current studies question the effectiveness and safety of cough suppressants, so you should check with your pediatrician before giving your child cough medicines or expectorants. Cough medicine isn't usually recommended to relieve cough caused by asthma.

- **Cold medicines.** Many cold medicines contain acetaminophen or ibuprofen. Always check the ingredients, especially if you're giving your child more than one medicine at the same time. If you're not careful, you could give your child too much of a certain kind of medicine, and it could lead to an overdose.

- **Cortisone/hydrocortisone cream.** Used to treat insect bites, mild skin rashes, poison ivy, and eczema. Ask your pediatrician how often you can apply it and if it's OK to use on your child's face. It should never be used for chickenpox, burns, infections, or open wounds or on broken skin.
- **Decongestant (liquid).** May relieve some cold symptoms. However, they can have many side effects. Children may become irritable, nervous, or restless. Current studies question the effectiveness of decongestants, so check with your pediatrician before giving your child these medicines.
- **Decongestant (nose drops).** Can help make breathing easier. However, they should never be given to an infant because too much of the medicine can be absorbed through the nose. Also, the more they are used, the less they work, and symptoms can return or even get worse. If your older child can't eat or sleep because of a stuffy nose, ask your pediatrician about decongestant nose drops. Don't give your child decongestant nose drops for more than 2 to 3 days unless your pediatrician says it's OK.
- **Saline nose drops.** May help if your child is having trouble eating or sleeping because of a stuffy nose. A bulb syringe may be used to suck out nasal mucus after saline drops are used. Put 1 to 2 drops into a nostril at a time. Use the bulb syringe to suck out the drops and mucus. Using a bulb syringe can irritate your child's nose, so try not to use it too often. If your child is sleeping and eating well, there's no need to treat a stuffy nose.
- **Stomach and intestinal problems medicine.** There are many OTCs for common stomach and intestinal problems such as heartburn, gas, constipation, and diarrhea. Most of these conditions go away by themselves. Sometimes a temporary change in diet helps. Before using any medicines for constipation or diarrhea, talk with your pediatrician. Repeated bouts of diarrhea or chronic constipation can be a sign of a more serious problem.

Remember to let your pediatrician know if your child has any side effects to any medicine.

Taking medicines the right way

For your child's medicine to work, it must be taken as directed. The following are important things to remember:

- **Stick with the schedule.** Don't skip a dose of your child's medicine. Ask your pediatrician or pharmacist what to do if a dose isn't given on time.
- **Give the right amount.** Measure carefully. Don't give your child more medicine because you think it may work better or faster. Giving your child more medicine than is needed may harm her. Follow the directions exactly.
- **Know your child's weight.** With OTCs, check the label to see how much medicine to give based on your child's weight. Age is not always an accurate measure of how much medicine to give your child.
- **Don't stop too soon.** Your child should finish *all* of her prescription medicine, even if she begins to feel better. The same goes for when she doesn't like the taste of the medicine or protests. This is especially true for antibiotics. The infection can come back if the medicine is stopped too soon.
- **Don't try to hide the medicine.** Even though most children's medicines come in flavors to make them taste better, your child may hate the taste and spit it out. It's not a good idea to try to hide the medicine in milk or food. This may affect how the medicine works. Your child may also only eat part of it, or it may settle to the bottom and never get into her mouth. Try giving an older child chewable tablets instead of liquids.

Liquid medicines

Many children's medicines come in liquid form because they are easier to swallow than pills. But they must be used the right way. Parents often misread the directions and give their children too much medicine. This can be very dangerous, especially if given over a period of several days. Always read the instructions carefully. Call your pediatrician if you aren't sure how much medicine to give your child or how often or for how long to give the medicine to your child. Use the measuring device that comes with the medicine (your tablespoons or teaspoons at home are usually not accurate).

- **Dosing spoons.** Works well for older children who can open their mouths and "drink" from the spoon.
- **Medicine cups.** These often come as caps on liquid cold and flu medicines. Make sure to use the cup that comes with the medicine— don't mix and match cups to other products.
- **Syringes and oral droppers.** Works well for infants. Simply squirt the medicine between your child's tongue and the side of her mouth (not the back of the throat). This makes it easier for her to swallow. If you have a syringe with a plastic cap, throw the cap into the trash so that it does not fall off in your child's mouth. Studies have shown that many parents think that the entire syringe or dropper needs to be filled with the medicine. This is not always true. Read the directions carefully and look at the numbers on the side of the dosing device.

Taking medicines safely

You can help prevent overdose or poisoning. The following are important safety tips:

- **Always use good light.** If the room is poorly lit, you may take the wrong medicine or give the wrong dose by mistake.
- **Recheck the label.** Read the label before you open the bottle and again before you give the medicine. Remember, "TBSP" is not the same as "T." TBSP is a *tablespoon;* T or TSP is a *teaspoon.*
- **Use safety caps.** Always use child-resistant caps. Medicines should be stored in a locked, child-proof cabinet.
- **Give the right dose.** Never guess how much to give your child. Also, extra medicine won't make your child feel any better any faster.

What if my child is poisoned?

If you think your child has swallowed any medicines or substances that might be harmful, stay calm and act fast. ***If your child is unconscious, not breathing, or having convulsions or seizures, call 911 or your local emergency number right away.*** If your child doesn't have these symptoms, call the poison center at 1-**800-222-1222.** A poison expert in your area is available 24 hours a day, 7 days a week.

Don't use syrup of ipecac. If you have syrup of ipecac in your home, flush it down the toilet and throw away the bottle. Syrup of ipecac is a drug that was used in the past to make children vomit if they swallowed poison. You shouldn't make a child vomit in any way.

- **Use the right measuring device.** Don't use a dosing cup labeled only with ounces if you need to measure the medicine in teaspoons.
- **Watch your child.** Never let your child take medicine by himself. Avoid calling medicine candy.
- **Check the package.** Before using any medicine, always check the package for cuts, tears, or other signs the package was opened.
- **Store your medicines in a cool, dry place.** Medicines can be affected by humidity, so don't store them in your bathroom.

Talk with your pediatrician if you have any questions or concerns about giving your child medicines. Always let your pediatrician know if your child is taking other medicines, if there are any changes in how your child is feeling, or if your child has any reactions to the medicines.

The information contained in this publication should not be used as a substitute for the medical care and advice of your pediatrician. There may be variations in treatment that your pediatrician may recommend based on individual facts and circumstances.

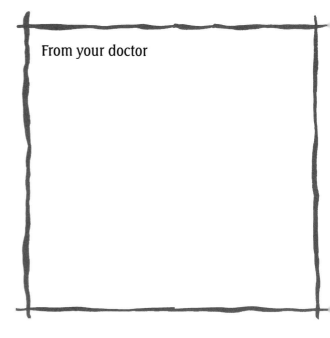

From your doctor

American Academy of Pediatrics

DEDICATED TO THE HEALTH OF ALL CHILDREN™

The American Academy of Pediatrics is an organization of 60,000 primary care pediatricians, pediatric medical subspecialists, and pediatric surgical specialists dedicated to the health, safety, and well-being of infants, children, adolescents, and young adults.

American Academy of Pediatrics
Web site—www.aap.org

Copyright © 2005
American Academy of Pediatrics, Updated 2/05

Playground Safety

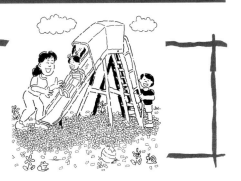

Each year, about 200,000 children get hurt on playground equipment with injuries serious enough to need treatment in the emergency department. About 15 children die each year from playground injuries. While many of these injuries happen on home equipment, most occur at school and public playgrounds.

Read on to find out how you can tell if the playground equipment at your home or child's school or in your neighborhood is as safe as possible.

How are children injured?

Most playground injuries occur when children fall off tall equipment like monkey bars. Other injuries happen when children

- Trip over equipment
- Get hit by equipment, such as a swing
- Get bruises, scrapes, or cuts from sharp edges
  Some injuries, such as head injuries, can be serious or even fatal. Other injuries may include broken bones, sprains, and wounds to the teeth and mouth.

How to prevent playground injuries

To check if play equipment is safe, ask yourself the following questions:

- Is the equipment the right size? For example, smaller swings are for smaller children and can break if larger children use them.
- Is the play equipment installed correctly and according to the manufacturer's directions?
- Can children reach any moving parts that might pinch or trap any body part?
- What's underneath the equipment? The best way to prevent serious injuries is to have a surface that will absorb impact when children land on it. This is especially needed under and around swings, slides, and climbing equipment. (See "What are safer surfaces?").
- Is wooden play equipment free of splinters and nails or screws that stick out?
  Here are some other things to check for.

Climbing structures

- Platforms higher than 30 inches above the ground intended for use by school-aged children should have guardrails or barriers to prevent falls.
- Vertical and horizontal spaces should be less than 3½ inches wide or more than 9 inches wide. This is to keep a small child's head from getting trapped.
- Rungs, stairs, and steps should be evenly spaced.
- Round rungs to be gripped by young hands should be about 1 to 1½ inches in diameter.

Slides

- Slides should be placed in the shade or away from the sun. Metal slides can get very hot from the sun and burn a child's hands and legs. Plastic slides are better because they do not get as hot, but they should still be checked before using.
- Slides should have a platform with rails at the top for children to hold. There should be a guardrail, hood, or other device at the top of the slide that requires the child to sit when going down the slide. Open slides should have sides at least 4 inches high.
- Make sure there are no rocks, glass, sticks, toys, debris, or other children at the base of a slide. These could get in the way of a child landing safely. The cleared area in front of the slide should extend a distance equal to the height of the slide platform, with a minimum of 6 feet and a maximum of 8 feet cleared.

Swings

- Swings should be clear of other equipment. Make sure there is a distance in front of and behind a swing that is twice the height of the suspending bar.
- Swing seats should be made of soft materials such as rubber, plastic, or canvas.
- Make sure open or "S" hooks on swing chains are closed to form a figure 8.
- Walls or fences should be located at least 6 feet from either side of a swing structure.
- Swing sets should be securely anchored according to the manufacturer's instructions to prevent tipping. Anchors should be buried deep enough so that children can't trip or fall over them.
- Swings should not be too close together. There should be at least 24 inches between swings and no more than 2 seat swings (or 1 tire swing) in the same section of the structure.
  Remember, even with these measures, children still need to be watched closely while they are playing.

The danger of wearing drawstrings and bicycle helmets on playground equipment

Drawstrings on clothing and bicycle helmets can strangle a child if they get caught on playground equipment. The best way to prevent this is to take drawstrings off jackets, shirts, and hats and shorten drawstrings on coats and jackets. Bicycle helmets should be worn while riding a bicycle, but *not* while playing on playground equipment.

What are safer surfaces?

Safer surfaces make a serious head injury less likely to occur if a child falls. This is because they are made to absorb the impact of a fall. Some examples of safer surfaces include the following:

- Wood chips, mulch, or shredded rubber—at least 9 inches deep for play equipment up to 7 feet high.
- Sand or pea gravel—at least 9 inches deep for play equipment up to 5 feet high.
- Rubber outdoor mats—make sure they are safety tested for playground equipment.

Check loose-fill surfaces often. They should be raked at least once a week to keep them soft. They also should be refilled often to keep the correct depth. Poured-in-place surfaces should be checked continually for wear. Concrete, asphalt, packed earth, and grass are *not* safe surfaces and should not be used under playground equipment.

No surface is totally safe. Many injuries are preventable, but they can sometimes occur even at the safest playgrounds and with the best supervision. Be prepared to handle an injury if it does occur.

For more information about playground safety and safer surfaces or to get a copy of the *Handbook for Public Playground Safety,* visit the US Consumer Product Safety Commission Web site at www.cpsc.gov.

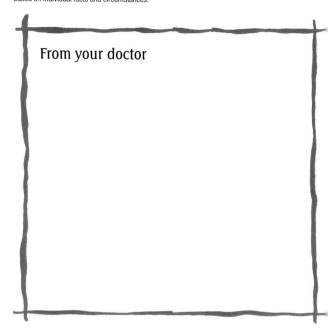

From your doctor

American Academy
of Pediatrics

DEDICATED TO THE HEALTH OF ALL CHILDREN™

The American Academy of Pediatrics is an organization of 60,000 primary care pediatricians, pediatric medical subspecialists, and pediatric surgical specialists dedicated to the health, safety, and well-being of infants, children, adolescents, and young adults.

American Academy of Pediatrics
Web site—www.aap.org

Copyright © 2006
American Academy of Pediatrics, Updated 10/05

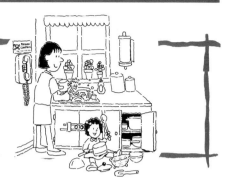

Protect Your Child From Poison

Children can get very sick if they come in contact with medicines, household products, pesticides, chemicals, cosmetics, or plants. This can happen at any age and can cause serious reactions. However, most children who come in contact with these things are not poisoned. And most who are poisoned are not permanently hurt if they are treated right away.

Read more to learn how to prevent poisonings and what to do if your child has been poisoned.

Prevention

Most poisonings occur when parents are not paying close attention. While you are busy cooking dinner, or planning tomorrow's schedule, your child may explore what's in the closet or under the bathroom sink.

Because children like to put things into their mouths and taste them, all dangerous items should be kept out of their reach. The best way to prevent poisonings is to lock up all dangerous items.

The most dangerous potential poisons in the home for young children are

- Medicines (iron medicines are one of the most serious causes of poisonings in children younger than 5 years)
- Cleaning products
- Antifreeze
- Windshield washer fluid
- Pesticides
- Furniture polish
- Gasoline, kerosene, lamp oil

Poison Help Line

Call **1-800-222-1222** if you have a poison emergency. A poison expert in your area is available 24 hours a day, 7 days a week. Also call if you have a question about a poison or about poison prevention. **1-800-222-1222** is a nationwide toll-free number that directs your call to your regional poison center.

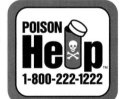

It also is important to store medicines and household products in their original containers. Many dangerous items look like food or drinks. For example, your child may mistake powdered dish soap for sugar or lemon liquid cleaner for lemonade.

Also, watch your child even more closely when you are away from home — especially at a grandparent's home where medicines are often left within a child's reach.

Read "How to poison-proof your home" for more safety tips. ➜

How to poison-proof your home

In the kitchen

- Store medicines, cleaners, lye, furniture polish, dishwasher soap, and other dangerous products in a locked cabinet.
- Lock medicines and poisons high, out of sight and reach of children.
- If you must store items under the sink, use safety latches that lock every time you close the cabinet (most hardware stores and department stores have them). Store medicines and household products in their original containers.

In the bathroom

- Buy and keep all medicines in containers with safety caps. But remember, these caps are child-resistant, not childproof, so store them in a locked cabinet.
- Discard any leftover prescription medicines by flushing them down the toilet.
- Store toothpaste, soap, shampoo, and other items used daily in a different cabinet from dangerous products.
- Take medicine where children cannot watch you; they may try to copy you.
- Call medicine by its correct name. You don't want to confuse your child by calling medicine candy.
- Check the label every time you give medicine. This will help you to be sure you are giving the right medicine in the right amounts to the right person. Mistakes are more common in the middle of the night, so always turn on a light when using any medicine.

In the garage and basement

- Keep paints, varnishes, thinners, pesticides, and fertilizers in a locked cabinet in their original, labeled containers.
- Read labels on all household products before you buy them. Try to find the safest ones for the job. Buy only what you need to use right away.
- Store products in their original containers. Never put poisonous products in containers that were once used for food, especially empty drink bottles, cans, or cups.
- Open the garage door before starting your car.
- Be sure that coal, wood, or kerosene stoves and appliances are in good working order. If you smell gas, turn off the stove or gas burner, leave the house, and call the gas company.

In the entire house

- Install smoke detectors and carbon monoxide detectors. Contact your local fire department for information on how many you need and where to install them.

Important information about syrup of ipecac

Syrup of ipecac is a drug that was used in the past to make children vomit after they had swallowed a poison. Although this may seem to make sense, this is not a good poison treatment. You should not make a child vomit in any way, including giving him syrup of ipecac, making him gag, or giving him saltwater. If you have syrup of ipecac in your home, flush it down the toilet and throw away the container.

Treatment

Swallowed poison

If you find your child with an open or empty container of a nonfood item, your child may have been poisoned. Stay calm and act quickly.

First, get the item away from your child. If there is still some in your child's mouth, make him spit it out or remove it with your fingers. Keep this material along with anything else that might help determine what your child swallowed.

Take the poison container with you to help the doctor determine what was swallowed. *Do not make your child vomit* because it may cause more damage.

If a child is unconscious, not breathing, having convulsions or having seizures, call 911 or your local emergency number right away.

If your child does not have these symptoms, call the poison center at **1-800-222-1222.** You may be asked for the following information:

- Your name and phone number.
- Your child's name, age, and weight.
- Any medical conditions your child has.
- Any medicine your child is taking.
- The name of the item your child swallowed. Read it off the container and spell it.
- The time your child swallowed the poison (or when you found your child), and the amount you think was swallowed.

If the poison is very dangerous, or if your child is very young, you may be told to take him right to the nearest hospital. If not, you will be told what to do at home.

Poison on the skin

If your child spills a dangerous chemical on her body, remove her clothes and rinse the skin with room temperature water for at least 15 minutes, even if your child resists. Then call the poison center at **1-800-222-1222.** Do not use ointments or grease.

Poison in the eye

Flush your child's eye by holding the eyelid open and pouring a steady stream of room temperature water into the inner corner. It is easier if another adult holds your child while you rinse the eye. If another adult is not around, wrap your child tightly in a towel and clamp him under one arm. Then you will have one hand free to hold the eyelid open and the other to pour in the water. Continue flushing the eye for 15 minutes. Then call the poison

center at **1-800-222-1222.** Do not use an eyecup, eyedrops, or ointment unless the poison center tells you to.

Poisonous fumes

In the home, poisonous fumes can come from

- A car running in a closed garage
- Leaky gas vents
- Wood, coal, or kerosene stoves that are not working right
- Space heaters, ovens, stoves, or hot water heaters that use gas

If your child is exposed to fumes or gases, have her breathe fresh air right away. If she is breathing, call the poison center at **1-800-222-1222** about what to do next. If she has stopped breathing, start cardiopulmonary resuscitation (CPR) and do not stop until she breathes on her own or someone else can take over. If you can, have someone call 911 right away. If you are alone, wait until your child is breathing, or after 1 minute of CPR, then call 911.

Remember

You can help make your home poison-safe by doing the following:

- Keep all medicines and household products locked up and out of your child's reach.
- Use safety latches on drawers and cabinets where you keep objects that may be dangerous to your child.
- Be prepared for a poisoning emergency. Post the poison help line number by every phone in your home. **1-800-222-1222** will connect you right away to your nearest poison center. (Be sure that your baby-sitter knows this number.)

The information contained in this publication should not be used as a substitute for the medical care and advice of your pediatrician. There may be variations in treatment that your pediatrician may recommend based on individual facts and circumstances.

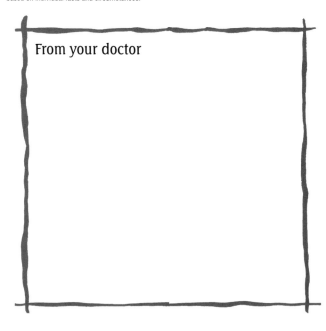

From your doctor

American Academy of Pediatrics

DEDICATED TO THE HEALTH OF ALL CHILDREN™

The American Academy of Pediatrics is an organization of 60,000 primary care pediatricians, pediatric medical subspecialists, and pediatric surgical specialists dedicated to the health, safety, and well-being of infants, children, adolescents, and young adults.

American Academy of Pediatrics
Web site — www.aap.org

Copyright © 2003
American Academy of Pediatrics, Updated 11/03

A Parent's Guide to Insect Repellents

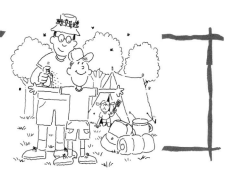

Mosquitoes, biting flies, and tick bites can make children miserable. While most children have only mild reactions to insect bites, some children can become very sick. Some insects carry dangerous illnesses such as West Nile virus, Lyme disease, and Rocky Mountain spotted fever.

One way to protect your child from biting insects is to use insect repellents. However, it's important that insect repellents are used safely and correctly.

Read more to learn about types of repellents, DEET, using repellents safely, and other ways to protect your child from insect bites. Also, read about West Nile virus, Lyme disease, and Rocky Mountain spotted fever.

Types of repellents

Insect repellents come in many forms including aerosols, sprays, liquids, creams, and sticks. Some are made from chemicals and some have natural ingredients. (See "Available Repellents.")

The following are types of repellents that are **not** effective:

- Wristbands soaked in chemical repellents
- Garlic or vitamin B_1 taken by mouth
- Ultrasonic devices that give off sound waves designed to keep insects away
- Bird or bat houses
- Backyard bug zappers (Insects may actually be attracted to your yard.)
  Keep in mind that insect repellents prevent bites from biting insects but not stinging insects. Biting insects include mosquitoes, ticks, fleas, chiggers, and biting flies. Stinging insects include bees, hornets, and wasps.

About DEET

DEET is a chemical used in insect repellents. The amount of DEET in insect repellents varies from product to product, so it's important to read the label of any product you buy. The amount of DEET may range from less than 10% to more than 30%.

Studies show that products with higher amounts of DEET protect people longer. For example, products with amounts around 10% may repel pests for about 2 hours, while products with amounts of about 24% last an average of 5 hours. But studies also show that products with amounts of DEET greater than 30% don't offer any extra protection.

The American Academy of Pediatrics (AAP) recommends that repellents should contain *no more than 30% DEET* when used on children. Insect repellents also are **not** recommended for children younger than 2 months.

Tips for using repellents safely

The following are guidelines on how to use insect repellents safely.

Dos

- Read the label and follow all directions and precautions.
- Only apply insect repellents on the outside of your child's clothing and on exposed skin.
- Spray repellents in open areas to avoid breathing them in.
- Use just enough repellent to cover your child's clothing and exposed skin. Using more doesn't make the repellent more effective. Avoid reapplying unless necessary.
- Assist young children when applying insect repellents on their own. Older children also should be supervised when using these products.
- Wash your children's skin with soap and water to remove any repellent when they return indoors, and wash their clothing before they wear it again.

Don'ts

- Never apply insect repellent to children younger than 2 months.
- Repellents should not be sprayed directly onto your child's face. Instead, spray a little on your hands first and then rub it on your child's face. Avoid the eyes and mouth.

Available Repellents

What's available	How well it works	How long it protects	Special precautions
Chemical repellents with **DEET** (N,N-diethyl-3-methylbenzamide)	Considered the best defense against biting insects.*	3 to 8 hours depending on how much DEET is in the product.	Caution should be used when applying DEET to children (see "Tips for using repellents safely").
Repellents made from **essential oils** found in plants such as citronella, cedar, eucalyptus, and soybean	Generally much less effective repellents; most give short-term protection only.	Usually less than 2 hours.	Allergic reactions are rare, but can occur.
Chemical repellents with **permethrin**	These repellents kill ticks on contact.	When applied to clothing, it lasts even after several washings.	Should only be applied to clothing, not directly to skin. May be applied to outdoor equipment such as sleeping bags or tents.

*In April 2005 the Centers for Disease Control and Prevention (CDC) recommended other repellents that may work as well as DEET: repellents with a chemical called picaridin and repellents with oil of lemon eucalyptus or 2% soybean oil. Currently these products have a duration of action that is comparable to that of about 10% DEET. Although these products are considered safe when used as recommended, long-term follow-up studies are not available. Also, more studies need to be done to see how well they repel ticks.

Diseases spread by insects

Diseases spread by insects are a major cause of illness to children and adults world-wide. Following is information about West Nile virus, Lyme disease, and Rocky Mountain spotted fever.

West Nile virus. In the United States, West Nile virus and outbreaks of various types of encephalitis get plenty of media coverage. These illnesses are carried by mosquitoes and transmitted to humans when the insects bite.

Most cases of West Nile virus are mild, with people showing no symptoms or having a fever, headache, and body aches. Other symptoms include the following:

- A mild rash
- Swollen lymph glands
- Severe headache
- High fever
- Stiff neck
- Confusion
- Seizures
- Sensitivity to light
- Muscle weakness
- Loss of consciousness

Lyme disease. In some areas of the United States, Lyme disease has been a major health problem. Deer ticks spread the disease. Deer ticks are tiny, black-brown, biting insects about the size of a poppy seed. The first and most obvious symptom of Lyme disease is a rash. It is a red spot surrounded by a light red ring that looks like a target. Other symptoms include the following:

- Headache
- Chills
- Fever
- Fatigue
- Swollen glands
- Aches and pains in the muscles or joints

Rocky Mountain spotted fever. Despite the name, Rocky Mountain spotted fever currently occurs mostly in other regions of the United States, including North and South Carolina, Oklahoma, and Tennessee. Ticks spread the disease. This is a serious disease in which patients develop the following symptoms:

- Fever
- Severe headache
- Confusion
- Nausea
- Vomiting
- Rash—Most also get a rash that starts as flat red spots that become purple over time. It begins on the palms and soles and then spreads to the arms and legs and then the trunk.

You don't need to be afraid to take your children outdoors. The chance of your children becoming infected with these diseases is quite low. The best way to protect yourself and your children is to follow the guidelines in this brochure for using repellents safely and avoiding areas where there may be a lot of biting insects.

If your child has been bitten by an insect and shows any of the above symptoms of West Nile virus, Lyme disease, or Rocky Mountain spotted fever, call your pediatrician.

- Insect repellents should not be applied on cuts, wounds, or irritated skin.
- Don't buy products that combine DEET with sunscreen. The DEET may make the sun protection factor (SPF) less effective. These products can overexpose your child to DEET because the sunscreen needs to be reapplied often.

Other ways to protect your child from insect bites

While you can't prevent *all* insect bites, you can reduce the number your child receives by following these guidelines.

- Tell your child to avoid areas that attract flying insects, such as garbage cans, stagnant pools of water, and flowerbeds or orchards.
- Dress your child in long pants, a lightweight long-sleeved shirt, socks, and closed shoes when you know your child will be exposed to insects. A broad-brimmed hat can help to keep insects away from the face. Mosquito netting may be used over baby carriers or strollers in areas where your baby may be exposed to insects.
- Avoid dressing your child in clothing with bright colors or flowery prints because they seem to attract insects.
- Don't use scented soaps, perfumes, or hair sprays on your child because they may attract insects.
- Keep door and window screens in good repair.

Reactions to insect repellents

If you suspect that your child is having a reaction, such as a rash, to an insect repellent, stop using the product and wash your child's skin with soap and water. Then call your local poison control center at 1-800-222-1222 or pediatrician for help. If you go to your pediatrician's office, take the repellent container with you.

- Check your child's skin at the end of the day if you live in an area where ticks are present and your child has been playing outdoors.
- Remember that the most effective repellent for *ticks* is permethrin. It should not be applied to skin but on your child's clothing.

Remember

Children need and love to be outdoors. You can make their time outdoors safer by reducing their exposure to biting insects that can carry dangerous diseases. If an insect bites your child and you are concerned about it, talk with your pediatrician.

The information contained in this publication should not be used as a substitute for the medical care and advice of your pediatrician. There may be variations in treatment that your pediatrician may recommend based on individual facts and circumstances.

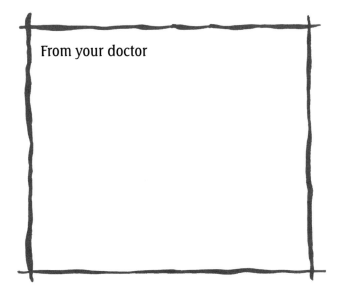

From your doctor

American Academy
of Pediatrics

DEDICATED TO THE HEALTH OF ALL CHILDREN™

The American Academy of Pediatrics is an organization of 60,000 primary care pediatricians, pediatric medical subspecialists, and pediatric surgical specialists dedicated to the health, safety, and well-being of infants, children, adolescents, and young adults.

American Academy of Pediatrics
Web site—www.aap.org

Copyright © 2005
American Academy of Pediatrics

Dangers of Secondhand Smoke

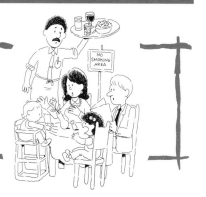

Even if you don't smoke, breathing in someone else's smoke can be deadly, too. Secondhand smoke causes about 3,000 deaths from lung cancer and tens of thousands of deaths from heart disease to nonsmoking adults in the United States each year.

Millions of children are breathing in secondhand smoke in their own homes. Secondhand smoke can be especially harmful to your children's health because their lungs still are developing. If you smoke around your children or they are exposed to secondhand smoke in other places, they may be in more danger than you realize.

Read more to learn about the dangers of secondhand smoke and how to create a smoke-free environment for your children.

What is secondhand smoke?

Secondhand smoke (also known as environmental tobacco smoke) is the smoke a smoker breathes out and that comes from the tip of burning ciga-rettes, pipes, and cigars. It contains about 4,000 chemicals. Many of these chemicals are dangerous; more than 50 are known to cause cancer. Anytime children breathe in secondhand smoke they are exposed to these chemicals.

Smoking and your developing baby

If you smoke when you're pregnant, your baby is exposed to harmful chemi-cals, too. Smoking when you're pregnant may lead to many serious health problems for your baby, including

- Miscarriage
- Premature birth (born not fully developed)
- Lower birth weight than expected (possibly meaning a less healthy baby)
- Sudden infant death syndrome (SIDS)
- Learning problems and attention-deficit/hyperactivity disorder (ADHD)

The health risks go up the longer a pregnant woman smokes and the more she smokes. Quitting anytime during pregnancy helps—of course, the sooner the better. All pregnant women should stay away from secondhand smoke and ask smokers not to smoke around them.

Secondhand smoke and your children's health

Infants have a higher risk of SIDS if they are exposed to secondhand smoke. Children, especially those younger than 2 years, have a higher risk of serious health problems, or problems may become worse. Children who breathe secondhand smoke can have more

- Ear infections
- Upper respiratory infections
- Respiratory problems such as bronchitis and pneumonia
- Tooth decay

Children of smokers cough and wheeze more and have a harder time getting over colds. Secondhand smoke can cause other symptoms including stuffy nose, headache, sore throat, eye irritation, and hoarseness.

Children with asthma are especially sensitive to secondhand smoke. It may cause more asthma attacks and the attacks may be more severe, requiring trips to the hospital.

Long-term effects of secondhand smoke

Children who grow up with parents who smoke are themselves more likely to smoke. Children and teens who smoke are affected by the same health problems that affect adults. Secondhand smoke may cause problems for children later in life including

- Lung cancer
- Heart disease
- Cataracts (an eye disease)

Secondhand smoke is everywhere

Children can be exposed to secondhand smoke in many places. Even if there are no smokers in your home, your children can still be exposed to secondhand smoke. Places include

- In a car or on a bus
- At child care or school
- At a babysitter's house
- At a friend's or relative's house
- In a restaurant
- At the mall
- At sporting events or concerts

Creating a smoke-free environment

The following tips may help keep your children from being exposed to secondhand smoke:

- **Set the example.** If you smoke, quit today! If your children see you smoking, they may want to try it, and they may grow up smoking as well. If there are cigarettes at home, children are more likely to experiment with smoking—the first step in developing the habit.
- **Make your home and car smoke-free.** Until you can quit, don't smoke around your children or in your home and car.
- **Remove your children from places where there are smokers.** Sit in nonsmoking sections in public places. Eat at smoke-free restaurants.
- **Ask people not to smoke in your home.** Don't put out any ashtrays. Remember, air flows throughout a house, so smoking in even one room allows smoke to go everywhere.
- **Ask people not to smoke in your car.** Opening windows isn't enough to clear the air.
- **Choose a babysitter who doesn't smoke.** If your babysitter does smoke, ask her not to smoke when she's caring for your children. Consider changing babysitters to find a smoke-free environment for your children.

- **Encourage smoke-free child care and schools.** Help your children's child care or school, including outdoor areas and teachers' lounges, become smoke-free. Get your children involved in the effort to make schools smoke-free!

An important choice

If you smoke, one of the most important things you can do for your own health and the health of your children is to stop smoking. Quitting is the best way to prevent your children from being exposed to secondhand smoke.

It may be hard to quit. Talk with your doctor if you need help. There are many over-the-counter and prescription medicines that may help you quit. Also, you may find it helpful to join a stop-smoking class. Contact the American Lung Association, American Heart Association, or American Cancer Society for more information about support groups where you live.

Parents need to make every effort to keep their children away from smokers and secondhand smoke. Parents who smoke should quit for their health and the health of their children.

Resources

For more information about tobacco use, read *Smoking: Straight Talk for Teens* and *The Risks of Tobacco Use: A Message to Parents and Teens* from the American Academy of Pediatrics. Other sources include

American Cancer Society
800/ACS-2345 (800/227-2345)
www.cancer.org

American Heart Association
800/AHA-USA-1 (800/242-8721)
www.americanheart.org

American Lung Association
800/LUNG-USA (800/586-4872)
www.lungusa.org

American Legacy Foundation (Great Start Program [quitting during pregnancy])
866/66-START (866/667-8278)
www.americanlegacy.org/greatstart

US Environmental Protection Agency (Smoke-Free Homes)
866/SMOKE-FREE (866/766-5337)
www.epa.gov/smokefree

Fire safety

Children can be burned or start fires when they play with lit cigarettes, lighters, or matches. Many of these fires are caused by children younger than 5 years. Cigarette lighters are especially dangerous. Although butane cigarette lighters have to be made child-resistant, they are *not* childproof.

Keep your children safe from injury by following these guidelines:
- Never allow anyone to smoke while holding a child.
- Never leave a lit cigarette, cigar, or pipe inside or outside.
- Keep matches and lighters out of your children's reach.
- Remember that child-resistant doesn't mean childproof.

Please note: Listing of resources does not imply an endorsement by the American Academy of Pediatrics (AAP). The AAP is not responsible for the content of the resources mentioned in this brochure. Phone numbers and Web site addresses are as current as possible, but may change at any time.

The information contained in this publication should not be used as a substitute for the medical care and advice of your pediatrician. There may be variations in treatment that your pediatrician may recommend based on individual facts and circumstances.

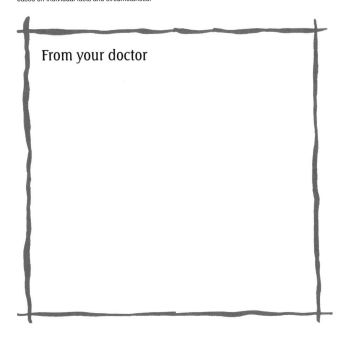

From your doctor

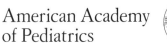

American Academy
of Pediatrics

DEDICATED TO THE HEALTH OF ALL CHILDREN™

The American Academy of Pediatrics is an organization of 60,000 primary care pediatricians, pediatric medical subspecialists, and pediatric surgical specialists dedicated to the health, safety, and well-being of infants, children, adolescents, and young adults.

American Academy of Pediatrics
Web site — www.aap.org

Copyright © 2004
American Academy of Pediatrics, Updated 01/04

Toy Safety

Part I Guidelines for Parents

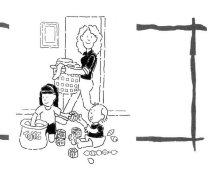

Few things make a child happier than a new toy or game. However, what seems to be harmless fun could result in a serious injury. Due to tough government regulations and efforts by US toy makers to test products, most toys on the market today are safe. Still, thousands of children suffer toy-related injuries every year. By knowing what to look for when buying toys and practicing a few simple ideas for safe use, you can often prevent problems before they occur.

How children are injured

Although most toy-related injuries are minor cuts, scrapes, and bruises, children can sometimes be seriously injured or even killed by dangerous toys or misuse of toys. Some common causes of injury are:

- **Abuse and misuse of toys.** Throwing toys, jumping on them, or taking them apart can be dangerous. When a toy breaks, sharp or pointed edges may be exposed that can cause a serious injury. Something as innocent as a doll or teddy bear may quickly become a hazard when your child pulls off an eye, removes a button, or exposes a sharp edge.
- **Small, loose, or broken toys and parts.** A small toy or part can easily become lodged in a child's ear, nose, or throat. Children can be seriously injured or killed from inhaling, swallowing, or choking on objects such as marbles, small balls, toy parts, or balloons. Small toys and parts intended for older children are also involved in choking deaths among toddlers.
- **Loose string, rope, ribbons, or cord.** These items can easily become tangled around your child's neck and strangle her. Dangling objects such as crib mobiles can be deadly if your child becomes entangled in them. Loose or long pieces of clothing, such as hood cords, can also strangle your child when the cords get tangled or caught on playground equipment. Strings or cords tied to pacifiers have been involved in numerous strangulation deaths in young children as well.
- **Toy guns.** Eye injuries often result from toys that shoot plastic objects or other flying pieces. Arrows, darts, or pellets can also be choking hazards. Very loud snapping or machine-gun noises can damage hearing. "Caps" are a hazard when used indoors or closer than 12 inches from your child's ear.
- **Riding Toys.** Injuries are caused not only when children fall off riding toys, but also when they ride them in the street when traffic is present or into swimming pools, ponds, and lakes.
- **Beach and pool toys** are usually not approved flotation devices. Never leave your child unattended at any time near a pool, beach, or pond. It only takes a few moments for a child to drown, even in very shallow water.
- **Electric plug-in toys.** Even if the label on a toy says it is UL-approved, burns and shocks can still result from frayed cords, misuse, or prolonged use of the toy.
- **Chemistry sets and hobby kits.** These kits can cause fires, explosions, or poisoning. They may contain chemicals that are often poisonous if swallowed, and they can catch fire or explode, causing serious burns and eye injuries.

- **Toy chests and other storage containers.** Toy chests can pinch, bruise, or break tiny fingers and hands if a lid closes suddenly. Death can even occur when a heavy lid without a safety support hinge traps and strangles a small child. Your child can also suffocate if trapped inside a toy chest. Open containers without lids are safest for toy storage.

Although children may like to play by themselves, injuries often occur when there is no proper supervision. Young children are more interested in having fun than in safety. As a result, improper play could lead to a serious toy-related injury. Proper supervision and teaching safe play are very important. Always supervise your child.

A word about...toy guns

It has been shown that toy guns can cause serious or fatal injuries to children. This is especially true for pellet and BB guns. Although these are often thought of as toys, they can be high-powered, lethal devices. Parents should also be aware that studies in recent years have raised questions about the effect playing with toy firearms has on a child's developing personality. Playing with toy weapons and firearms may cause more aggressive, violent behavior in some children. Playing with toy firearms may also make it easier for a child to mistake a real firearm for a toy.

Tips for buying toys

Use the following guidelines to choose safe and appropriate toys for your child.

1. **Read the label** before buying the toy. Warning labels provide important information about how to use a toy, what ages the toy is safe for, and whether adult supervision is recommended. Be sure to show your child how to use the toy properly.
2. **Think LARGE** when it comes to choosing toys. Make sure all toys and parts are larger than your child's mouth to prevent choking. Avoid small toys intended for older children that could fit into your child's mouth. This will decrease the risk of choking.
3. **Avoid toys that shoot small objects into the air.** They can cause serious eye injuries or choking.
4. **Avoid toys that make loud or shrill noises** to help protect your child's hearing. Ask to try the toy in the store. Check the loudness of the sound it makes. Don't buy toys that may be too loud for your child's sensitive hearing.
5. **Look for sturdy toy construction.** When buying a soft toy or stuffed animal, make sure the eyes, the nose, and any other small parts are secured tightly. Make sure it is machine washable. Check to see that seams and edges are secure. Remove loose ribbons or strings to avoid strangulation. Avoid toys containing small bean-like pellets or stuffing that can cause choking or suffocation if swallowed.

Age recommendations

Age recommendations printed on toy packages are very important. They reflect the safety of a toy based on four categories. These include:

- The safety aspects of the toy and any possible choking hazards
- The physical ability of the child to play with the toy
- The ability of a child to understand how to use a toy
- The needs and interests at various levels of a child's development

These recommendations are based on general developmental levels of each age group. However, every child is different. What is right for one child may not suit the skills and needs of another. Match the toy to your child's abilities. A toy that is too advanced or too simple for your child may be misused, which could lead to an injury.

6. **Watch out for sharp points or edges** and toys made from thin plastic or other material that may break easily. Don't buy toys with metal parts for a baby or toddler. If your older child plays with darts or arrows, make sure they have blunt tips made of soft rubber or flexible plastic. Tips should be securely fastened.
7. **Avoid toxic items and materials** that could cause poisoning. Look for paint sets, crayons, and markers that are labeled nontoxic. Small batteries are not only toxic, they also can pose a choking or swallowing hazard.
8. **Avoid hobby kits and chemistry sets** for any child younger than 12 years old. If these kits are purchased for older children (12 to 15 years of age), make sure you provide proper supervision and store them out of reach of young children.
9. **Electric toys should be "UL Approved"** Check the label to make sure the toy is approved by the Underwriters Laboratories.
10. **Be careful when buying crib toys.** Strings or wires that hang in a crib should be kept short. They may pose a serious strangulation hazard when a child begins to crawl or stand. Remove crib gyms and mobiles as soon as your child can push up on her hands and knees.
11. **Choose a toy chest carefully.** Look for smooth, finished edges that are nontoxic. If it has a lid, make sure it is sturdy, with locking supports and safe hinges. It should stay open in any position and hinges should not pinch your child's skin. The chest should also have ventilation holes to prevent suffocation if your child becomes trapped inside. The best toy chest is a box or basket without a lid.

How to prevent toy injuries

Use the following guidelines to keep your child safe:

Supervise your child's play

Injuries can happen despite your best efforts to choose the safest toy for your child. Supervision is the best way to prevent injuries.

- Keep all toys with small parts away from your young child until she learns not to put them in her mouth, usually by about the age of 5 years.
- Do not allow your child to play with a toy that was intended for an older child. Watch older children too, as they might put things in a smaller child's mouth.

- Keep uninflated and broken balloons away from children of all ages, as they are a serious choking hazard. When a child tries to inflate a balloon, he can easily inhale it. Also, never allow a child to place an inflated balloon in his mouth.
- To prevent injuries, stop reckless or improper play. Make sure your child never plays with toys near stairs, traffic, or swimming pools.

Store toys properly

- Store toys on a shelf or in a toy chest. They should be out of the way and off the floor, to avoid being stepped on or tripped over. A toy designed for an older child should be stored far out of reach of a curious toddler.
- Teaching your child to pick up and put toys away will help her learn to become responsible for her belongings.
- Never store a toy in its original packaging. Staples can cause cuts and plastic wrap can lead to choking or suffocation. To avoid injuries, immediately discard toy packaging before giving a new toy to your baby or toddler.

Keep toys in good condition

- Make sure you examine toys regularly. Look for damaged or broken parts that may pose a hazard. Look for splinters on wooden toys, loose eyes or small parts on dolls, rips or exposed wires in stuffed animals, or rust on metal toys.
- Never leave metal toys outside overnight. Rain, snow, or even dew may cause them to rust. Repair or replace any broken parts.
- If you're ever in doubt about a toy's safety, throw it away.

Playtime should be fun...and safe

Playing with toys is an important part of your child's development and growth. Choosing toys carefully will assure that playtime is educational, fun, and, most importantly, safe. By using the guidelines listed above, you can help prevent toy-related injuries. If you're not sure about a toy's safety or proper use, call the manufacturer. Your child's pediatrician can also help you decide which toys are safe and appropriate for your infant, toddler, or young child.

The information contained in this publication should not be used as a substitute for the medical care and advice of your pediatrician. There may be variations in treatment that your pediatrician may recommend based on individual facts and circumstances.

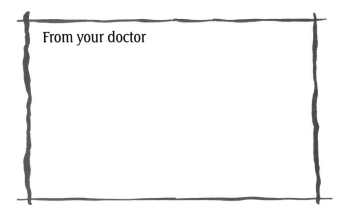

From your doctor

American Academy
of Pediatrics

DEDICATED TO THE HEALTH OF ALL CHILDREN™

The American Academy of Pediatrics is an organization of 60,000 primary care pediatricians, pediatric medical subspecialists, and pediatric surgical specialists dedicated to the health, safety, and well-being of infants, children, adolescents, and young adults.

American Academy of Pediatrics
Web site—www.aap.org

Copyright ©1994
American Academy of Pediatrics, Updated 12/98

Toy Safety

Part II Age-Appropriate Toys and Toys to Avoid

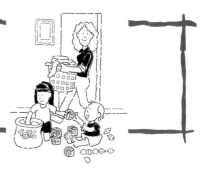

Age-appropriate toys

The following is a list of toys that the American Academy of Pediatrics recommends for specific age groups. Use these recommendations when shopping for toys. Keep in mind, these are only guidelines. All toys can be dangerous when they are not used properly or are in poor condition. Parents should continue to watch out for mislabeled toys and always provide proper supervision for young children.

Newborn to 1-year-old baby

Choose brightly-colored, lightweight toys that appeal to your baby's sight, hearing, and touch.

1. Cloth, plastic, or board books with large pictures
2. Large blocks of wood or plastic
3. Pots and pans
4. Rattles
5. Soft, washable animals, dolls, or balls
6. Bright, movable objects that are out of baby's reach
7. Busy boards
8. Floating bath toys
9. Squeeze toys

1 to 2-year-old toddler

Toys for this age group should be safe and be able to withstand a toddler's curious nature.

1. Cloth, plastic, or board books with large pictures
2. Sturdy dolls
3. Kiddy cars
4. Musical tops
5. Nesting blocks
6. Push and pull toys (remember—no long strings)
7. Stacking toys
8. Toy telephones (without cords)

2 to 5-year-old preschooler

Toys for this age group can be creative or imitate the activity of parents and older children.

1. Books (short stories or action stories)
2. Blackboard and chalk
3. Building blocks
4. Crayons, non-toxic finger paints, clay
5. Hammer and bench
6. Housekeeping toys
7. Outdoor toys: sandbox (with a lid), slide, swing, playhouse
8. Transportation toys (tricycles, cars, wagons)
9. Tape or record player
10. Simple puzzles with large pieces
11. Dress-up clothes
12. Tea party utensils

5 to 9-year-old children

Toys for this age group should help your child develop new skills and creativity.

1. Blunt scissors, sewing sets
2. Card games
3. Doctor and nurse kits
4. Hand puppets
5. Balls
6. Bicycles with helmets
7. Crafts
8. Electric trains
9. Paper dolls
10. Jump ropes
11. Roller skates with protective gear
12. Sports equipment
13. Table games

10 to 14-year-old boys and girls

Hobbies and scientific activities are ideal for this age group.

1. Computer games
2. Sewing, knitting, needlework
3. Microscopes/telescopes
4. Table and board games
5. Sports equipment
6. Hobby collections

Toys to avoid

Infants and toddlers should never be given toys with the following:

- Parts that could pull off and/or fit into a child's mouth, nose, or ear
- Exposed wires and parts that get hot
- Lead paint
- Toxic materials
- Breakable parts
- Sharp points or edges
- Glass or thin parts
- Springs, gears, or hinged parts that could pinch tiny fingers or become caught in your child's hair

To check whether a toy is unsafe or to report a toy-related injury, call the Consumer Product Safety Commission at 800/638-2772 or visit their Web site at www.cpsc.gov

The information contained in this publication should not be used as a substitute for the medical care and advice of your pediatrician. There may be variations in treatment that your pediatrician may recommend based on individual facts and circumstances.

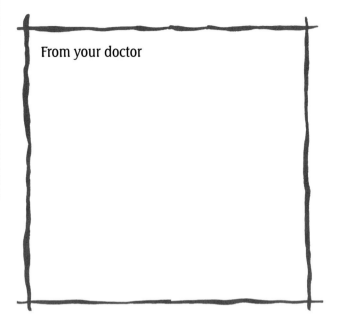

From your doctor

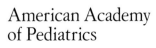

American Academy of Pediatrics

DEDICATED TO THE HEALTH OF ALL CHILDREN™

The American Academy of Pediatrics is an organization of 60,000 primary care pediatricians, pediatric medical subspecialists, and pediatric surgical specialists dedicated to the health, safety, and well-being of infants, children, adolescents, and young adults.

American Academy of Pediatrics
Web site—www.aap.org

Copyright © 1994
American Academy of Pediatrics, Updated 12/98

Trampolines

Trampolines often are described as fun for kids and a way to get exercise. However, an estimated 100,000 people were injured on trampolines in 1999. That is almost triple the number of people injured in 1991. Most of these injuries happened on home trampolines.

The American Academy of Pediatrics recommends that trampolines *never* be used at home, in routine gym classes, or on playgrounds.

Trampolines can be very dangerous

Almost two thirds of the people injured from trampolines are children ages 6 through 14 years. Common injuries include the following:
- Broken bones (sometimes needing surgery)
- Concussions and other head injuries
- Sprains/strains
- Bruises, scrapes, and cuts
  Neck and spinal cord injuries that can result in permanent paralysis or death also occur.

How children are hurt

Children can be hurt on trampolines in many ways. Most injuries result from the following:
- Landing wrong while jumping
- Attempting stunts
- Colliding with another person on the trampoline
- Falling or jumping off the trampoline
- Landing on the springs or frame of the trampoline
  Adult supervision will not adequately prevent injuries on home trampolines. Trampolines should be used only in supervised training programs for gymnastics, diving, or other competitive sports. A professional trained in trampoline safety should always supervise the use of trampolines.

Don't risk it! Parents should find out if their children's friends have trampolines before sending their children over to play. Children and teenagers should never use trampolines at their home or another person's home, in routine gym classes, or on the playground!

The information contained in this publication should not be used as a substitute for the medical care and advice of your pediatrician. There may be variations in treatment that your pediatrician may recommend based on individual facts and circumstances.

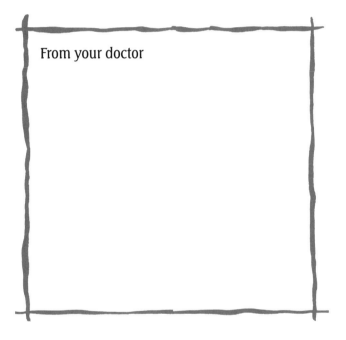

From your doctor

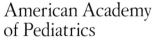

American Academy of Pediatrics

DEDICATED TO THE HEALTH OF ALL CHILDREN™

The American Academy of Pediatrics is an organization of 60,000 primary care pediatricians, pediatric medical subspecialists, and pediatric surgical specialists dedicated to the health, safety, and well-being of infants, children, adolescents, and young adults.
American Academy of Pediatrics
Web site—www.aap.org

Copyright ©1999 Rev 0501
American Academy of Pediatrics

A Parent's Guide to Water Safety

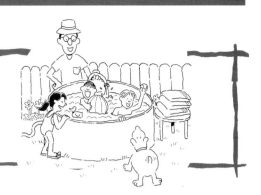

Drowning is one of the top causes of injury and death in children. Children can drown in pools, rivers, ponds, lakes, or oceans. They can even drown in a few inches of water in bathtubs, toilets, and large buckets. Read more about how to help keep your children safe around water.

Water safety at home

Parents need to keep a close eye on infants and young children, especially as they learn to crawl. *To keep your child safe, make sure you*

- **Always stay within arm's reach of your child when she is in the bathtub.** Many bathtub drownings happen (even in a few inches of water) when a parent leaves a small child alone or with another young child. Your child is always more important than answering the telephone or taking care of household chores.
- **Empty all buckets and other large containers.** The weight of a bucket filled with liquid can be heavy, and a child may not be able to tip it over and get out if she falls in.
- **Keep bathroom doors closed.** Install doorknob covers or a hook-and-eye latch or other lock that is out of the reach of your small child.
- **Keep toilets closed.** Always close the toilet lid, and consider using a toilet lid latch.
- **Watch your child when using a bath seat or ring.** Bath seats and rings are meant to be bathing aids. They are not substitutes for adult supervision and will not keep your child from drowning.

Water safety at the pool

An adult should actively watch children at all times while they are in a pool. Use "touch supervision." This means an adult is never more than an arm's length away, or is able to touch the child, at all times. Remember, supervision by an older child, and even the presence of a pool lifeguard, isn't a safe substitute for adult supervision.

Pool rules

If you have a pool, insist that the following rules are followed:
- Keep toys away from the pool when the pool is not in use.
- Empty blow-up pools after each use.
- No tricycles or other riding toys at poolside.
- No electrical appliances near the pool.
- No diving in a pool that is not deep enough.
- No running on the pool deck.

Pool fences

To prevent a small child from entering the pool area on his own, there should be a fence that completely surrounds the pool or spa. Combined with the watchful eyes of an adult, a fence is the best way to protect your child *and* other children who may visit or live nearby.

A pool fence should be climb-resistant and should not have anything alongside it (such as lawn furniture) that can be used to climb it.

Pool fences should also
- Completely surround the pool, separating it from the house and the rest of the yard.
- Be at least 4 feet high and have no footholds or handholds that could help a child climb it.
- Have no more than 4 inches between vertical slats. Chain-link fences are very easy to climb and are not recommended as pool fences. If they must be used, the diamond shape should not be bigger than 1¾ inches.
- Have a gate that is well maintained and is self-closing and self-latching. It should only open away from the pool. The latches should be higher than a child can reach.
- Keep children away from steps or ladders (for above-ground pools). If not, the steps or ladders should be locked or removed to prevent access by children.

WRONG!

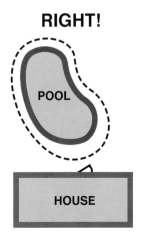

RIGHT!

In an emergency

The following are ways to be ready for an emergency:

- **Learn CPR.** Anyone caring for or watching children should know CPR (cardiopulmonary resuscitation). CPR can save a life and help reduce injury after a near drowning. The American Red Cross, the American Heart Association, and your local hospital or fire department offer CPR training.
- **Always have a phone near the pool.** Clearly post your local emergency phone number (usually 911).
- **Post safety and CPR instructions at poolside.**
- **Make sure all rescue equipment is nearby.** This includes a shepherd's hook, safety ring, and rope.

The following are things to do in an emergency:

- **Yell for help.** Carefully lift the child out of the water.
- **Start CPR right away.** Have someone call the emergency medical service (911).
- **Call your pediatrician.** Even if the child seems normal when revived, call your pediatrician right away.

Additional protection products, when used with a 4-sided fence, are also important; however, these are not substitutes for adequate fencing. These may include the following:

- Automatic pool covers (motorized covers operated by a switch). Pool covers should cover the entire pool so that a child can't slip under them. Make sure there is no standing water on top of the pool cover. Be aware that floating solar covers are *not* safety covers.
- Door alarms
- Doors to the house that are self-closing/self-latching
- Window guards
- Pool alarms

Swimming lessons

Children are generally not developmentally ready for formal swimming lessons until after their fourth birthday. Also, swimming lessons for infants and toddlers do not necessarily make them safer in or around the water and are not a recommended means of drowning prevention at these ages.

If you want to put your small child in a swimming program, choose one that doesn't require him to put his head under water (swallowing too much water can make your child sick). Also, find a program that lets you swim with your child. Once your child is ready (generally after his fourth birthday) he should be taught how to swim. However, remember that teaching your child to swim does not mean he is safe in the water. Even a child who knows how to swim can drown a few feet from safety. Also remember that even a child who knows how to swim needs to be watched at all times. No one, adult or child, should ever swim alone.

Older children and teens are also at risk from drowning, even if they know how to swim. They often drown while swimming in unsupervised places such as water-filled quarries, rivers, or ponds. Although many teens can swim well, they often encounter risky situations that they might not recognize, such as rough currents, surf, and sharp rocks. Alcohol is also a factor in many drownings among teens.

Diving

Serious spinal cord injuries, permanent brain damage, and death can occur to swimmers who dive into shallow water or spring upward on the diving board and hit it on the way down.

Keep safe by following these simple common-sense diving rules.

- Check how deep the water is. Enter the water feet first, especially when going in for the first time.
- Never dive into above-ground pools; they are usually not deep enough.
- Never dive into the shallow end of a pool.
- Never dive through inner tubes or other pool toys.
- Learn how to dive properly by taking classes.

Water safety in other bodies of water

Swimming in a pool is different from swimming in other bodies of water. In addition to rules for pool safety, parents and children should know the rules for swimming in oceans, lakes, ponds, rivers, and streams. *These include*

- Never swim without adult supervision.
- Never dive into water unless an adult who knows the depth of the water says it's OK.
- Never try water sports such as skiing, scuba diving, or snorkeling without instructions from a qualified teacher.
- Always use an approved personal flotation device (life jacket) when boating, riding on a personal watercraft, fishing, waterskiing, or playing in a river or stream.
- Never swim around anchored boats, in motor boat lanes, or where people are water skiing.
- Never swim during electrical storms.
- If you swim or drift far from shore, stay calm and tread water, or float on your back until help arrives.
- Water wings and other blow-up swimming aids should not be used in place of life vests.
- Other water hazards found near many homes include canals, ditches, post holes, wells, fish ponds, and fountains. Watch your child closely if your child is playing near any of these areas.

Life jackets and life preservers

If your family enjoys spending time on the water, make sure everyone wears an approved personal flotation device or life jacket. Some people think life jackets are hot, bulky, and ugly. However, today's models look and feel better and protect better. Many states require the use of life jackets and life preservers. They must be present on all boats traveling in water supervised by

Don't drink and swim

Swimmers are at serious risk of drowning when they drink alcohol or use other drugs while swimming, diving, and playing water sports. These activities require clear thinking, coordination, and the ability to judge distance, depth, speed, and direction. Alcohol impairs all of these skills. People who are supervising other swimmers should not be using alcohol or drugs.

the US Coast Guard. Remember, without wearing a life jacket, your child is not protected.

Keep the following tips in mind:

- A life jacket should not be used in place of adult supervision.
- Choose a life jacket that fits your child's weight and age. It should be approved by the US Coast Guard and tested by Underwriters Laboratories (UL). Check the label to be sure. The label should also say whether the jacket is made for an adult or a child.
- Teach your child how to put on her own life jacket and make sure it is worn the right way.
- Blow-up water wings, toys, rafts, and air mattresses should never be used as life jackets or life preservers.

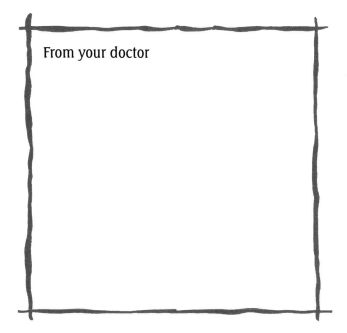

From your doctor

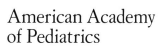
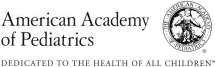

American Academy of Pediatrics

DEDICATED TO THE HEALTH OF ALL CHILDREN™

The American Academy of Pediatrics is an organization of 60,000 primary care pediatricians, pediatric medical subspecialists, and pediatric surgical specialists dedicated to the health, safety, and well-being of infants, children, adolescents, and young adults.

American Academy of Pediatrics
Web site — www.aap.org

Copyright © 2005
American Academy of Pediatrics, Updated 5/05

Adolescents and School-aged Children

Tips for Parents of Adolescents

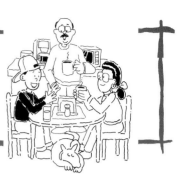

Adolescence is a time of change and challenge for your preteen or teenager. The changes that occur during adolescence are often confusing not only for your son or daughter, but for you as well. Though these years can be difficult, the reward is watching your child become an independent, caring, and responsible adult. The American Academy of Pediatrics (AAP) offers the following tips to help you face the challenges of your child's adolescence:

1. **Spend *family* time with your adolescent.** Although many preteens and teens may seem more interested in friends, this does not mean they are not interested in family.

2. **Spend time *alone* with your adolescent.** Even if your teen does not want time alone with you, take a moment here and there to remind him that your "door is always open," and you are always there if he needs to talk. Remind him often.

3. **When your adolescent talks**
   - Pay attention.
   - Watch, as well as listen.
   - Try not to interrupt.
   - Ask him to explain things further if you don't understand.
   - If you don't have time to listen when your child wants to talk, set a time that will be good for both of you.

4. **Respect your adolescent's feelings.** It's okay to disagree with your child, but disagree respectfully, not insultingly. Don't dismiss her feelings or opinions as silly or senseless. You may not always be able to help when your child is upset about something, but it is important to say, "I want to understand" or "Help me understand."

5. **When rules are needed, set and enforce them.** Don't be afraid to be unpopular for a day or two. Believe it or not, adolescents see setting limits as a form of caring.

6. **Try not to get upset if your adolescent makes mistakes.** This will help him take responsibility for his own actions. Remember to offer guidance when necessary. Direct the discussion toward solutions.

   "I get upset when I find clothes all over the floor,"

   is much better than, *"You're a slob."*

   Be willing to negotiate and compromise. This will teach problem solving in a healthy way. Remember to choose your battles. Some little annoying things that adolescents do may not be worth a big fight — let them go.

7. **Criticize a behavior, not an attitude.**
   For example, instead of saying,

   "You're late. That's so irresponsible. And I don't like your attitude,"

   try saying,

"I worry about your safety when you're late. I trust you, but when I don't hear from you and don't know where you are, I wonder whether something bad has happened to you. What can we do together to help you get home on time and make sure I know where you are or when you're going to be late?"

8. **Mix criticism with praise.** While your teen needs to know how you feel when she is not doing what you want her to do, she also needs to know that you appreciate the positive things she *is* doing. For example,

   "I'm proud that you are able to hold a job and get your homework done. I would like to see you use some of that energy to help do the dishes after meals."

9. **Let your child be the adolescent he wants to be,** not the one you wish he was. Also, try not to pressure your adolescent to be like you were or wish you had been at that age. Give your teen some leeway with regard to clothes, hairstyle, etc. Many teens go through a rebellious period in which they want to express themselves in ways that are different from their parents. However, be aware of the messages and ratings of the music, movies, and video games to which your child is exposed.

10. **Be a parent first, not a pal.** Your adolescent's separation from you as a parent is a normal part of development. Don't take it personally.

11. **Don't be afraid to share with your adolescent that you have made mistakes** as a parent. A few parenting mistakes are not crucial. Also, try to share with your teen mistakes you made as an adolescent.

12. **Talk to your pediatrician** if you are having trouble with your adolescent. He or she may be able to help you and your child find ways to get along.

The following is additional information you may find helpful in understanding some of the life changes and pressures your adolescent may be experiencing.

Dieting and body image

"My daughter is always trying new diets. How can I help her lose weight safely?"

We live in a society that is focused on thinness. Adolescents see many role models in fashion magazines, on television, and in the movies that emphasize the importance of being thin. This concern about weight and body image leads many adolescents, especially girls, to resort to extreme measures to lose weight. Be aware of any diet or exercise program with which your child is involved. Be watchful of how much weight your child loses, and make sure the diet program is healthy. Eating disorders such as anorexia nervosa and bulimia nervosa can be very dangerous. If you suspect your child has an eating disorder, talk to your pediatrician right away.

Nutrition

The growth rate during adolescence is one of the most dramatic changes the body ever goes through. It is very important for your adolescent to have a proper diet. Follow these suggestions to help keep your teen's diet a healthy one

- Limit fast food meals. Discuss the options available at fast food restaurants, and help your teen find a good balance in her diet. Fat should not come from junk food but from healthier foods such as cheese or yogurt. Vegetables and fruit are also important.
- Keep the household supply of "junk food" such as candy, cookies, andpotato chips to a minimum.
- Stock up on low-fat healthy items for snacking such as fruit, raw vegetables, whole-grain crackers, and yogurt.
- Check with your pediatrician about the proper amounts of calories, fat, protein, and carbohydrates for your child.
- As a parent, model good eating habits.

Many diets are unhealthy for adolescents because they do not have the nutritional value that bodies need during puberty. If your teen wants to lose weight, urge her to increase physical activity and to take weight off slowly. Let her eat according to her own appetite, but make sure she gets enough fats, carbohydrates, protein, and calcium.

Make sure your teen is not confusing a "low-fat" diet with a "no fat" diet. Teens need 30% of their calories from fat, and cutting fat out of the diet altogether is not healthy. A low-fat diet should still include 30 to 50 grams of fat daily. Many teens choose vegetarian diets. If your child decides to become a vegetarian, make certain she reads about it and becomes an educated vegetarian. She may need to see her pediatrician or a nutritionist to ensure that she is getting enough fat, calories, protein, and calcium.

Many adolescents are uncomfortable with their bodies. If your adolescent is unhappy with the way she looks, encourage her to start a physical activity program. Physical activity will stop hunger pangs, create a positive self-image, and take away the "blahs". Unfortunately, some teens may try to change their bodies by dangerous means such as unhealthy dieting (as discussed previously) or with drugs such as anabolic steroids. Encourage *healthy* exercise. If your child wants to train with weights, she should check with her pediatrician, as well as a trainer, coach, or physical education teacher. Help create a positive self-image by praising your child about her appearance. Set a good example by practicing what you preach. Make exercise and eating right a part of your daily routine also.

Dating and sex education

"With all the sex on television, how can I teach my son to 'wait' until he is ready?"

There are constant pressures for your adolescent to have sex. These pressures may come from the movies, television, music, friends, and peers. Teens are naturally curious about sex. This is completely normal and healthy. Talk to your adolescent to understand his feelings and views about sex. Start early and provide your teen with access to information that is accurate and appropriate. Delaying sexual involvement could be the most important decision your child can make. Talk to your teen or preteen about the following things he needs to think about before becoming sexually active:

Medical and physical risks, like unwanted pregnancy and STDs (sexually transmitted diseases) such as

- Gonorrhea
- Chlamydia
- Hepatitis B
- Syphilis
- Herpes
- HIV, the virus that causes AIDS

Emotional risks that go along with an adolescent having sex before he is ready. The adolescent may regret the decision when he is older or feel guilty, frightened, or ashamed from the experience. Have your adolescent ask himself, "Am I ready to have sex?" "What will happen after I have sex?"

Methods of contraception — Anyone who is sexually active needs to be aware of the various methods of contraception that help prevent unintended pregnancies, as well as ways to protect against sexually transmitted diseases. Remember to tell your teen that latex condoms should always be used *along with* a second method of contraception to prevent pregnancy and STDs.

Setting limits — Make sure your adolescent has thought about what his limits are *before* dating begins.

Most importantly, let your adolescent know that he can talk to you and his pediatrician about dating and relationships. Offer your guidance throughout this important stage in your teen's life.

Smoking and tobacco

"My daughter smokes behind my back. How do I convince her to quit?"

Smoking can turn into a lifelong addiction that can be extremely hard to break. Discuss with your adolescent some of the more undesirable effects of smoking, including bad breath, stained teeth, wrinkles, a long-term cough, and decreased athletic performance. Addiction can also lead to serious health problems like emphysema and cancer.

"Chew" or "snuff" can also lead to nicotine addiction and causes the same health problems as smoking cigarettes. Mouth wounds or sores also form and may not heal easily. Smokeless tobacco can also lead to cancer.

If you suspect your teen or preteen is smoking or using smokeless tobacco, talk to your pediatrician. Arrange for your child to visit the pediatrician, who will want to discuss the risks associated with smoking and the best ways to quit before it becomes a lifelong habit. Smokers young and old often are more likely to listen to advice from their doctor than from others.

If you smoke…quit

If you or someone else in the household smokes, now is a good time to quit. Watching a parent struggle through the process of quitting can be a powerful message for a teen or preteen who is thinking about starting. It also shows that you care about your health, as well as your child's.

Alcohol

"I know my son drinks once in a while, but it's just beer. Why should I worry?"

Alcohol is the most socially accepted drug in our society, and also one of the most abused and destructive. Even small amounts of alcohol can impair judgment, provoke risky and violent behavior, and slow down reaction time. An intoxicated teenager (or anyone else) behind the wheel of a car is a lethal weapon. Alcohol-related car crashes are the leading cause of death for young adults, aged 15 to 24 years.

Though it's illegal for people under age 21 to drink, we all know that most teenagers are no strangers to alcohol. Many of them are introduced to alcohol during childhood. If you choose to use alcohol in your home, be aware of the example you set for your teen. The following suggestions may help:

- Having a drink should never be shown as a way to cope with problems.
- Don't drink in unsafe conditions — driving the car, mowing the lawn, using the stove, etc.
- Don't encourage your child to drink or to join you in having a drink.
- Never make jokes about getting drunk; make sure that your children understand that it is neither funny nor acceptable.
- Show your children that there are many ways to have fun without alcohol. Happy occasions and special events don't have to include drinking.
- Do not allow your children to drink alcohol before they reach the legal age and teach them never, ever to drink and drive.
- Always wear your seatbelt (and ask your children to do the same.)

Drugs

"I am afraid some of my daughter's friends have offered her drugs. How can I help her make the right decision?"

Your child may be interested in using drugs other than tobacco and alcohol, including marijuana and cocaine, to fit in or as a way to deal with the pressures of adolescence. Try to help your adolescent build her self-confidence or self-esteem. This will help your child resist the pressure to use drugs. Encourage your adolescent to "vent" emotions and troubles through conversations and physical activity rather than by getting "high."

Set examples at home. Encourage your adolescent to participate in leisure and outside activities to stay away from the peer pressure of drinking and drugs. Talk with your children about healthy choices.

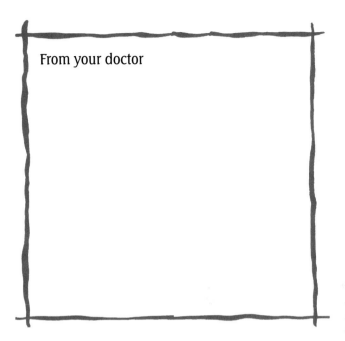

From your doctor

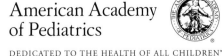

American Academy of Pediatrics

DEDICATED TO THE HEALTH OF ALL CHILDREN™

The American Academy of Pediatrics is an organization of 60,000 primary care pediatricians, pediatric medical subspecialists, and pediatric surgical specialists dedicated to the health, safety, and well-being of infants, children, adolescents, and young adults.

American Academy of Pediatrics
Web site — www.aap.org

Copyright © 1995
American Academy of Pediatrics, Updated 2/00

Health Care for College Students
What Your Pediatrician Wants You to Know

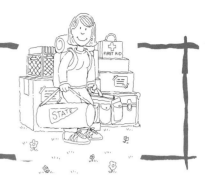

Starting college is an exciting time in your life. New worlds are opening up to you, and there are many choices to make: what classes to take, what to major in, what kind of work you want to do when you graduate. All of these choices are now *yours*. This is both a great freedom and a huge responsibility.

In much the same way, you are now largely in charge of your health and well-being. You probably have a lot of questions about keeping healthy while in college. This brochure will answer some of your questions about how to take care of yourself.

Your pediatrician and the student health service

Your pediatrician will not abandon you just because you are starting college. He or she may give you a physical before you start school (some colleges require you to have a physical before you can attend classes). Your pediatrician will also make sure that all your immunizations are up-to-date and all your medical records are complete. You will still be able to call your pediatrician if you have any questions. If you continue to live near your pediatrician, you may still want to see him or her for your care. But if you are going to live on campus, and the school provides a student health service, it may be the first place you go for health care. If one is not available, most schools will provide you with a list of health services in the community.

What is a student health service?

The student health service is an important part of the college or university you are about to attend. It is there for you when you need medical care, advice, information, or counseling. Student health services are not Band-Aid stations. Their medical, nursing, and counseling staffs are familiar with the problems and needs of college students. They also know pediatricians and other physicians in the community in case you need additional care.

Yet, if you are used to going to your pediatrician for your health care, the student health service may seem a bit strange at first. You may see a team of health care providers, which may include doctors, nurse practitioners, therapists, and health educators. This system will work best if you keep open the lines of communication between yourself, your parents, the student health service, and your pediatrician.

Things to do before you go

Get your medical and immunization records. Make sure the student health service has the following information about your medical history:

1. A complete list of every medication you take, including its dosage and strength
2. A list of your allergies, significant past medical problems (including surgeries and hospitalizations), and special needs (such as chronic conditions and disabilities)
3. A record of any mental health problems

4. Relevant family medical history
5. A record of which immunizations you have received, including type of vaccine, date given, and any reaction

Make sure you have health insurance. If you will still be on your parents' policy, take a copy of the insurance card with you. Find out what type of plan you have (HMO, PPO, etc), what the policy covers, how to file claims, and what to do in case of an emergency. Talk this over with your parents. Remember that if you are on your parents' insurance policy, they will be notified each time the insurance company is billed for something.

Take extras of any prescription medications you need. Also, find out the name of a pharmacy near your school and how to obtain prescription refills when you need them.

Get a book. Everyone should own a book on personal health care.

Things to take with you

A good first aid kit is a useful thing to have in case you do not feel well or you have a small emergency. Your first aid kit should contain the following:

- Bandages for small cuts and scrapes
- Gauze and adhesive tape
- An elastic bandage for wrapping sprains
- Liquid soap
- Antibacterial/antibiotic ointment
- A digital (not mercury) thermometer
- An ice pack or chemical cold pack
- Medicine for an upset stomach
- Acetaminophen or ibuprofen for aches, pains, and fever
- Medicine for diarrhea
- Medicine for allergies
- Sore throat lozenges or spray

The basics of staying healthy

There are many things you can do on your own to keep yourself healthy.

Rest

College students often skimp on rest because there is so much to do. However, trying to get by on too little sleep can cause some serious problems.
What happens when you do not get enough sleep?
- You may be more likely to catch colds and other minor illnesses. Your body cannot fight off germs as well when you are tired and run-down.
- You are more likely to feel stressed or become depressed.
- You may have a hard time staying awake in class.
- You may have trouble concentrating on papers and tests.
Young adults often need a bit more sleep than older adults—sleeping about 8 to 9 hours a night is necessary for most 18-year-olds.

Nutrition

Eating well is just as important as getting enough rest. This means eating enough fruits and vegetables every day; eating lean meats, fish, and poultry; and limiting fried and processed foods. Watching your intake of junk food, fatty foods, sugar, and salt is important. Also, it is important to consume enough food that is high in calcium, such as low-fat dairy products, to help maintain bone mass and strength.

It is possible to eat a healthy vegetarian diet at college. However, this may require some additional planning to make sure you get all the nutrients you need.

Exercise

Another important part of staying healthy is getting enough exercise.

There are 3 basic types of exercise, and ideally everyone should do all 3.

- **Aerobic** exercise strengthens your heart and lungs (good examples are biking, running, fast walking, swimming, aerobic dancing, and rowing). Three times a week you should get some type of aerobic exercise for at least 20 minutes.
- **Strengthening** exercise tones and builds muscles and bone mass (you can do this by doing sit-ups, push-ups, and leg lifts, or by working out with weights or resistance bands).
- **Stretching** exercise, like yoga, improves your flexibility or range of motion.

There are a number of ways to sneak more exercise into your day. Instead of driving or taking a bus to run errands, walk or ride a bike (wear a helmet when biking). Walking to class can be good exercise, too. Even in-line skating around campus can be a good workout (but make sure you wear a helmet, wrist guards, and knee pads). If you are not used to exercising or if you have a chronic health problem, you may want to talk with your pediatrician or a doctor at the student health service before starting an exercise program.

Sexual health

College is often a time when young people begin to explore their sexuality. This does not mean that all college students are sexually active. In fact, many are not. If you have decided to wait to have sex, you are not alone. Remember, the decision as to when to have sex is yours and yours alone. Do not let yourself be pressured into having sex if you do not want to.

If you are sexually active or are thinking about it, you owe it to yourself to make responsible decisions about sex. Make sure you can talk to your partner about the quality of your relationship and about sexual issues. Discuss whether you will date other people. Find out your partner's sexual history, including exposure to sexually transmitted diseases (STDs). If you are in a heterosexual relationship, talk about birth control and what you would do if it failed. If you cannot talk about these issues with your partner, you should think about whether you should have a sexual relationship with him or her.

College may also be a time for sorting out your sexual identity. If you are questioning your sexual identity, talking with a counselor may help. Many colleges have support and social groups for gay, lesbian, and bisexual students. These groups can help students feel less isolated.

Sexual relationships expose you to the risk of STDs and viruses that can cause cancer and acquired immunodeficiency syndrome (AIDS). The more sexual partners you have, the greater your risk. There are more than 25 diseases that are spread through sexual contact. Some of them are easy to treat, but when left untreated they can cause serious health problems. Others, like herpes, have no cure. AIDS, also sexually transmitted, can kill you. Not having sex is the only sure way to prevent STDs. If you do have sex, the safest way is to have sex with only one person who has no STDs and no other sex partners. Use a latex condom *every time* you have sex.

Common health problems

There are times when you should contact the student health service immediately. Call the health service if you have any of the following:

- A fever of 102.5°F or higher
- A headache accompanied by a stiff neck
- Pain with urination
- An unusual discharge from your penis or vagina
- A change in your menstrual cycle
- Pain in the abdomen that will not go away
- A persistent cough, chest pain, or trouble breathing
- Pain or any other symptoms that worry you or last longer than you think they should

Respiratory infections

Illnesses like colds, the flu, and sore throats are hard to escape while in college. With students living together in dormitories and apartments, eating together in large cafeterias, and sitting together in classrooms, these respiratory infections spread easily. Washing your hands often will help you avoid these illnesses. Dust allergy and exposure to cigarette smoke will make you more likely to get cold symptoms.

How you treat a respiratory infection will depend on whether it is caused by bacteria or a virus. **Colds and flu** are caused by viruses. There is really nothing you can do to get rid of them quickly—the most you can do is rest, drink a lot of fluids, and treat the symptoms. How can you tell a cold from the flu? Colds usually cause milder symptoms than the flu. Coughing, sneezing, watery eyes, and mild fevers are common cold symptoms. The flu, on the other hand, is more serious. You will probably have a fairly high fever, body aches, and a dry cough with the flu. You may also have an upset stomach or vomit. If you are vomiting, drink liquids such as sports drinks, water, or tea.

Over-the-counter cold and flu medications may help relieve your symptoms. Read labels when buying medications for colds and flu to make sure you are getting the right medicine for your symptoms.

Some types of the flu can be treated with antiviral agents if given in the first day or two of the illness. This can speed recovery. Under some circumstances, antiviral agents can be taken before exposure to the flu and can

---

The truth about mononucleosis ("mono")

College students often worry about a disease called **"mono"**—also known as "the kissing disease." Mono, a viral infection, is not as common or usually as serious as most people think. Symptoms include fever, sore throat, headache, swollen glands, and extreme tiredness. If you seem to have a sore throat or bad flu that does not go away in a week to 10 days, the problem might be mono. See your doctor. Mono is diagnosed by a blood test called the "mono spot." Even if the test confirms that you have mono, there is no specific treatment, except to get plenty of rest and eat a healthy diet. However, you may need to restrict your activity to prevent possible serious injury. The good news is that most people are better within a month. If you have had a documented case of mono, you cannot get it again.

prevent illness. Consider getting the influenza vaccine when it becomes available each fall. Safe and effective vaccines are available to protect against the flu.

Strep throat and some sinus and ear infections are caused by bacteria. These are treated with antibiotics. If you have a very sore throat, pain in your ears or sinuses, or a persistent fever, go to the student health service. The staff will be able to tell you what the problem is and give you antibiotics if you need them. If your doctor does give you antibiotics, *take them exactly as you are told, and be sure to take all of them.* If you do not, bacteria can become resistant to the antibiotics and result in a more serious infection.

Meningococcal disease

College students, particularly freshmen living in dormitories, are at an increased risk of contracting meningococcal disease. A common form of this is meningitis. This disease can infect the brain, spinal cord, and/or blood. Symptoms include a high fever; stiff neck; severe headache; a flat, pink to red to purple rash; nausea; vomiting; and sensitivity to light. It is important to seek medical treatment immediately. The disease can be fatal or may result in permanent brain damage or lifelong problems with the nervous system.

Safe vaccines are now available to prevent the forms of meningococcal disease that are most common among college students. If you plan to live in a dormitory, ask your pediatrician about immunization against meningococcal disease before you leave for college.

Bruises, sprains, and strains

Bruises, sprains, and strains are very common and usually are not very serious.

- **Bruises** are injuries to the skin that cause the surface of the skin to turn purple, brown, or red in color.
- **Strains** are injuries to the muscles and tendons that result from too much or sudden stretching.
- **Sprains** are injuries to the ligaments, the connecting tissue between bones. Bruises, strains, and sprains should be treated with
- **Rest**—especially for the first 24 hours.
- **Ice**—put ice packs or cold gel packs on the injury for 20 minutes every 4 hours.
- **Compression**—wrap the injured body part in an elastic bandage.
- **Elevation**—for example, if you have sprained your ankle, prop your foot up on pillows to keep it at a level higher than your heart.

Visit the student health service if your pain or swelling does not get better in a day or two.

Taking care of your mental health

Starting college brings with it many new stresses. You may be away from home for the first time in your life and may miss your family and friends. You will have more schoolwork to do, and it may take more time and effort than in high school. It may take you a while to find people with whom you have things in common. All these things can make you feel alone, overworked, and stressed out.

Friends

Friends usually become your main support system while in college. In fact, college friends often become close friends for life.

You may be worried about how you will make new friends. You will probably meet some people you like in the first few days of school, and you will meet more in your classes, in clubs or sports, and through other friends. If it takes a while to find people you click with, do not worry—it will happen.

Roommates can be terrific friends or great sources of stress. Even roommates who like each other will have conflicts over things like cleaning, bedtimes, and music. Talk these things over early on, and you will be less likely to have problems later. If you and your roommate just cannot get along, talk to a resident counselor. He or she can offer advice on how to handle your roommate problem.

Homesickness

Homesickness is very common among students away from home—even those who had previously been away at overnight camp or traveled far away. There is a difference between being away from home for 8 weeks and being gone for 8 months. There is also a difference between leaving home for a while (knowing you will be going back) and the start of leaving for good (knowing your returns may never be the same again). Feeling homesick does not make you less mature or mean you are not ready to be on your own. If you feel homesick, talk to your friends at school about it. Chances are they are feeling the same way. Keep in touch with family and friends back home, but make sure you develop new relationships at school. If your homesickness just will not go away and does not seem to be getting better after a few months at school, speaking with a counselor might help. Also, remember that going home for the first visit may be difficult because of changes in yourself or your family. Old conflicts do not just disappear once you go to college, and new ones may surface. Again, if things are too stressful for you to handle alone, talk to a counselor.

Depression

There will be days when you feel down, when the pressures of college life really get to you. Those feelings are normal and will pass in time. When you feel down, take some time out for yourself and do something that makes you feel good. Spend time with friends. Exercise. Read a good book.

Sometimes, though, feeling down can turn into depression. Depression is a serious illness that can be treated. If you have had any of the following symptoms for 2 weeks or more, see a counselor right away:

- Sad mood
- Hopeless, helpless, worthless, or guilty feelings
- Loss of pleasure in things you usually enjoy
- Sleep problems
- Eating problems
- Low energy, extreme tiredness, lack of concentration
- Thoughts of death or suicide
- Physical symptoms such as headaches, stomachaches, or body aches that do not respond to treatment

Do not think you can handle depression on your own. If one of your friends seems depressed, suggest that he or she see a counselor as soon as possible.

Drinking and violence

Drinking is a huge problem on most college campuses. The majority of college students drink, and a large number drink to excess. More than half of all male college students are binge drinkers (those who have 5 or more drinks at one sitting), and more than one third of female students are binge drinkers. Heavy or binge drinking can lead to physical illness (or death), long-term drinking problems, and aggression and violence. Drinking is known to increase sexual aggressiveness, which can lead to sexual harassment and date rape. Drinking also clouds your judgment and may make you more likely to engage in unsafe sexual practices, which in turn may lead to STDs and unintended pregnancies.

The legal drinking age in the United States is 21. The best way to prevent drinking-related problems is to avoid drinking altogether. If you are of legal age and choose to drink, be responsible. Stop after 1 or 2 drinks. *Do not* drink and drive, *do not* let friends drink and drive, and *do not* ride with someone who has been drinking. Follow the designated driver rule. Do not drink with people you do not know. If you feel you need to cut down on your drinking, if friends comment on the amount of drinking you do, or if you ever feel guilty about something you have done while drinking, see a counselor at school.

Just some friendly advice...

- Poor study habits are the primary reason students do poorly in college. College means increased freedom, with less time spent in the classroom and more time spent studying independently. Learn to budget your time and use it wisely.
- Violence, crime, racism, sexism, and cults are alive and well on every college campus. A college campus is no safer than your hometown. Lock your doors and take care of yourself.
- Sorority and fraternity life can offer many advantages, but it can also isolate students from the rest of the college experience. Make sure you thoroughly investigate any sorority or fraternity that you are considering. College life will present many opportunities and challenges. Take care of yourself, and enjoy your college years.

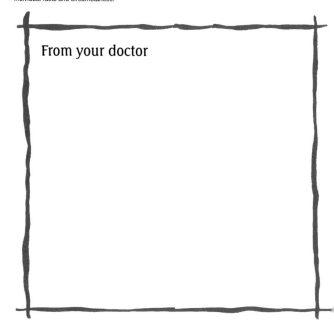

Health record card
Use this card to keep track of important health information.

Name:

Address:

Phone:

Date of Birth:

Pediatrician's Name:

Office Address:

Telephone/Fax:

Allergies:

Chronic Medical Conditions:

Blood Type:

The information contained in this publication should not be used as a substitute for the medical care and advice of your pediatrician. There may be variations in treatment that your pediatrician may recommend based on individual facts and circumstances.

From your doctor

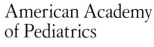

American Academy of Pediatrics

DEDICATED TO THE HEALTH OF ALL CHILDREN™

The American Academy of Pediatrics is an organization of 60,000 primary care pediatricians, pediatric medical subspecialists, and pediatric surgical specialists dedicated to the health, safety, and well-being of infants, children, adolescents, and young adults.

American Academy of Pediatrics
Web site — www.aap.org

Copyright © 1997
American Academy of Pediatrics, Updated 1/02

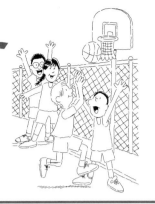

Lactose Intolerance and Your Child

After drinking milk or eating ice cream, does your child have stomach cramps or get diarrhea? If so, your child may have lactose intolerance.

Lactose intolerance can make your child quite uncomfortable, but small changes in your child's diet may help treat the problem.

Read more to learn about what lactose intolerance is and how to help your child live with it.

What is lactose intolerance?

Lactose intolerance occurs in people who can't digest lactose. *Lactose* is the sugar found in milk. It also is found in other dairy products, such as ice cream and soft cheeses. People who are lactose intolerant don't make enough *lactase*. Lactase is a natural enzyme made by your intestinal tract that digests lactose. When there isn't enough lactase, lactose that is eaten isn't digested and stays in the intestines causing gas, bloating, stomach cramps, and diarrhea.

Many parents confuse the terms *lactose intolerance* and *milk allergy*. While they may share similar symptoms, they are entirely different conditions. Lactose intolerance is a digestive problem, while milk allergy involves the immune system. Your child can be tested for milk allergy or lactose intolerance.

Who gets lactose intolerance?

Between 30 and 50 million people in the United States are lactose intolerant. If your child is lactose intolerant, you may see symptoms around the time he starts school or during the teen years.

One cause of lactose intolerance is genetic. Certain ethnic groups are more likely to become lactose intolerant. About 90% of Asian Americans, 80% of African Americans, 62% to 100% of American Indians, 53% of Mexican Americans, and 15% of people of northern European descent are lactose intolerant.

Lactose intolerance also can occur in people who have a disease affecting the small intestine, such as celiac disease or Crohn disease.

Temporary lactose intolerance

It's rare for a baby to be born with lactose intolerance. However, after a bout of severe diarrhea, which can temporarily affect the ability to produce lactase, a toddler or older child may have trouble digesting milk for 1 to 2 weeks. Drinking milk or eating certain dairy foods may result in the common symptoms of lactose intolerance and more diarrhea.

If your toddler or older child wants milk and has these symptoms, use only lactose-reduced or lactose-free milk for 1 to 2 weeks. Yogurt and aged cheeses usually are digestible because the lactose is broken down when they're made.

Other foods that may contain lactose

You *and* your child must become expert label-readers to know what foods contain lactose. The following words on a food label may mean that the food contains lactose:
- Whey
- Curds
- Milk by-products
- Dry milk solids
- Non-fat dry milk powder

Lactose also may be added to many non-dairy and prepared foods. If your child has a very low tolerance for lactose, she may be sensitive to the following food products that may contain lactose:
- Bread, baked goods
- Breakfast cereals and drinks
- Instant potatoes and soups
- Margarine
- Lunch meat (not including kosher meat)
- Salad dressing
- Candy
- Snack foods
- Dry mixes for pancakes, biscuits, and cookies
- Powdered coffee creamer
- Non-dairy whipped topping

What are the symptoms?

Common symptoms of lactose intolerance include
- Stomach cramps
- Bloating
- Gas
- Diarrhea
- Nausea

These symptoms usually begin about 30 minutes to 2 hours after drinking or eating foods containing lactose.

How do I know if my child is lactose intolerant?

One way to check if your child has trouble digesting lactose is to take all milk products out of your child's diet for 2 weeks and see if symptoms improve. After 2 weeks, slowly reintroduce them in small amounts each day to see if symptoms return.

Because many non-dairy and prepared foods contain lactose, it may be hard to remove all of these food from your child's diet. (See "Other foods that may contain lactose.")

If you think your child is lactose intolerant, talk with your pediatrician. Your child may need to be tested. The most common test for lactose intolerance is the *lactose breath test*. It's also called the hydrogen breath test. This test measures hydrogen levels in the breath after a lactose solution is swallowed. Normally, hydrogen is found only in low levels in a person's breath. However, when lactose isn't digested, it ferments in the intestines and produces hydrogen, which then will be exhaled through the lungs.

Your pediatrician may refer you to a specialist. If needed, a specialist can measure lactase and other enzymes from a small intestine sample. The sample usually is obtained during a diagnostic endoscopy. This procedure lets doctors view the inside of the intestines and obtain tissue samples.

What changes can help my child?

There is no cure for lactose intolerance. However, if your child is lactose intolerant, diet changes can make a big difference. You can help decide what changes are best for your child.

- **By trial and error.** In time your child will learn, by trial and error, how much milk or milk-based foods she can handle. Younger children with lactose intolerance should avoid foods containing lactose. These foods include milk, ice cream, and soft cheeses, such as cottage cheese, American cheese, and mozzarella. Older children usually can eat small amounts of lactose-containing foods, particularly if the foods are eaten as part of a meal and not alone. Many children can keep eating yogurt and aged cheeses, such as Swiss, cheddar, and Parmesan.
- **Over-the-counter lactase.** Give your child over-the-counter lactase right before each meal. This may help her body digest foods that contain lactose.
- **Lactose-free or lactose-reduced.** Offer your child lactose-free or lactose-reduced milk and other dairy products. Lactose-reduced milk retains all the ingredients of regular milk. You can store it in the refrigerator the same length of time.

Remember

Lactose intolerance doesn't have to make your child's life miserable. There are many options for children who are lactose intolerant. Talk with your pediatrician about what products or diet changes would be best for your child.

Other sources of calcium

In the rare cases in which all milk and dairy products have to be avoided, it's important that your child get other sources of calcium. A variety of calcium-rich foods include

- Broccoli
- Pinto beans
- Sweet potatoes
- Turnips
- Collard greens
- Lettuce greens such as spinach and kale
- Canned fish with bones such as sardines, salmon, and tuna
- Tofu
- Oranges
- Juices with added calcium

If your child isn't getting the daily recommended amount of calcium (see chart), your pediatrician may recommend a calcium supplement.

Age group	Recommended Daily Amount of Calcium
1–3 years	500 mg
4–8 years	800 mg
9–18 years	1,300 mg

The information contained in this publication should not be used as a substitute for the medical care and advice of your pediatrician. There may be variations in treatment that your pediatrician may recommend based on individual facts and circumstances.

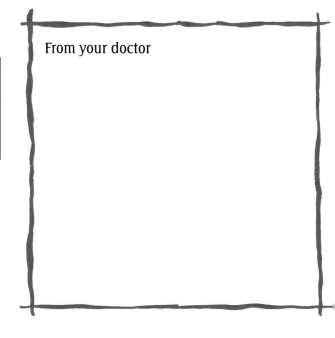

From your doctor

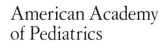

American Academy
of Pediatrics

DEDICATED TO THE HEALTH OF ALL CHILDREN™

The American Academy of Pediatrics is an organization of 60,000 primary care pediatricians, pediatric medical subspecialists, and pediatric surgical specialists dedicated to the health, safety, and well-being of infants, children, adolescents, and young adults.

American Academy of Pediatrics
Web site—www.aap.org

Copyright © 2004
American Academy of Pediatrics

puberty—ready or not
expect some big changes

Puberty is the time in your life when your body starts changing from that of a child to that of an adult. At times you may feel like your body is totally out of control! Your arms, legs, hands, and feet may grow faster than the rest of your body. You may feel a little clumsier than usual.

Compared to your friends you may feel too tall, too short, too fat, or too skinny. You may feel self-conscious about these changes, but many of your friends probably do too.

Everyone goes through puberty, but not always at the same time or exactly in the same way. In general, here's what you can expect.

When?

There's no "right" time for puberty to begin. **But girls start a little earlier than boys**—usually between 8 and 13 years of age. Puberty for boys usually starts at about 10 to 14 years of age.

What's happening?

Chemicals called hormones will cause many changes in your body.

Breasts!

Girls. The first sign of puberty in most girls is breast development—small, tender lumps under one or both nipples. The soreness goes away as your breasts grow. Don't worry if one breast grows a little faster than the other. By the time your breasts are fully developed, they usually end up being the same size.

When your breasts get larger, you may want to *start wearing a bra.* Some girls are excited about this. Other girls may feel embarrassed, especially if they are the first of their friends to need a bra. Do what is comfortable for you.

Boys. During puberty, boys may have swelling under their nipples too. If this happens to you, you may worry that you're growing breasts. *Don't worry—you're not.* This swelling is very common and only temporary. But if you're worried, talk with your pediatrician.

Hair, where?!

Girls & Boys. During puberty, soft *hair starts to grow* in the pubic area (the area between your legs and around your genitals—vagina or penis). This hair will become thick and very curly. You may also notice hair under your arms and on your legs. Boys might get hair on their faces or chests. Shaving is a personal choice. If you shave, remember to use your own clean razor or electric shaver.

Zits!

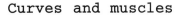

Girls & Boys. Another change that happens during puberty is that your skin gets **oilier** and you may start to sweat more. This is because your glands are growing too. It's important to wash every day to keep your skin clean. Most people use a deodorant or antiperspirant to keep odor and wetness under control. **Don't be surprised,** even if you wash your face every day, that you still get pimples. This is called acne, and it's normal during this time when your hormone levels are high. Almost **all teens** *get acne* at one time or another. Whether your case is mild or severe, **there are things you can do to keep it under control.** For more information on controlling acne, talk with your pediatrician.

Curves and muscles

Girls. As you go through puberty, you'll get taller, your hips will get wider, and your waist will get smaller. Your body also begins to build up fat in your belly, bottom, and legs. This is normal and gives your body the curvier shape of a woman.

Boys. As you go through puberty, you'll get taller, your shoulders will get broader, and as your muscles get bigger, your weight will increase.

Sometimes the weight gain of puberty causes girls and boys to feel so uncomfortable with how they look that they try to lose weight by throwing up, not eating, or taking medicines. This is not a healthy way to lose weight and may make you very sick. If you feel this way, or have tried any of these ways to lose weight, please talk with your parents or your pediatrician.

Does size matter?

Boys. During puberty, the penis and testes get larger. There's also an increase in *sex hormones.* You may notice you get erections (when the penis gets stiff and hard) more often than before. This is normal. Even though you may feel **embarrassed,** try to remember that unless you draw attention to it, most people won't even notice your erection. **Also, remember that** the size of your penis has nothing to do with manliness or sexual functioning.

Wet dreams

Boys. During puberty, your testes begin to produce sperm. This means that during an erection, you may also ejaculate. This is when semen (made up of sperm and other fluids) is released through the penis. This could happen while you are sleeping. You might wake up to find your sheets or pajamas are wet. This is called a nocturnal emission or "wet dream." This is normal and will stop as you get older.

Periods

Girls. Your *menstrual cycle,* or "period," starts during puberty. Most girls get their periods 2 to 2½ years after their breasts start to grow (between 10–16 years of age). During puberty, your ovaries begin to release eggs. If an egg connects with sperm from a man's penis (fertilization), it will grow inside your uterus and develop into a baby. To prepare for this, a thick layer of tissue and blood cells builds up in your uterus. If the egg doesn't connect with a sperm, the body does not need these tissues and cells. They turn into a blood-like fluid and flow out of your vagina. Your period is the monthly discharge of this fluid out of the body. A girl who has **started having periods is able to get pregnant,** even if she doesn't have a period every month.

You will need to wear some kind of sanitary pad and/or tampon to absorb this fluid and keep it from getting on your clothes. Most periods last from 3 to 7 days. Having your period does not mean you have to avoid any of your normal activities like swimming, horseback riding, or gym class. Exercise can even help get rid of cramps and other discomforts that you may feel during your period.

Voice cracking?

Boys. Your **voice** will get deeper, but it doesn't happen all at once. It usually starts with your voice cracking. As you keep growing, the cracking will stop and your voice will stay at the lower range.

New feelings

In addition to all the physical changes you will go through during puberty, there are many **emotional changes** as well. For example, you may start to care more about what other people think about you because you want to be accepted and liked. Your relationships with others may begin to change. Some become more important and some less so. You'll start to *separate more from your parents* and identify with others your age. You may begin to **make decisions** that could affect the rest of your life.

At times you may not like the attention of your parents and other adults, but they too are trying to adjust to the changes that you're going through. Many teens feel that their parents don't understand them—**this is a normal feeling.** It's usually best to let them know (politely) how you feel and then talk things out together. Also, it's normal to lose your temper more easily and to feel that nobody cares about you. **Talk about your feelings** with your parents, another trusted adult, or your pediatrician. You may be surprised at how much better you will feel.

Sex and sexuality

During this time, many young people also become more aware of their **feminine** and **masculine** sides. A look, a touch, or just thinking about someone may make *your heart beat faster*

and produce a warm, tingling feeling all over. Talking with your parents or pediatrician is a good way to get information and to help you think about how these changes affect you.

You may ask yourself...

- When should I start dating?
- When is it OK to kiss?
- Is it OK to masturbate (stimulate your genitals for sexual pleasure)?
- How far would I go sexually?
- When will I be ready to have sexual intercourse?
- Will having sex help my relationship?
- Is oral sex really sex?

Some answers...

Masturbation is normal and won't harm you. Many boys and girls masturbate, many don't. Deciding to become sexually active, however, can be **very confusing.** On the one hand, you hear so many warnings and dangers about having sex. On the other hand, movies, TV, magazines, even the lyrics in songs all seem to be telling you that having sex is OK.

The fact is, sex is a part of life and, like many parts of life, **it can be good or bad.** It all depends on you and the choices you make. Take dating, for example. If you and a friend feel ready to start dating and it's OK with your parents, that's fine. You may find yourself in a more serious relationship. But if one of you wants to stop *dating,* try not to hurt the other person's feelings—just be honest with each other. After a breakup both partners may be sad or angry, but keeping on with normal activities and talking it over with a trusted adult is usually helpful.

Getting close to someone you like is OK too. Holding hands, hugging, and kissing may happen, but they *don't have to lead to having sex.* Deciding whether to have sex is one of the most important decisions you will ever make. Some good advice is in a brochure called *Deciding to Wait* that your pediatrician can give you. Why not **take your time** and think it through? Talk with your parents about your family's values. Waiting to have sex until you are older, in a serious relationship, and able to **accept the responsibilities** that come along with it is a great idea! And you can avoid becoming pregnant, getting someone pregnant, or getting deadly diseases.

There is only one way to avoid pregnancy and infections related to sex, and **that is by not having sex.** And remember that oral sex is sex. You don't have to worry about pregnancy with oral sex, but you do have to worry about infections like herpes, gonorrhea, and HIV (the virus that causes AIDS).

However, if you decide to have sex, talk with your pediatrician about which type of birth control is best for you and how to **protect yourself** against sexually transmitted diseases.

Taking care of yourself

As you get older, there will be many decisions that you will need to make to ensure that you **stay healthy.** Eating right, exer-

...cising, and **getting enough rest** are important during puberty because your body is going through many changes. It's also important to `feel good about yourself` and the decisions you make. Whenever you have questions about your health or your feelings, don't be afraid to share them with your parents and pediatrician.

From your doctor

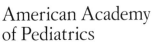

American Academy
of Pediatrics

DEDICATED TO THE HEALTH OF ALL CHILDREN™

The American Academy of Pediatrics is an organization of 60,000 primary care pediatricians, pediatric medical subspecialists, and pediatric surgical specialists dedicated to the health, safety, and well-being of infants, children, adolescents, and young adults.

American Academy of Pediatrics
Web site — www.aap.org

Copyright © 2005
American Academy of Pediatrics

School Health Centers and Your Child

School health centers are becoming more and more common. Most handle medical emergencies, provide health screenings and refer students to doctors for health problems. A growing number of these centers also offer health services such as immunizations and physical examinations. Therapies for children with special needs may also be available.

School health centers can provide important health care to students who need it. However, it is important that your child's pediatrician stay involved in that care. While school-based centers are convenient, your child's own pediatrician remains his or her best source for health supervision and medical care.

Many parents assume that because a school health clinic and the regular school health office exist side-by-side, that they communicate and work together well. Unfortunately this is not always what occurs. Parents need to stay involved.

What you can do:

- Make sure that your child's school nurse, counselor or health center staff routinely contact your pediatrician about his medical care.
- Check with your school's regular health office and your school's clinic to be sure that they work together. Give them permission to exchange health information that is important for keeping your child healthy in school. Be certain that they keep you informed.
- Continue to take your child to his pediatrician for regular preventive health care. This is important even if he or she has many of his or her health needs met at school.
- Stay involved in the health education, the health services and the supervision that your child receives at school.

Your Child Needs A Medical Home

All children and teens need a "medical home." This means health care that is available 24 hours a day, 7 days a week. This care is coordinated by one team of pediatric health care professionals.

A medical home is family centered. Your pediatrician knows you and your child. Mutual trust develops.

When your child or teen has a medical home, she or he receives ongoing medical care. Care is provided based on your child's medical history. If she or he graduates or transfers to another school, her or his medical home remains the same.

Signs of a Good School Health Program

- The staff works in partnership with other community health and social service programs.
- Students and parents sit on its administrative board. This board makes group decisions about the health care that is provided.
- The center helps students who do not have a medical home find one.
- The center assists in arranging health insurance for students who need it.
- It is easily accessible for all students.
- It provides quality health care that focuses on the long-term needs of each student.

This information is based on the American Academy of Pediatrics' policy statement School Health Centers and Other Integrated School Health Services, published in January 2001. Parent Pages offers parents relevant facts that explain current policies about children's health.

The information contained in this publication should not be used as a substitute for the medical care and advice of your pediatrician. There may be variations in treatment that your pediatrician may recommend based on individual facts and circumstances.

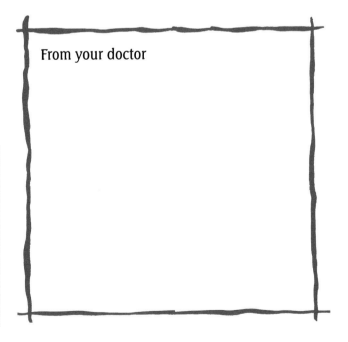

From your doctor

American Academy
of Pediatrics

DEDICATED TO THE HEALTH OF ALL CHILDREN™

The American Academy of Pediatrics is an organization of 60,000 primary care pediatricians, pediatric medical subspecialists, and pediatric surgical specialists dedicated to the health, safety, and well-being of infants, children, adolescents, and young adults.

American Academy of Pediatrics
Web site — www.aap.org

Copyright © 2003
American Academy of Pediatrics

Students With Chronic Health Conditions:
Guidance for Families, Schools, and Students

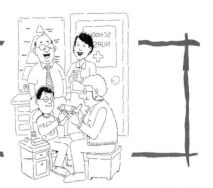

School is more than a place to gain knowledge and skills. It also is a place where children meet new friends and learn about themselves and other important life lessons. Because children spend many hours in school, it is important that it be a safe and supportive environment for all children.

Ten percent to 15% of children in our nation's schools have a chronic health condition (such as asthma, allergies, diabetes, and seizure disorders). Parents, school staff, and pediatricians need to work together to make sure children with chronic illnesses have the same educational opportunities as other students.

Read more to learn how parents, schools, students, and pediatricians can create a safe and supportive place for students with chronic health conditions.

Parent responsibilities

If your child has a chronic illness, how he is cared for and treated at school is important. You will need to work with the school to make sure his health care needs are being met at school, and that he is given the same opportunities to participate in school activities as other students.

The following are ways you can help your child receive the education and services he or she needs to succeed in school:

- **Talk to the school.** Don't be afraid to tell the school about your child's condition. Some parents worry about sharing this information, but the more informed teachers and other school staff are, the better prepared they will be to help your child. If the school staff don't have all the facts, they may make wrong assumptions about your child's behavior or performance.
- **Make a health plan.** Ask your pediatrician to help you write down exactly what the school should do if your child has certain health needs. School staff should know how to reach you or your pediatrician in case there is an emergency. Remember to call the school right away when contact information has changed.

  Also, try to plan her medicine or treatment schedule at a time that interferes the least with her classes; the best time may be during lunch or a study break. If your child takes medicine at school, ask about the school's policies for storage and self-usage. For example, if appropriate, schools may let some students with asthma carry their inhalers and use them if needed. Make sure your child is able to take her medicine in a comfortable place, and that the school is provided with an adequate supply. Remember to call the school right away if there are any changes in your child's condition.
- **Give your consent.** Encourage open communication between your pediatrician and the school staff so that everyone who cares for your child has all the facts about his condition. If the school staff have any questions, they should call your pediatrician. You will have to sign a release form that gives the school permission to contact your pediatrician. Also, your pediatrician will need your written permission to discuss your child's condition with the school. If your child requires medicine or special procedures, the school must receive written instructions from your pediatrician.

What does the school need to know?

If your child has special health needs, the school should have a written document outlining a health care and emergency plan. The following information should be in the document:

- A brief medical history
- The child's special needs
- Medicine or procedures required during the school day
- Special dietary needs
- Transportation needs
- Possible problems, special precautions
- Pediatrician's name
- Emergency plans and procedures (including whom to contact)

- **Plan ahead.** Meet with your child's teachers regularly to talk about how your child is doing at school. During parent-teacher conferences, ask if your child's health condition is affecting her schoolwork or behavior. If your child is missing a lot of school due to illness, talk with her teacher about ways to help her keep up with her work. For example, when your child misses school, plan how homework will be sent home.
- **Teach others.** A number of school systems have programs that teach students about chronic illnesses and disabilities. The programs hope to increase awareness and sensitivity among students. If your child is old enough, is willing, and has the school's support, he may want to share his experience with his class. If you're interested, you can find ways to participate in school curriculum committees or with the PTA to help educate parents and students about classmates with chronic health conditions.
- **Know the law.** By law, your child is entitled to an education that will help her develop to her full potential. Schools may be required to provide additional services that will assist in both in-school programs and after-school events. Federal laws such as the Individuals with Disabilities Education Act (IDEA) and the Americans with Disabilities Act (ADA) state that every child should be allowed to attend school in the "least restrictive" setting possible.

  Get to know these laws so you are aware of all the services your child is entitled to. For example, if she needs speech therapy, psychological counseling, or physical therapy to do well in school, the school *must* determine if she is qualified for them and, if so, must then provide them. She also may be eligible for home-based education, *if* the home is the least restrictive setting. Schools only are required to provide health-related services that affect your child's education or are required at school for safety reasons. Parents and health care systems are responsible for the rest.

If your child's educational needs are not being met, the following are some steps you can take:

- **Work with the school.** Ask the teacher and other school staff to meet with your pediatrician to create guidelines to help your child succeed at school. These guidelines should clearly state what the school would do for your child.
- **Know the guidelines for resolving complaints.** There are procedures (spelled out by every school district) through which you can appeal and try to solve any problems. Ask the school for a written copy of these guidelines for resolving complaints.
- **Contact the local board of education.** If you still are not satisfied, contact the local board of education or the regional office of the US Department of Education.

School responsibilities

By law, school districts are required to offer programs that provide children with chronic health conditions with the full range of educational opportunities. Federal laws designed to ensure this happens include the following:

- **ADA (Americans with Disabilities Act)** prohibits discrimination against students in education programs or activities that receive federal funds based on disability.
- **IDEA (Individuals with Disabilities Education Act)** allows children with disabilities to remain in regular classrooms with regular teachers if the student can learn optimally in that environment.
- **Section 504** is a civil rights law that prohibits discrimination against people with disabilities—children with disabilities should be given equal access to education.
- **FERPA (Family Educational Rights and Privacy Act)** is a federal law that protects the privacy of students. Schools are required to obtain written permission from parents before a child's education record can be released. The law also requires schools to release a child's education record to a parent, if requested. Schools may disclose, without consent, "directory" information such as a student's name, address, phone number, birth date and place of birth, honors and awards, and attendance dates.
- **State or local laws and district policies** may require schools to provide different services for students with chronic illnesses. These services often vary by state and school district.

Once the school is informed a student has a chronic health condition, a meeting is often scheduled to discuss what services may be needed. The meeting should include parents, the student (if old enough), school health staff, the coordinator of special needs services, student aids, and the child's primary teacher. Health care providers, such as the child's pediatrician, also should be invited or asked to provide information in writing.

One goal of this meeting is to develop a written plan that clearly describes the services the student needs. Depending on the child's needs, this plan may be described as a 504 Plan or an Individualized Education Program (IEP). This legal document outlines exactly what services the child will receive and sets short- and long-term goals for the child. The plan should be reviewed regularly to ensure it continues to meet the child's needs.

Other school responsibilities include the following:

- **Provide staff training and support.** Schools should provide their staff the training and tools necessary to ensure students' health and educational needs are met. Staff members should be prepared to handle emergencies. There should be a staff member available who is properly trained to give medicine or other emergency care during the school day and at all school-related activities regardless of time or location. Schools should ensure that case management is provided as needed.
- **Promote a supportive environment.** Schools should promote a supportive learning environment that views students with chronic illnesses as the same as other students. Schools should make it as easy as possible for students with chronic illnesses to participate in such school activities as physical education, recess, after-school programs, and field trips. Schools should promote good general health, personal care, nutrition, and physical activity.
- **Provide a safe environment.** Schools should make sure that students can take their prescribed medicine in a safe, reliable, and effective manner, and that it's available when needed.
- **Keep parents informed.** Schools should communicate regularly with parents and with the student's pediatrician (if permission is given).
- **Keep information confidential.** Schools should make sure proper records are kept and that confidentiality is maintained.

Student responsibilities

Include your child as much as possible in all discussions and plans that affect his school experience. This will help your child learn to be an active participant in the care and management of his health. Also, make sure your child has an adult to go to if he has any concerns or needs during the school day. Talk to your child regularly about how he feels his health condition is being managed at school and if any improvements or changes need to be made.

Pediatrician's role

Your pediatrician cares about your child's health and can be an excellent resource regarding school issues. The following are ways your pediatrician can be involved in enhancing your child's school experience.

- **Answer the school's questions.** Your pediatrician should have on file any permission forms that allow her to talk directly to your child's school. Make sure the forms are updated at the beginning of each school year. This is extremely important if the school needs specific medical information about your child's condition. It also can relieve you of having to carry messages back and forth between school personnel and your pediatrician.
- **Provide the school with medical information.** Ask your pediatrician to provide the school with a description of your child's medical, developmental, and safety needs. This should include special precautions the school should take in an emergency.
- **Help the school develop a plan.** Invite your pediatrician to work directly with school staff as they explore ways to meet any special needs your child may have. Pediatricians may not be aware of all options that are available in each school to meet a child's needs, but your pediatrician's input and point of view makes her a valuable member of the school's team.

- **Help improve your child's school attendance.** At your child's check-ups, talk with your pediatrician about your child's school attendance and involvement in school activities (such as physical education programs). For example, while you may think missing 2 or 3 school days each month due to your child's asthma is OK, your pediatrician may be able to help reduce the amount of time your child misses school.

The information contained in this publication should not be used as a substitute for the medical care and advice of your pediatrician. There may be variations in treatment that your pediatrician may recommend based on individual facts and circumstances.

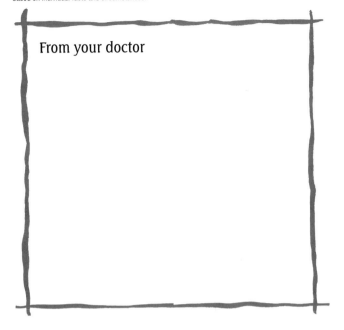

From your doctor

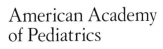

American Academy
of Pediatrics

DEDICATED TO THE HEALTH OF ALL CHILDREN™

The American Academy of Pediatrics is an organization of 60,000 primary care pediatricians, pediatric medical subspecialists, and pediatric surgical specialists dedicated to the health, safety, and well-being of infants, children, adolescents, and young adults.

American Academy of Pediatrics
Web site—www.aap.org

Copyright © 2004
American Academy of Pediatrics

For Today's Teens:
A Message From Your Pediatrician

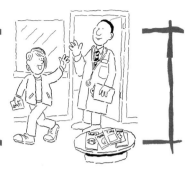

Your pediatrician may have cared for you since you were a small child. As you continue to grow and change, you will have new health needs. Even though you are becoming an adult, your pediatrician can still help you stay healthy.

When you are 11 or 12 years old, most pediatricians will speak with you and your parent or guardian at your checkup and suggest that you spend some time alone with him or her during future health care visits. What you talk about during these visits will remain confidential. This way you will begin to learn how to take care of your own health.

Growing up is often confusing. Your body is changing and you may feel differently than you did a few years ago. The changes you feel now may leave you wondering what's happening to your mind and body. You may have questions about these changes and how you should take care of yourself. Your pediatrician can answer questions about the following:

- eating right
- your height and weight
- exercise and sports
- acne
- dating
- body changes
- school performance
- alcohol and other drugs
- other concerns you may have

Why do teens need a pediatrician?

Some teenagers only visit their pediatrician when they are sick or hurt, but staying healthy means more than just seeing a doctor when something is wrong. As you become an adult, you need to take charge of your own health. This means preventing problems before they start. A first step might be to see your pediatrician once a year, just to make sure everything is OK and any problems are prevented from becoming serious.

You should also see your pediatrician when you are sick or concerned about what is happening to your body. Most likely, your concerns are normal. Growing up may also trigger changes in how you think and feel. You may feel sad, angry, or nervous at times. You should feel free to talk to your pediatrician about these things. After all, these emotions are a part of being healthy too.

What health services do pediatricians offer?

The following is a partial list of different things that you can talk about with your pediatrician:

Sports or school physicals:

Many schools ask students to get a physical before joining a team sport. It's important for you to talk about your health with your pediatrician before you participate in any sport. Your pediatrician can help you avoid injuries and stay healthy and fit.

Treatment of illnesses or injuries:

It is important for you to tell your pediatrician about any illnesses or injuries you have. Let your pediatrician know about pain you have or changes in the way you feel, even if you think they aren't serious. This is the only way your pediatrician can help you stay healthy.

A word about...privacy

Talking about personal things with your family and friends can sometimes be difficult. When you feel uncomfortable talking about certain things with your parents, you can always ask your pediatrician. Getting answers about how your body works, how you can take care of yourself, how to handle your emotions, and how to stay healthy, will help you make the right decisions about your health.

Your pediatrician will respect you as a patient. Because the pediatrician is your doctor, he or she will keep your discussions private whenever possible. However, your parents are obviously very concerned about your health and well-being, and your pediatrician will want to keep them informed of extreme situations; for example, if your life, or someone else's, is in danger. In most cases though, the information you share with your pediatrician will stay between you and your pediatrician.

Growth and development:

Your body is probably changing fast and you might want to talk to your pediatrician about what to expect as you grow. For example, you may be wondering about the following:

- Will you be as tall as your parents?
- Is your sexual development normal?
- Will your acne clear up?
- Will your body fill out more?
- Should you be worried about your weight?

These are all things you can discuss openly and freely with your pediatrician. Just ask.

Personal and/or family problems:

Sometimes you might have a hard time dealing with problems with friends or family. Feeling like your parents don't understand you, losing a best friend, getting teased at school, pressure from friends- all these things can get the best of you once in a while. If you don't know where to turn, remember that your pediatrician is there to help.

School problems:

As a student, you may worry sometimes about your grades and your future. No matter what you try, it may be hard to keep up with school, a job, sports, or other activities. Maybe you find it difficult to get along with others at school or to concentrate on your studies. Your pediatrician may be able to help you through this busy time of your life.

Alcohol and drug use:

You may be tempted to take risks as you make new friends. You may also get a lot of pressure from your friends. Remember, what's right for them might not always be right for you. Becoming an adult means more than just physical growth. It also means determining what is right for you. This is especially important since many people you know may be using cigarettes, alcohol, or other drugs. Instead of going along with the crowd, you need to decide what is the best choice for you. Your pediatrician can explain how smoking, drinking, or taking other drugs can affect you.

Sexual relationships:

During visits with your pediatrician, you'll have a chance to ask questions about dating, sexual activity, and infections. Your pediatrician also can talk to you confidentially about postponing sex and how to protect yourself against sexually transmitted diseases (STDs) and pregnancy. It's important to make smart choices about sex now. The wrong choice could affect the rest of your life.

Conflicts with parents:

At times, It might be hard to get along with your family and this could lead to problems at home. Maybe it seems like no one understands you or respects your ideas. You're not alone. If you have a problem that your parents may not understand, talk with your pediatrician. Sometimes an outside person can give a better view of these difficult situations.

Referrals to other doctors for special health needs:

You may have a medical problem that will require you to see another doctor or specialist. In that case, your pediatrician can refer you to another doctor who can take care of your needs. A referral may involve an ophthalmologist (eye doctor) for vision, a psychologist or psychiatrist for stress or depression, or other doctors that handle specific medical needs. Even though you may need to see a specialist for a special problem, you should continue to see your pediatrician for regular checkups or illnesses. After all, he or she is still your doctor and will want to keep up with your general needs.

Educational brochures, magazines, or videos on health topics:

In addition to talking about your health with your pediatrician, you also may be able to learn more about how to take better care of yourself by reading brochures or by watching videos. The American Academy of Pediatrics offers free material covering health topics that might interest you, such as acne, sports and fitness, sexuality, substance abuse, eating disorders, and more. Ask your pediatrician for more information.

What you can do to stay healthy

Use the following list to take care of yourself and stay healthy:

- **Eat right and get plenty of sleep.**
- **Know how to handle minor injuries,** such as cuts and bruises, as well as minor illnesses like colds.
- **Know how to seek medical attention** for problems such as vomiting, headache, high fever, earache, sore throat, diarrhea, or abdominal pain.
- **Take care of your mental health** and ask for help if you have sleep problems, sadness, family stress, school problems, problems with alcohol or other drugs, or trouble relating to friends, family, or teachers.
- **Avoid alcohol, cigarettes, smokeless tobacco (chew), and other drugs.**
- **Delay having sexual relations** or use protection if you choose to have sex.
- **Exercise regularly,** with help from an adult who knows what is right for your body.
- ***Always* wear your seat belt** when you are in a car or truck.

As you become an adult, you'll face many challenges. With help from your pediatrician, you'll learn how to make the right decisions that will help you grow up healthy.

The information contained in this publication should not be used as a substitute for the medical care and advice of your pediatrician. There may be variations in treatment that your pediatrician may recommend based on individual facts and circumstances.

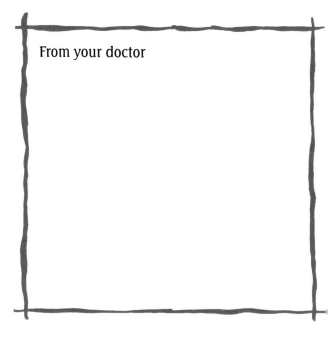

From your doctor

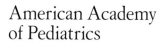

© 2007 American Academy of Pediatrics

Behavioral and Psychosocial Issues

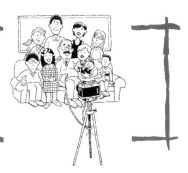

Adoption:
Guidelines for Parents Part I | Adopting a Young Child

If you have recently adopted or soon will be adopting a child, you are probably experiencing many different emotions. The excitement and delight of a new addition to the family is often mixed with concern or even fear of what lies ahead.

There are many different types of adoption. Children often are adopted by a relative or a stepparent. More and more families are adopting children of another race, country, or culture. Many families adopt older children from foster homes, but most children who are adopted come into their new families as infants or very young children. The fact is, children of any age or background who are adopted will bring special issues and challenges to your family that biological parents never face.

By better understanding the role adoption plays in your child's growth and development, you can help your child accept his own uniqueness and learn to be proud of who he is and how he helped form your family.

Better early than never

Talk to your child about her adoption as soon as she is able to understand—usually between ages 2 and 4. The word adopted should become a part of your child's vocabulary early on. These early discussions give you practice in talking about adoption and show your child that it is OK to bring up the topic. If you are uneasy that your child is not biologically yours, she will feel it.

Just as any child delights in the story of the day she was born, a child who is adopted will treasure details of how she came into the family. While going through the adoption process, keep a scrapbook or journal the same way an excited mother does during pregnancy. Keep track of important dates and steps in the process. Take pictures of the people and places involved in your child's earlier life. Details about your child's earlier life and the adoption process will help make both easier to understand.

Share with your child the joy you felt at bringing her home that very first day. Many families even celebrate the arrival or adoption date every year, in addition to a birthday. It shows that the child came to the family in a different way, but is just as valued and loved.

The longer you wait to discuss adoption with your child, the harder it will be. Any level of openness you can build when your child is very young will help as your child grows and begins to ask more difficult questions about her adoption.

If talking with your child about adoption is difficult, talk to your pediatrician. He or she can be a valuable source of support and understanding.

Is anything different?

As he grows into adulthood, your child may be asked questions by other people that he will not be able to answer. They may be simple, innocent questions such as, "Where did you get those big, blue eyes?" or "Do you look more like your mom or your dad?"

They could be questions on a form to be filled out at the doctor's office or when joining an athletic team at school, such as, "Has any blood relative ever had cancer? Diabetes?" or "What is your ethnic background?"

The most painful questions may be the ones the child asks himself. "Who am I?" "Where did I come from?" "Why did my parents give me away?"

Sooner or later, these questions or others like them will come up. Many children who are adopted simply don't have the answers.

Being adopted can play a vital role in the development of your child's self-image. It becomes a basic part of who he is. Some children who are adopted grow up feeling different from other children. Those differences are real. Many adopted children have two sets of parents. Some may have been denied affection or even basic nutrition or medical care. Whatever the circumstances, it is important to recognize that your child's life experience has been quite different from that of other children.

Keep no secrets

As the years pass, your child will become more concerned about his place in your family. This may be especially true around ages 9 through 12, when most children become very worried about appearance and fitting in. Your child may begin to ask questions about his own appearance, his background, and the adoption and its circumstances. The following are some common questions your child may ask:

- "Did I grow in your body, Mommy?"
- "Why did my birth mother give me away?"
- "Did she and my birth father love each other?"
- "What was my name before I was adopted?"
- "What nationality am I?"
- "Do I have brothers or sisters?"
- "How much did it cost to adopt me?"

- **Do your best to answer questions honestly and in a way that will be easy for your child to understand at her age.** They may be painful questions for you to think about, but it is normal for children who are adopted to ask them. It is important to develop trust between you and your child. The more your child trusts you, the easier it will be for her to come to you with questions. If your child feels that talking about these questions makes you uncomfortable, she may keep them inside. She may then wonder, imagine, and perhaps fear the worst. Your child may also seek the answers elsewhere, perhaps from a relative or friend who may not give accurate information. Dealing with these issues openly is very important for your child. Be honest and as informative as you can. You may not know the answers for some questions. Be honest about that too.

- **Avoid responding with your own worries** like "Why do you want to know?" or "Are you unhappy with our family?" Your child's curiosity is healthy and natural. It should not be discouraged or seen as a threat to you—it's normal. Questioning your child's loyalties may only confuse him further. If your child believes talking about his adoption will hurt you, he will avoid it.

- **Don't force the issue on your child**. Some children are curious from the very beginning. Others may be afraid to bring it up. The best you can do is create an atmosphere in the family that lets your child know it is OK to talk about adoption. In a loving, supportive environment, when your child is ready to know more, she will ask.

Relatives, friends, and strangers

Even when adoption is handled well at home, there may be relatives who are not quite as understanding. This is particularly important when the child is from a different race or country. Some friends or relatives may disapprove of or even resist accepting your child into the family.

Explain to your relatives that your child is as much a part of the family as anyone else. You may not change their minds or correct old thinking, but it is important to show loyalty to your child. For a child to feel loved and welcomed, he needs to be treated like a full member of the family. Do not settle for anything less.

Questions from strangers can also be tricky. When a stranger innocently asks, "Where did he get those big blue eyes?," and everyone in the family has small brown eyes, tell the truth. Say simply, "From his mother." It may not be necessary to share personal information with a stranger, but don't lie. If your child hears you lying to a stranger, he may assume there is something about being adopted that he should be ashamed of, something that needs to be covered up.

You do not have to introduce your child as "my adopted son." He is simply your son. However, if a question comes up about differences in appearance or ethnicity, offer a simple, but honest explanation. When you are proud of your child's identity, he too, will learn to appreciate his own value.

Facing the past

It can be very difficult to talk with your child about the past. It may be painful to think about or acknowledge your child's other identity. Children who are adopted need to belong and to feel connected to their roots. Having kind and loving adoptive parents does not erase the past. Sooner or later, many adopted children want to know where they came from and why they were placed for adoption.

As your child gets older, make sure she knows where to look for information about the adoption. It is a good idea to keep copies of your child's important papers accessible to her at any time. She may want to look them over in private and in her own time. Someday, she may want to read through them with you. In some cases, she may never have the desire to see the papers at all. But it is important that the choice be hers and that the option be available to her.

Preparing for the future

As your child grows into adulthood, he may begin thinking about searching for his birth family. He may begin to feel less dependent on you, and more able to search for information on his own. Some states have programs available to help adults who were adopted get information about their adoption. Only a few states have open records. Check with your state government to find out about the laws concerning adoption records.

Birth mothers and fathers also may conduct searches. The pain or guilt of giving up a child may become too much to bear over the years. Many have gone on to raise other children and may feel a need for information about the child they placed for adoption.

It is important for you to consider the possibility that the birth parents may one day play a role in your child's life. By establishing an open, loving, and supportive relationship with your child, the issues that may emerge in the teen and adult years will often be much easier to manage. Search and reunion can bring pain and joy for everyone involved. The child, no matter what age, needs the continuing love and support of his adoptive family.

Your family, your child

Raising a family today is difficult. Raising a child who is adopted can present unique challenges. If the child misbehaves, gets into trouble, or has problems at school, it is tempting to blame adoption. The fact is, all children sometimes misbehave or get into trouble. It is possible your child's problems have nothing to do with adoption at all. They may simply be a normal part of growth.

As your child grows, he is influenced by family, the community, friends, school, and society in general. He is also influenced by the genes passed to him from his birth mother and father. There is no research that can tell us which is more important, but we know that both are powerful. Adoption is an important part of who your child is, but keep in mind that many other factors will affect who he becomes.

Helping your child accept the fact that he is different, yet just like everyone else, may not sound easy, but it is important to try. Talking openly and truthfully with your child about his adoption, his birth parents, and his feelings is the key. Adoption gives both you and your child a tremendous gift—the gift of each other. With love, honesty, and patience, you and your child will form a relationship that is as deep and meaningful as any bond between a parent and child.

The information contained in this publication should not be used as a substitute for the medical care and advice of your pediatrician. There may be variations in treatment that your pediatrician may recommend based on individual facts and circumstances.

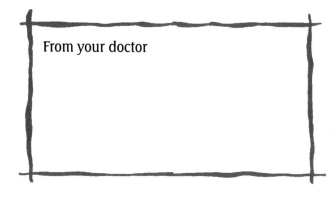

From your doctor

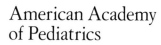

American Academy
of Pediatrics

DEDICATED TO THE HEALTH OF ALL CHILDREN™

The American Academy of Pediatrics is an organization of 60,000 primary care pediatricians, pediatric medical subspecialists, and pediatric surgical specialists dedicated to the health, safety, and well-being of infants, children, adolescents, and young adults.

American Academy of Pediatrics
Web site—www.aap.org

Copyright © 1999
American Academy of Pediatrics

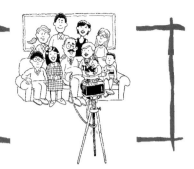

Adoption:
Guidelines for Parents Part II Adopting an Older Child

If you have recently adopted or soon will be adopting a child, you are probably experiencing many different emotions. The excitement and delight of a new addition to the family is often mixed with concern or even fear of what lies ahead.

There are many different types of adoption. Children often are adopted by a relative or a stepparent. More and more families are adopting children of another race, country, or culture. Many families adopt older children from foster homes, but most children who are adopted come into their new families as infants or very young children. The fact is, children of any age or background who are adopted will bring special issues and challenges to your family that biological parents never face.

By better understanding the role adoption plays in your child's growth and development, you can help your child accept his own uniqueness and learn to be proud of who he is and how he helped form your family.

Adopting the older child

Becoming a new parent is tough, but becoming a new parent of a school-age child or adolescent can be tougher.

An older child may bring problems from the past into his new family. He may have lived in a number of foster homes, each affecting him in some way. He may have lived with one or both birth parents for a time. There may be a history of drug, alcohol, physical, or sexual abuse. He may have been separated from siblings. Many factors could have affected your child's life before he came to your home. Following are some suggestions that will help you deal with them:

- **Learn as much as you can about your child's background** and that of his birth parents. The adoption agency can help you gather as much information as possible. By learning everything you can about your child and his past, you may become more aware of problems that may lie ahead. Keep in mind, it is impossible for you or the adoption agency to know everything your child may have gone through.

- **Keep a connection to your child's past.** It is important that your child feel connected in a positive way to the life she had before coming to your home. Keep in touch with someone she knew; a grandparent, relative, friend, or neighbor. If possible, put together a "life book" by collecting mementos and photos of your child's previous home, school, and people she was close to. These things will be important as your child adjusts to her new life.

- **Don't be afraid to seek help.** Adoptive parents should understand that an older child with serious problems may need professional help to resolve these issues. Constant and persistent love can work wonders for most children, however, in some cases, love may not be enough.

- **Don't blame yourself.** An older child may rebel against his new family. This anger is usually because of the child's past losses. These problems are not your fault. Remind yourself that you are part of the solution as you help your child work out his issues. Most of all, be patient.

- **Talk to your pediatrician.** He or she may be able to help or suggest counselors or support groups.

Relatives, friends, and strangers

Even when adoption is handled well at home, there may be relatives who are not quite as understanding. This is particularly important when the child is from a different race or country. Some friends or relatives may disapprove of or even resist accepting your child into the family.

Explain to your relatives that your child is as much a part of the family as anyone else. You may not change their minds or correct old thinking, but it is important to show loyalty to your child. For a child to feel loved and welcomed, he needs to be treated like a full member of the family. Do not settle for anything less.

Questions from strangers can also be tricky. When a stranger innocently asks, "Where did he get those big blue eyes?," and everyone in the family has small brown eyes, tell the truth. Say simply, "From his mother." It may not be necessary to share personal information with a stranger, but don't lie. If your child hears you lying to a stranger, he may assume there is something about being adopted that he should be ashamed of, something that needs to be covered up.

You do not have to introduce your child as "my adopted son." He is simply your son. However, if a question comes up about differences in appearance or ethnicity, offer a simple, but honest explanation. When you are proud of your child's identity, he too, will learn to appreciate his own value.

Facing the past

It can be very difficult to talk with your child about the past. It may be painful to think about or acknowledge your child's other identity. Children who are adopted need to belong and to feel connected to their roots. Having kind and loving adoptive parents does not erase the past. Sooner or later, many adopted children want to know where they came from and why they were placed for adoption.

As your child gets older, make sure she knows where to look for information about the adoption. It is a good idea to keep copies of your child's important papers accessible to her at any time. She may want to look them over in private and in her own time. Someday, she may want to read through them with you. In some cases, she may never have the desire to see the papers at all. But it is important that the choice be hers and that the option be available to her.

Preparing for the future

As your child grows into adulthood, he may begin thinking about searching for his birth family. He may begin to feel less dependent on you, and more able to search for information on his own. Some states have programs available to help adults who were adopted get information about their adoption. Only a few states have open records. Check with your state government to find out about the laws concerning adoption records.

Birth mothers and fathers also may conduct searches. The pain or guilt of giving up a child may become too much to bear over the years. Many have gone on to raise other children and may feel a need for information about the child they placed for adoption.

It is important for you to consider the possibility that the birth parents may one day play a role in your child's life. By establishing an open, loving, and supportive relationship with your child, the issues that may emerge in the teen and adult years will often be much easier to manage. Search and reunion can bring pain and joy for everyone involved. The child, no matter what age, needs the continuing love and support of his adoptive family.

Your family, your child

Raising a family today is difficult. Raising a child who is adopted can present unique challenges. If the child misbehaves, gets into trouble, or has problems at school, it is tempting to blame adoption. The fact is, all children sometimes misbehave or get into trouble. It is possible your child's problems have nothing to do with adoption at all. They may simply be a normal part of growth.

As your child grows, he is influenced by family, the community, friends, school, and society in general. He is also influenced by the genes passed to him from his birth mother and father. There is no research that can tell us which is more important, but we know that both are powerful. Adoption is an important part of who your child is, but keep in mind that many other factors will affect who he becomes.

Helping your child accept the fact that he is different, yet just like everyone else, may not sound easy, but it is important to try. Talking openly and truthfully with your child about his adoption, his birth parents, and his feelings is the key. Adoption gives both you and your child a tremendous gift—the gift of each other. With love, honesty, and patience, you and your child will form a relationship that is as deep and meaningful as any bond between a parent and child.

The information contained in this publication should not be used as a substitute for the medical care and advice of your pediatrician. There may be variations in treatment that your pediatrician may recommend based on individual facts and circumstances.

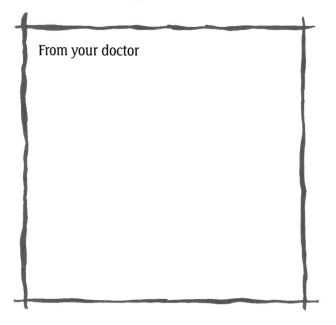

From your doctor

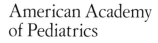

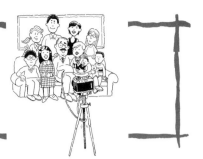

Adoption:
Guidelines for Parents Part III Additional Resources

"Who are my real parents?"

Early on, many parents find themselves dealing with the question of who the child's "real" or "natural" parents are. Relatives or friends may ask if you have met the child's "real" parents. Your child herself may even ask about her "real" mother or father. Let your child know that the words mother and father have more than one meaning.

A mother is someone who gives birth to a child, but a mother is also someone who loves, nurtures, and guides a child to adulthood. She takes care of the child's needs every day, changes the diapers, and dries the tears. Being a father also can have different meanings.

Find other words that everyone in your family is comfortable with. The terms birth mother and father are very common. Biological parents is also used frequently. Remember, both sets of parents are "real" and deserve to be recognized for who they are and the roles they have played in the child's life.

A note from your pediatrician...
international adoptions

Parents who adopt children from other countries need to be aware of the special medical needs their child may have. Your pediatrician recommends the following:

- Immunizations should meet US standards.
- Test for infectious diseases (such as HIV, hepatitis B and C, syphilis, tuberculosis, and parasites) and nutritional disorders (such as lead poisoning, anemia, rickets, and iodine deficiency), even if testing was done in another country before the adoption.
- Have your child's vision, hearing, and developmental abilities (such as language) assessed as soon as possible.

"You are special because..."

Adoptive parents often tell their child she is special because she was "chosen" or that she was "given up out of love." Though the parents mean well, these statements may be confusing to the child.

For most parents, adoption is not the first choice. Most adoptions in the United States are by parents who first tried to conceive and were unable to do so. Sooner or later, children learn this. Telling the child she is even more special because she is "chosen" may be recognized by the child as bending the truth. Some children may feel that being chosen means they must always be the best at everything.

Being told she was given up out of love may raise questions about what love is and whether others who love her will leave too.

The most important thing for your child to know is that she is wanted —not any more than a biological child would be and not any less. Any attempt to make the adopted child feel more special than a biological child may have quite a different, unintended effect.

Every child in the family should be treated the same by you, your spouse, the siblings, and your relatives. Children who are adopted may feel different from other members of the family. Her appearance, her performance in school, or her athletic ability may be quite different. But she is, first and foremost, your child. What makes her special is not that she was adopted, but that she is yours.

A word about...open adoptions

When there is contact between birth parents and adoptive parents during the adoption process, it is considered an "open adoption." This can mean simply exchanging names and addresses or, in fully open adoptions, the birth parents may have ongoing communication with or even visit the child.

In an open adoption, your young child may not understand the relationships between the two sets of parents. There are fewer secrets in an open adoption, but just as many difficult questions. It is important to address the issues mentioned in this brochure and provide your child with the guidance and support she needs.

For more information

There are many quality resources available to find out more about adoption. The following are just a few:

Books

Adopting the Hurt Child: Hope for Families with Special-Needs Kids; by Gregory C. Keck, Regina M. Kupecky (Pinon Press, 1998)

The Adoption Triangle; by Arthur D. Sorosky, Annette Baran, and Reuben Pannor (Corona, 1989)

Being Adopted; The Lifelong Search for Self; by David M. Brodzinsky, Marshall Schechter, and Robin Marantz Henig (Anchor, 1993)

Birthmothers: Women Who Have Relinquished Babies for Adoption Tell Their Stories; by Merry Bloch Jones (Chicago Review, 1993)

How It Feels to Be Adopted; by Jill Krementz (Knopf, 1988)

Journey of the Adopted Self; by Betty Jean Lifton (BasicBooks, HarperCollins, 1995)

Let's Talk About It: Adoption; by Fred Rogers (Paper Star, 1998)

Raising Adopted Children; by Lois R. Melina (HarperCollins, 1998)

Real Parents, Real Children; by Holly van Gulden and Lisa M. Bartels-Rabb (Crossroad, 1995)

Talking With Young Children About Adoption; by Mary Watkins, Susan Fisher (Yale University Press, 1995)

Organizations

Adoptive Families of America (AFA)
2309 Como St
St Paul, MN 55108
800/372-3300
http://www.AdoptiveFam.org

American Adoption Congress (AAC)
1000 Connecticut Ave, NW
Suite 9
Washington, DC 20036
202/483-3399
http://www.american-adoption-cong.org

Child Welfare League of America (CWLA)
440 First Street, NW
Third Floor
Washington, DC 20001
202/638-2952
http://www.cwla.org

North American Council on Adoptable
   Children (NACAC)
970 Raymond Ave, Suite 106
St Paul, MN 55114-1149
651/644-3036
E-mail: NACAC@aol.com

These resources were chosen to represent a broad range of viewpoints. Inclusion on this list does not imply an endorsement by the American Academy of Pediatrics. The Academy is not responsible for the content of the resources mentioned above. Addresses and phone numbers are as current as possible, but may change at any time.

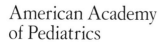

American Academy
of Pediatrics

DEDICATED TO THE HEALTH OF ALL CHILDREN™

The American Academy of Pediatrics is an organization of 60,000 primary care pediatricians, pediatric medical subspecialists, and pediatric surgical specialists dedicated to the health, safety, and well-being of infants, children, adolescents, and young adults.

American Academy of Pediatrics
Web site — www.aap.org

Copyright © 1999
American Academy of Pediatrics

Healthy Communication With Your Child

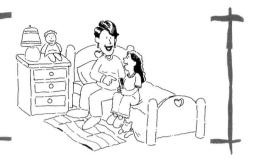

Healthy communication with your child is one of the most important and rewarding skills that you can develop as a parent. It also makes the tough parts of parenting (such as disciplining your child) much easier and more effective. Good communication is a two-way street, meaning that listening to your child is just as important as talking to him.

When you talk in a calm and caring manner, you let your child know what you expect of him and give him information that he needs. You also show him that when you ask him to calm down and control his temper, you are practicing what you preach.

Listening to your child helps you learn more about what is going on with your child. You can learn his thoughts about a subject, how he is getting along socially, what problems he may be having, and whether your child is getting the message that you are trying to communicate.

Good communication is needed so that you can be a good teacher for your child and know what is happening in your child's life.

Why is healthy communication important?

Healthy communication is important because it helps your child
- Feel cared for and loved
- Feel safe and not all alone with her worries
- Learn to tell you what she feels and needs directly in words
- Learn how to manage her feelings safely so that she does not act on feelings without thinking
- Talk to you openly
- Learn to listen to you

Healthy communication also helps *you*
- Feel close to your child
- Know your child's needs
- Know you have powerful tools to help your child develop and grow
- Manage your own stress and frustrations with your child

What are the building blocks of healthy communication?

Here are a few important ways to build healthy communication
- **Be available.** Make time in everyone's busy schedule to stop and talk about things. Even 10 minutes a day without distractions for you and your child to talk can make a big difference in forming good communication habits. Turn off the television or radio. Give your undivided attention to your child. Sit down and look at your child while you talk. Those few minutes a day can be of great value.
- **Be a good listener.** When you listen to your child, you help your child feel loved and valued. Ask your child about his feelings on a subject. If you are not clear about what your child is saying, repeat what you are hearing to be sure that you understand what your child is trying to say. You do not

have to agree with what your child is saying to be a good listener. Sharing his thoughts with you helps your child calm down, so later he can listen to you.
- **Show empathy.** This means tuning in to your child's feelings and letting him know you understand. If your child is sad or upset, a gentle touch or hug may let him know that you understand those sad or bad feelings. Do not tell your child what he thinks or feels. Let him express those feelings. And be sure not to minimize these feelings by saying things like, "It's silly to feel that way," or "You'll understand when you get older." His feelings are real to him and should be respected.
- **Be a good role model.** Remember, children learn by example. Use words and tones in your voice that you want your child to use. Make sure that your tone of voice and what you do send the same message. For example, if you laugh when you say, "No, don't do that," the message will be confusing. Be clear in your directions. Once you get the message across, do not wear out your point. If you use words to describe your feelings, it will help your child to learn to do the same. When parents use feeling words, such as, "It makes me feel sad when you won't do what I ask you to do," instead of screaming or name calling, children learn to do the same.

Keys to healthy communication

Do
- Give clear, age-appropriate directions such as, "When we go to the store I expect you to be polite and stay with me." Make sure your child understands what you have said. Sometimes children do not fully understand the meanings of words they hear and use.
- Praise your child whenever you can.
- Calmly communicate your feelings.
- Be truthful.
- Listen carefully to what your child says.
- Use your talking times as teachable moments – do not miss opportunities to show your child healthy communication.
- Model what you want your child to do – practice what you preach.
- Make sure that when you are upset with your child, she knows that it is her behavior that is the problem, not the child herself.

Don't
- Give broad, general instructions such as, "You'd better be good!"
- Name call or blame. "You are bad" should be replaced with "I don't like the way you are acting."
- Yell or threaten.
- Lie or tell your child half-truths.
- Use silence to express strong feelings. Long silences frighten and confuse children.

Discipline is not punishment

Part of a parent's job is to discipline a child. Discipline is not punishment. Discipline is actually a form of communication. It means teaching children appropriate behavior and correcting inappropriate behavior.

How do you change a child's behavior? The most effective way is through healthy communication. Make sure to teach your child what positive behavior is and praise him when he behaves the way you want him to. Focus on the things he does right and he will be less likely to do things you do not want him to do.

No matter how old your child is, he needs you to calmly and clearly explain (in language that he can fully understand) what you expect from him and what the consequences will be (for example, taking away a privilege) if he acts inappropriately. Then, if the child does misbehave, follow through on the consequences you and he have already discussed. This way, you are not reacting purely out of anger or frustration.

Keeping your cool

There are times when all parents feel that they are out of patience. However, it is always important to find ways to help your child to behave without hurting her feelings. Here are a few ways to calm yourself when you feel stressed, before you try to talk with your child.

- Take a few deep breaths very slowly.
- Wait 5 minutes before starting to talk to your child.
- Try to find a word to label what you are feeling (such as "disappointment"). Say it to yourself and be sure that it is appropriate for you child.
- Share your feelings of frustration with your spouse or a friend.
- Do not hold grudges. Deal only with the present.
- Seek professional help if you feel that you have lost control.

Quick ways to offer praise

A smile and a short phrase can communicate valuable information. Here are just a few phrases that will go a long way.

- Outstanding!
- Nice work!
- Terrific!
- You made my day!
- You are so responsible.
- Good for you.
- You are really growing up!
- I like the way you share.
- Awesome!
- You figured it out on your own.
- I like the way you took care of that.
- What a good listener you are!
- You are so important to me.
- I love you so much!
- Bravo!

The information contained in this publication should not be used as a substitute for the medical care and advice of your pediatrician. There may be variations in treatment that your pediatrician may recommend based on individual facts and circumstances.

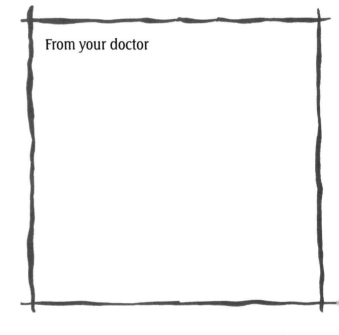

From your doctor

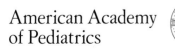

American Academy of Pediatrics

DEDICATED TO THE HEALTH OF ALL CHILDREN™

The American Academy of Pediatrics is an organization of 60,000 primary care pediatricians, pediatric medical subspecialists, and pediatric surgical specialists dedicated to the health, safety, and well-being of infants, children, adolescents, and young adults.

American Academy of Pediatrics
Web site—www.aap.org

Copyright © 2003
American Academy of Pediatrics, Updated 9/03

Surviving: Coping With Adolescent Depression and Suicide

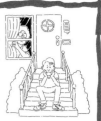

A 19-year-old college sophomore finished his term paper, asked his roommate to hand it in, and then drove himself to a park and rigged his car's exhaust pipe with a hose to the inside of his car. He died of carbon monoxide poisoning, leaving a note that asked his family for forgiveness because he "could not go on."

Like many other teens he seemed happy, well-adjusted, and high achieving. But inside him was an unhappiness and depression so great that the only solution he could see was suicide.

This is not an isolated incident. Children, teenagers, and young adults are killing themselves at rising rates. Suicide is the third leading cause of death among young people 15 to 24 years old, and it appears to be on the rise. According to a 1991 Centers for Disease Control and Prevention study, 27% of high school students thought about suicide, 16% had a plan, and 8% made an attempt. The Alcohol, Drug Abuse and Mental Health Administration has declared adolescent suicide as a national mental health problem.

Why do teens kill themselves? Experts cite divorce, family violence, the breakdown of the family unit, stress to perform and achieve, and even the threat of AIDS as factors that contribute to the higher suicide rate. More than 50% of teens who commit suicide also have a history of alcohol and drug use. Stressful life events, such as the loss of a significant person or school failure, often trigger suicides among teens.

Depression plays a role

To better understand the cause of adolescent suicide, one must look past the surface to figure out what is going on inside the suicidal teen's head. Many teens who are considering suicide suffer from depression. People who work with depressed teens see a common theme of unhappiness, as well as feelings of inner turmoil, chaos, and low self-worth. Also hopelessness and anger often contribute to adolescent suicide.

One study found that 90% of suicidal adolescents believed that their families did not understand them. These teens felt alone and anonymous. They also believed that their parents either denied or ignored their attempts to communicate feelings of unhappiness, frustration, or failure. Some parents view depression and complaining as weaknesses, so they encourage their children to be strong and not to show their emotions. Suicidal teens often feel that their emotions are played down, not taken seriously, or met with hostility by the people around them.

One pediatrician who counsels suicidal adolescents said they often talk about how hopeless everything seems. They often feel that they are not in control, as an example, not in control over the direction of their lives.

Depressed teens may be drawn to others who feel as they do forming a bond of hopelessness and despair. Some popular music reflects these feelings of alienation, self-destructive rage, and thoughts about suicide.

Adolescents need to learn that with treatment, depression ends. However, a teen who is experiencing deep depression for the first time may not be able to focus on that. Something that may seem trivial to a parent or teacher may crush an adolescent who is already in a fragile emotional state—so much so that he or she is unable to think clearly and see a way out of the problem. The teen may then see suicide as the only choice.

Adolescent suicide is treatable and preventable

People who are depressed and thinking about suicide often show changes in their behavior. These changes in behavior are usually an outgrowth of depression and are warning signs. If your teen shows these warning signs, please talk to her about her concerns and have her get help if the warning signs continue.

- Noticeable changes in eating or sleeping habits
- Unexplained, or unusually severe, violent or rebellious behavior
- Withdrawal from family or friends
- Running away
- Persistent boredom and/or difficulty concentrating
- Drug and/or alcohol abuse
- Unexplained drop in the quality of schoolwork
- Unusual neglect of appearance
- Drastic personality change
- Complaints of physical problems that are not real
- A focus on themes of death
- Giving away prized possessions
- Talking about suicide or making plans, even jokingly
- Threatening or attempting to kill oneself

Before committing suicide, people often threaten to kill themselves. These threats should always be taken seriously, as should previous suicide attempts. Most people who commit suicide have made at least one previous attempt.

Asking your teen whether he is depressed or is thinking about suicide lets him know that someone cares. You're not putting thoughts of suicide into his head. Instead you're giving your teen the chance to talk about his problems.

Remember that depression and suicidal feelings are treatable mental disorders. The first step is to listen to your adolescent. A professional must then diagnose your teen's illness and determine a proper treatment plan. Your teen needs to share her feelings, and many suicidal teens are pleading for help in their own way. Your teen needs to feel that there is hope-that people will listen, that things will get better, and that she can overcome her problems.

Parents and friends can help a depressed teen through the following strategies:

1. Talk, ask questions, and be willing to really listen. Don't dismiss your teen's problems as unimportant. Parents and other influential adults should never make fun of or ignore an adolescent's concerns, especially if they matter a great deal to her and are making her unhappy.
2. Be honest. It you're worried about your teen, say so. You will not spark thoughts of suicide just by asking about it.

3. Share your feelings. Let your teen know he's not alone. Everyone feels sad or depressed at times.

4. Get help for your teen and yourself. Talk to your pediatrician, teacher, counselor, clergy, or other trained professional. Don't wait for the problem to "go away." Although feelings of sadness and depression can disappear as quickly as they came, they can also build to the point that an adolescent thinks of suicide as the only way out. Be careful not to assume that your teen's problems have been so easily solved.

A teen attempting suicide should immediately be taken to a hospital emergency room for a psychiatric evaluation. If a depressed adolescent is assessed to be safe to go home, it's a good idea to remove from your home any lethal, accessible means to commit suicide, such as medications, firearms, razors, knives, etc.

Sources of help

There are many sources of information to help troubled teens and their families. Often a pediatrician, who has charted the adolescent's physical and emotional progress since infancy, is in the best position to detect and help treat adolescent depression. Your teen may, however, need additional counseling.

Check the *Yellow Pages* in your city for the phone numbers of local suicide hot lines, crisis centers, and mental health centers.

The following organizations can also supply information on suicide prevention:

American Academy of Child and Adolescent Psychiatry
3615 Wisconsin Ave, NW,
Washington, DC 20016
202/966-7300

American Association of Suicidology
4201 Connecticut Ave, NW, Suite 310,
Washington, DC 20008
202/237-2280

American Psychiatric Association
1400 K St, NW, Suite 501,
Washington, DC 20005
202/682-6000

American Psychological Association
750 1st St, NE,
Washington, DC 20002
202/336-5700

National Mental Health Association
1021 Prince St,
Alexandria, VA 22314-2971
800/969-6642

With professional treatment and support from family and friends, teens who are suicidal can become healthy again.

The information contained in this publication should not be used as a substitute for the medical care and advice of your pediatrician. There may be variations in treatment that your pediatrician may recommend based on individual facts and circumstances.

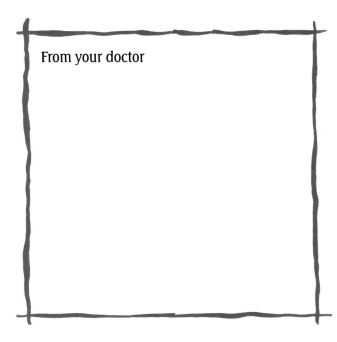

From your doctor

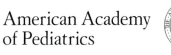

American Academy
of Pediatrics
DEDICATED TO THE HEALTH OF ALL CHILDREN™

The American Academy of Pediatrics is an organization of 60,000 primary care pediatricians, pediatric medical subspecialists, and pediatric surgical specialists dedicated to the health, safety, and well-being of infants, children, adolescents, and young adults.

American Academy of Pediatrics
Web site—www.aap.org

Copyright © 1990
American Academy of Pediatrics, Updated 2/95

Discipline and Your Child

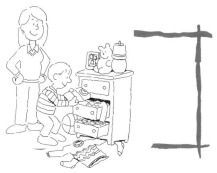

As a parent, it is your job to teach your child the difference between acceptable and unacceptable behavior. But getting your child to behave the way you want is not as hard as you think. This brochure will help you learn effective ways to discipline your child.

Because learning takes time, especially for a young child, you may find that it takes several weeks of working on a behavior before you see a change. Try not to get frustrated when you do not see the results of your efforts right away.

Discipline vs punishment

Many parents think discipline and punishment are the same thing. However, they are really quite different. Discipline is a whole system of teaching based on a good relationship, praise, and instruction for the child on how to control his behavior. Punishment is negative; an unpleasant consequence for doing or not doing something. Punishment should be only a very small part of discipline.

Effective discipline should take place all the time, not just when children misbehave. Children are more likely to change their behavior when they feel encouraged and valued, not shamed and humiliated. When children feel good about themselves and cherish their relationship with their parents, they are more likely to listen and learn.

Encourage good behavior from infancy

You can begin laying the groundwork for good behavior from the time your child is born. When you respond to your infant's cries, you are teaching her that you are there, you can be counted on when she needs you, and that she can trust you. When your child is about 2 months of age, start to modify your responses and encourage your baby to establish good sleeping patterns by letting her fall asleep on her own. By keeping a reasonably steady schedule, you can guide her toward eating, sleeping, and playing at times that are appropriate for your family. This lays the groundwork for acceptable behavior later on.

Once your baby starts to crawl (between 6 and 9 months of age) and as she learns to walk (between 9 and 16 months of age), safety is the most critical discipline issue. The best thing you can do for your child at this age is to give her the freedom to explore certain things and make other things off-limits. For example, put childproof locks on some cabinets, such as those that contain heavy dishes or pots, or poisonous substances like cleaning products. Leave other cabinets open. Fill the open cabinets with plastic containers or soft materials that your child can play with. This feeds your baby's need to explore and practice, but in safe ways that are acceptable to you.

You will need to provide extra supervision during this period. If your child moves toward a dangerous object, such as a hot stove, simply pick her up, firmly say, "no, hot" and offer her a toy to play with instead. She may laugh at first as she tries to understand you but, after a few weeks, she will learn.

Discipline issues become more complex at about 18 months of age. At this time, a child wants to know how much power she has and will test the limit of that power over and over again. It is important for parents to decide— together—what those limits will be and stick to them. Parents need to be very clear about what is acceptable behavior. This will reduce the child's confusion and her need to test. Setting consistent guidelines for children when they are young also will help establish important rules for the future.

If you and your partner disagree, discuss it with each other when you are not with your child. Do not interfere with each other when your child is present. This upsets the child or teaches her to set the adults up against each other which can cause more problems.

Tips to avoid trouble

One of the keys to effective discipline is avoiding power struggles. This can be a challenge with young children. It is best to address only those issues that truly are important to you. The following tips may help:

- **Offer choices whenever possible.** By giving acceptable choices, you can set limits and still allow your child some independence. For example, try saying, "Would you like to wear the red shirt or the blue one?"
- **Make a game out of good behavior.** Your child is more likely to do what you want if you make it fun. For example, you might say, "Let's have a race and see who can put his coat on first."
- **Plan ahead.** If you know that certain circumstances always cause trouble, such as a trip to the store, discuss with your child ahead of time what behavior is acceptable and what the consequences will be if he does not obey. Try to plan the shopping trip for a time when your child is well rested and well fed, and take along a book or small toy to amuse him if he gets bored.
- **Praise good behavior.** Whenever your child remembers to follow the rules, offer encouragement and praise about how well he did. You do not need any elaborate system of rewards. You can simply say, "Thank you for coming right away," and hug your child. Praise for acceptable behavior should be frequent, especially for young children.

Strategies that work

Of course you cannot avoid trouble all of the time. Sooner or later your child will test you. It is your child's way of finding out whether you can be trusted and really will do what you say you will do if she does not listen to you.

When your child does not listen, try the following techniques. Not only will they encourage your child to cooperate now, but they will teach her how to behave in the future as well.

Natural consequences. When a child sees the natural consequences of her actions, she experiences the direct results of her choices. (But be sure the consequences do not place her in any danger.) For example, if your child drops her cookies on purpose, she will not have cookies to eat. If she throws and breaks her toy, she will not be able to play with it. It will not be long before your child learns not to drop her cookies and to play carefully with her toys.

When you use this method, resist the urge to lecture your child or to rescue her (by getting more cookies, for example). Your child will learn best when she learns for herself and will not blame you for the consequences she receives.

Logical consequences. Natural consequences work best, but they are not always appropriate. For example, if your child does not pick up her toys, they may be in the way. But chances are she will not care as much as you do. For older children, you will need to step in and create a consequence that is closely connected to her actions. You might tell her that if she does not pick up her toys, then you will put them away where she will not be allowed to play with them again for a whole day. Children less than 6 years of age need adult help picking up yet can be asked to assist with the task. If your child refuses your request for help, take her by the hand as you silently finish the job. This insistence that your child participate, along with your silence, becomes a clear consequence for your child.

When you use this method, it is important that you mean what you say and that you are prepared to follow through *immediately*. Let your child know that you are serious. You do not have to yell and scream to do this. You can say it in a calm, matter-of-fact way.

Withholding privileges. In the heat of the moment, you will not always be able to think of a logical consequence. That is when you may want to tell your child that, if she does not cooperate, she will have to give something up she likes. The following are a few things to keep in mind when you use this technique:

- Never take away something your child truly needs, such as a meal.
- Choose something that your child values that is related to the misbehavior.
- For children younger than 6 or 7 years of age, withholding privileges works best if done immediately following the problem behavior. For instance, if your young child misbehaves in the morning and you withhold television viewing for that evening, your child probably will not connect the behavior with the consequence.
- Be sure you can follow through on your promise.

Time-out. Time-out should be your last resort and you should use it only when other responses do not work. Time-outs work well when the behavior you are trying to punish is clearly defined and you know when it occurred. Time-outs also can be helpful if you need a break to stay calm. You can use a time-out with a child as young as 1 year old. Follow these steps to make a time-out work:

1. Choose a time-out spot. This should be a boring place with no distractions, such as a chair. Remember the main goal is to separate the child from the activity and people connected with the misbehavior. It should allow the child to pause and cool off. (Keep in mind that bathrooms can be dangerous and bedrooms may become playgrounds.) Decide which 2 or 3 behaviors will be punished with time-out and explain this to your child.
2. When your child does something she knows will result in a time-out, you may warn her once (unless it is aggression). If it happens again, send her to the time-out spot *immediately*. Tell her what she did wrong in as few words as possible. A rule of thumb is 1 minute of time out for every year of your child's age. (For example, a 4-year-old would get a 4-minute time-out.) But even 15 seconds will work. If your child will not go to the spot on her own, pick her up and carry her there. If she will not stay, stand behind her and hold her gently but firmly by the shoulders or restrain her in your lap and say, "I am holding you here because you have to have a time-out." Do not discuss it any further. It should only take a couple of weeks before she learns to cooperate and will choose to sit quietly rather than be held down for time-out.
3. Once your child is capable of sitting quietly, set a timer so that she will know when the time-out is over. If fussing starts again, restart the timer. Wait until your child stops protesting before you set the timer.

4. When the time is up, help your child return to a positive activity. Your child has "served her time." Do not lecture or ask for apologies. If you need to discuss her behavior, wait until later to do so.

Tips to make discipline more effective

You will have days when it seems impossible to get your child to behave. But there are ways to ease frustration and avoid unnecessary conflict with your child.

- **Be aware of your child's abilities and limitations.** Children develop at different rates and have different strengths and weaknesses. When your child misbehaves, it may be that he simply cannot do what you are asking of him or he does not understand what you are asking.
- **Think before you speak.** Once you make a rule or promise, you will need to stick to it. Be sure you are being realistic. Think if it is really necessary before saying "no."
- **Remember that children do what "works."** If your child throws a temper tantrum in the grocery store and you bribe him to stop by giving him candy, he will probably throw another tantrum the next time you go. Make an effort to avoid reinforcing the wrong kinds of behavior, even with just your attention.
- **Work toward consistency.** No one is consistent all of the time. But try to make sure that your goals, rules, and approaches to discipline stay the same from day to day. Children find frequent changes confusing and often resort to testing limits just to find out what the limits are.
- **Pay attention to your child's feelings.** If you can figure out why your child is misbehaving, you are one step closer to solving the problem. It is kinder and helps with cooperation when you let your child know that you understand. For example, "I know you are feeling sad that your friend is leaving, but you still have to pick up your toys." Watch for patterns that tell you misbehavior has a special meaning, such as your child is feeling jealous. Talk to your child about this rather than just giving consequences.
- **Learn to see mistakes—including your own—as opportunities to learn.** If you do not handle a situation well the first time, don't despair. Think about what you could have done differently, and try to do it the next time. If you feel you have made a real mistake in the heat of the moment, wait to cool down, apologize to your child, and explain how you will handle the situation in the future. Be sure to keep your promise. This gives your child a good model of how to recover from mistakes.

Set an example

Telling your child how to behave is an important part of discipline, but *showing* her how to behave is even more significant. Children learn a lot about temper and self-control from watching their parents and other adults interact. If they see adults relating in a positive way toward one another, they will learn that this is how others should be treated. This is how children learn to act respectfully.

Even though your children's behavior and values seem to be on the right track, your children will still challenge you because it is in their nature and is a part of growing up. Children are constantly learning what their limits are, and they need their parents to help them understand those limits. By doing so, parents can help their children feel capable and loved, learn right from wrong, develop good behavior, have a positive approach toward life, and become productive, good citizens.

Why spanking is not the best choice

The American Academy of Pediatrics recommends that if punishment is needed, alternatives to spanking should be used.

Although most Americans were spanked as children, we now know that it has several important side effects.

- It may seem to work at the moment, but it is no more effective in changing behavior than a time-out.
- Spanking increases children's aggression and anger instead of teaching responsibility.
- Parents may intend to stay calm but often do not, and regret their actions later.
- Because most parents do not want to spank, they are less likely to be consistent.
- Spanking makes other consequences less effective, such as those used at child care or school. Gradually, even spanking loses its impact.
- Spanking can lead to physical struggles and even escalate to the point of harming the child.
- Children who continue to be spanked are more likely to be depressed, use alcohol, have more anger, hit their own children, approve of and hit their spouses, and engage in crime and violence as adults.
- These results make sense since spanking teaches the child that causing others pain is justified to control them—even with those they love.

If you are having trouble disciplining your child or need more information on alternatives to spanking, talk to your pediatrician.

The information contained in this publication should not be used as a substitute for the medical care and advice of your pediatrician. There may be variations in treatment that your pediatrician may recommend based on individual facts and circumstances.

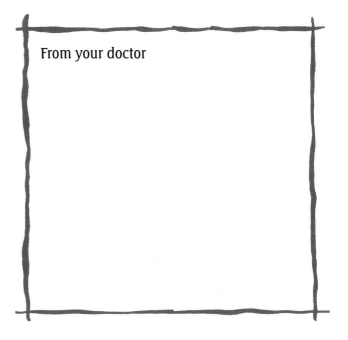

From your doctor

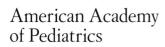

American Academy of Pediatrics

DEDICATED TO THE HEALTH OF ALL CHILDREN™

The American Academy of Pediatrics is an organization of 60,000 primary care pediatricians, pediatric medical subspecialists, and pediatric surgical specialists dedicated to the health, safety, and well-being of infants, children, adolescents, and young adults.

American Academy of Pediatrics
Web site — www.aap.org

Copyright © 1998
American Academy of Pediatrics, Updated 1/02

Divorce and Children

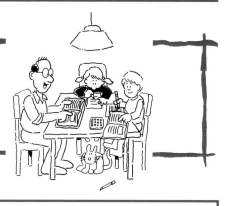

Every year, more than one million children in the United States experience the divorce of their parents. The average divorce takes place within the first 7 years of marriage, so many of these children are under the age of 6. For many children, divorce can be as difficult as the death of a parent. The entire family is faced with the challenge of adjusting to a new way of life. When this happens, children need the guidance, patience, and love of both parents to help them through.

Put your child first

The most important factor in how divorce affects a child's life is how parents treat each other and their children during and after the divorce. Keep in mind, divorce is a major event in your child's life, one that she has no control over. Parents must work together to make the changes as easy as possible for everyone. Even as the marriage ends, your role as a parent continues. In fact, it becomes more important than ever. Set aside your differences with your child's other parent and *put your child first*, by following these suggestions:

- **Never force your child to take sides.** Every child will have loyalties to both parents.
- **Do not involve your child in arguments** between the two of you.
- **Do not criticize each other in front of your child** or when your child might be listening to a conversation you are having with someone else. Even if you find out the other parent is saying bad things about you, explain to your child that when people get angry they sometimes say things that are hurtful.
- **Discuss your concerns and feelings with your child's other parent** when and where your child cannot hear.
- **Avoid fighting in front of your child.**

Making it easier

As a parent, there are many things you can do to help your child adjust to the changes in your family, including the following:

Talk with your child early and often

This is a very important way for you to help your child through difficult times. Being able to share his fears, worries, and feelings with you can make your child feel safe and special. The earlier you tell him what is happening and the more often you talk, the more comfortable he will feel. When talking with your child about the divorce, follow these guidelines:

- **Be completely honest and open** about the circumstances. Talk about the divorce in simple terms. For example, "Your dad and I are having some trouble getting along" or "Your mother and I are thinking we may need to separate."

How children react to divorce

Reactions to a divorce can vary depending on your child's age, sex, temperament, past experiences, and family support. The following are normal ways that your child may react to a separation or divorce. If any of these behaviors become excessive, talk to your pediatrician.

Children under 3 years of age may:
- Be sad
- Be afraid of others
- Not want to be separated from one parent
- Have problems eating or sleeping
- Have trouble with toilet training
- Have outbursts or tantrums
- Blame themselves for the divorce—especially children between 3 and 5 years of age.

School-age children may:
- Be moody or angry
- Have problems eating or sleeping
- Seem distracted and faraway
- Not do as well in school
- Have tantrums
- Be more aggressive or angry
- Express their sadness and wish for parents to get back together
- Worry about divided loyalty to their parents

Adolescents may:
- Withdraw emotionally from family and/or friends
- Become aggressive or angry
- Engage in risky behaviors such as sexual experimentation or use of drugs
- Worry about the financial effects of divorce on the family
- Have problems eating or sleeping
- Feel depressed

- **Make sure your child knows he is not responsible.** Children will often think it is their fault that one parent has left. They may blame themselves or feel alone, unwanted, or unloved. Let your child know the changes are not his fault, that you love him and will not leave him.
- **Try not to blame your ex-spouse** or show your anger. Explain that parents sometimes make adult decisions to live separately.

- **Be patient with questions.** You do not have to have all the answers. Sometimes just carefully listening to your child's concerns is more helpful than talking. Following are questions you might expect from your child:
  - –Why are you getting divorced?
  - –Will you ever get back together again?
  - –Where am I going to live?
  - –Will we move?
  - –Will I have to change schools?
  - –Was the divorce my fault?
  - –How often will I see Daddy/Mommy?
  - –Are we going to be poor?

Give your child the reassurance he needs to feel safe and loved. If needed, don't hesitate to get help from your pediatrician or a family counselor.

A word about....custody

Custody arrangements can be one of the most difficult issues in a divorce. Today, parents are able to work out a wide variety of custody and visitation arrangements. *Physical custody* defines where the child lives and can be split between both parents. Even if physical custody remains with one parent, the other parent can share *legal custody*. Legal custody allows a parent to share in key decisions such as a child's schooling, medical treatment, and religion.

Although mothers are still more likely to maintain custody of the child, more and more fathers are now taking on this role. While there is no evidence that one form of custody is better than another, all children need a stable place where they feel secure.

Even more important than custody is that both parents remain as involved as possible. Ideally, both parents should play a role in the child's life by helping with homework, attending athletic or other after-school events, and contributing emotional and financial support. The parents should work together to arrange a flexible schedule for visits. Neither parent should be prevented from taking part in raising the child. Make sure your child knows that it is OK to love both parents.

If you are having custody disagreements, consider calling a mediator to help settle disagreements. Mediators can be found by contacting a lawyer or family court.

Allow your child to be a child

Resist using your child as a replacement for your ex-spouse. Avoid pressuring children with statements like, "You are the man in the family now" or "Now I have to depend on you." Children have a right to enjoy childhood and grow up at a normal pace. As they grow older, they will be able to take on more responsibility and help around the house. Don't expect too much too soon.

Child support

According to the US Department of Health and Human Services, millions of female-headed households do not receive child support. In some cases, one parent does not want money from the other parent. In others, the parent may not be able or willing to pay or perhaps cannot even be found. Many times, the parent with custody simply does not enforce the child support agreement.

The financial burden of raising a child should not fall on one parent alone. Both parents have a financial obligation to their child. However, even when child support is paid, money issues may still be a problem between parents. Remember, if either parent uses money as a weapon, it is the child who is caught in the cross fire.

Contact your state's child support enforcement agency for guidelines on what parents *must* pay for child support. If your child's other parent will not cooperate, your state or local government may take action to force payment. State agencies can also help if your child's other parent has suddenly moved and you do not know where he or she is living. In most cases, it is often helpful to talk with an attorney.

For more information, contact:
Department of Health and Human Services
Office of Child Support Enforcement
370 L'Enfant Promenade, SW
Washington, DC 20447
202/401-9373

Web site: http://www.acf.dhhs.gov/
programs/cse/index.ht

Respect the relationship between your child and the other parent

Allow your children to spend time with their other parent without making them feel guilty or disloyal to you. When a parent leaves, many children are afraid the other one may leave too. Reassure your children that you both still love them even though they may only be living with one parent at a time. It is important to let your children show their love to both parents. Unless your ex-spouse is unfit to parent, try not to let your differences keep your children away from him or her. Remember, one of the most important ways to help your children cope with a separation or divorce is to help them maintain a strong, loving relationship with both parents.

Keep your child's daily routine simple and predictable

Many divorced parents feel guilty that the divorce has upset their children. They find it hard to discipline the children when they need it. Making rules, setting a good example, and providing emotional support can be difficult. Giving in to your child's demands will not help. Anger or difficult behavior may be part of your child's attempts to cope with the divorce. Set sensible limits. Schedule meals, chores, and bedtime at regular times so that your child knows what to expect each day. Parents living separately should agree on a set of consistent rules for both households. It is also very important to live up to your promises to visit or spend time with your child. A routine weekly or monthly schedule may be comforting to your child.

Use help from the outside

Children often turn to neighbors, grandparents, and peers for comfort and attention. These relationships can offer support and stability to children as well as needed relief to a parent. Teachers or school social workers who are aware of the divorce and understand the child's problems may also be able to give a helping hand.

For parents too, the changes are not easy. Many adults going through a divorce experience depression. If you are suffering from anxiety or depression as a result of a divorce or separation, don't be afraid to see a counselor. It is important for parents to be healthy so they can be available to their children during this difficult time. Social agencies, mental health centers, women's centers, and support groups for divorced or single parents are helpful. There are also many informative books and articles about divorce for both parents and children (see "For More Information"). Your pediatrician is very aware of the effects that separation and divorce may have on emotions and behavior. He or she can help you find ways to cope with the stress you and your children are feeling.

Adjusting to a new life

Children have great strength and the ability to bounce back from rough times. After a divorce, children may even develop much closer relationships with each parent. In time, most children learn to accept the changes brought on by divorce. The challenge becomes much easier though, when both parents provide the understanding, support, and love that all children need from their mothers and fathers, even after they separate.

For more information

There are many excellent books available on coping with divorce for both you and your children. Here are just a few to look for at your local library or bookstore. Please note: Not all of these materials have been reviewed by the American Academy of Pediatrics.

Preschoolers:

The Dinosaurs Divorce: A Guide for Changing Families
    by Laurene Krasny Brown and Marc Brown (Little Brown & Co, 1988)

It's Not Your Fault, Koko Bear
    by Vicki Lansky (Book Peddlers, 1998)

School-age kids:

The Boys and Girls Book About Divorce
    by Richard Gardner (Bantam, 1970)

How It Feels When Parents Divorce
    by Jill Krementz (Knopf, 1988)

Why Are We Getting a Divorce?
    by Peter Mayle (Crown Publishers, 1988)

Parents:

Caring for Your Baby and Young Child:Birth to Age 5
    from the American Academy of Pediatrics (Bantam, 1998)

Caring for Your School-Age Child:Ages 5–12
    from the American Academy of Pediatrics (Bantam, 1995)

Caring for Your Adolescent: Ages 12–21
    from the American Academy of Pediatrics (Bantam, 1991)

Vicki Lansky's Divorce Book for Parents
    by Vicki Lansky (Book Peddlers, 1996)

The American Academy of Pediatrics also offers a brochure called *Single Parenting: What You Need to Know* that you might find helpful. Please ask your pediatrician.

From your doctor

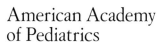

American Academy of Pediatrics

DEDICATED TO THE HEALTH OF ALL CHILDREN™

The American Academy of Pediatrics is an organization of 60,000 primary care pediatricians, pediatric medical subspecialists, and pediatric surgical specialists dedicated to the health, safety, and well-being of infants, children, adolescents, and young adults.
American Academy of Pediatrics
Web site — www.aap.org
Copyright © 1994
American Academy of Pediatrics, Updated 3/99

eating disorders: anorexia and bulimia

Most people enjoy eating.

But for people with an eating disorder, it brings about very different feelings. They become **obsessed** with thoughts of eating and have an intense fear of gaining weight. These thoughts disrupt their daily activities.

The 2 most well-known eating disorders are *anorexia nervosa* and *bulimia nervosa*. **Anorexia** is self-starvation. **Bulimia** is a disorder in which a person eats large amounts of food *(binges)* and then tries to undo the effects of the binge in some way, usually by ridding the body of the food that was eaten. Some people have symptoms of both anorexia and bulimia. (A quick note about people with *binge-eating disorder:* they eat large amounts of food in a short time and feel intense guilt afterward, but unlike people with bulimia, they don't purge themselves.)

What **causes** eating disorders?

There is **no single cause** of eating disorders. But many factors can lead to an eating disorder. Genetics are now felt to play an important role. Although each person's situation is different, people with eating disorders may **share many of the same traits,** such as

- Feeling insecure
- An excessive desire to be in **control**
- A **distorted** body image (feeling fat even when they're not)
- A family **history of depression** or an eating disorder
- Severe **family problems**
- A history of **sexual or physical abuse**
- **Pressure** from activities that place a high value on body size such as running, gymnastics, wrestling, or ballet

What is anorexia?

People with anorexia have a distorted image of their bodies and such an intense fear of becoming fat that they hardly eat and become **dangerously thin.** Many people with anorexia also vomit and overexercise, and they may abuse diet pills to keep from gaining weight. If the condition gets worse, they can die from suicide, heart problems, or starving to death.

People with anorexia focus all of their energy on staying thin. Much of their time is spent thinking about food. For example, people with anorexia may

- **Eat only a small number of "safe" foods,** usually those low in calories and fat.
- Cut up food into tiny pieces.
- Spend more time *playing with food* than eating it.
- Cook food for others but not eat it.

- Exercise compulsively.
- Wear baggy clothes to **hide their bodies,** or complain that normal clothes are too tight.
- Spend more time **alone** and **isolated** from friends and family.
- Become more withdrawn and *secretive.*
- Seem depressed or anxious.
- Have a decrease in activities, motivation, or energy level.
- Do things to keep their minds off their hunger, such as chewing food 30 times before swallowing.

What does anorexia do to the body?

Over time, anorexia can lead to kidney and liver damage, bone damage, and heart problems. When the **body is starved of food,** many physical changes occur like

- The constant feeling of being **cold** because the body has lost the fat and muscle it needs to keep warm. (People with anorexia may **exercise** even more to try to get warm).
- Dizziness, **fainting,** or near-fainting.
- **Bones sticking out** and skin shrinking around the bones. The stomach may look like it's sticking out (often causing anorexics to think they're still fat).
- **Hair loss.**
- *Brittle hair* and *fingernails.*
- Dry and rough skin.
- **Menstrual periods stopping** (or not starting at all if a girl developed anorexia before her first period). This condition is called **amenorrhea.**
- Stomach **pain,** constipation, and bloating.
- Stunted growth that could be permanent.
- **Anemia** (low red blood cells) causing tiredness, weakness, and dizziness.
- **Loss of sexual function** in *boys.*

Who is at risk of developing anorexia?

Most people with anorexia are **girls** in their teens or even younger. But **boys** can be anorexic, too. Teens who develop anorexia usually are good students, even overachievers. They get along well with others, tend to be **perfectionists,** and don't like to admit they need help with anything. They may appear to be in **control.** However, they actually are insecure, self-critical, and have **low self-esteem.** They are very concerned about being liked and focused on pleasing others.

Most people who develop anorexia start by dieting. Dieting becomes more severe and strict over time. They may think that losing weight will make them feel better about themselves. Dieting also might be a response to a major life change like puberty or going away to college. Because people with anorexia have low self-esteem, they have a hard time coping with these changes and feel like they're **losing control.** Over time, dieting is no longer about losing weight, but a way to feel in control.

When should a person get help?

It's important to know the **early signs of anorexia** before it's too late. The earlier an eating disorder is recognized, the better chance there is of recovery. If someone is having physical symptoms caused by weight loss or answers "yes" to any of the following, that person should get help right away.

- "I can't stop dieting, even though I've been told that I've lost too much weight."
- "Even though I've lost a lot of weight, when I look in the mirror, I still think I'm fat."
- "I can't stop exercising."

What is bulimia?

Bulimia is another eating disorder that is harmful to a person's physical and mental health. Bulimia and anorexia share some of the same symptoms.

- As with anorexia, food and staying thin become an obsession, but instead of avoiding food, people with bulimia eat large amounts of food in a short time (binge).
- Guilt and fear then cause them to **get rid of the food** (purge) by vomiting or other means such as overexercising.

People with bulimia have a difficult time controlling their eating behavior. They may be afraid to eat in public or with other people because they are afraid they won't be able to control their urges to **binge and purge.** Their fear may cause them to avoid being around people. They also may

- Become very **secretive** about eating food.
- Spend a lot of time thinking about and planning the next binge, set aside certain times to binge and purge, or avoid social activities to binge and purge.
- **Steal food or hide it** in strange places, like under the bed or in closets.
- Binge on **foods with distinct colors** to know when the food is later thrown up.
- Exercise to "purge" their bodies of food consumed.

People with bulimia often suffer from other problems as well, such as

- Depression and thoughts of suicide
- Substance abuse

What are bingeing and purging?

Bingeing

- During a binge, people with bulimia eat large amounts of food, often in less than a few hours.
- **Eating during a binge is almost mindless.** They eat without paying attention to what the food tastes like or if they are hungry or full.
- Binges usually end when there is no more food to eat, their stomachs hurt from eating, or something such as a phone call breaks their concentration on bingeing.

Purging

- After bingeing, people with bulimia **feel guilty** and are **afraid of gaining weight.** To ease their guilt and fear, they purge the food from their bodies by vomiting or other means.
- They also may turn to extreme exercise or strict dieting.
- This period of "control" lasts until the next binge, and then **the cycle starts again.** Bulimia becomes an attempt to control 2 very strong impulses—the desire to eat and the desire to be thin.

What does bulimia do to the body?

Like anorexia, bulimia damages the body. For example,

- Teeth start to **decay** from contact with stomach acids during vomiting.
- Weight goes up and down.
- Menstrual periods become irregular or stop.
- The face and throat look puffy and swollen.
- Periods of **dizziness** and blackouts occur.
- **Dehydration** caused by loss of body fluids occurs (treatment in a hospital may be needed).
- Constant upset stomach, constipation, and sore throat may be present.
- **Damage** to vital organs such as the liver and kidneys, heart problems, and death can occur.

Who gets bulimia?

Most people with bulimia are girls in their **teens** and **young adult women.** But **boys** can be bulimic, too. People with bulimia often have a hard time controlling impulses, stress, and anxieties. As with anorexia, people with bulimia aren't happy with their bodies and **think they are fat.** This leads to dieting. Then in response to anxiety and other emotions or hunger, they give in to their **impulses and cravings** for food by bingeing. People with bulimia may be underweight, overweight, or of average weight.

How are eating disorders **treated?**

The **earlier** an eating disorder is recognized, the higher the chances are of treatment working. Treatment depends on many things, including the person's willingness to make changes, **family support,** and the stage of the eating disorder.

Successful treatment of eating disorders involves a team approach. The team includes many health care professionals working together, each treating a certain aspect of the disorder. Treatment should begin with a visit to a pediatrician to see how the eating disorder has affected the body. If the effects are severe, the person may need medical treatment or even need to be hospitalized.

In treating anorexia, increasing the person's weight is crucial. If this person refuses to eat, hospitalization may be needed so that adequate nutrition can be ensured. People with bulimia also may need to be hospitalized to treat medical complications, replace needed nutrients in the body, or **stop the cycle** of bingeing and purging.

Counseling is an important part of treatment. Counseling helps people with eating disorders understand how they use food as a way to deal with problems and feelings. It helps them improve their self-images and develop the **confidence** to take control of their lives. Family therapy usually is needed to help **family** members understand the problem, how to be encouraging and supportive, and how to help manage the symptoms. Nutrition counseling with a registered dietitian also is recommended to assist patients and families in returning to healthy eating habits.

Living with an eating disorder is very hard on teens and their families! The wear and tear on the body is tremendous. Without help, a person with an eating disorder can have serious health problems, become very sick, and even die. However, with treatment, **a person can get well and go on to lead a healthy life.**

Where can I find more information?

National Eating Disorders Association
www.nationaleatingdisorders.org
800/931-2237

National Association of Anorexia Nervosa and Associated Disorders
www.anad.org
847/831-3438

American Anorexia/Bulimia Association
www.uvm.edu/~jlbrink/index.html
212/575-6200

From your doctor

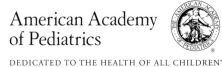

American Academy
of Pediatrics

DEDICATED TO THE HEALTH OF ALL CHILDREN™

The American Academy of Pediatrics is an organization of 60,000 primary care pediatricians, pediatric medical subspecialists, and pediatric surgical specialists dedicated to the health, safety, and well-being of infants, children, adolescents, and young adults.

American Academy of Pediatrics
Web site—www.aap.org

Copyright © 2005
American Academy of Pediatrics

Responding to Children's Emotional Needs During Times of Crisis: Information for Parents

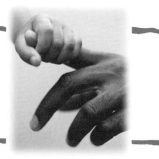

Pediatricians are often the first responders for children and families suffering emotional and psychological reactions to terrorism and other disasters. As such, pediatricians have a unique opportunity to help parents and other caregivers communicate with children in ways that allow them to better understand and recover from traumatic events such as terrorist attacks or other disasters. Pediatricians also can help to facilitate timely referral to mental health services, as appropriate, for these children and their families.

Important tips for parents and other caregivers include:

- Take care of yourself first. Children depend on the adults around them to be and feel safe and secure. If you are very anxious or angry, children are likely to be more affected by your emotional state than by your words. Find someone you trust to help with your personal concerns.
- Watch for unusual behavior that may suggest your child is having difficulty dealing with disturbing events. Stress-related symptoms to be aware of include depressed or irritable moods; sleep disturbances, including increased sleeping, difficulty falling asleep, nightmares or nighttime waking; changes in appetite, either increased or decreased; social withdrawal; obsessive play, such as repetitively acting out the traumatic event, which interferes with normal activities; and hyperactivity that was not previously present.
- Talk about the event with your child. To not talk about it makes the event even more threatening in your child's mind. Silence suggests that what has occurred is too horrible to even speak of.
- Start by asking what your child has already heard about the events and what understanding he or she has reached. As your child explains, listen for misinformation, misconceptions, and underlying fears or concerns.
- Explain—as simply and directly as possible—the events that occurred. The amount of information that will be helpful to a child depends on his or her age. For example, older children generally want and will benefit from more detailed information than younger children. Because every child is different, take cues from your own child as to how much information to provide.
- Limit television viewing of terrorist events or other disasters, especially for younger children. When older children watch television, try to watch with them and use the opportunity to discuss what is being seen and how it makes you and your child feel.
- Encourage your child to ask questions, and answer those questions directly. Like adults, children are better able to cope with a crisis if they feel they understand it. Question-and-answer exchanges help to ensure ongoing support as your child begins to understand the crisis and the response to it.

- Don't force the issue with your child. Instead, extend multiple invitations for discussion and then provide an increased physical and emotional presence as you wait for him or her to be ready to accept those invitations.
- Recognize that your child may appear disinterested. In the aftermath of a crisis, younger children may not know or understand what has happened or its implications. Older children and adolescents, who are used to turning to their peers for advice, may initially resist invitations from parents and other caregivers to discuss events and their personal reactions. Or, they may simply not feel ready to discuss their concerns.
- Reassure children of the steps that are being taken to keep them safe. Terrorist attacks and other disasters remind us that we are never completely safe from harm. Now more than ever it is important to reassure children that, in reality, they should feel safe in their schools, homes, and communities.
- Consider sharing your feelings about the event or crisis with your child. This is an opportunity for you to role model how to cope and how to plan for the future. Before you reach out, however, be sure that you are able to express a positive or hopeful plan.
- Help your child to identify concrete actions he or she can take to help those affected by recent events. Rather than focus on what could have been done to prevent a terrorist attack or other disaster, concentrate on what can be done now to help those affected by the event.
- If you have concerns about your child's behavior, contact your child's pediatrician, other primary care provider, or a qualified mental health care specialist for assistance.

For additional information, please visit the American Academy of Pediatrics' Children, Terrorism & Disasters Web site at www.aap.org/terrorism.

The recommendations in this publication do not indicate an exclusive course of treatment or serve as a standard of medical care. Variations, taking into account individual circumstances, may be appropriate.

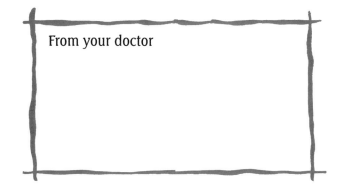

From your doctor

American Academy of Pediatrics

DEDICATED TO THE HEALTH OF ALL CHILDREN™

The American Academy of Pediatrics is an organization of 60,000 primary care pediatricians, pediatric medical subspecialists, and pediatric surgical specialists dedicated to the health, safety, and well-being of infants, children, adolescents, and young adults.

American Academy of Pediatrics
Web site — www.aap.org

Copyright © 2000
American Academy of Pediatrics

Gambling: NOT A SAFE THRILL

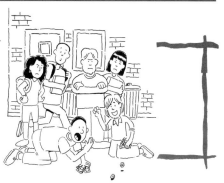

Gambling has become a form of entertainment for many Americans. However, for young people, gambling may become a serious addiction. The chances of a young gambler getting "hooked" are far greater than those of an adult.

Consider the following numbers:

- There are nearly 8 million compulsive gamblers in the United States today. More than 1 million of them are teens.
- Two thirds of all students from ages 12 to 18 gamble regularly.
- About 90% of high school seniors have gambled at least once.

Gambling should not be seen as a "safe thrill." Parents need to be aware of the danger gambling poses to young people and the warning signs of problem gambling. Compulsive gambling, considered by some experts to be the "addiction of the 90s," has entered the new millennium.

What is compulsive gambling?

When gambling moves beyond fun and games and starts becoming the focus of a person's life, it is considered compulsive gambling. There are three phases of compulsive gambling.

The Winning Phase

- Gambling is fun and exciting.
- Winning makes the gambler feel like a "big shot."
- Losses are thought of as "bad luck."
- All the gambler thinks about is gambling.
- The gambler thinks gambling is the most exciting thing in life.
- Free time, lunch breaks, or recess are often spent gambling.

The Losing Phase

- The gambler starts to lose, often borrowing money to cover losses.
- Self-esteem decreases.
- The gambler may lie to friends and family about gambling.
- The gambler may begin to sell possessions to cover bets.
- The gambler begins to miss school, work, or other important events to gamble.

The Desperation Phase

- The gambler becomes obsessed with gambling.
- Severe mood swings, lying, cheating, and stealing may occur.
- School failure is common.
- Nothing or nobody comes before a bet.
- Suicide may be attempted as a way out.

Who is the typical teen gambler?

Today, many communities rely on gambling casinos as a major source of income. Teens in these communities may be at greater risk for developing problems with gambling than other teens. However, teen gambling can be found anywhere — in cities and small towns, among the wealthy and the poor.

It is not easy to "spot" teen gamblers. They look no different than their friends. They often are very outgoing and social. In addition, teen gamblers tend to be

- Highly motivated, energetic
- Smart
- Competitive, risk takers
- Good students, hard working
- Perfectionists
- Confident

Teens who develop problems with gambling may have other issues, such as difficulties with their family or friends, problems with other addictions like alcohol or drugs, or engaging in other high-risk behaviors.

How do teens gamble?

Any game of chance or skill that is played for money is gambling. Most forms of gambling are illegal for anyone under the age of 18. However, teens find their own ways to gamble, including the following:

- Playing cards or dice games for money
- Playing games of skill for money (pool, basketball)
- Buying lottery tickets and scratch cards
- Playing casino- and arcade-type games (like pull tabs and slot machines)
- Placing bets on sports events
- Gambling on the Internet

Why do teens gamble?

Gambling is promoted as fun and exciting; an easy way to "strike it rich." Many young people hope that if they can win big money, all their problems will be solved. As legalized gambling spreads to almost every community, it is easy for young people to get caught up in the promises of wealth and power. Adults do, too. In the United States, 80% of adults participate in some form of gambling. Teens who gamble may be copying their parents' behavior.

How can I tell if my son or daughter is having a problem with gambling?

Look for the following warning signs:

- Finding gambling "stuff" like lottery tickets, betting sheets, casino chips
- Excessive TV sports watching and an overly intensive interest in the outcome of sports events
- Visits to a casino, despite being underage
- Excessive "checking in" or spending time on the Internet
- Unexplained debts
- Flaunting large amounts of money or buying expensive items
- Absences from school or work
- Anxiety and nervousness
- Stealing for gambling money

What parents can do

You are the best role model for your children. Take a close look at your own attitudes and habits. Do you spend your last dollar on lottery tickets? Do you make frequent visits to the casino with hopes of striking it rich? While gambling may be okay for you, you may be sending a message to your teen that gambling is a safe and healthy activity.

Talk to your children about gambling. Remind them that gambling is illegal for teens. Be clear about how you feel about gambling, and let them know what you expect of them. Help your children develop ways to resist gambling and develop interests in other activities. Avoid using recreational activities offered at casinos for child care while parents gamble.

Identifying a gambling problem early is the key to successful treatment. If you feel your teen may have a problem, there are people in your community who can help, including the following:

- Pediatricians
- Counselors
- Teachers
- Elders or Clergy

Compulsive gambling is like other addictions. Outside help may be the only way a person can stop. Talk to your pediatrician for information about treatment options, like individual counseling or family therapy, that can give compulsive gamblers the strength they need to quit.

Resources

For more information on treatment options, support groups, or other educational materials, contact

North American Training Institute
314 W Superior St, Suite 702
Duluth, MN 55802
218/722-1503
www.nati.org
www.wannabet.org (a Web site for kids on gambling)

Gambler's Anonymous
International Service Office
PO Box 17173
Los Angeles, CA 90017
213/386-8789
www.gamblersanonymous.org

The National Council on Problem Gambling, Inc
Nationwide Helpline
800/522-4700
208 G Street
NE 2nd Floor
Washington, DC 20002
http://www.ncpgambling.org/

Please note: Inclusion on this list does not imply an endorsement by the American Academy of Pediatrics. The Academy is not responsible for the content of the resources mentioned above. Addresses, phone numbers, and Web site addresses are as current as possible, but may change at any time.

The information contained in this publication should not be used as a substitute for the medical care and advice of your pediatrician. There may be variations in treatment that your pediatrician may recommend based on individual facts and circumstances.

A few questions for teens

Give this brochure to your son or daughter. Ask your child to think about the questions below. Talk about your answers together. Can your teen answer "yes" to many of these questions? If so, it may be time to look for help.

1. Do you think gambling is the most exciting activity you do?
2. Do you often spend your free time involved in gambling activities?
3. Do you try to prevent your family and friends from knowing how much you gamble?
4. Do your friends gamble? Are you considered to be part of the "gambling crowd"?
5. Do you often daydream about gambling?
6. Do you often gamble during lunch breaks, recess, after school hours, or on weekends?
7. Do you miss school or other important events due to gambling activities?
8. Do you ever lie about whether you gamble or how much you lose?
9. Is gambling the main source of what you do to feel good about yourself?
10. Do you gamble alone?
11. Do you gamble with money that is supposed to be used for other reasons (such as lunch money, bus fare, or clothes)?
12. Have you ever borrowed money to gamble?
13. Have you ever stolen money or property in order to gamble or pay gambling debts?
14. Do you get upset or irritable if you are unable to gamble?
15. Do you most want to gamble when you are upset?
16. Do you often feel sad or guilty because you lost money gambling?
17. Is it hard for you to stop gambling after you lose money?
18. Do you often gamble longer than you wanted to and lose more money than you intended?
19. When gambling, do you tend to lose track of time or forget about everything else?
20. Do you find that thinking about gambling makes it hard for you to do schoolwork?

Excerpted with permission from the North American Training Institute's book, Wanna Bet?™ Everything You Ever Wanted to Know About Teen Gambling but Never Thought to Ask © 1995, 1997. Web site: www.wannabet.org or www.nati.org

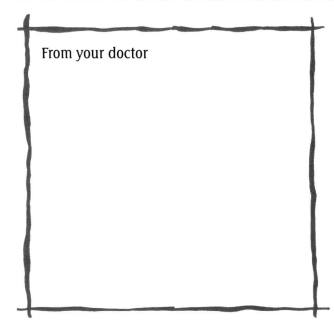

From your doctor

American Academy of Pediatrics

DEDICATED TO THE HEALTH OF ALL CHILDREN™

The American Academy of Pediatrics is an organization of 60,000 primary care pediatricians, pediatric medical subspecialists, and pediatric surgical specialists dedicated to the health, safety, and well-being of infants, children, adolescents, and young adults.

American Academy of Pediatrics
Web site—www.aap.org

Copyright © 1999
American Academy of Pediatrics, Updated 8/01

© 2007 American Academy of Pediatrics

Media History

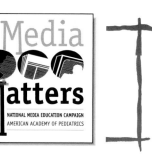

Please check one answer for each question. If the question does not apply to your family (ie, you do not own a VCR, video game player, or computer), leave that section blank.

Child's Name _____

Date _____

Television

Does your child watch more than 1 to 2 hours of TV per day? ☐ Frequently ☐ Sometimes ☐ Never

Do you watch TV with your child or know what your child is watching? ☐ Frequently ☐ Sometimes ☐ Never

Do you discuss TV shows with your child? ☐ Frequently ☐ Sometimes ☐ Never

Does your child have a TV in his or her room? ☐ Yes ☐ No

Do you limit your child's watching of TV shows that often contain violence, sex, foul or explicit language, or images of tobacco or alcohol use? ☐ Frequently ☐ Sometimes ☐ Never

Do you have rules about when TV can be watched? ☐ Yes ☐ No

Do you allow your child to eat meals or snacks while watching TV? ☐ Yes ☐ No

Does your child ask you to buy products he or she sees advertised on TV? ☐ Frequently ☐ Sometimes ☐ Never

Movies and Videos

Do you allow your child to watch movies or videos that are R-rated? ☐ Frequently ☐ Sometimes ☐ Never

Do you read movie reviews to know the content of PG-13 movies? ☐ Frequently ☐ Sometimes ☐ Never

Does your child have nightmares or trouble sleeping after watching movies? ☐ Frequently ☐ Sometimes ☐ Never

How often does your child watch music videos on TV? ☐ Frequently ☐ Sometimes ☐ Never

Radio, CDs, Cassette Tapes

Are you familiar with the type of music your child listens to? ☐ Yes ☐ No

Have you talked to your child about lyrics that you object to? ☐ Yes ☐ No

Do you set limits on the types of music your child listens to? ☐ Yes ☐ No

Video and Computer Games

Are you familiar with the types of games your child plays? ☐ Yes ☐ No

Do you check a game's rating before you rent or buy it? ☐ Yes ☐ No

Do you allow your child to own or rent games with violent content? ☐ Frequently ☐ Sometimes ☐ Never

Do you limit the number of hours your child plays these games? ☐ Frequently ☐ Sometimes ☐ Never

Internet and Computer On-line Services

Do you monitor Internet and on-line computer use? ☐ Frequently ☐ Sometimes ☐ Never

Does your child have a computer in his or her room? ☐ Yes ☐ No

Are you familiar with the types of chat rooms and Web sites your child visits? ☐ Yes ☐ No

Do you talk to your child about the best use of the Internet? ☐ Frequently ☐ Sometimes ☐ Never

Have you purchased blocking software that prevents your child from visiting inappropriate/pornographic Web sites? ☐ Yes ☐ No

Books

Do you read to your child or does your child read at least once a day? ☐ Yes ☐ No

Do you provide your child with a variety of reading materials? ☐ Yes ☐ No

Do you talk to your child about the books that you read together or that your child is reading on his or her own? ☐ Frequently ☐ Sometimes ☐ Never

Behavioral and Psychosocial Issues

Do you have any specific concerns about:

Your child's use of tobacco, alcohol, or illicit drugs? ☐ Yes ☐ No

Your child's own sense of body image or sexuality? ☐ Yes ☐ No

Displays of aggressive behavior or use of foul language? ☐ Yes ☐ No

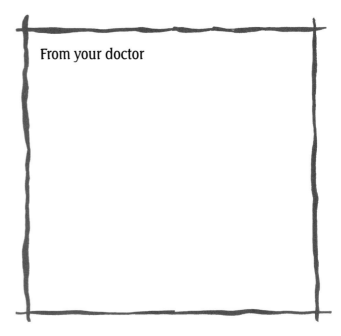

From your doctor

American Academy of Pediatrics
DEDICATED TO THE HEALTH OF ALL CHILDREN™

The American Academy of Pediatrics is an organization of 60,000 primary care pediatricians, pediatric medical subspecialists, and pediatric surgical specialists dedicated to the health, safety, and well-being of infants, children, adolescents, and young adults.

American Academy of Pediatrics
Web site—www.aap.org

Copyright © 2000
American Academy of Pediatrics

© 2007 American Academy of Pediatrics

Medicine and the Media:
How to Make Sense of the Messages

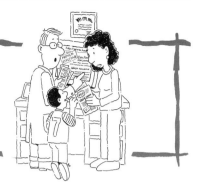

Your child is sick or hurt and the first thought on your mind is, "How can I make my child better?" That's natural. No parent wants his or her child to suffer. So how do you decide what medicines to give or treatments to try?

Aside from your pediatrician, what sources can you trust? Commercials and magazine ads claim products help and heal. Web sites claim to have "cutting-edge" health information. TV programs and newspapers report on the "latest" studies showing which treatments work and don't work.

One challenge of parenting is sorting through all available information about children's health. Some sources can be trusted, while others should be questioned. Read more to learn about the language of advertisers, good science, questioning your sources, using the Internet, Web site addresses, and evaluating new treatments or medicines.

The language of advertisers

Advertisers try many ways to get you to buy the products they are selling. They may use certain words or phrases to interest you, such as

- **"#1 Pediatrician Recommended" or "Doctor Recommended"**
  These are marketing terms that try to get you to buy a product. Although the product may be recommended by a group of doctors, what the advertisers don't tell you is how many doctors or how long ago the recommendation was made. It could be 5 or 100 doctors surveyed 10 years ago.
- **"Patented Design"**
  A patent means that the maker or inventor of a product has proven to the government that he or she was the first to create the product. In return, the government gives a patent and says that only the patent holder can make or sell the product for a certain period. A patent doesn't necessarily mean that the product is the best, is safe, or will work.
- **"Clinically Shown"**
  This phrase means that the product was tested on patients as part of a study to see if the product worked. There are many ways to conduct studies. However, if the people doing the study don't follow strict scientific rules for doing research, the study results may have little meaning.

Good science

Scientific studies require careful planning. Researchers need to follow specific procedures and processes. Studies must follow certain rules to be considered scientifically credible, including the following:

- The testing must take place in carefully **controlled conditions.** Researchers have to make sure to control factors that could affect the results. For example, if researchers want to know how a medicine affects a child, they have to make sure the child isn't taking any other medicines at the same time.

- Researchers need to determine how many people should be included in the study. **Study size** varies according to the kind of study and number of people needed to demonstrate an effect.
- The group of people receiving treatment should be compared to a **control group** to truly test if the treatment has any effect. A control group doesn't receive the new treatment, but instead may be given a placebo (sugar pill) or an alternative treatment.
- Good clinical studies should be **replicated.** That means other researchers should be able to do the same study again using different subjects and get similar results. We know we can trust the findings when different studies come to the same conclusions.
- Well-done, scientifically sound studies should go through **peer review.** This means other experts on the topic being studied should review each study and make sure that all proper scientific standards were met.

Questioning your sources

It's important to ask the following questions when evaluating a source:
1. **What is the source?**
   In general, sources you can trust include accredited medical schools, government agencies, professional medical associations, and recognized national disorder/disease-specific organizations. However, don't rely mainly on the name of the organization—do your own research.
2. **Who is the expert?**
   The doctors or researchers being interviewed may sound like experts, but what are their credentials? What expertise and experience do they have? They may be doctors, but are they experts on the particular issue being talked about? Are there conflicts of interest? Are they working for a company that may benefit from their "expert" support? Are they being paid for their support of a product? If so, this could influence what information these experts choose to share.
3. **What are the facts?**
   Know the difference between preliminary and confirmed findings—a "breakthrough" finding may seem promising but still has to be replicated and reviewed over time. Don't let a headline make you think that "new study" is the same as "proven." Another word of caution: "new" doesn't mean improved. Sometimes newer medicines are not an improvement over older medicines and cost much more.

Using the Internet

The Internet can be a valuable source of medical information and advice, but you can't trust everything you read. The Internet also is the source of a lot of health-related theories and opinions that haven't been proven.

Begin your search for information with the most reliable, general-information Web sites and expand from there. The Web site for the American Academy of Pediatrics (AAP), www.aap.org, is a good starting point.

Web site addresses

The last 3 letters in a Web site address can tell you what type of organization or company set up the site.

- **.gov**—Government Web sites often provide large amounts of information for the general public.
- **.org**—Nonprofit organization Web sites may contain useful information. However, not all organizations put out reliable materials. Search for information on nonprofit Web sites that you have heard of and have good reputations.
- **.edu**—Academic or education-based Web sites may have educational materials for parents.
- **.com**—Commercial Web sites often are designed to sell you something. They are not necessarily a source of reliable information.

Evaluating new treatments or medicines

When you come across a new treatment or medicine, ask yourself the following questions:

1. **Will it work for my child?**

   Be suspicious if the information describing the treatment or medicine
   - Claims it will work for everyone.
   - Uses a story about one person's experience or testimonials as proof that it works.
   - Cites only one study as proof.
   - Cites a study without a control (comparison) group.

2. **How safe is it?**

   Be suspicious if the treatment or medicine
   - Comes without directions for proper use.
   - Doesn't list contents or ingredients.
   - Has no information or warnings about side effects.
   - Is described as "harmless" or "natural." Remember, most medication is made from natural sources. A "natural" treatment doesn't necessarily work and, worse yet, actually may be harmful to your child. Being "natural" does not necessarily mean it is good or safe.
   - Isn't approved by the Food and Drug Administration (FDA).
   - Appears on an infomercial.

3. **How is it promoted?**

   Be suspicious if the ad for the treatment or medicine
   - Claims it's based on a secret formula.
   - Claims it works immediately and permanently.
   - Claims it's a "miraculous" or an "amazing" breakthrough.
   - Claims it is a "cure."
   - Indicates it's available from only one source.

Remember

You shouldn't trust everything that you read or hear. Make sure that your pediatrician knows about your questions and concerns; share the information you've found. You and your pediatrician are partners in your child's health.

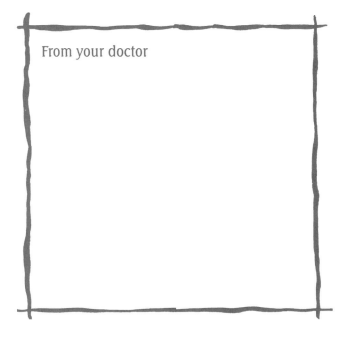

From your doctor

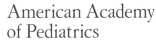

American Academy of Pediatrics

DEDICATED TO THE HEALTH OF ALL CHILDREN™

The American Academy of Pediatrics is an organization of 60,000 primary care pediatricians, pediatric medical subspecialists, and pediatric surgical specialists dedicated to the health, safety, and well-being of infants, children, adolescents, and young adults.

American Academy of Pediatrics
Web site—www.aap.org

Copyright © 2004
American Academy of Pediatrics

The Ratings Game:
CHOOSING YOUR CHILD'S ENTERTAINMENT

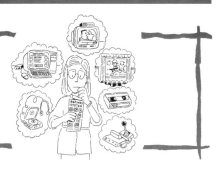

Even before reaching middle school age, your child will spend tens of thousands of hours watching television, movies, and videos; listening to the radio, CDs, and cassettes; playing video and computer games; and surfing the Internet. But TV, movies, music, games, and the Internet are much more than entertainment. They are a source of information, and they help teach our children about the world in which we live. As children have more and more entertainment options to choose from, it becomes even more important for parents to become involved in making choices.

To help parents make informed choices, many entertainment companies are now using *ratings systems.* Movies have used ratings for years, but ratings are now being given to TV programs, video and computer games, and music. Ratings are designed to give parents more information about the content of the program, movie, music, or game. The ratings are usually based on the amount of violence, sex, nudity, strong language, or drug use your child will see or hear.

Why do we need ratings?

Ratings have become more common because research has shown how much children are influenced by what they see and hear, especially at very young ages. The effects don't seem to go away as the child gets older. One study of 8-year-old boys found that those who watched violent TV programs growing up were most likely to be involved in aggressive, violent behavior by age 18 and serious criminal behavior by age 30.

Young children who see violent acts in movies, shows, and games may not be able to tell the difference between "make-believe" and real life. They may not understand that *real* violence hurts and kills people. When the "good guys" or heroes use violence, children may learn that it is okay to use force to solve problems. Younger children may even become more afraid of the world around them.

Most entertainment companies are now providing ratings for their products. However, it is up to you to protect your child from the effects of exposure to violence, as well as sex, drug use, and even strong language. Look for ratings and warning labels. Use them to make smart decisions about what your child sees and hears. Ratings can be useful tools, but watch and listen *with* your child to discuss the content and meaning of the shows they watch, music they hear, or games they play.

Movies

When you think of ratings systems, the one used by the Motion Picture Association of America (MPAA) probably comes to mind. Though movie producers are not required to use the rating system, most movies that make it to the big screen have one of the following MPAA ratings:

G GENERAL AUDIENCES All Ages Admitted — Contains very little violence; no nudity, sex, or drug use. May contain some tobacco or alcohol use.

PG PARENTAL GUIDANCE SUGGESTED SOME MATERIAL MAY NOT BE SUITABLE FOR CHILDREN — May contain adult themes, alcohol and tobacco use, some profanity, violence, or brief nudity.

PG-13 PARENTS STRONGLY CAUTIONED Some Material May Be Inappropriate for Children Under 13 — Contains more intense themes, violence, nudity, sex, or language than a PG film, but not as much as an R. May contain drug use scenes.

R RESTRICTED UNDER 17 REQUIRES ACCOMPANYING PARENT OR ADULT GUARDIAN — Contains adult material. May include graphic language, violence, sex, nudity, and drug use.

NC-17 NO ONE 17 AND UNDER ADMITTED — Children should not be admitted. Contains violence, sex, drug abuse, and other behavior that most parents would consider off-limits to children.

This is the oldest, most well-known, and widely used rating system for any form of media, but it is not perfect. For example, the ratings divide children into three age groups (under 13, 13 to 17, and over 17). However, a PG movie that contains some violence or nudity will have a much different effect on a 5-year-old child than it would a 12-year-old. Find out as much as you can about a movie before letting your child watch. Read reviews, check the Internet, talk to friends who have seen it. Choose carefully when considering movies with PG-13, PG, and sometimes even G ratings. If you aren't sure, see the movie first, and decide if it is appropriate for your child.

Videos

Along with cable television, the use of VCRs and video-taped movies in the home has made it much more difficult to control your child's viewing. Children have easier access to R-rated movies than ever before. Most video stores have no way to prevent a child from renting or buying inappropriate material. Younger children are also more likely to watch the same movies many times. Just as a young child will sit and watch her favorite television show every day, she is just as likely to watch the same videotape over and over.

Movies from the video store are rated with the same system used for movies in the theater. Read the package and pay attention to the rating. Decide what movies are appropriate for your child depending on her age and maturity. Set rules and apply them at home, as well as at the theater. Talk to the manager of your local video store about setting stricter rules for renting videos rated anything more than G. For suggestions of quality children's videos, contact the Coalition for Quality Children's Media at 505/989-8076 or on the Web at http://www.cqcm.org.

Keep in mind, *children under 17 years of age should not be allowed to view R-rated movies.* The rating states that children under 17 should not view these films without a parent or guardian; however, these films often contain graphic violence, drug use, sex, nudity, and inappropriate language. Even though the rating system seems to suggest a younger child may watch an R-rated movie when a parent is present, it is *not* recommended they watch at all. *No child 17 years of age or under should be allowed to watch a movie rated NC-17.*

Television

The television industry has adopted a set of ratings called the TV Parental Guidelines to help parents select programs for their children. Channels that have agreed to use the ratings show them for 15 seconds at the start of a program. They may also be found in your local TV listings. The ratings apply to all TV programs, *except news and sports.* (Keep in mind that news programs often contain violence that may be inappropriate for viewing by young children.) Instead of flipping through channels, use the following ratings to help you and your child choose TV shows:

 The program is suitable for all children. Whether animated or live-action, it is designed for a young audience, including ages 2 to 6. The program is not expected to frighten younger children.

 The program is suitable for children aged 7 and older who can tell the difference between make-believe and reality. The program may contain mild fantasy or comedic violence that could frighten children under 7.

 The program is suitable for children aged 7 and older who can tell the difference between make-believe and reality. The program contains fantasy violence more intense or combative than TV-Y7. Violence is the central theme of the program and the fighting is presented in an exciting way. Violent acts are glorified, and violence is used as an acceptable, effective way to solve a problem. Programs can be cartoons, live-action, or a combination of both.

 General Audience. Most parents would find this program suitable for all ages. There is little or no violence, no strong language, and little or no sexual content.

  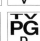 **Parental guidance is suggested.** The program contains material that parents may find unsuitable for younger children. It may have an inappropriate theme, and it may contain moderate violence (V), some sexual content (S), and strong language (L) or suggestive dialogue between characters (D).

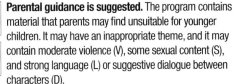 **Parents are strongly cautioned.** The program contains some material that many parents would find unsuitable for children under 14. It contains intense violence (V), sexual content (S), and strong language (L) or intensely suggestive dialogue (D).

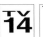 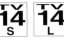 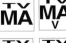 **Mature Audience.** The program may be unsuitable for children under age 17. It contains graphic violence (V), strong sexual content (S), and/or crude, indecent language (L).

Starting in 2000, all new television sets with screens **13 inches or larger** will have a computer device called the *v-chip*. The v-chip allows parents to block programs from their televisions. TVs with screens smaller than 13 inches will not have the v-chip. If your child is allowed to watch TV alone, choose a set that is at least 13 inches so you can use the v-chip to block programs.

TV for toddlers

The first two years of your child's life are especially important in the growth and development of your child's brain. During this time, children need good, positive interaction with other children and adults. Too much television can negatively affect early brain development. This is especially true at younger ages, when learning to talk and play with others is so important.

Until more research is done about the effects of TV on very young children, the American Academy of Pediatrics does not recommend television for children aged 2 or younger. For older children, the Academy recommends no more than 1 to 2 hours per day of educational, nonviolent programs.

Computer games

The Entertainment Software Rating Board (ESRB) assigns ratings* to games for personal computers and home video systems. The ratings are as follows:

 Early Childhood. Suitable for ages 3 and older. Does not contain inappropriate material.

 Everyone. Suitable for ages 6 and older. May contain minimal violence, some comic mischief (such as slapstick comedy), or some crude language. (E is a new rating. Older games may still carry the rating K-A, Kids to Adults, which is also suitable for ages 6 and older.)

 Teen. Suitable for ages 13 and older. May contain violence, mild or strong language, or suggestive themes.

 Mature. Suitable for ages 17 and older. May contain more intense violence, language, or sexual themes.

 Adults Only. Suitable only for adults. May contain graphic sex or violence. Not intended to be rented or sold to anyone under the age of 18.

 Rating Pending. Game has not yet been rated.

On the back of the game package, the ESRB also includes a brief description of the content to give parents more information about the game. For example, an EC rating might come with the description "Edutainment," which means educational entertainment. Other content descriptors include the following:

- Informational
- Suggestive themes
- Comic mischief
- Mature sexual themes
- Mild violence
- Strong sexual content
- Violence
- Mild language
- Realistic violence
- Strong language
- Nudity
- Hate speech
- Use of tobacco and alcohol
- Strong hate speech

* Please be advised that the ESRB rating icons, "EC," "K–A," "E," "T," "M," "AO," "RP" are copyrighted works and certifiication marks owned by the Interactive Digital Software Association and the Entertainment Software Rating Board and may only be used with their permission and authority. Under no circumstances may the rating icons be self-applied to any product that has not been rated by the ESRB. For information regarding whether a product has been rated by the ESRB, please call the ESRB at (212) 759-0700 or 1-800-771-3772.

A word about…the Internet

The rapid growth of the Internet has placed knowledge and information at your child's fingertips. However, not all information on the Internet is appropriate for children. Anyone can set up a Web site and post information on any topic. You might be surprised how easy it is for your child to locate information that contains graphic sex, violence, or drug use.

Internet companies are still in the process of creating a universal ratings system for material posted on the Net. Until a system is created, there are many options available to parents. The Recreational Software Advisory Council on the Internet (RSAC*i*) offers a system to Web site developers on a voluntary basis. Most Internet browsers are already set up to use RSAC*i*. For more information, visit the Web site at http://www.rsac.org. The Entertainment Software Rating Board offers a rating system as well. Visit http://www.esrb.org to find out more.

There also are many services and software products available that allow parents to block or filter inappropriate Web sites and material. Ask your Internet service provider about site blocking, restrictions on e-mail, and other controls for parents.

It is very important that your child have your help and supervision when using the Internet. Even if your child is an experienced computer user, he needs your involvement and your supervision.

Computer game companies rate their games voluntarily, but most now use the ESRB system. Some games may also carry a rating by the Recreational Software Advisory Council (RSAC). Their system assigns a score based on a scale of 0 to 4 in the categories of Violence, Sex, Nudity, and Language. The rating score appears on the front of the game package.

Coin-operated video games

All new coin-operated video games are labeled with a Parental Advisory Disclosure Message that appears in the artwork of the game or on a color sticker on the machine. The labels come in the following colors:

Green — Suitable for all ages
Yellow — Mild
Red — Strong

Yellow and red stickers indicate content in one of the following four categories:

- Animated violence
- Life Like violence
- Sexual content
- Language

For example, a yellow sticker with the description "Sexual Content Mild" means the game contains sexually suggestive references or material. A red sticker that reads "Life Like Violence Strong" means the game contains scenes involving human-like characters in combat situations that may result in pain, injury, or death to one or many characters.

Music

The Recording Industry Association of America has a Parental Advisory Program that is also voluntary. Each record company uses its own guidelines to determine which recordings will be labeled with a parental advisory.

If a record company decides to use the advisory, it is required to use a standard black and white logo reading

 The logo is smaller than 1-inch square and should be located on the front of the CD, cassette, album, or videocassette.

If you have any doubt about the content of lyrics in the music your child chooses, listen to the music before allowing your child to buy it. Many music stores will allow you to listen to CDs before buying. Check out the Internet too. Most record companies and recording artists have their own Web sites where you may be able to read song lyrics or even hear samples of recent recordings.

Protect your child

Your child will be exposed to all forms of entertainment and media at a very young age. By helping your child develop the skills to question what they see and hear in the media, you can protect your child from the many negative messages in movies, television, music, and games. Follow these guidelines:

1. **Use the ratings.** Help children and teens choose movies, shows, videos, music, Web sites, and computer and video games that are appropriate for their ages and interests. Get into the habit of checking the content ratings and parental advisories for all media. Use the ratings as a guide, but watching and listening yourself are the best ways to decide which movies, shows, games, or CDs are suitable for your child. *Keep in mind that companies do not have to use ratings. Beware of products that have no ratings, and find out more about them before letting your child watch, play, or listen.*

2. **Set time limits.** Limit your child's total screen time to no more than 1 or 2 hours per day. This includes TV, movies, video and computer games, and surfing the Internet. Consider using a timer to enforce the rule.

3. **Watch *with* your child.** Whenever possible, participate in your child's TV, video game, music, or computer time, and discuss what she sees and hears. When you share your child's experiences, you can talk to her about the messages she is receiving. Discuss how the messages compare with the values you are teaching your child.

4. **Keep TV sets, VCRs, video games, and computers out of your child's bedroom.** Instead, put them where you can be involved and monitor the activity. Do not let your child watch TV while doing homework or eating meals.

5. **Know how much is too much.** It is easy to overlook the messages children are getting from media. There are signs that TV, movies, or games may be having too much of an impact on your child's behavior. If your child has a problem with any of the following behaviors, talk to your pediatrician, and take a look at how much TV, movies, or computer games may be affecting him:
   - Poor school performance
   - Hitting or pushing other kids often
   - Aggressively talking back to adults
   - Frequent nightmares
   - Increased eating of unhealthy foods
   - Smoking, drinking, or other drug use

6. **Voice your opinion.** Let the people who produce children's entertainment know how you feel about their products. Networks, sponsors, and game companies pay attention to letters and calls from the public. If you think a product or program is offensive, let them know about it. Encourage publishers of television guides to print ratings.

7. **Give your child other options.** Watching TV or playing video games can become a habit for your child. Help your child find other things to do with his time, such as the following:
   - Playing
   - Reading
   - Physical activity and sports
   - Learning a hobby, sport, instrument, or an art
   - Other activities with family, friends, or neighbors

8. **Set a good example.** You are the most important role model in your child's life. Limiting your own TV and movie viewing and choosing programs carefully will help your child do the same.

9. **Get more information.** The following people and places can provide you with more information:
   - **Your pediatrician.** Ask about the following brochures from the American Academy of Pediatrics (AAP):
     Television and the Family
     The Internet and Your Family
     Understanding the Impact of Media on Children and Teens
   - **Your local Parent/Teacher Association (PTA)**
   - **Public service groups** publish newsletters that review programs and games and give tips on how to make entertainment a positive experience for you and your child. Check with your pediatrician or the AAP Web site.
   - **Parents of your child's friends and classmates** can also be helpful. Talk with other parents and agree to enforce similar rules about entertainment.

   For more information on the AAP Media Matters campaign, visit the AAP Web site at http://www.aap.org. Or, contact any of the following organizations:

Coin-Operated Video Games
American Amusement Machine Association (AAMA)
450 E Higgins Rd, Suite 201
Elk Grove Village, IL 60007
847/290-9088
Web site: http://www.coin-op.org

Amusement and Music Operators Association (AMOA)
450 E Higgins Rd, Suite 202
Elk Grove Village, IL 60007
847/290-5320
Web site: http://www.amoa.com

International Association of Family Amusement Centers (IAFAC)
36 Symonds Rd
Hillsboro, NH 03244
603/464-6498

Computer games
Entertainment Software Rating Board (ESRB)
845 Third Ave
New York, NY 10022
212/759-0700
Web site: http://www.esrb.org

Internet
Recreational Software Advisory Council (RSAC)
3460 Olney-Laytonsville Rd, Suite 202
Olney, MD 20832
301/260-8669
Web site: http://www.rsac.org

Movies
Motion Picture Association of America (MPAA)
15503 Ventura Blvd
Encino, CA 91436
818/995-6600
Web site: http://www.mpaa.org

Music
Recording Industry Association of America (RIAA)
1330 Connecticut Ave NW, Suite 300
Washington, DC 20036
202/775-0101
Web site: http://www.riaa.com

Television
National Association of Broadcasters (NAB)
1771 N St NW
Washington, DC 20036
202/429-5300
Web site: http://www.nab.org

TV Parental Guidelines Monitoring Board
PO Box 14097
Washington, DC 20004
202/879-9364
Web site: http://www.tvguidelines.org

Note: The mention and description of any rating system in this brochure does not imply endorsement by the American Academy of Pediatrics. The Academy is not responsible for the content of any of the Web sites mentioned above.

The information contained in this publication should not be used as a substitute for the medical care and advice of your pediatrician. There may be variations in treatment that your pediatrician may recommend based on individual facts and circumstances.

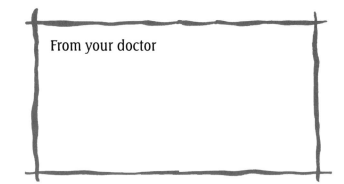

From your doctor

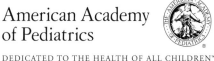

American Academy
of Pediatrics

DEDICATED TO THE HEALTH OF ALL CHILDREN™

The American Academy of Pediatrics is an organization of 60,000 primary care pediatricians, pediatric medical subspecialists, and pediatric surgical specialists dedicated to the health, safety, and well-being of infants, children, adolescents, and young adults.

American Academy of Pediatrics
Web site—www.aap.org

Understanding the Impact of Media on Children and Teens

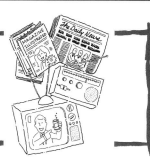

In a matter of seconds, most children can mimic a movie or TV character, sing an advertising jingle, or give other examples of what they have learned from media. Sadly, these examples may include naming a popular brand of beer, striking a "sexy" pose, or play fighting. Children only have to put a movie into the VCR, open a magazine, click on a Web site, or watch TV to experience all kinds of messages. It really is that easy.

Media offer entertainment, culture, news, sports, and education. They are an important part of our lives and have much to teach. But some of what they teach may not be what we want children to learn.

This brochure gives an overview of some of the messages media send young people that could be negative or harmful to their health. You will learn how you can teach your children to better understand the media messages they see and hear in print, over airwaves, on networks, and on-line.

The power of media messages

Sometimes you can see the impact of media right away, such as when your child watches superheros fighting and then copies their moves during play. But most of the time the impact is not so immediate or obvious. It occurs slowly as children see and hear certain messages over and over, such as the following:

- Fighting and other violence used as a way to "handle" conflict
- Cigarettes and alcohol shown as cool and attractive, not unhealthy and deadly
- Sexual action with no negative results, such as disease or unintended pregnancy

Media messages: good or bad?

Whatever form they take (ads, movies, computer games, music videos), messages can be good or bad for your child. Just as you would limit certain foods in your child's diet that may be unhealthy, you also should limit her media diet of messages. Some examples of these follow.

Use of cigarettes and alcohol

Messages about tobacco and alcohol are everywhere in media. Kids see characters on screen smoking and drinking. They see signs for tobacco and alcohol products at concerts and sporting events. Advertising and movies send kids the message that smoking and drinking make a person sexy or cool and that "everyone does it." Advertising also sways teens to smoke and drink. Teens who see a lot of ads for beer, wine, liquor, and cigarettes admit that it influences them to want to drink and smoke. It is not by chance that the three most advertised cigarette brands are also the most popular ones smoked by teens.

Advertisers of tobacco and alcohol purposely leave out the negative information about their products. As a result, young people often do not know what the health risks are when they use these products. Sometimes TV broadcasts and print articles do the same thing. For example, a magazine might do a story about the common causes of cancer but not mention smoking as a top cause. Does your child know why? The answer may be that the magazine publisher takes money to publish tobacco ads or even owns another company that makes cigarettes.

Fatty foods and thin bodies

Media heavily promote unhealthy foods while at the same time telling people they need to lose weight and be thin. Heavy media use can also take time away from physical activity.

Studies show that girls of all ages worry about their weight. Many of them are starting to diet at early ages. Media can promote an unrealistic image of how people look. Often, the thin and perfect-looking person on screen or in print is not even one whole person but parts of several people! This "person" is created by using body doubles, airbrushing, and computer-graphics techniques.

Violence

Children learn their attitudes about violence at a very young age and these attitudes tend to last. Although TV violence has been studied the most, researchers are finding that violence in other media impacts children and teens in many of the same harmful ways.

- From media violence children learn to behave aggressively toward others. They are taught to use violence instead of self-control to take care of problems or conflicts.
- Violence in the "media world" may make children more accepting of real-world violence and less caring toward others. Children who see a lot of violence from movies, TV shows, or video games may become more fearful and look at the real world as a mean and scary place.

Although the effects of media on children might not be apparent right away, children are being negatively affected. Sometimes children may not act out violently until their teen or young-adult years.

Media education basics

Parents need to set limits and be actively involved with the TV shows, computer games, magazines, and other media that children use. But this is only one step in helping media play a positive role in children's lives. Because media surround us and cannot always be avoided, one way to filter their messages is to develop the skills to question, analyze, and evaluate them. This is called *media literacy* or *media education*.

Just as a print-literate child learns to be critical of the things he reads, he should also be able to do the same with moving pictures and sounds. Your child can learn to understand both the obvious and hidden messages in all media. Once children learn media education skills, they will begin to ask questions and think about the media messages they watch, read, and hear. And they usually will enjoy doing it!

Following are basic media education points your child should know:
- **People create media messages.** Any media message, whether it's a magazine article or a TV talk show, is created by a team of people. Those people write it, decide what pictures to use, and what to leave out. All of these things give the message a purpose.
- **Each media form uses its own language.** Newspapers make headlines large to attract readers to certain stories. Media with sound may use music to make people feel a range of emotions. When children learn about these techniques they are able to understand how a message is delivered instead of only being affected by it.
- **No two people experience the same media message in exactly the same way.** How a person interprets a message depends on things unique to that person's life. These can include age, values, memories, and education.
- **Media messages have their own values and points of view.** These are built into the message itself. Children should compare the promoted values against their own values. It is important for children to learn that they have a *choice* in whether to accept the values that are being promoted in any media message.

Everyday media education ideas

Besides asking how and why media messages are created, children of various ages can do everyday activities with you or other adults to help build media education skills. Make a game out of the following:
- Play "Spot the Commercials." Help your child learn to tell the difference between a regular program and the commercials that support it. This may be tricky during children's shows because many commercials advertise toys based on TV characters.
- Do a taste test to compare a heavily advertised brand with a generic or other nonadvertised brand. Try products such as cereals or soft drinks. See whether your child and his friends can tell the difference and whether advertising influenced their guesses.
- Look at the headlines, photos, and placements of articles in a newspaper. How do these affect which stories your child wants to read? Read a few stories and compare their content with their headlines and photos.
- When you see a movie, video, or video game with your child, talk about whether what happens on screen would happen in the "real" world. For example, would a person *really* be able to drive a car super fast, down narrow streets, without crashing?
- While shopping, compare products with advertisements your child has seen. Look at the ingredients, label, or packaging. Is any of this information in the ad? Does the ad give any specific information about the product itself? How is the product different than it seemed from the ad or packaging?
- How many brands of beer, cigarettes, or other such products can your child name? If she can name even one, this is a great way to begin talking about the power of advertising. Discuss the health risks of using these products and how the ads leave out that information.

- Watch a music video with your child. What stories are the pictures telling? Does the story on screen match the meaning of the words in the song? How does the video make your child feel? Can your child note any stereotypical, violent, or sexual images in the video? Is there any tobacco, alcohol, or drug use? Watch a music video with the sound off and see how it is different.

How a media message is created

The exercise that follows is a fun way for older children to think about who puts together a media message and why.

Have your child choose a media message and then answer the following questions about it. Television commercials are easy to practice with because they are short and often contain powerful words, images, and music. You could also pick a video game, the packaging for a children's toy, or a music video. The choices are endless.

1. **Describe the kinds of people involved in creating the message.** These can include writers, photographers, designers, special effects people, or stunt people.
2. **Depending on the media message you choose, talk about the visual effects that were used** (lighting, camera angles, computer-generated images, etc). Also discuss the sound (the words that are spoken, who says them, music, special effects, and other sounds). How do these different things affect the power and meaning of the message?
3. **Discuss the purpose of the message.** Are the people who made the message trying to give you information? Do they want you to do something (such as buy a product)? Or is the message just to entertain you? Many times the true meaning of a message is hidden below the surface—it is not always stated in the message. As children gain more experience questioning how messages are put together, they will be able to get at the true meaning of any message.
4. **What does your child think about the message?** Does she agree with it or disagree with it, and why? One reason to accept or reject a message could be to decide whether it is realistic or agrees with her values.

Set the home stage for media education

Starting when children are very young, most of their media use takes place in the home. Parents can help their children make better use of media by doing the following:

Make a media plan. Schedule media times and choices in advance, just as you would other activities. A media plan helps everyone to choose and use media carefully.

Set media time limits. Limit children's total screen time. This includes time watching TV and videotapes, playing video and computer games, and surfing the Internet. One way to do this is to use a timer. When the timer goes off, your child's media time is up, no exceptions. The American Academy of Pediatrics recommends no more than 1 to 2 hours of quality TV and videos a day for older children and no screen time for children under the age of 2.

Set family guidelines for media content. Help children and teens choose shows, videos, and video games that are appropriate for their ages and interests. Get into the habit of checking the content ratings and parental advisories for all media. Use these ratings to decide what media are suitable for your child.

Be clear and consistent with children about media rules. If you do not approve of their media choice, explain why and help them choose something more appropriate.

Keep TV sets, VCRs, video games, and computers out of children's bedrooms. Instead, put them where you can be involved and monitor children's use. If children or teens are allowed to have a TV set or other media in their bedrooms, know what media they are using and supervise their media choices. If you have Internet access, supervise your children while they are on-line.

Make media a family activity. Whenever possible, use media with your children and discuss what they see, hear, and read. When you share your children's media experiences, you can help them analyze, question, and challenge the meaning of messages for themselves. During a media activity, help children "talk back," or question what they see. Do this during a violent act, an image or message that is misleading, or an advertisement for an unhealthy product.

"Talking back," or asking questions about media messages, builds the life-long skills your child needs to be a critical media consumer. Discuss how the media messages compare with the values you are teaching your child.

Look for media "side effects." Unless they come clearly labeled as containing violence, sex, or graphic language, parents often overlook the messages children are getting from media. Instead, be aware of the media children and teens use and the impact it could be having. This is especially important if your child shows any of the following behaviors:

- Poor school performance
- Hitting or pushing other kids often
- Aggressively talking back to adults
- Frequent nightmares
- Increased eating of unhealthy foods
- Smoking, drinking, or drug use

Talk to your child's pediatrician about any behavior that is a concern. Your pediatrician may take a media history of your child. This can help uncover whether certain behavioral problems exist or could develop based on how much and what kind of media your child uses. If there are problems or you think they could develop, work with your child to change his media use.

Voice your opinion. Let people who profit from the media and set guidelines about content know how you feel about media messages.

- In a phone call, letter, or e-mail message, tell companies and advertisers what you like and what you do not like. Have your kids voice their opinions too. One letter or call can make a difference.
- When media content and advertisers do not support your family's values, voice your opinion with your buying power. Do not buy their products, and tell them why.
- Support media literacy education in your child's school.

It's up to parents like you. You can learn more about media's impact by talking with your child's pediatrician and reading about media education. Schools, hospitals, and community groups may hold free workshops on topics such as taking control of kids' TV watching.

You can make a difference in the way media impacts your kids. If you limit, supervise, and share media experiences with children, they have much to gain. When you help your children understand how their media choices affect them, they actively control their media use rather than giving in to the influence of media without thinking about it.

Visiting the on-line world

Spend time with your child on the Internet and monitor where she goes and who she "talks" to on-line. Children need to be protected on-line. They are "clicks" away from being exploited by advertisers and exposed to violence, sex, adult language, and substance use.

Check for on-line ratings to help you assess violence, sex, language, and "adult" material. Use Internet-blocking programs as one way to protect your child on-line.

Make it a rule to never give out personal information on-line. This includes your child's name, address, phone number, school name or location, facts about parents and siblings, or favorite products.

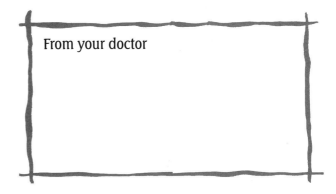

From your doctor

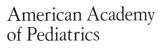

American Academy of Pediatrics

DEDICATED TO THE HEALTH OF ALL CHILDREN™

The American Academy of Pediatrics is an organization of 60,000 primary care pediatricians, pediatric medical subspecialists, and pediatric surgical specialists dedicated to the health, safety, and well-being of infants, children, adolescents, and young adults.

American Academy of Pediatrics
Web site—www.aap.org

Copyright © 1999
American Academy of Pediatrics

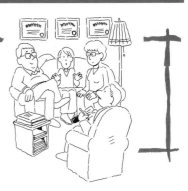

Your Child's Mental Health:
When to Seek Help and Where to Get Help

Have you noticed a recent change in your child's behavior? Is he having trouble getting along with friends? Is he failing school? Is his new behavior affecting your family?

Your pediatrician may suggest that your child see a mental health or behavioral specialist. In many cases, a child psychiatrist, psychologist, clinical social worker, counselor, or pediatric developmental and behavioral specialist can help your child.

In the United States, 1 in 10 children and teens has serious emotional and behavioral problems. Many others have symptoms that may lead to problems that are more serious if not treated.

Read more to learn about getting help, risk factors, mental health professionals, insurance and payment issues, ways to talk with your child, and additional resources. The result can be less stress and greater happiness for you, your child, and your family.

When to seek help

Let your pediatrician know if your child has one or more of the following signs or symptoms:
- Poor or delayed language development
- Problems listening or behaving
- Excessive activity (hyperactivity)
- Difficulty concentrating
- Difficulty with friends and other children
- Chronic sadness, irritability, or grumpiness
- Difficulty sleeping or excessive sleeping
- Eating disorder (eating too much or too little)
- Frequent worrying and fearfulness
- Extreme shyness
- Reluctance to attend school
- Suicidal thoughts
- Substance abuse
- Aggressive and/or risky behavior
- Sudden change in behavior or school performance

Risk factors

Almost always, no one is to blame for a child's mental health difficulties. However, certain situations may increase a child's risk for emotional problems. These include
- Family stress, such as a move, job loss, or birth of a baby
- Chronic sickness or medical condition in the child or another family member
- Grief and loss caused by death, parental separation, or divorce
- Remarriage and stepparenting
- Exposure to violence, either within or outside the family
- Foster care

- Frustration with schoolwork
- Peer pressures

Where to get help

Successful treatment for your child depends on appropriate health care, as well as the involvement and support of the entire family.

There are many types of professionals trained to help children and their families with emotional and behavioral problems. Your pediatrician can help you select the best type of care for your child. With your permission, your pediatrician can also coordinate care to make sure that the needs of your child and family are met, especially when a mental health professional is involved in treatment.

Mental health professionals include the following (license and practice requirements may differ from state to state):
- **Child and adolescent psychiatrists.** Licensed physicians trained in psychiatry. These doctors have additional special training in treating children, teens, and families. They can evaluate your child, prescribe medicine if necessary, and provide a full range of treatments for emotional and behavioral problems, as well as psychiatric disorders.
- **Child and adolescent clinical psychologists.** Licensed doctoral (PhD)-level specialists trained to diagnose and treat children and teens with learning, behavioral, and emotional difficulties. These specialists have advanced training and experience in treating depression, anxiety, conduct disorders, and complications related to medical illnesses or treatment.
- **Master's-level psychologists or mental health counselors.** Master's-level specialists who can administer psychological tests. They can also provide individual and family counseling. In some states, these specialists may be independently licensed to practice and are known as "psychologists." In other states, they may practice only under the supervision of a doctoral-level licensed psychologist or psychiatrist.
- **School psychologists.** Specialists with a doctoral or master's degree who work with children at school. School psychologists evaluate and counsel children with learning, emotional, and behavioral problems.
- **Licensed clinical social workers.** Master's- or doctoral-trained mental health professionals who specialize in diagnosis and treatment of behavioral and emotional problems. Social workers also provide counseling to children and families. They help families deal with physical, mental, or emotional illness and disability, and improve their problem-solving and coping skills.
- **Developmental-behavioral pediatricians.** Pediatricians trained to help children with developmental, learning, and behavioral disorders, as well as emotional and physical growth. They can also help children and families manage problems that involve childhood illness or disability. They can prescribe medicine, if needed, and typically work with other doctors and counselors to meet families' needs.

Talking to your child about therapy

Your child may not want to see another doctor or counselor, or understand why. She may feel fearful, embarrassed, or defensive about her problems ("It's not my fault!" "I'm not crazy, am I?").

It's important to talk with your child before her first visit to a new doctor or counselor. If your pediatrician has made the referral, it's natural for this discussion to occur in the doctor's office with your child. If not, you should talk about it at home. How much information your child needs and when you share it will depend on her age and maturity. A younger child will need only a little information, 1 to 2 days before the first appointment, to reduce "worry time."

Your teen may need more information, either at home or in the pediatrician's office. Let her know that you are aware of her struggles. Also, tell her that counseling will make her life easier. For instance, she'll get along better with friends and classmates and experience less stress, fear, and other symptoms. Make sure she knows that what she tells her doctor or counselor is private and will remain confidential.

It's important that your child not feel that the problem is hers alone or her fault. Let her know that the entire family will support her and help her get well. Sometimes counseling can and should begin with the entire family, not the child alone. This may be especially helpful if your child is resistant. In any case, it's usually best to talk about the appointment as something that will happen; if you ask if she would "like to go," she may feel she has the chance to refuse.

Tell your child that seeking help is a great sign of strength—it says, "I deserve to feel better." Let her know that mental health professionals don't solve problems; instead they build on a person's strengths, empowering them to manage their own problems.

- **Child neurologists.** Licensed physicians with specialized training in diagnosing and treating children with problems of the nervous system. These specialists assist in determining whether a child has a brain condition that affects learning and behavior and in choosing treatment for this type of condition. Child neurologists can prescribe medicine and are very helpful when a child needs medicine for both a brain condition and a behavioral problem.
- **Psychopharmacologists.** Physicians or nurses with specialized training in the prescription of psychotropic medicine for the treatment of children with mental illness or severe behavioral problems. They may be child psychiatrists, child neurologists, pediatricians, or nurse clinicians with a special interest in children with severe behavioral problems.
- **Other mental health professionals.** Counselors, nurses with specialized training, and family therapists who have expertise in helping children and teens with mental health problems. They can also help families provide support and care for their children.
- **Community mental health resources.** Mental health professionals and services offered through health departments, public mental health programs, religious organizations, non-profit counseling agencies, colleges, and medical centers.
- **Family organizations and support groups.** Local and national organizations offering a range of resources including brochures, books, or information posted on the Internet; public speakers and conferences; and support and advocacy groups.

Insurance and payment issues

It's important that you know exactly how much your insurance company will pay. Your insurance package may provide limited coverage for mental health services. It may help to ask your insurance company the following questions:

- Does my pediatrician need to formally recommend that my child see a mental health professional before the cost of the visit is covered? Or do I need approval through a separate process specifically for mental health services?
- Do I have to choose a doctor or counselor from an approved list? Does the list include professionals with expertise in children and their families?
- Are certain disorders excluded from coverage?
- Is there a lifetime or annual limit for mental health coverage? If so, what is it?
- Exactly how much of the cost of mental health services will I need to pay?

More resources for you and your child

Your pediatrician may direct you to other resources if you don't have health insurance, if your health care plan doesn't cover mental health care, or if your health care plan doesn't provide enough mental health coverage to meet your family's needs.

In some communities, mental health centers or family service agencies charge based on what you are able to pay. Medicaid or the State Children's Health Insurance Program (SCHIP)—publicly funded programs to cover the medical costs of low-income children—also covers some mental health costs. In some states and for some diagnoses, these or other funds may be available, even if you have private insurance, for mental health services not covered by your health insurance.

If you have trouble obtaining or filling out a Medicaid or SCHIP application, ask your pediatrician's office for help. For more information about Medicaid or SCHIP contact the Centers for Medicare & Medicaid Services at 877/267-2323 or www.cms.hhs.gov.

Self-help organizations may also offer counseling and support to children and their families. These organizations operate drop-in centers and sponsor gatherings for group discussions on specific topics, such as substance abuse or attention and learning problems. Your child's school may have guidance counselors and other professionals with training in behavioral health assessment and treatment. Clergy can also provide help. It's important to talk about each of these options with your pediatrician.

Privacy issues

The law protects your privacy related to mental health but allows your doctor to share information with other professionals involved in your child's and family's treatment.

Tips on dealing with insurance companies

When speaking with or writing to an insurance company, keep these 5 points in mind
1. Don't be afraid to ask questions.
2. Keep good communication records, including with whom you spoke and on what day and time.
3. Be polite.
4. Be patient.
5. Be persistent.

Remember

Parents and pediatricians play an important role in a child's mental health care.

It's common for parents and families to feel as if their child's problems are their fault. Many people are also afraid or embarrassed about a child's need for mental health treatment. While these feelings are normal, it's important that you not blame yourself for your child's problems. Your pediatrician, along with one or more mental health professionals, can help you better understand your child's behavior. They can guide you and other members of your family to help in the healing process.

If you are separated or divorced from your child's other parent, it's important to establish a plan for including the other parent in your child's assessment and treatment. Your pediatrician will help you decide whether scheduling visits together or separately, sharing reports, or making phone calls can best do this.

It's very helpful for you to continue to talk with your pediatrician and with the doctor or mental health professional who is working with your child.

In some cases, you will need to sign special forms authorizing the release of information. This may include medical, family, school, and social history records. You can decide whether to give out this information.

At a certain age (which varies by state), your child may legally consent to or refuse care. Your pediatrician can help explain these laws and how they affect your child and your family.

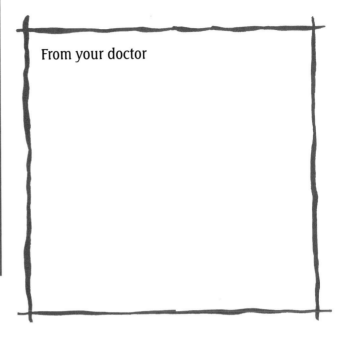

From your doctor

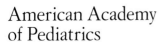

American Academy of Pediatrics

DEDICATED TO THE HEALTH OF ALL CHILDREN™

The American Academy of Pediatrics is an organization of 60,000 primary care pediatricians, pediatric medical subspecialists, and pediatric surgical specialists dedicated to the health, safety, and well-being of infants, children, adolescents, and young adults.

American Academy of Pediatrics
Web site — www.aap.org

Copyright © 2003
American Academy of Pediatrics

Sibling Relationships

Part I Siblings, Step-siblings, Half-siblings, and Twins

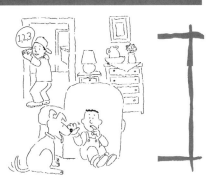

Siblings are very important to many of us. Almost 80% of children grow up with at least one brother or sister. Even though they may not get along all the time, siblings play very positive roles in each other's lives. Brothers and sisters learn their first lessons about getting along with others from one another. They are friends, playmates, and keepers of secrets. They help one another learn to relate to the outside world. They even protect and watch out for each other.

When brothers and sisters do not get along, their arguments can cause a parent to feel frustrated and angry. Each child also makes different demands on you. Your relationship with one child may lead the other to feel that you are playing favorites.

It may be hard to keep the peace in your family. This brochure offers information that may help you understand why your children get along the way they do, and how you can help them learn to live together in peace.

Why siblings get along the way they do

Many things affect relationships between brothers and sisters. Some of these are:

- Personality
- Age
- Number of years between siblings (spacing)
- Gender
- Birth order

Personality similarities and differences

Parents often wonder how children growing up in the same home with the same parents can be so different. The fact is that siblings are usually more different than alike.

Two factors affect your children's personalities—nature (what they were born with) and nurture (their experiences). Even though they have the same parents, each child's genetic makeup is different. Their experiences are also not the same. As a result, each child develops his own personality.

Some parents feel it is important to always treat each child the same way. They do not want one child to think they love the other more. Treating your children differently does not have to mean you are playing favorites. Each child is an individual, and you should treat him that way. Doing so is part of what makes each child a unique person. It is a way of showing that you appreciate how special he is.

Age, gender, birth order, and spacing

Your children's ages make a big difference in how you treat them and in how well they get along. For example, you may hug and kiss your toddler more than your school-age child. As a result, your older child may think that you love the younger sibling more. Parents should treat younger children differently than older ones, however. A toddler's needs are not the same as those of a school-age child.

Gender affects your children's relationships with each other, as well. Many parents find that children of different genders tend to get along better than do children of the same gender. Siblings of the same sex tend to compete with each other more than they do with opposite-sex siblings.

Birth order and family size also affect how children behave. The experience of an only child is different from that of a child in a larger family. Also, an older child's experience is different from a younger one's: The older child has a younger sibling, while the younger child has an older sibling. A third child has two older siblings, and so on. Because of birth order, family size, and individual experiences, no two children view the family the same way.

How your children are spaced affects how well they get along, too. Children who are less than 2 years apart often have more conflict than children who are spaced further apart. This may be because they compete over the same "turf." You might want to keep this in mind when you are planning your family.

Understanding sibling rivalry

Few things are more upsetting than children who do not get along. No matter how hard you try to keep the peace, your children are likely to fight over toys, pick on or tattle on one another, and tease and criticize each other. You may wonder, "What have I done wrong?" The answer is probably nothing. Sibling rivalry is a natural part of growing up.

Sibling rivalry between children who are under 4 years of age tends to be at its worst when they are less than 3 years apart. This is largely because preschool children still depend on their parents a great deal and have not

---

Step-siblings and half-siblings

Step-families create another type of sibling rivalry. With current high divorce and remarriage rates, the number of step-siblings and half-siblings is growing. This creates new conflicts. When two families become one, children who barely know each other may all of a sudden share bedrooms and bathrooms. This can cause fights over toys, space, and what to watch on TV. At the same time, children are trying to get used to their parents' new marriage, new step-parents, and maybe a new house. Also, parents may decide to have more children, introducing half-siblings into the family. It is not always an easy adjustment.

Here are some ideas to cut down on problems in step-families and families with half-siblings:

- Do not expect step-siblings to spend all of their time together.
- Each child should spend some time alone with his or her own parent.
- Whenever possible, step-siblings and half-siblings should have their own rooms. If they have to share a room, however, each youngster should have her own toys and other possessions; do not force children to turn all their things into community property.
- If you and your new spouse decide to have a child together, you should be open and honest about it with your older children. Reassure them that your decision to have a child together does not mean you will love them less. Involve them in planning for the new baby as much as possible.
- Both parents should be involved in parenting each child.

---

made friends or gotten close to other adults yet. Children who are 2 and 3 years old are also very self-centered and have a very hard time sharing their parents with siblings.

Competition between brothers and sisters can heat up as children grow older. It is often at its worst when children are between 8 and 12 years old. Siblings close in age or those who have the same interests tend to compete more.

Sometimes, especially when children are several years apart, the older one accepts and protects the younger sibling. Once the younger one grows and develops more skills and talents, however, the older child may feel "shown up" by the younger one. The older child may feel threatened or embarrassed. He may then begin to compete with the younger child, or become more aggressive toward him. The younger child, too, may become jealous about the privileges his big brother or sister gets as he or she gets older. Though you may think you know, it is often hard to tell which child is causing the problem.

In many cases, the oldest child in the family feels a greater sense of rivalry than the younger ones. A younger child may look up to his older brother or sister, but the oldest child may think his siblings disturb his privacy or threaten his special status in the family.

Preteens and teenagers can pose other problems. Younger children may resent the older ones' freedoms and privileges, and older ones may resent being asked to watch over their younger siblings. Parents should explain that there are different rules for each child based on age and degree of maturity. Although you will do your best to be fair, things may not always be *equal* for the siblings. Explain to your younger child that he will have the same privileges when he gets older. At the same time, do not make your preteen or teenager take his little brother or sister along everywhere he goes.

What parents can do about sibling rivalry

Here are some tips on managing conflict between your children:

- **Do not compare your children in front of them.** It is natural to notice differences between your children. Just try not to comment on these in front of them. It is easy for a child to think that he is not as good or as loved as his sibling when you compare them. Remember, each child is a special individual. Let each one know that.
- **As much as possible, stay out of your children's arguments.** You may have to step in and settle a spat between toddlers or preschoolers. For example, if they are arguing over blocks, you might need to split the blocks into piles for each of them. Older children will probably settle an argument peacefully if left alone. If your children try to involve you, explain that they are both responsible for creating the problem and for ending it. Do not take sides. Set guidelines on how your children can disagree and resolve their conflicts. Of course, you must get involved if the situation gets violent. Make sure your children know that you will not stand for such behavior. If there is any reason to suspect that your children may become violent, watch them closely when they are together. Preventing violence is always better than punishing after the fact, which often makes the rivalry worse. Praise your children when they solve their arguments, and reward good behavior.
- **Be fair.** Divide household chores fairly. If you must get involved in your children's arguments, listen to all sides of the story. Make a "no tattling"

rule. Give children privileges that are right for their ages, and try to be consistent. If you allowed one child to stay up until 9 o'clock at 10 years of age, the other should have the same bedtime when she is 10.

- **Respect your child's privacy.** When it is necessary to punish or scold, do it with the child alone in a quiet, private place. When possible, do not embarrass one child by scolding him in front of the others. This will only make the other child tease the one you punished.
- **Use regular family meetings for all family members to express their thoughts and feelings, as well as to plan the week's events. Give positive recognition and rewards (allowances, special privileges).**

Sibling relationships are very special. We form our earliest bonds with our brothers and sisters. No one else shares the same family history. By helping your children learn to value, love and respect their siblings, you are giving them a great gift—the gift of a lifelong friend.

Raising twins

From the very start it is important that you treat your twin babies as individuals. If they are identical, it is easy to treat them as a "package," giving them the same clothing, toys, and attention. But although they may look alike, emotionally they are very different. In order to grow up happy and secure as individuals, they need you to support their differences.

Identical and fraternal twins compete with each other and depend on each other as they grow. Sometimes one twin acts as the leader and the other the follower. Either way, most twins develop very close relationships early in life simply because they spend so much time with each other.

If you also have other children, your twin newborns may make your older children doubly jealous. Twins need huge amounts of your time and energy, and will get a lot of extra attention from friends, relatives, and strangers on the street. You can help your other children accept this by offering them "double rewards" for helping with the new babies. If you have twin newborns, it is even more important that you spend some very special time alone with the other children, doing their favorite things.

As your twins get a little older, especially if they are identical, they may choose to play only with each other. This may make their other siblings feel left out. To keep the twins from leaving other children out, urge them to play separately with other children. Also, you or their babysitter might play with just one twin, while the other plays with a sibling or friend.

The information contained in this publication should not be used as a substitute for the medical care and advice of your pediatrician. There may be variations in treatment that your pediatrician may recommend based on individual facts and circumstances.

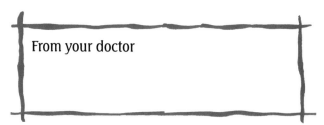

From your doctor

American Academy of Pediatrics

DEDICATED TO THE HEALTH OF ALL CHILDREN™

The American Academy of Pediatrics is an organization of 60,000 primary care pediatricians, pediatric medical subspecialists, and pediatric surgical specialists dedicated to the health, safety, and well-being of infants, children, adolescents, and young adults.

American Academy of Pediatrics
Web site — www.aap.org

Copyright © 1996
American Academy of Pediatrics

Sibling Relationships

Part II Preparing for a New Baby

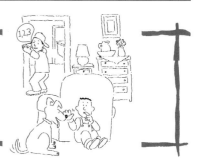

Preparing your children for a new baby

A new baby brings both joys and challenges to a family. Parents are excited but they are also nervous about how their older children will react to the newborn. All sorts of questions come up: how should we tell our older children that they are going to have a baby brother or sister? Will they be jealous of the new baby? How can we make sure they will get along as they get older?

How your children react to a new baby depends largely on their ages at the time the baby is born. Knowing what to expect from each age group will make it easier to handle the changes in your family.

Ages 2 to 4

Toddlers and preschoolers may have a hard time adjusting to a new baby, especially if they are between 2 and 3 years old. At this age, your child is still very attached to you and does not yet understand about sharing you with others. Your child also may be very sensitive to changes going on around her, and may feel threatened by the idea of a new family member. Here are some suggestions for how to ease your preschooler into being a big brother or big sister.

- **Wait a while before telling your preschooler that you are going to have a baby, but do not wait too long.** A child younger than 4 will have a hard time understanding an abstract concept like an unborn baby. You should explain it to your child when you start buying nursery furniture or baby clothes, or when she starts to ask about mom's growing "stomach." Picture books for preschoolers can be very helpful. So can sibling preparation classes (ask your hospital if they offer them). Try to tell your child before she hears about the new baby from someone else.
- **Be honest.** Do not promise that things will be the same after the baby comes, because they will not be, no matter how hard you try. Explain that the baby will be cute and cuddly, but will also cry and take a lot of your time and attention. Also, make sure that your older child knows that the baby will not be an instant playmate. Let your preschooler know that you will love her just as much after the baby is born as you do now.
- **Involve your preschooler in planning for the baby.** This will make her less jealous. Let her shop with you for baby items. Show her pictures of herself as a newborn. If you are going to use some of her old baby things, let her play with them a bit before you get them ready for the new baby.
- **Do not make major changes in your preschooler's routine until after the baby is born.** You should complete making any changes such as toilet training or switching from a crib to a bed before the baby arrives. If that is not possible, put them off until after the baby is settled in at home. Otherwise, your preschooler may feel overwhelmed by trying to learn new things on top of all the changes caused by the new baby.

- **Expect your child to "regress" a little.** Do not worry too much if news that a baby is coming or if the baby's arrival makes your preschooler start acting like a baby again. For example, your toilet-trained child might suddenly start having "accidents," or she might want to take a bottle. This is normal and is your older child's way of making sure she still has your love and attention. Instead of telling her to act her age, let her have the attention she needs. Praise her when she acts more "grown-up."
- **Prepare your child for when you are in the hospital.** Toddlers and preschoolers may be confused when you leave for the hospital. Explain to your child that you will be back with the new baby in a few days.
- **Set aside some special time for your older child.** No matter how busy you are with the new baby, make sure you save some special time each day just for you and your older child. Read, play games, listen to music, or simply talk together. Show her that you want to know what she is doing, thinking, and feeling—not only about the baby but about everything else in her life. Also, make her feel a part of things by having her cuddle next to you when you feed the baby.
- **Encourage visitors to give attention to your older child.** Visitors can make such a fuss over a new baby that your older child might feel left out. Ask family and friends to spend a little time with your older child when they come to see the new baby. They might also give her a small gift when they bring gifts for the baby.
- **Have your older child spend time with dad.** A new baby presents a great opportunity for fathers to spend time alone with older children.

School-age children

Children older than 5 are usually not as threatened by a newborn as younger children are. This is particularly true if the school-age child has good self-esteem and feels loved and valued. Even so, your older child may resent the attention the baby gets. To prepare your school-age child for a new baby:

- **Tell your child about what is happening in language she can understand.** Explain what having a new brother or sister means, noting that the changes may affect her—both the good and the not-so-good. **Make your firstborn feel like a part of the process.** Have your older child help get the house ready for the new sibling by fixing up the baby's bedroom, picking out a new crib, buying diapers. If there is time, have her come to the hospital soon after the delivery so that she feels part of the growing family. Then, when you bring the baby home, make your older child feel that she has a role to play in caring for the baby. Tell her she can hold the baby, although she must ask you first. Praise her when she is gentle and loving toward the baby.

- **Make sure your older child feels listened to.** Do not overlook your older child's needs and activities. Let her know she can talk about her feelings. Tell her: "A new baby means a lot more work for me. If you ever feel that I am not spending enough time with you, let me know so I can give you plenty of extra love." Make an effort to spend some time alone with her each day; use that as a chance to make her feel like the most important person in your life.

What parents can do about sibling rivalry

It is important not to get too upset when your children are jealous of each other, especially if the older child is a preschooler. It takes time for a youngster to learn that his parents do not love him any less because they have another child to love.

Here are some tips on managing conflict between your children:

- **If your older child starts imitating the baby, do not make fun of or punish him.** Let him drink from a bottle or climb in the crib once or twice, but make it very clear that he does not have to act like a baby to get your attention. Praise him when he acts "grown up" and give him chances to be a "big brother." It should not take long for him to see that he gets more attention by acting his age than by acting like a baby.

- **If your older child is between 3 and 5 years old, try to cut down on conflicts over space by setting aside an area just for her.** Giving your older child her own space and keeping her things apart from shared ones will cut down on quarrels.

- **Do not compare your children in front of them.** It is natural to notice differences between your children. Just try not to comment on these in front of them. It is easy for a child to think that he is not as good or as loved as his sibling when you compare them. Remember, each child is a special individual. Let each one know that.

- **As much as possible, stay out of your children's arguments.** You may have to step in and settle a spat between toddlers or preschoolers. For example, if they are arguing over blocks, you might need to split the blocks into piles for each of them. Older children will probably settle an argument peacefully if left alone. If your children try to involve you, explain that they are both responsible for creating the problem and for ending it. Do not take sides. Set guidelines on how your children can disagree and resolve their conflicts. Of course, you **must** get involved if the situation gets violent. Make sure your children know that you will not stand for such behavior. If there is any reason to suspect that your children may become violent, watch them closely when they are together. Preventing violence is always better than punishing after the fact, which often makes the rivalry worse. Praise your children when they solve their arguments, and reward good behavior.

- **Be fair.** Divide household chores fairly. If you must get involved in your children's arguments, listen to all sides of the story. Make a "no tattling" rule. Give children privileges that are right for their ages, and try to be consistent. If you allowed one child to stay up until 9 o'clock at 10 years of age, the other should have the same bedtime when she is 10.

- **Respect your child's privacy.** When it is necessary to punish or scold do it with the child alone in a quiet, private place. When possible, do not embarrass one child by scolding him in front of the others. This will only make the other child tease the one you punished.

- **Use regular family meetings for all family members to express their thoughts and feelings, as well as to plan the week's events. Give positive recognition and rewards (allowances, special privileges).**

Sibling relationships are very special. We form our earliest bonds with our brothers and sisters. No one else shares the same family history. By helping your children learn to value, love and respect their siblings, you are giving them a great gift—the gift of a lifelong friend.

The information contained in this publication should not be used as a substitute for the medical care and advice of your pediatrician. There may be variations in treatment that your pediatrician may recommend based on individual facts and circumstances.

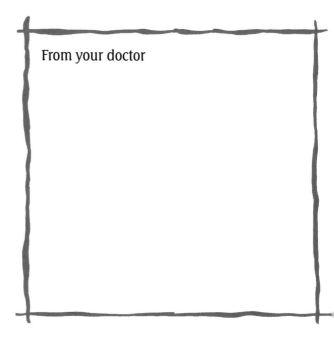

From your doctor

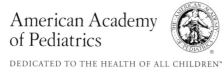

American Academy of Pediatrics

DEDICATED TO THE HEALTH OF ALL CHILDREN™

The American Academy of Pediatrics is an organization of 60,000 primary care pediatricians, pediatric medical subspecialists, and pediatric surgical specialists dedicated to the health, safety, and well-being of infants, children, adolescents, and young adults.

American Academy of Pediatrics
Web site—www.aap.org

Copyright © 1996
American Academy of Pediatrics

Single Parenting

Part I What You Need to Know

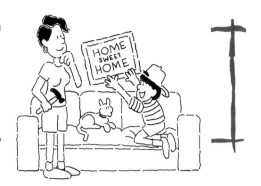

Single-parent families are more and more common in today's society. One of every four American children lives in a single-parent home. While most single-parent homes are the result of divorce, many parents are raising children alone for other reasons as well. Some parents may be alone due to the death of a spouse. Others choose to have or adopt a child without a partner. Whatever the circumstances, single parents cope with unique issues and challenges.

A death in the family

Losing a parent is one of the most traumatic events that can happen to a child. A child under 5 years of age cannot understand that death is permanent. Older children may have an understanding, but will have many questions they may be afraid to ask. Where did Daddy go when he died? Why did he die? Who will take care of me if you die? Children can react to death in many ways. Some will be quiet and sad. Others may be angry, guilty, or refuse to believe the parent is gone. It's important to accept your child's response, whatever it is. If signs of sadness or anger continue, talk to your pediatrician. He or she may recommend professional counseling to help get the healing process back on track.

Unplanned pregnancy

An unplanned pregnancy brings great change. The job of caring for a new baby is not easy, especially for single parents. Those who work may feel they aren't able to spend enough time at home with the baby. Money can be tight. Finding affordable child care might be hard. Be aware that help is available. Family, friends, and religious and community leaders are your best resources for support. If you need to find a job, employment agencies and temporary services can help. You may also qualify for government programs such as Head Start, Temporary Assistance for Needy Families (TANF), Women, Infants, and Children Supplemental Feeding Program (WIC), and Earned Income Credit (EIC).

Single-parent adoption

It is increasingly common for a single person to adopt a child on his or her own. Adoption can bring special challenges to parents. The child may be a baby just a few days old, or she could be school age. The adopted child may be of another country, race, culture, or from an abusive background. As a result, adoptive families can easily feel different from other families. The differences are real, but the rewards of working through these issues can be great. Working with your pediatrician to prevent and solve problems can be very important to your child's happiness and success.

Divorce and separation

Nearly two thirds of all single-parent families are the result of a divorce or separation. For a child, divorce can be just as hard as the death of a parent. A long period of grief and mourning can be expected. The age of the child also plays a role. A preschooler may regress in such things as toilet training, and may develop new fears or nightmares. A school-age child is more likely to show anger and feel guilty or sad. He may also do poorly in school. A teenager may worry about moving away from friends or not having money for college. No matter the age, some children feel responsible for the divorce of their parents and dream about getting them back together.

Divorce or separation often leaves parents angry with each other. During disagreements with your child's other parent, stop and ask yourself: How will this affect my child? You may disagree with each other, but try to set aside your differences for your child's sake. Use the following tips to avoid problems:

- **Never force your child to take sides.** Every child will have loyalties to both parents.
- **Don't involve your child in arguments** between the two of you.
- **Don't criticize each other in front of your child.** Even if you find out the other parent is saying bad things about you, explain to your child that people sometimes say mean things when they are angry.
- **Discuss your concerns and feelings with your child's other parent** when and where your child cannot hear.
- **Don't fight in front of the children,** especially about them.

If you are considering separation or divorce, you may find it helpful to discuss it with your pediatrician or ask for a copy of the American Academy of Pediatrics brochure *Divorce and Children*. A visit with a counselor may also help by giving you and your child a chance to talk about any problems and to plan for the changes ahead.

Talking with your child

Talking with your child is a very important way for you to help each other through tough times. Being able to share her fears, worries, and feelings with you can make your child feel safe and special. The more often you talk, the more comfortable she will feel. Be patient as you listen to her questions. You don't have to have all the answers. Sometimes just listening is more helpful than giving advice. If needed, don't hesitate to get help from your pediatrician or a family counselor. The following suggestions may be useful in talking with your child about the changes in your family.

- **Be honest with your child.** If your spouse has died, your young child may not understand what has happened. Be careful what you say. Young children often see death as a temporary situation. It is very important not to talk about death as "going away" or "going to sleep." Your child may believe that the deceased parent will come back, wake up, or the child may think that she will die while asleep. If you are going through a divorce, talk about it in simple terms. Try not to blame your ex-spouse or show your anger. Explain that parents sometimes choose to live separately. Give your child all the comfort she needs to feel safe and loved.
- **Make sure your child knows he is not the cause.** Children will often think that it's their fault that one parent has left. After a separation, divorce, or a death of a parent, children may blame themselves. They may feel alone, unwanted, or unloved. Let him know the changes are not his fault, that you love him and won't leave him.
- **Talk to your child about his fears.** Confusion about a parent leaving or dying can be scary for your child. In your child's mind, if one parent can leave, maybe the other one can too. He may think being away from a parent is temporary and that if he behaves, the parent will return. It is important to discuss these fears with your child, and to be as reassuring as possible.

Find good child care

Good child care is essential for your child's well-being and your peace of mind. If you are a working parent, finding quality child care may be one of the most difficult tasks you will face.

Never leave a child home alone. Find someone you trust to take care of your children while you are working. Don't rely on older brothers and sisters to babysit for younger siblings. Even the most reliable brother or sister does not have the maturity to be responsible for a younger sibling on a daily basis. Also, be careful about asking new friends or partners to watch your children, even for a short time. They may not have the patience, especially if the child's behavior becomes difficult. Children need to be cared for by an adult with proven experience in child care. The best way to make sure your child is getting good care is to visit the child care center or watch your babysitter when he or she is with your child.

Your pediatrician can offer advice on finding the best child care for your family. The local city or county government in your area may also have a list of licensed child care centers or homes. Ask your pediatrician for the brochure *Child Care: What's Best for Your Family* from the American Academy of Pediatrics. It includes a checklist of what to ask and what to look for when choosing child care services. You may also find the AAP book *Caring for Your Baby and Young Child: Birth To Age 5* helpful.

Custody

All children need a place where they can feel truly at home. Although the parent who lives with the child takes care of the day-to-day needs, the parent without custody should remain as involved as possible. He or she can still help with homework, go to athletic or other after-school events, and contribute support.

Cooperation between parents is very important for a child's long-term well-being. Remember, it's the job of both parents to stay involved in their child's life. Work together to arrange a flexible schedule for visits. Neither parent should be kept from taking part in raising the child. Make sure your child knows that it is okay to love both parents.

Dating and the single parent

Be choosy about which dates you introduce to your children. Try to form a solid relationship before bringing someone new into your home. Particularly, overnight guests may confuse your child. If you are dating someone special, you may not know how to present him or her to your child. Talk to your friend about your child before they meet. When you feel the time is right, let your child meet your new partner. Don't expect them to be close right away. Give them time to become friends.

If your new partner is new to child-rearing, he or she may feel awkward with your family. Observe how your friend gets along with your child. He or she should be patient and understanding. Before you leave your child with a new partner, be sure that he or she can be trusted.

A new life

Raising a child on your own isn't easy. Single parents face unique problems, but children in single-parent homes can grow up just as happy as children in two-parent homes. Providing a loving, supportive home for your children is the most important factor in helping them grow up well-adjusted and happy. By seeking out the information provided here, you've taken the first step to adapting to the changes in your life. Making the right choices for you and your children will help all of you live a new and rewarding life together as a family.

The information contained in this publication should not be used as a substitute for the medical care and advice of your pediatrician. There may be variations in treatment that your pediatrician may recommend based on individual facts and circumstances.

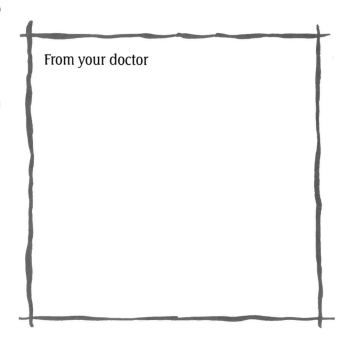

From your doctor

Single Parenting

Part II Additional Resources

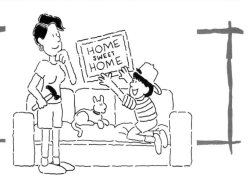

10 ways to reduce stress

Single-parenthood brings added pressure and stress to the job of raising children. With no one to share day-to-day responsibilities or decision-making, parents must provide greater support for their children while they themselves may feel alone. The following suggestions may help reduce stress in your family:

1. **Get a handle on finances.** Finances are often a problem for single parents. Learn how to budget your time and money. Know when your paycheck or other income will arrive, and keep track of household bills. If you write down monthly bills and due dates, they will be easier to manage. Do what you can to improve your finances. Contact employment and temporary agencies for help finding a job. Consider getting your high school diploma, a college degree, or other special training.

2. **Talk early and often.** Don't leave your child in the dark about the changes in the family. She will handle her problems much better by talking about her feelings. Sit quietly with your child just before bedtime. It may be a great time for her to talk with you.

3. **Find support and use it.** Don't try to handle everything by yourself. Get help whenever you can. It is difficult when a single parent must hold down a job and care for children at the same time. Try not to feel guilty about things you can't do or can't provide without a partner. You will need the support that family and friends can give. Get to know other single parents through support groups. Your pediatrician can also be a great source of help and information.

4. **Take time for family.** Working every day, fixing dinner, cleaning the house, and paying the bills can be overwhelming. Set aside some time each day to enjoy your children and your relationship with them. Spend quiet time playing, reading, working on arts-and-crafts projects, or just listening to music together. Time spent together is one of the most important things you can give to your child.

5. **Take time for yourself.** Whether you are reading, relaxing, or visiting with friends, time spent away from your children is important for you, and for them. Go to a movie. Find a hobby. Do things that interest you. Being a single parent doesn't mean you can't have an adult life.

6. **Keep a daily routine.** Making rules, setting a good example, and providing support is tough, but giving in to your child's demands will not help. Schedule meals, chores, and bedtime at regular times so that your child knows what to expect each day. A routine will help your child feel more secure.

7. **Maintain consistent discipline.** If others help in the care of your child, talk to them about your own methods of discipline. Divorced or separated parents should work together to use the same way of disciplining their children. Discipline doesn't have to mean physical punishment. You can teach a child to behave in ways that are good for both himself and those around him. Many good methods have been developed. Check your local library for helpful books on parenting. Local hospitals, the YMCA, and church groups often sponsor parenting classes. Learning good ways to handle your child's behavior will reduce stress for both of you.

8. **Treat kids like kids.** Children have a right to enjoy childhood and grow up at their own pace. Though single parenting can get lonely, resist treating your children like substitutes for a partner. Avoid expressing your frustration to them. Try not to rely on them for comfort or sympathy. As children grow older, they will be able to take on more responsibility and help around the house. Don't expect too much too soon.

9. **Stay positive.** The pain of a separation, divorce, or death will ease over time. Be aware that your children will always be affected by your mood and attitude. They will need your praise and your love through hard times. It's okay to be honest about your own feelings of sadness and loss, but let them know better times lie ahead for both of you.

10. **Take care of yourself.** This is a difficult time for you, too. Exercising regularly, maintaining a proper diet, and getting enough rest can help you better deal with stress. Visit your own doctor on a regular basis. Ask your pediatrician not only about help for your child, but also about help for yourself.

A word about...child support

In a divorce, separation, or unplanned pregnancy, both parents have a continuing financial obligation to the child. If you have custody of your child, seek child support. According to the US Department of Health and Human Services, millions of single-parent households do not receive child support. In some cases, one parent doesn't want money from the other parent. In others, the parent may not be able or willing to pay or perhaps cannot even be found. Many times, the parent with custody simply does not try to get child support.

Contact your state child support enforcement agency for guidelines on what parents must pay for child support. If your child's other parent has disappeared or won't cooperate, your state or local government may be able to help.

For more information, contact:
Department of Health and Human Services
Office of Child Support Enforcement
370 L'Enfant Promenade, SW
Washington, DC 20447
202/401-9373
Web site: www.acf.dhhs.gov/programs/cse/index.html

The information contained in this publication should not be used as a substitute for the medical care and advice of your pediatrician. There may be variations in treatment that your pediatrician may recommend based on individual facts and circumstances.

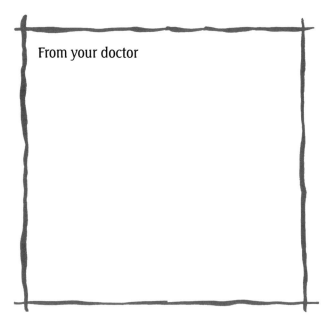

From your doctor

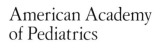

American Academy
of Pediatrics

DEDICATED TO THE HEALTH OF ALL CHILDREN™

The American Academy of Pediatrics is an organization of 60,000 primary care pediatricians, pediatric medical subspecialists, and pediatric surgical specialists dedicated to the health, safety, and well-being of infants, children, adolescents, and young adults.

American Academy of Pediatrics
Web site — www.aap.org

Copyright © 1994
American Academy of Pediatrics, Updated 12/98

Television and the Family

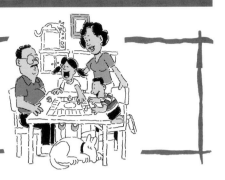

Family is the most important influence in a child's life, but television is not far behind. Television can inform, entertain, and teach us. However, some of what TV teaches may not be what you want your child to learn. TV programs and commercials often show violence, alcohol or drug use, and sexual content that are not suitable for children or teenagers. Studies show that TV viewing may lead to more aggressive behavior, less physical activity, altered body image, and increased use of drugs and alcohol. By knowing how television affects your children and by setting limits, you can help make your child's TV-watching experience less harmful, but still enjoyable.

How TV affects your child

There are many ways that television affects your child's life. When your child sits down to watch TV, consider the following:

Time

Children in the United States watch about 4 hours of TV every day. Watching movies on tape or DVD and playing video games only adds to time spent in front of the TV screen. It may be tempting to use television, movies, and video games to keep your child busy, but your child needs to spend as much time exploring and learning as possible. Playing, reading, and spending time with friends and family are much healthier than sitting in front of a TV screen.

Nutrition

Studies show that children who watch too much television are more likely to be overweight. They do not spend as much time running, jumping, and getting the exercise they need. They often snack while watching TV. They also see many commercials for unhealthy foods, such as candy, snacks, sugary cereals, and drinks. Commercials almost never give information about the foods children should eat to keep healthy. As a result, children may persuade their parents to buy unhealthy foods.

Violence

If your child watches 3 to 4 hours of noneducational TV per day, he will have seen about 8,000 murders on TV by the time he finishes grade school. Children who see violence on television may not understand that real violence hurts and kills people. They become numb to violence. If the "good guys" use violence, children may learn that it is okay to use force to solve problems. Studies show that even children's cartoons contain a significant amount of violence.

Research also shows a very strong link between exposure to violent TV and violent and aggressive behavior in children and teenagers. Watching a lot of violence on television can lead to hostility, fear, anxiety, depression, nightmares, sleep disturbances, and post-traumatic stress disorder. It is best not to let your child watch violent programs and cartoons.

A word about...TV for toddlers

Children of all ages are constantly learning new things. The first 2 years of life are especially important in the growth and development of your child's brain. During this time, children need good, positive interaction with other children and adults to develop good language and social skills. Learning to talk and play with others is far more important than watching television.

Until more research is done about the effects of TV on very young children, the American Academy of Pediatrics (AAP) does not recommend television for children younger than 2 years of age. For older children, the AAP recommends no more than 1 to 2 hours per day of quality screen time.

Sex

Television exposes children to adult behaviors, like sex. But it usually does not show the risks and results of sexual activity. On TV, sexual activity is shown as normal, fun, exciting, and without consequences. In commercials, sex is often used to sell products and services. Your child may copy what she sees on TV to feel more grown up.

Alcohol, tobacco, and other drugs

Young people today are surrounded by messages that say drinking alcohol and smoking cigarettes or cigars are normal activities. These messages do not say that alcohol and tobacco harm people and may lead to death. Beer and wine are some of the most advertised products on television. TV programs and commercials often show people who drink and smoke as healthy, energetic, sexy, and successful. It is up to you to teach your child the truth about the dangers of alcohol, tobacco, and other drugs.

Commercials

The average child sees more than 40,000 commercials each year. Commercials are quick, fast-paced, and entertaining. After seeing the same commercials over and over, your child can easily remember a song, slogan, or catchy phrase. Commercials try to convince your child that having a certain toy or eating a certain food will make him happy or popular. Older children can begin to understand how ads use pictures, music, and sound to entertain. Kids need to know that ads try to convince people to buy things they may not need.

Learning

Television affects how your child learns. High-quality, nonviolent children's shows can have a positive effect on learning. Studies show that preschool children who watch educational TV programs do better on reading and math tests than children who do not watch those programs. When used carefully, television can be a positive tool to help your child learn.

321

10 things parents can do

As a parent, there are many ways you can help your child develop positive viewing habits. The following tips may help:

1. **Set limits**
   Limit your child's use of TV, movies, and video and computer games to no more than 1 or 2 hours per day. Do not let your child watch TV while doing homework. Do not put a television in your child's bedroom.

2. **Plan your child's viewing**
   Instead of flipping through channels, use a program guide and the TV ratings to help you and your child choose shows. Turn the TV on to watch the program you chose and turn it off when the program is over.

3. **Watch TV with your child**
   Whenever possible, watch TV with your child and talk about what you see. If your child is very young, she may not be able to tell the difference between a show, a commercial, a cartoon, or real life. Explain that characters on TV are make-believe and not real.

   Some "reality-based" programs may appear to be "real," but most of these shows focus on stories that will attract as many viewers as possible. Much of their content is not appropriate for children. News broadcasts also contain violent or other inappropriate material. If your schedule prevents you from watching TV with your child, talk to her later about what she watched. Better yet, record the programs so that you can watch them *with* your child at a later time.

4. **Find the right message**
   Even a poor program can turn out to be a learning experience if you help your child find the right message. Some television programs may portray people as stereotypes. Talk with your child about the real-life roles of women, the elderly, and people of other races that may not be shown on television. Discuss ways that people are different and ways that we are the same. Help your child learn tolerance for others. Remember, if you do not agree with certain subject matter, you can either turn off the TV or explain why you object.

5. **Help your child resist commercials**
   Do not expect your child to be able to resist ads for toys, candy, snacks, cereal, drinks, or new TV programs without your help. When your child asks for products advertised on TV, explain that the purpose of commercials is to make people want things they may not need. Limit the number of commercials your child sees by watching public television stations (PBS). You can also record programs and leave out the commercials or buy or rent children's videos or DVDs.

6. **Look for quality children's videos and DVDs**
   There are many quality videos and DVDs available for children that you can buy or rent. Check reviews before buying or renting programs or movies. Information is available in books, newspapers, and magazines, as well as on the Internet.

7. **Give other options**
   Watching TV can become a habit for your child. Help your child find other things to do with his time, such as playing; reading; learning a hobby, a sport, an instrument, or an art; or spending time with family, friends, or neighbors.

TV Parental Guidelines and the v-chip

In 1996, Congress passed a law that helps parents control what their children watch on television. The law called for a rating system to be developed. The ratings, known as the TV Parental Guidelines, help parents know which programs contain sex and violence. Parents can use a computer device in their televisions called the v-chip to block programs according to these ratings. The law requires all new television sets with screens 13" or larger that were made in the United States after January 1, 2000, to have the v-chip.

The ratings apply to all TV programs except news and sports. They appear for 15 seconds at the start of a program. When the rating appears on the screen, an electronic signal sends the rating to the v-chip in your television set.

The ratings are as follows:

TV-Y   **For all children**

TV-Y7   **For children age 7 and older.** The program may contain mild violence that could frighten children younger than age 7.

TV-Y7-FV   **For children age 7 and older.** The program contains fantasy violence that is glorified and used as an acceptable, effective way to solve a problem. It is more intense than TV-Y7.

TV-G   **For general audience.** Most parents would find this program suitable for all ages. There is little or no violence, no strong language, and little or no sexual content.

TV-PG   **Parental guidance is suggested.** Parents may find some material unsuitable for younger children. It may contain moderate violence, some sexual content, or strong language.

TV-14   **Parents are strongly cautioned.** The program contains some material that many parents would find unsuitable for children younger than age 14. It contains intense violence, sexual content, or strong language.

TV-MA   **For mature audience.** The program may not be suitable for children younger than age 17. It contains graphic violence, explicit sexual activity, or crude language.

Additional letters may be added to the ratings to indicate violence (V), sexual content (S), strong language (L), or suggestive dialogue (D).

This ratings system was created to help parents choose programs that are suitable for children, even without the use of the v-chip. The ratings are usually included in local TV listings. Before watching, check your local TV listings to find out if a program contains violence, sexual content, or strong language. Remember that ratings are not used for news programs, which may not be suitable for young children. Also, TVs with screens smaller than 13" will not have the v-chip.

More information is available at the following Web sites:
- www.fcc.gov/vchip
- www.vchipeducation.org

8. **Set a good example**
   You are the most important role model in your child's life. Limiting your own TV viewing and choosing programs carefully will help your child do the same.

The Children's Television Act of 1990

The Children's Television Act ensures that TV stations pay attention to the needs of children from age 2 to 16. Under this law, stations must air at least 3 hours of educational and informational shows for children each week. They must also limit advertising during children's shows to 12 minutes per hour on weekdays and 10.5 minutes per hour on weekends. Stations that do not follow the law risk losing their license.

Keep tabs on TV stations in your community. TV stations file quarterly Children's Television Programming Reports with the Federal Communications Commission (FCC). You can access these reports on the FCC's Web site at svartifoss2.fcc.gov/prod/kidvid/prod/kidvid.htm

You can also file complaints with the FCC. More information is available at

Federal Communications Commission
Consumer Information Bureau
Consumer Complaints
445 12th St SW
Washington, DC 20554
Phone: 888/225-5322 (toll-free)
Fax: 202/418-0232
www.fcc.gov/cib

Toppling TVs pose a hazard

Newer televisions with larger, heavier screens in smaller casings can present a danger to toddlers. Small children are being seriously injured and, in some cases, killed when these front-heavy models fall on them. More than 2,000 children end up in the emergency room each year due to injuries from falling televisions, according to the US Consumer Product Safety Commission.

The following safety tips can be used to prevent such injuries:

- Place your television set on low furniture that is the proper size and is designed to support your TV model.
- Use braces or anchors to secure televisions and supporting furniture to the wall.
- Do not place remote controls, videos, or other objects that children might try to reach on top of the television.
- Do not allow children to play with or climb on the television set.

You can also help by encouraging manufacturers to design models that are more stable and to provide methods for tethering TVs to the wall.

---

9. Express your views

When you like or do not like something you see on television, make yourself heard. Write to the TV station, network, or the program's sponsor. Stations, networks, and sponsors pay attention to letters from the public. If you think a commercial is misleading, write down the product name, channel, and time you saw the commercial and describe your concerns. Call your local Better Business Bureau if the commercial is for a local business or product. For national advertising, send the information to

Children's Advertising Review Unit
Council of Better Business Bureau
845 Third Ave
New York, NY 10022

Encourage publishers of TV guides to print ratings and feature articles about shows that are educational for children.

10. Get more information

The following people and places can provide you with more information about the proper role of TV in your child's life:

- **Your pediatrician** may have information about TV or can help you get it through the AAP. Information from the AAP is also available on the Internet at www.aap.org.
- **Public service groups** publish newsletters that review programs and give tips on how to make TV a positive experience for you and your child.
- **The parent organization at your child's school.**

- **Parents of your child's friends and classmates** can also be helpful. Talk with other parents and agree to enforce similar rules about TV viewing.

When used properly, television can inform, educate, and entertain you and your family. By taking an active role in your child's viewing, you can help make watching TV a positive and healthy experience.

Please note: Listing of resources does not imply endorsement by the American Academy of Pediatrics (AAP). The AAP is not responsible for the content of the resources mentioned in this brochure. Phone numbers, addresses, and Web site addresses are as current as possible, but may change at any time.

The information contained in this publication should not be used as a substitute for the medical care and advice of your pediatrician. There may be variations in treatment that your pediatrician may recommend based on individual facts and circumstances.

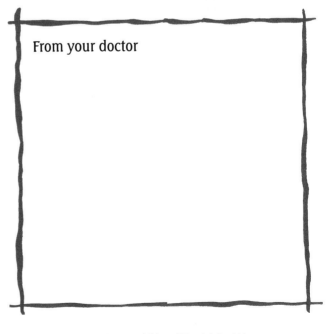

From your doctor

**American Academy
of Pediatrics**

DEDICATED TO THE HEALTH OF ALL CHILDREN™

The American Academy of Pediatrics is an organization of 60,000 primary care pediatricians, pediatric medical subspecialists, and pediatric surgical specialists dedicated to the health, safety, and well-being of infants, children, adolescents, and young adults.

American Academy of Pediatrics
Web site—www.aap.org

Copyright © 1991
American Academy of Pediatrics, Updated 12/01

Temper Tantrums:
A NORMAL PART OF GROWING UP

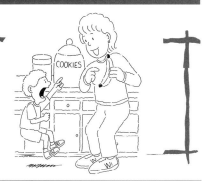

Strong emotions are hard for a young child to hold inside. When children feel frustrated, angry, or disappointed, they often express themselves by crying, screaming, or stomping up and down. As a parent, you may feel angry, helpless, or embarrassed. Temper tantrums are a normal part of your child's development as he learns self-control. In fact, almost all children have tantrums between the ages of 1 and 3. You've heard them called "the terrible twos." The good news is that by age 4, temper tantrums usually stop.

Why do children have tantrums?

Your young child is busy learning many things about her world. She is eager to take control. She wants to be independent and may try to do more than her skills will allow. She wants to make her own choices and often may not cope well with not getting her way. She is even less able to cope when she is tired, hungry, frustrated, or frightened. Controlling her temper may be one of the most difficult lessons to learn.

Temper tantrums are a way for your child to let off steam when she is upset. Following are some of the reasons your child may have a temper tantrum:

- Your child may not fully understand what you are saying or asking, and may get confused.
- Your child may become upset when others cannot understand what she is saying.
- Your child may not have the words to describe her feelings and needs. After 3 years of age, most children can express their feelings, so temper tantrums taper off. Children who are not able to express their feelings very well with words are more likely to continue to have tantrums.
- Your child has not yet learned to solve problems on her own and gets discouraged easily.
- Your child may have an illness or other physical problem that keeps her from expressing how she feels.
- Your child may be hungry, but may not recognize it.
- Your child may be tired or not getting enough sleep.
- Your child may be anxious or uncomfortable.
- Your child may be reacting to stress or changes at home.
- Your child may be jealous of a friend or sibling. Children often want what other children have or the attention they receive.
- Your child may not yet be able to do the things she can imagine, such as walking or running, climbing down stairs or from furniture, drawing things, or making toys work.

How to help prevent temper tantrums

As a parent, you can sometimes tell when tantrums are coming. Your child may seem moody, cranky, or difficult. He may start to whine and whimper. It may seem as if nothing will make him happy. Finally, he may start to cry, kick, scream, fall to the ground, or hold his breath. Other times, a tantrum may come on suddenly for no obvious reason. You should not be surprised if your child has tantrums only in front of you. This is one way of testing your rules and

A word about...safety

Many times, you will have to tell your child "no" to protect her from harm or injury. For example, the kitchen and bathroom can be hazardous places for your child. Your child will have trouble understanding why you will not let her play there. This is a common cause of a tantrum. "Childproof" your home and make dangerous areas or objects off-limits.

Keep an eye on your child at all times. After telling your child "no," never leave her alone in a situation that could be hazardous. Take away dangerous objects from your child immediately and replace them with something safe. It is up to you to keep your child safe and teach her how to protect herself from getting hurt. Be consistent and clear about safety.

limits. Many children will not act out their feelings around others and are more cautious with strangers. Children feel safer showing their feelings to the people they trust.

You will not be able to prevent all tantrums, but the following suggestions may help reduce the chances of a tantrum:

- **Encourage your child to use words** to tell you how he is feeling, such as "I'm really mad." Try to understand how he is feeling and suggest words he can use to describe his feelings.
- **Set reasonable limits** and don't expect your child to be perfect. Give simple reasons for the rules you set, and don't change the rules.
- **Keep a daily routine** as much as possible, so your child knows what to expect.
- **Avoid situations that will frustrate your child,** such as playing with children or toys that are too advanced for your child's abilities.
- **Avoid long outings or visits** where your child has to sit still or cannot play for long periods of time. If you have to take a trip, bring along your child's favorite book or toy to entertain him.
- **Be prepared with healthy snacks when your child gets hungry.**
- **Make sure your child is well rested,** especially before a busy day or stressful activity.
- **Distract your child** from activities likely to lead to a tantrum. Suggest different activities. If possible, being silly, playful, or making a joke can help ease a tense situation. Sometimes, something as simple as changing locations can prevent a tantrum. For example, if you are indoors, try taking your child outside to distract his attention.
- **Be choosy about saying "no."** When you say no to every demand or request your child makes, it will frustrate him. Listen carefully to requests. When a request is not too unreasonable or inconvenient, consider saying yes. When your child's safety is involved, do not change your decision because of a tantrum.

- **Let your child choose whenever possible.** For example, if your child resists a bath, make it clear that he will be taking a bath, but offer a simple decision he can make on his own. Instead of saying, "Do you want to take a bath?" Try saying, "It's time for your bath. Would you like to walk upstairs or have me carry you?"
- **Set a good example.** Avoid arguing or yelling in front of your child.

What to do when tantrums occur

When your child has a temper tantrum, follow the suggestions listed below:

1. Distract your child by calling his attention to something else, such as a new activity, book, or toy. Sometimes just touching or stroking a child will calm him. You may need to gently restrain or hold your child. Interrupt his behavior with a light comment like, "Did you see what the kitty is doing?" or "I think I heard the doorbell." Humor or something as simple as a funny face can also help.
2. Try to remain calm. If you shout or become angry, it is likely to make things worse. Remember, the more attention you give this behavior, the more likely it is to happen again.
3. Minor displays of anger such as crying, screaming, or kicking can usually be ignored. Stand nearby or hold your child without talking until he calms down. This shows your support. If you cannot stay calm, leave the room.
4. Some temper tantrums cannot be ignored. The following behaviors should not be ignored and are *not* acceptable:
   - Hitting or kicking parents or others
   - Throwing things in a dangerous way
   - Prolonged screaming or yelling

   Use a cooling-off period or a "time-out" to remove your child from the source of his anger. Take your child away from the situation and hold him or give him some time alone to calm down and regain control. For children old enough to understand, a good rule of thumb for a time-out is 1 minute of time for every year of your child's age. (For example, a 4 year old would get a 4-minute time-out.) But even 15 seconds will work. If you cannot stay calm, leave the room. Wait a minute or two, or until his crying stops, before returning. Then help him get interested in something else. If your child is old enough, talk about what happened and discuss other ways to deal with it next time.

   For more information, ask your pediatrician about the American Academy of Pediatrics brochure *Discipline and Your Child*.

   You should never punish your child for temper tantrums. He may start to keep his anger or frustration inside, which can be unhealthy. Your response to tantrums should be calm and understanding. As your child grows, he will learn to deal with his strong emotions. Remember, it is normal for children to test their parents' rules and limits.

Do not give in by offering rewards

Do not reward your child for stopping a tantrum. Rewards may teach your child that a temper tantrum will help her get her way. When tantrums do not accomplish anything for your child, they are less likely to continue.

You may also feel guilty about saying "no" to your child at times. Be consistent and avoid sending mixed signals. When parents don't clearly enforce certain rules, it is harder for children to understand which rules are firm and which ones are not. Be sure you are having some fun each day with your child. Think carefully about the rules you set and don't set too many. Discuss with those who care for your child which rules are really needed and be firm about them. Respond the same way every time your child breaks the rules.

When temper tantrums are serious

Your child should have fewer temper tantrums by the middle of his fourth year. Between tantrums, his behavior should seem normal and healthy. Like every child, yours will grow and learn at his own pace. It may take time for him to learn how to control his temper. When the outbursts are severe or happen too often, they may be an early sign of emotional problems. Talk to your pediatrician if your child causes harm to himself or others during tantrums, holds his breath and faints, or if the tantrums get worse after age 4. Your pediatrician will make sure there are no serious physical or psychological problems causing the tantrums. He or she can also give you advice to help you deal with these outbursts.

It is important to realize that temper tantrums are a normal part of growing up. Tantrums are not easy to deal with, and they can be a little scary for you and your child. Using a loving and understanding approach will help your child through this part of his development.

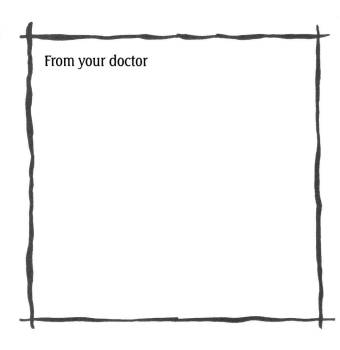

From your doctor

American Academy
of Pediatrics

DEDICATED TO THE HEALTH OF ALL CHILDREN™

The American Academy of Pediatrics is an organization of 60,000 primary care pediatricians, pediatric medical subspecialists, and pediatric surgical specialists dedicated to the health, safety, and well-being of infants, children, adolescents, and young adults.

American Academy of Pediatrics
Web site—www.aap.org

Copyright © 1989
American Academy of Pediatrics, Updated 3/99

SECTION EIGHT

Sexual Health and Sexuality

Breast Self-Exam

Once a month, right after your period, you should examine your breasts. Although breast cancer is rare in young women, it usually can be cured if found early, and a breast self-exam is the best way to find it.

Do the following to examine your breasts:

1. Stand in front of your mirror with your arms at your sides and see if there are any changes in the size or shape of your breasts. Look for any puckers or dimples, and press each nipple to see if any fluid comes out. Raise your arm above your head and look for changes in your breasts from this position.

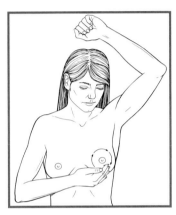

2. Lie down and place a towel or pillow under your right shoulder. Place your right hand under your head. Hold your left hand flat and feel your right breast with little, pressing circles. Think of each breast as a pie divided into 4 pieces. Feel each piece and then feel the center of the "pie" (the nipple area).

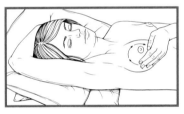

3. Now put your right arm down at your side, and do the same thing on the outside of the breast, starting under the armpit.
4. Repeat steps 2 and 3 for the other breast.

Most women have some lumpiness or texture to their breasts; breasts are not just soft tissue. Get to know your breasts, then be alert for any lumps or other changes should they ever appear. Remember, most lumps and changes are not cancerous. However, if you think you have found a lump or notice any other changes, don't press or squeeze it; see your pediatrician.

The information contained in this publication should not be used as a substitute for the medical care and advice of your pediatrician. There may be variations in treatment that your pediatrician may recommend based on individual facts and circumstances.

Illustrations by Lauren Shavell

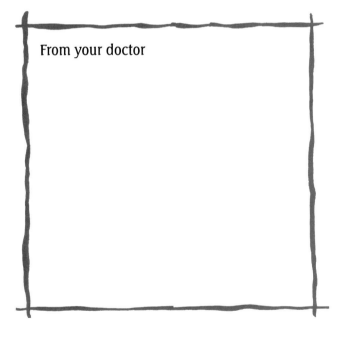

From your doctor

American Academy of Pediatrics

DEDICATED TO THE HEALTH OF ALL CHILDREN™

The American Academy of Pediatrics is an organization of 60,000 primary care pediatricians, pediatric medical subspecialists, and pediatric surgical specialists dedicated to the health, safety, and well-being of infants, children, adolescents, and young adults.

American Academy of Pediatrics
Web site — www.aap.org

Copyright © 1999
American Academy of Pediatrics

emergency contraception

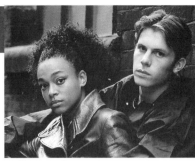

If you have had sex in the last 5 days

- Did you or your partner **use any form of birth control** to prevent pregnancy? If no, there's a chance you could get pregnant.
- If you and your partner used a condom as your only method of birth control, did it `rip or slip` during sex? If yes, there's a chance you could get pregnant.
- If you did use a method of birth control (birth control pills and condoms) to prevent pregnancy, **did you use it correctly?** If no, there's a chance you could get pregnant.

You could be at risk of getting pregnant if...

1. You had unprotected intercourse in the last 5 days.

   OR

2. You had a problem with or concern about how well your birth control method might have worked. For example,
   - You **did not plan to** have sex and used nothing to prevent pregnancy.
   - You were **forced to have sex** and nothing was used to prevent pregnancy.
   - You used a **condom but it broke** or slipped during sex and nothing else was used to prevent pregnancy.
   - You're taking **birth control pills** but *missed* taking 2 or more pills in a row and you had unprotected sex.
   - You're using the **birth control patch** but it was *off for more than 24 hours* during the 3 weeks when it was supposed to be on your skin and you had unprotected sex.
   - You're using the **birth control ring** but took it *out for more than 3 hours* during the 3 weeks when it was supposed to be in your vagina and you had unprotected sex.
   - You're using the `Depo-Provera shot` but it has been **more than 2 weeks** since you should have gotten your next shot and you had unprotected sex.

Remember, **"withdrawal"** of the penis **does not work** to prevent pregnancy.

What is emergency contraception?

Emergency contraception is a **type of birth control** used to prevent pregnancy after unprotected sex.

How do the pills work?

Emergency contraception pills can prevent
- An egg from being released from the ovary (ovulation). This is the main way it works.

Emergency contraception pills may also prevent
- An egg from being fertilized by the sperm (fertilization)
- A fertilized egg from attaching itself to the wall of the uterus (implantation)

Emergency contraception pills are NOT the same as RU-486 or Mifepristone, also called the abortion pill.
- Emergency contraception pills use the same hormones as regular birth control pills.
- If you're already pregnant and take emergency contraception pills, they won't cause a miscarriage or abortion.
- If you've taken emergency contraception but find out later that you were already pregnant, the pills won't cause birth defects if you continue the pregnancy.
- Emergency contraception pills do not prevent sexually transmitted diseases (STDs).

What types of pills can I take?

Your pediatrician may prescribe one of the following:
- **Plan B® progestin-only pills.** These pills are specifically made for emergency contraception. Call the pharmacy before you go to see if they have the medicine in stock, what the cost is, and if the pills are covered by your insurance.
- **Special dose of regular birth control pills.** These pills can have the same effects as emergency contraception pills if taken as your pediatrician tells you.

Pills need to be taken within 5 days of unprotected sexual intercourse. Take them as soon as possible after unprotected sex.
- **Plan B progestin-only pills**—Take both pills at one time.
- **Special dose of regular birth control pills**—Take each dose 12 hours apart. *You may also want to take medicine that prevents nausea before you take the special dose of pills.* The pills work about 80% of the time to prevent pregnancy if taken around the time of ovulation. They won't work if you're already pregnant.

Some people have nicknamed emergency contraception pills the "morning after pill," but this information is wrong. There's more than 1 pill and the pills are not always taken the morning after. They can be taken up to 5 days after unprotected sex. However, the sooner you take them, the better they work.

Are the pills safe?

Emergency contraception pills are `safe` but as with all medicines **there can be side effects. Nausea** and **vomiting** may occur but are less likely with the Plan B progestin-only pill. Other side effects include *fatigue, tender breasts, headache, stomach pain, and dizziness.* These side effects usually last less than 24 hours. You may **notice changes in your next period.** Your period may come earlier or later, or be lighter or heavier than you're used to. The pills won't hurt your ability to get pregnant in the future. Because the pills won't protect you from getting pregnant the next time you have sex, you must still use your usual form of birth control.

Call your pediatrician if you vomit within 30 to 60 minutes after taking the pills, or if you have any other concerns. It is critical to call your pediatrician for an appointment within 2 weeks after taking emergency contraception. At the visit you can get a pregnancy test to make sure you did not get pregnant and a test for STDs.

Remember

If you're going to have sex…

- ***Talk with your pediatrician about which type of regular birth control is best for you.*** The choice to become sexually active is yours. Choosing not to have sex is the only way to avoid all STDs and avoid getting pregnant. Emergency contraception pills shouldn't be your regular form of birth control. However, you may want to have them on-hand just in case you need them to prevent pregnancy.

- **Always use a condom to reduce the risk of getting an STD.** Condoms work best when they are used the right way. No other form of birth control, including emergency contraception, can protect you from getting an STD.

- **Make sure that you are checked for an STD.** If you had unprotected sex, not only can you become pregnant, you could also get an STD. Often a simple urine test can screen for STDs.

- **Don't be afraid to say NO if you've changed your mind and don't want to have sex.** It's best to stay away from situations that can lead to sex when you don't feel ready. Drinking alcohol and using drugs may lead to you having sex when you don't mean to. It's never OK for someone to pressure you to have sex.

Where can I find more information?

Always feel free to share your concerns and questions with your pediatrician. If you'd like to do some reading on your own, you may want to contact one of the following sources:

The American College of Obstetricians and Gynecologists
www.acog.org

DuraMed Pharmaceuticals
800/330-1271
www.go2planB.com

Emergency Contraception Hot Line
888/NOT-2-LATE

Emergency Contraception Web Site
http://ec.princeton.edu

International Consortium for Emergency Contraception
www.cecinfo.org

Managing Contraception
www.managingcontraception.com

The National Women's Health Information Center
800/994-WOMAN (800/994-9662)
www.4woman.gov

Planned Parenthood
www.plannedparenthood.org

Please note: Inclusion on this list does not imply endorsement by the American Academy of Pediatrics (AAP). The AAP is not responsible for the content of the resources mentioned in this brochure. Phone numbers and Web site addresses are as current as possible, but may change at any time.

Note: Products are mentioned for informational purposes only and do not imply endorsement by the AAP.

The information contained in this publication should not be used as a substitute for the medical care and advice of your pediatrician. There may be variations in treatment that your pediatrician may recommend based on individual facts and circumstances.

The persons whose photographs are depicted in this publication are professional models. They have no relation to the issues discussed. Any characters they are portraying are fiictional.

From your doctor

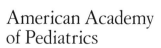

American Academy of Pediatrics

DEDICATED TO THE HEALTH OF ALL CHILDREN™

The American Academy of Pediatrics is an organization of 60,000 primary care pediatricians, pediatric medical subspecialists, and pediatric surgical specialists dedicated to the health, safety, and well-being of infants, children, adolescents, and young adults.

American Academy of Pediatrics
Web site—www.aap.org

Copyright © 2005
American Academy of Pediatrics

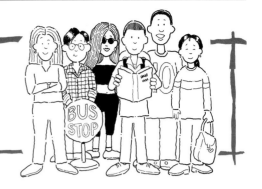

Gay, Lesbian, and Bisexual Teens:
Facts for Teens and Their Parents

The teenage years are filled with new experiences, changes, and a growing sense of who you are. But for teenagers who feel "different" from their peers, these years can be confusing, frustrating, and even scary.

It is important for everyone to understand more about the diversity in people's sexual orientation. If you are a teenager, this brochure provides information to help as you discover more about yourself, your friends, and your place in the world. There also is information that may help your parents understand you better.

"Am I gay?"

Many gay and lesbian adults remember their late childhood or early teenage years as the time when they first began to wonder about their sexual orientation. Unfortunately, because we live in a society that is not always accepting of gay, lesbian, and bisexual people, dealing with the possibility that they may be gay can be a very difficult thing for teens.

How do you know if you are gay? Many young people go through an anxious stage during which they wonder, "Am I gay?" It is normal to feel this way as your sexual identity is taking shape. Maybe you feel attracted to someone of the same gender or you have had some same-sex activity. This is normal and does not necessarily mean that you are gay, lesbian, or bisexual.

Sexual *behavior* is not always the same as sexual *orientation*. Many people have had same-sex experiences but do not consider themselves gay, lesbian, or bisexual. Others call themselves gay without having had any sexual experience.

Sexual orientation develops as you grow and experience new things. It may take time to figure it all out. Do not worry if you are not sure. If over time you find you feel romantic attraction to members of the same sex, and these feelings continue to grow stronger as you get older, you probably are gay or bisexual. It is not a bad thing, it is just who you are.

Definitions

Gay (or *homosexual*): People who have sexual and/or romantic feelings for people of the same gender. Men are attracted to men and women are attracted to women.

Lesbian: Gay woman.

Straight (or *heterosexual*): People who have sexual and/or romantic feelings for people of the opposite gender. Men are attracted to women and women are attracted to men.

Bisexual (or *bi*): People who have sexual and/or romantic feelings for both men and women.

Sexual orientation: How an individual is physically and emotionally attracted to other males and females.

You are not alone

Some estimates say that about 10% of the population is gay. You cannot tell by looking at people whether they are gay. Gay people are all shapes, sizes, and ages. They have many types of racial and ethnic backgrounds.

Pay no attention to stereotypes. Just because a boy has some feminine qualities or a girl acts somewhat masculine does not mean that he or she is gay. Most gay males and females look and act just like their straight peers.

"Am I normal?"

First, homosexuality is not a mental disorder. The American Psychiatric Association confirmed this in 1974. The American Psychological Association and the American Academy of Pediatrics agree that homosexuality is not an illness or disorder, but a form of sexual expression.

No one knows what causes a person to be gay, bisexual, or straight. There probably are a number of factors. Some may be biological. Others may be psychological. The reasons can vary from one person to another. The fact is, you do not choose to be gay, bisexual, or straight.

Talking about it

Most people find that it is hard to start talking about their sexual feelings and attractions, but in the long run it feels better if you do not keep these important feelings a secret. You do not have to *know* that you are lesbian, gay, or bisexual before you talk to people about your feelings. Remember that the process of sharing what you are feeling is different for every person. Start with people you trust the most. This may include the following:

- Close friends
- Gay, lesbian, or bisexual friends
- Parents
- Close family members
- Your pediatrician
- A teacher, school counselor, coach, or other adult mentor
- A minister, priest, rabbi, or spiritual advisor
- A local gay, lesbian, and bisexual support group

The important thing is to find someone you trust with whom you can talk about your thoughts and worries.

Coming out

Because of the negative feelings some people have about homosexuality, "coming out of the closet," or revealing your sexual orientation, can be difficult. Some people wrestle with revealing their identity for years before finally deciding to do so. Others keep their sexual orientation a secret for their entire lives.

Talk to other gay friends about their "coming out" experiences. This may help you know what to expect. Gay youth organizations also can be a great source of support. See the end of this brochure for a list of such groups.

If you do know that you are gay, lesbian, or bisexual, do not feel pressured to "come out" before you are ready. On the other hand, keeping your identity a secret can be a burden. It is up to you to decide the best time to share your sexual orientation with your family and friends.

Telling your family and friends that you are gay probably will not be easy. Your family may respond well. But most parents picture a traditional future for their child. News that their child is gay may require them to rethink a whole new future.

Choose a good time and place to tell your family. If this information comes out during a family conflict or crisis, it may be even harder for your parents to accept it.

Be prepared for a variety of reactions including shock, denial, anger, guilt, sadness, and even rejection. Remember, you have had time to accept your identity. Give your family and friends time, too. Keep in mind that you can help them by being open, honest, and patient.

Often family and friends will be relieved that you have helped them to understand you better. Whether right away, or after some time, they may be happy to help you sort out your sexual orientation and how it affects your life.

Health concerns for gay and lesbian youth

Gay, lesbian, and bisexual teens are not the only ones who need to be concerned about their health. All teens need to be aware of what can happen if they are sexually active, use drugs, or engage in other risky behaviors.

Sexual activity: You do not have to have sex to be aware of your sexual identity. Most teenagers, whether they are gay, lesbian, bisexual, or straight, are not sexually active. In fact, not having sex is the *only* way to protect yourself completely against sexually transmitted diseases (STDs). But if you choose to have sex, make sure you know the risks and how to protect yourself.

- Gay and bisexual males must be particularly careful and always use latex condoms. Using condoms is the only way to protect against human immunodeficiency virus (HIV)/acquired immune deficiency syndrome (AIDS) and many other diseases that are spread during anal, vaginal, or oral intercourse. Condoms also help to prevent pregnancy during vaginal intercourse.
- Lesbians and bisexual females also must *always* use protection such as latex dental dams and condoms to avoid sexually transmitted diseases and unplanned pregnancies.
- Avoid risky sexual practices like using alcohol and drugs before or during sex, having unknown sexual partners, or having sex in unfamiliar or public places.
- Regular health examinations are crucial. Ask your pediatrician if you have questions or concerns about STDs or other health issues.
- Make sure all of your immunizations are up-to-date. Check that you have had three doses of the hepatitis B vaccine. Hepatitis B is a virus that can make you very sick. It can be spread through contact with infected blood or other body fluids. This can happen during sexual intercourse or when drug users share needles.

Substance use: Being a gay or lesbian teen in our society can be very difficult. Avoid using drugs or alcohol to relieve depression, anxiety, and low self-esteem. Doing so can lead to addiction.

In many communities, bars are popular places for gay and lesbian people to socialize. This increases the pressure to drink and use other drugs. Drug and alcohol use can lead to unsafe sex. Adopt a drug-free lifestyle and look for other ways to socialize and meet new people.

Mental health: Isolation, peer rejection, ridicule, harassment, depression, and thoughts of suicide — any teen may feel these things at some time. However, gay and lesbian youth are more than twice as likely to attempt suicide than straight teenagers. About 30% of those who try to kill themselves actually die.

A message to parents: when your teenager is gay, lesbian, or bisexual

Each year some parents learn that their son or daughter is gay, lesbian, or bisexual. This news is sometimes difficult. Most parents dream that their child's future will include a traditional marriage and grandchildren. Keep in mind that your son or daughter still can find lifelong companionship and become a parent.

Parents also often have to deal with their own guilt. They may ask themselves questions like, "Did I do anything to cause this?" "Should we have done something differently when he was a child?" "Is it my fault?" Questions like these are common, but do not help.

Rejecting your child also is not a good response. When gay, lesbian, and bisexual teens make their sexual orientation known, some families reject them. Perhaps that is how you think you would react. But that is the wrong response. It may be very difficult for your teenager to come to terms with her or his sexuality. Your child may find it devastating if you reject her or him at the same time. Your child needs you very much!

So take a deep breath and think. Take a little time to come to grips with your child's sexual orientation. You may need to readjust your dreams for your child's future. You may have to deal with your own negative stereotypes of gay, lesbian, and bisexual people. But you must not reject your teenager for his or her sexual orientation. He or she is still your child and needs your love and support.

Many parents find that it helps to talk to other parents whose children are lesbian, gay, or bisexual. Check the end of this brochure for information about support groups for parents.

Your teenager did not choose to be gay, lesbian, or bisexual. Accept her or him and be there to help with any problems that arise. Your pediatrician may be able to help you with this new challenge or suggest a referral for counseling.

Gay and lesbian youth who fear rejection or discovery may not know whom to turn to for support. Try your pediatrician, parents, a trusted teacher, or a counselor. Members of the gay, lesbian, and bisexual community, or gay and lesbian youth groups, also can be helpful. They can be a real source of support and a place to find healthy role models.

Counseling may be helpful for you if you feel confused about your sexual identity. Avoid any treatments that claim to be able to change a person's sexual orientation, or treatment ideas that see homosexuality as a sickness.

Discrimination and violence: Gay and lesbian youth are at high risk for becoming victims of violence. Studies have found that 30% to 70% of gay youth have experienced verbal or physical assaults in school. They also may be called names, harassed by others, or rejected by friends and family.

There are things you can do to avoid becoming a victim of violence, especially at school.

- Talk to a trusted school counselor, administrator, or teacher about any harassment or violence you have experienced at school. You have the right to attend a safe school that is free from discrimination, harassment, violence, and abuse.
- Get involved in gay/straight alliances at your school (or help form one). These groups can help promote better understanding between gay, lesbian, and bisexual youth, and other students and teachers.
- Join a gay youth support group in your community.
- Encourage your parents to join a support group for parents and family members of gay and lesbian teenagers.

Resources

Hetrick-Martin Institute for the Protection of Gay and Lesbian Youth
2 Astor Pl
New York, NY 10003
212/674-2400
www.hmi.org

Lambda Youth OUTreach
www.lambda.org

National Gay and Lesbian Task Force
1700 Kalorama Rd NW
Washington, DC 20009-2624
202/332-6483
www.ngltf.org

National Youth Advocacy Coalition
1638 R St NW
Suite 300
Washington, DC 20009
202/319-7596
Fax: 202/319-7365
www.nyacyouth.org

OutProud, the National Coalition for Gay, Lesbian, Bisexual and
   Transgender Youth
369 Third St
Suite B-362
San Rafael, CA 94901-3581
www.outproud.org

Parents, Families and Friends of Lesbiansand Gays (PFLAG)
1726 M St NW
Suite 400
Washington, DC 20036
202/467-8180
www.pflag.org

Youth Guardian Services, Inc
8665 Sudley Rd
#304
Manassas, VA 20110-4588
877/270-5152
www.youth-guard.org

Youth Resource
A Project of Advocates for Youth
1025 Vermont Ave NW
Suite 200
Washington, DC 20005
202/347–5700
www.youthresource.com

The information contained in this publication should not be used as a substitute for the medical care and advice of your pediatrician. There may be variations in treatment that your pediatrician may recommend based on individual facts and circumstances.

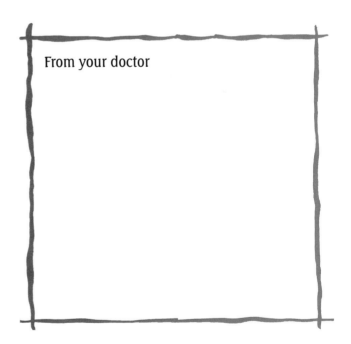

From your doctor

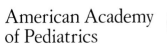

American Academy
of Pediatrics

DEDICATED TO THE HEALTH OF ALL CHILDREN™

The American Academy of Pediatrics is an organization of 60,000 primary care pediatricians, pediatric medical subspecialists, and pediatric surgical specialists dedicated to the health, safety, and well-being of infants, children, adolescents, and young adults.
American Academy of Pediatrics
Web site — www.aap.org

Gay, Lesbian, or Bisexual Parents:
Information for Children and Parents

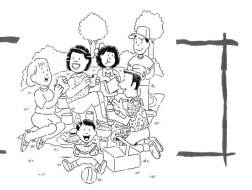

Millions of children have one or more gay and/or lesbian parents. For some children, having a gay or lesbian parent is not a big deal. Others may find it hard to have a family that is different from most families. Being different in any way can be confusing, frustrating, and even scary. But what really matters is that children can talk to their parents about how they feel and that there is love and support in the family.

The following are answers to some common questions from children (first part) and parents (second part). If you know someone who has a lesbian or gay parent (or 2 parents), you might be interested in reading this too.

Questions from children

Q: Why do some people think having homosexual parents is wrong?

A: Many years ago homosexuality was considered to be an illness. Despite the fact that a lot of research shows that this isn't true, some people still think that there is something wrong with being homosexual. Because of these beliefs, gay and lesbian parents and their children often face disapproval and stress. They may have less support from family and friends than heterosexual parents do.

Q: What if other people don't understand?

A: In almost every way your family is just like your friends' families. But not everyone will accept your parents' sexual orientation. People may tease or judge you because of it. Though your parents did not choose to be gay, they did choose to have a family and love their children. Some people may not accept this, even people you expect to be tolerant and accepting. It's OK if you don't want to talk about having gay parents or answer people's questions. Remember, you don't have to accept other people's opinions about your family. Many people will respect and support you and your family.

Nevertheless, it can be hard for you when others think badly about your parents or tease you about your family. This is why it's important to talk with your parents about how you feel. You also may find it helpful to talk with other adults. Focus on the positive things people say. Spend time with friends who accept you as you are, and who respect your parents for who they are.

Q: If my parents are gay or lesbian does that mean that I will be too?

A: Many people worry that children whose parents are homosexual won't have a chance to learn about heterosexual relationships. Research has shown that although children and teens whose parents are gay or lesbian know about what it's like to be homosexual, most of them discover that they are heterosexual.

Definitions

Sexual orientation: Whether a person is attracted to a person of the same sex or a different sex. For example,

Straight (or heterosexual): People who have sexual and/or romantic feelings for people of the opposite sex. Men are attracted to women and women are attracted to men.

Gay (or homosexual): People who have sexual and/or romantic feelings for people of the same sex. Men are attracted to men and women are attracted to women.

Lesbian: Gay woman.

Bisexual (or bi): People who have sexual and/or romantic feelings for both men and women.

Q: What should I tell people if they ask me about my parents?

A: Talk with your parents about what they would like you to tell people about them. They can help you think about how to answer questions from friends, teachers, and other people in your community. Think about who you want to talk to and what you would like to tell people about your family and your parents' sexual orientation. Like any other personal topic, you can choose to discuss your family with whomever you want.

Questions from parents

Q: When and how should I "come out" to my children?

A: The "right" time depends on when you and your child are ready. Each child is different and may understand things at different times. Some children may be surprised, confused, or even angry when you tell them about your sexual orientation; others may be relieved to understand you better. Some studies have suggested that children who were told that their parents were gay, lesbian, or bisexual early in childhood found the news easier to accept than those who were first told when they were teens. More research needs to be done in this area. In general, open and honest communication is important. There are many books written to help parents teach children about sexual orientation and family diversity.

Keep in mind that children may be teased or criticized by others about your sexual orientation, and may even get critical comments from your divorced spouse or other family members. It is important to be as open as possible with your children. Let them know that even though your family is different in some ways from other families, there are many ways in which your family is just like any other family, and you love them just the same.

Q: How will my child(ren) be affected?

A: Studies have shown that children with gay and/or lesbian parents are ultimately just as happy with themselves and their own gender as are their friends with heterosexual parents. Children whose parents are homosexual show no difference in their choice of friends, activities, or interests compared to children whose parents are heterosexual. As adults, their career choices and lifestyles are similar to those of children raised by heterosexual parents.

Research comparing children raised by homosexual parents to children raised by heterosexual parents has found no developmental differences in intelligence, psychological adjustment, social adjustment, or peer popularity between them. Children raised by homosexual parents can and do have fulfilling relationships with their friends as well as romantic relationships later on.

Q: What questions and concerns should I expect?

A: Your children will probably have different concerns and questions depending on their age, personality, and your family's decisions. For example, all children whose parents have separated or divorced need to know that the separation was not their fault, and that both parents will continue to love and care for them. Children and teens may be interested in the implications for them of whether their same-sex parents are married or united in a civil union.

Children are interested in and affected by their parents' thoughts, feelings, and decisions. It's important that you answer your children's questions as honestly as you can, being sensitive to their developmental needs at the different stages in their lives.

- **Preschool-aged children** often are very curious about their family background, so they may ask many questions about a mother or a father whom they don't know or who isn't always around. It's best to answer their questions simply and honestly. Expect more questions as new ideas occur to your child.
- **School-aged children** will become more aware that their family is different and may want to know about their family background. They may think of new questions as they meet other children from different family backgrounds.
- **Young and older teens** are aware that they are different. Some teens who didn't care before may become self-conscious and even embarrassed about their parents. Some teens may become concerned about their own sexual orientation but may be reluctant to talk with others for fear of being teased or criticized. This may be a good time to talk more about your sexual orientation and life choices.

Q: What can I do to support my children?

A: The following are ways all parents can support their children:
- **Show unconditional love.** Reassure your children that no matter what, you will always love them.
- **Have fun together.** Find activities that you all enjoy, and be sure to save time for your children.
- **Talk with your children.** Be open and honest with your children. This is the most important thing. Let them know that even though your family might be different from other families in some ways, there are many ways your family is similar to others. Remind them that all families have problems and disagreements. One way to strengthen your family bond

is to find positive ways to talk to each other and to work together to deal with problems.
- **Teach your children.** Use books, Web sites, and other materials to help your children learn that there are other families like your family. Encourage your children to tell you if they are teased or left out because of your homosexuality. Use such experiences to teach your children about understanding and valuing differences among people, and about how to cope with people who may not approve.
- **Teach the schools.** Work with your children's schools to make sure that family diversity is talked about and valued. Suggest books that should be available in the library that describe families like yours.
- **Find other families like yours.** Your children may benefit from meeting other children who have gay or lesbian parents. You might find a local group of families, or your children might be interested in joining an e-mail list or finding a pen pal.

Resources

You may wish to contact the following organizations for more information:

Children of Lesbians and Gays Everywhere (COLAGE)
415/861-KIDS (415/861-5437)
www.colage.org

Family Pride Coalition (formerly Gay and Lesbian Parents Coalition)
202/331-5015
www.familypride.org

Gay, Lesbian and Straight Education Network (GLSEN)
212/727-0135
www.glsen.org

Parents, Families & Friends of Lesbians & Gays (PFLAG)
202/467-8180
www.pflag.org

Rainbow Families
612/827-7731
www.rainbowfamilies.org

Please note: Inclusion in this list does not imply an endorsement by the American Academy of Pediatrics (AAP). The AAP is not responsible for the content of the resources mentioned in this brochure. Phone numbers and Web site addresses are as current as possible, but may change at any time.

The information contained in this publication should not be used as a substitute for the medical care and advice of your pediatrician. There may be variations in treatment that your pediatrician may recommend based on individual facts and circumstances.

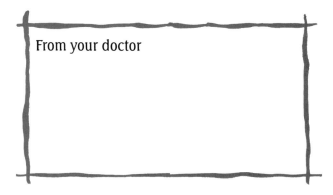

From your doctor

American Academy of Pediatrics

DEDICATED TO THE HEALTH OF ALL CHILDREN™

The American Academy of Pediatrics is an organization of 60,000 primary care pediatricians, pediatric medical subspecialists, and pediatric surgical specialists dedicated to the health, safety, and well-being of infants, children, adolescents, and young adults.

American Academy of Pediatrics
Web site—www.aap.org

Copyright © 2005
American Academy of Pediatrics

Know the Facts About HIV and AIDS

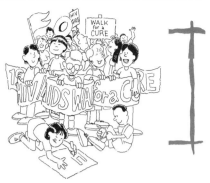

AIDS, which stands for **acquired immune deficiency syndrome,** is a very serious disease that affects children, teens, and adults. It is caused by a virus called the human immunodeficiency virus (HIV). The virus is **acquired** and causes a **deficiency** in the body's **immune** system. AIDS has rapidly become a leading cause of death in young adults and children in many areas in the United States. Although there is treatment available, there is no cure for AIDS. The disease can be prevented by educating yourself and your children about AIDS and HIV, including the behaviors that can increase the risk of getting AIDS.

What are HIV and AIDS?

HIV is the virus that causes AIDS. When someone is infected with HIV, it means the virus is attacking the immune system. The immune system is the body's way of fighting infections and helping to prevent some types of cancer. Damage to the immune system from HIV can occur over months, as sometimes happens in infants. Sometimes it occurs slowly over years, as more often happens in adults. AIDS is diagnosed in an HIV-infected person when the immune system is severely damaged or when certain other serious infections or cancer occurs.

Many people do not know they are infected with HIV because it can take many years for serious symptoms to develop. However, even if an infected person shows no symptoms, the infection can be spread to others. Many people with HIV infection look and act healthy. You cannot tell just by looking at people whether they are infected with HIV. A blood test for HIV is the only way to be sure.

How is HIV spread?

HIV is spread from one person to another through certain body fluids. These fluids include blood and blood products, semen (sperm), fluid from the vagina, and breast milk. The following are ways HIV can be spread:

- **By sexual intercourse (vaginal, anal, or oral) with a person who is infected with HIV.** Both males and females can spread HIV. Latex condoms can help prevent the spread of HIV and other sexually transmitted diseases (STDs). The safest way to prevent these diseases is to abstain from all forms of sexual intercourse until married or in a long-term mature relationship with an uninfected partner.
- **Through contact with an infected person's blood.** Sharing syringes or needles for drug use or for other activities such as tattooing or ear piercing can spread HIV. Accidental injuries from contaminated needles can also cause HIV infection. This can happen if a person comes into contact with used needles that have been thrown away. Rarely, HIV has been spread by an infected person's blood directly contacting the mucous membranes, cuts, scrapes, or open sores of another person.

- **To a baby by an HIV-infected mother** during pregnancy, labor, delivery, or breastfeeding.
- **Through blood or blood products from blood transfusions, organ transplants, or artificial insemination.** This occurs very rarely because donors of blood, sperm, tissue, and organs in the United States are tested routinely for HIV.

How is HIV *not* spread?

It is very important to know how HIV is ***not*** spread. Fear and wrong information about HIV and AIDS cause suffering to those who have been infected with HIV. Make sure you and your children understand that HIV ***cannot*** be spread through casual contact with someone who has AIDS or is infected with HIV. You *cannot* get HIV in the following ways:
- Shaking hands
- Hugging
- Sitting next to someone
- Sharing bathrooms
- Eating food prepared by an HIV-infected person

Also, you ***cannot*** get HIV from the following:
- The air
- Insect bites
- Giving blood
- Swimming pools

Teaching your young child about HIV and AIDS

Children need to learn about HIV and AIDS at a very early age. By the time your children are 3 or 4 years old, make sure you have clearly explained the following to them:
- They should never touch anyone else's blood or open sores.
- They should never touch needles or syringes. If they see someone who is bleeding or if they find a needle or syringe, they should tell an adult. Remind your children never to touch a needle or syringe if they find one in the garbage or on the ground.
- AIDS cannot be caught by playing with HIV-infected children.

By grade-school age, your child should begin to have a better understanding of illness and body parts. Your child should begin to learn more about how HIV can and cannot be spread.

Teaching your preteen or teenager about HIV and AIDS

To avoid being infected with HIV through sexual contact, preteens and teenagers need to know that the ***best*** way to protect themselves against HIV and AIDS is to refrain from having any type of sexual intercourse. Urge your teenager to postpone sexual intercourse until married or in a long-term, mature relationship with an uninfected partner. Neither person should have any other sexual partners.

If teenagers do not postpone having sexual intercourse, then proper use of latex condoms and limiting the relationship to one partner will help them avoid HIV infection. This will also lower the risk of getting other sexually transmitted diseases (STDs) such as syphilis, gonorrhea, Chlamydia infection, and genital warts. Adolescents should also know about other types of birth control. However, it should be emphasized that other forms of birth control do ***not*** prevent HIV infection or other STDs.

For more information for you and your adolescent, ask your pediatrician about the following brochures from the American Academy of Pediatrics:

- *Making the Right Choice: Facts for Teens on Preventing Pregnancy*
- *Deciding to Wait*
- *The Correct Use of Condoms: A Message to Teens*

HIV and drug use

Adolescents also need to know about the extremely high risk of being infected with HIV if they use drugs, especially intravenous (IV) drugs that are injected with needles. Sharing a needle or syringe spreads blood from one person to another. People who do not use drugs themselves but are having sexual intercourse with an HIV-infected drug user can also be infected with HIV. Sharing needles for non-drug use, such as for tattoos, ear piercing, intentional scarring or cutting with a razor or needle, or injecting drugs like steroids, can also spread HIV.

When talking to your adolescent about drugs, make sure your adolescent understands that using drugs is very dangerous. The risk of getting HIV increases even when non-IV drugs like alcohol or cocaine are used. This is because drugs affect a person's judgment and can lead to risky behaviors, such as having sex without a latex condom or having sex with multiple partners.

See the following brochures from the American Academy of Pediatrics for more information on drug use (including alcohol and tobacco) and children:

- *Marijuana: Your Child and Drugs*
- *Cocaine: Your Child and Drugs*
- *Alcohol: Your Child and Drugs*
- *The Risks of Tobacco Use: A Message to Parents and Teens*
- *Smoking: Straight Talk for Teens*

If your preteen or teenager is using drugs or alcohol or is involved in risky sexual behaviors, he is at higher risk of HIV infection. If you think your adolescent or child is at risk of becoming infected with HIV, it is very important to discuss this with your pediatrician.

Who should be tested for HIV?

Anyone involved in the risky behaviors mentioned previously *should* get an HIV test. Anyone who wants to know whether or not they have HIV can be tested. However, a negative test does not mean a person is uninfected if the risky behaviors took place only a few months before the test.

The following symptoms may suggest a need for HIV testing:

- Persistent fevers
- Loss of appetite
- Frequent diarrhea
- Poor weight gain or rapid weight loss
- Chronic lymph node swelling
- Persistent or recurring extreme tiredness or lethargy
- White spots in the mouth
- Recurring or unusual infections

While there is no cure for HIV or AIDS, there are medications that can help delay symptoms, help prevent the spread of HIV to an unborn baby, and help prevent additional infections in HIV-infected people.

HIV and AIDS are important issues to think about and discuss. Educating yourself and your family about HIV and AIDS is the best way to keep your family healthy. If you need more information, talk to your pediatrician. Most importantly, talk to your child or adolescent. Make sure she knows the facts about this serious yet preventable disease.

The information contained in this publication should not be used as a substitute for the medical care and advice of your pediatrician. There may be variations in treatment that your pediatrician may recommend based on individual facts and circumstances.

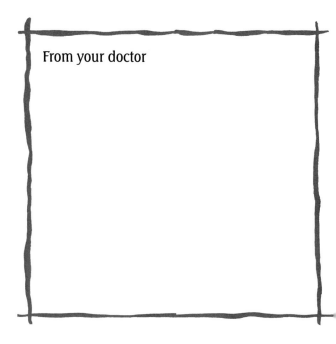

From your doctor

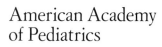

American Academy
of Pediatrics

DEDICATED TO THE HEALTH OF ALL CHILDREN™

The American Academy of Pediatrics is an organization of 60,000 primary care pediatricians, pediatric medical subspecialists, and pediatric surgical specialists dedicated to the health, safety, and well-being of infants, children, adolescents, and young adults.

American Academy of Pediatrics
Web site—www.aap.org

Copyright © 1995
American Academy of Pediatrics, Updated 5/99

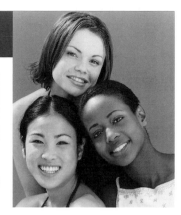

the pelvic exam

Pelvic exams are an important way to take care of your health. You should **get a pelvic exam** if you have ever had sex (even one time) or are having any problems with your periods.

Most women have questions and concerns about their first pelvic exam, but knowing what to expect can help you to feel more at ease. The pelvic exam only **takes about 5 minutes,** and your pediatrician will talk you through it and answer any questions you may have.

Why do I need a pelvic exam?

"Is a pelvic exam right for me now? If not now, when?" These are good questions to ask your pediatrician.

Basically, a pelvic exam is the best way for your pediatrician to **check** your reproductive system, which includes your vulva, vagina, cervix, ovaries, fallopian tubes, and uterus. The exam also includes **lab tests** that can check for problems like diseases that are easily treated if found early. Sometimes the pelvic exam includes tests for sexually transmitted diseases (STDs). However, for many patients with no symptoms a simple urine test can determine if you have 2 common STDs: chlamydia or gonorrhea.

The Female Reproductive System

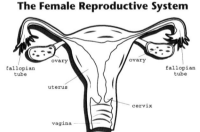

It's also a **great time to talk** with your pediatrician about things you may be thinking about, such as

- **Changes** in your body
- Your breasts
- Your **periods** (menstruation)
- **Sex**
- Pregnancy and birth control
- STDs
- Vaginal discharge
- Anything that hurts or bothers you

First a **mini-checkup**

Before the exam, your pediatrician may check your height, weight, blood pressure, lungs, heart, breasts, and stomach. You may be asked to give a small sample of urine and to empty your bladder so the pelvic exam is more comfortable.

There are **2 main parts** of your exam: the interview and the pelvic exam.

Part 1— The interview

Before the pelvic exam, your pediatrician will **ask you questions** about your **health** and your periods. So don't be surprised if you're asked questions like

- When did you get your first period?
- When was your last period?
- Do you have your periods regularly? How often?
- How long do they last?
- Do you have any pain, cramps, headaches, or mood swings with your periods?
- Do you use tampons, pads, or both?
- Have you ever had vaginal itching, discharge, or problems urinating?
- Do you douche? If yes, how often?

Don't be surprised if your pediatrician asks you about **sex.** You may be embarrassed or feel like your sex life is nobody else's business, but your pediatrician needs to know these things to help you protect your health. So be honest! And don't forget, whatever you say to your pediatrician is **confidential** and won't be discussed with anyone else without your permission (unless it's something life threatening, of course). These questions may include

Have you ever had any type of sexual intercourse (oral, anal, or vaginal)? **If yes,**

- When was the first time you had sex?
- Did you want to have sex, or were you forced to have sex?
- Have you had sex with more than 1 person? If yes, how many people?
- Have you had sex with men, women, or both men and women?
- How old were the people you had sex with?
- Do you use condoms or other types of birth control?

Remember, you can ask questions too. In fact, this is a great time to ask any questions you may have about your period, tampon use, sex, and other stuff. **Your pediatrician has lots of good information** and can give you advice on making good decisions, the benefits of not having sex (abstinence), and preventing pregnancy and diseases.

So don't be afraid to ask!

Part 2— The pelvic exam

OK, so now it's time for the pelvic exam. You'll be left alone to undress and put on a gown. There will also be an extra sheet that you can use to cover yourself. Remember, **the entire exam only takes about 5 minutes.** Some girls think that having a pelvic exam will mean they are no longer virgins, but that's not true. The pelvic exam **doesn't change whether you are a virgin.** It's also not true that the pelvic exam is a "test" to see if you are a virgin. The exam can be done even if you have never had sexual intercourse, because the opening to your vagina is large enough to allow for the exam.

3 simple steps

Your pediatrician will describe each step of the exam. If you have any questions or feel uncomfortable, let your pediatrician know. Your pediatrician will have a nurse or assistant in the room during the exam. You can ask your mom, sister, or friend to join you if it makes you more at ease—it's up to you.

Step 1: The vulva (outside of your vagina and surrounding areas)

Your pediatrician will begin by looking at the outside of your vagina and surrounding areas to make sure everything looks normal.

Step 2: Inside your vagina

Then your pediatrician will use an instrument called a *speculum* to look inside your vagina. Specula are about the size of a tampon, made of disposable plastic or sterilized metal, and have no sharp edges.

- The speculum will be gently inserted into your vagina. You will feel some pressure, but it shouldn't hurt. Take **deep breaths** and try to **relax.** This will help relax your vaginal muscles and make this part of the test easier.

- Once the speculum is inside the vagina, it is opened so that your pediatrician can see your cervix.

- Then your pediatrician will use a cotton-tipped swab or a plastic brush to take a small sample of cells from your cervix. Samples are sent for tests, such as the **Pap smear,** which tests for abnormalities of the cervix. You may also be checked for diseases like gonorrhea and chlamydia with a second cotton swab.

- Once everything is collected, the speculum is gently removed. It's normal to have a little bit of spotting after the Pap smear.

Step 3: Uterus and ovaries

The last step of the exam checks your uterus and ovaries. Your pediatrician will gently insert 1 or 2 gloved fingers into your vagina and press on the outside of your abdomen with the other hand. It's quick and may feel a little funny, but shouldn't hurt.

That's it! Most women are surprised when their pelvic exam is over because it really is that quick.

Your sexual health

The following are 4 important things concerning your sexual health:

- **Having sexual feelings is normal.** Whether you decide to have sex is your choice. Talk with your partner about how you feel.

- **Not everyone your age is having sex,** including oral sex and intercourse. More than half of all teens **choose to wait** until they're older to have sex. Abstinence (not having sex, including oral, anal, and vaginal sex) means you won't become pregnant, become a teen parent, or get an STD.

- If you're going to have sex, using condoms is the best way to avoid getting STDs or becoming pregnant.

- To make sure you stay healthy, get regular medical checkups, urine testing for STDs, and a pelvic exam.

If your pediatrician finds a disease or any other problem, you may be referred to an OB/GYN (obstetrician/gynecologist). This type of doctor specializes in women's reproductive health.

Remember, the pelvic exam is an important part of taking care of your health. Ask your pediatrician if it's right for you.

From your doctor

American Academy of Pediatrics

DEDICATED TO THE HEALTH OF ALL CHILDREN™

The American Academy of Pediatrics is an organization of 60,000 primary care pediatricians, pediatric medical subspecialists, and pediatric surgical specialists dedicated to the health, safety, and well-being of infants, children, adolescents, and young adults.

American Academy of Pediatrics
Web site — www.aap.org

Copyright © 2005
American Academy of Pediatrics

Child Sexual Abuse:
What It Is and How To Prevent It

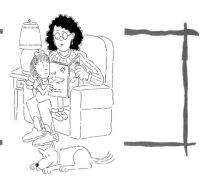

Sexual abuse of children is more common than most people realize. At least 1 out of 5 adult women and 1 out of 10 adult men report having been sexually abused in childhood. By educating yourself and your children about sexual abuse, you can help prevent it from happening to your children and better cope with it if it does.

What is child sexual abuse?

Sexual abuse is when an adult or an older child forces sexual contact on a younger child. The abuser may use physical abuse, bribery, threats, tricks, or take advantage of a younger child's lack of knowledge. Any of the following acts by an adult or older child are sexual abuse:

- Fondling a child's genitals
- Getting a child to fondle their genitals
- Mouth to genital contact with a child
- Rubbing their genitals on a child
- Penetrating a child's vagina or anus
- Showing their genitals to a child
- Showing pornographic or "dirty" pictures or videotapes to a child
- Using a child as a model to make pornographic materials

Could my child be sexually abused? By whom?

Children are abused most often by adults or older children whom they know and who can influence their behavior by exerting power over them. In 8 out of 10 reported cases, the abuser is someone the child knows. The abuser is often an authority figure whom the child trusts or loves.

How would I know if my child is being sexually abused?

Many parents expect their son or daughter to tell them or another trusted adult about being sexually abused. Abusers often threaten or convince the child not to tell anyone about it. The child may believe that the abuse is his fault and that he will be punished if someone finds out. A child's first statements about abuse may be vague and incomplete. He may just hint about the problem to see if he would get in trouble. Abused children may tell a friend about it. The friend may then tell an adult. Children may tell about abuse after a personal safety program at their school. Parents may suspect abuse because of the child's behavior. You should be aware of the following behavioral changes in your child that may be symptoms of sexual abuse:

- Noticeable, new fear of a person (even a parent) or certain places
- Unusual or unexpected response from the child when asked if she was touched by someone
- Drawings that show sexual acts
- Abrupt changes in behavior, such as bed-wetting or loss of bowel control
- Sudden awareness of genitals
- Sexual acts and words shared with other children or animals

- Questions about sexual activity that are beyond the child's development
- Changes in sleep habits, such as nightmares in young children
- Constipation, or refusal to have bowel movements

Physical signs of abuse may include the following:

- Anal or genital redness, pain, or bleeding
- Unusual discharge from the anus or vagina
- Sexually transmitted diseases such as gonorrhea, chlamydia, or genital warts
- Repeated urinary tract infections in females
- Pregnancy, in older females

What should I do if my child reveals sexual abuse to me?

Children tend to ignore things that make them feel uncomfortable, rather than recognize them as warning signs. If your child talks about abuse, listen carefully and take it very seriously. When a child's plea for help is ignored, not believed, or punished, she may not risk telling again. As a result, the child could remain a victim of abuse for months or years. Teach your child that it is OK to talk about uncomfortable feelings.

If your child reveals abuse, you should take the following steps:

1) **Face the issue.** Listen to your child's reasons for revealing the abuse. Tell your child the abuse is not her fault. Give her extra love, comfort, and reassurance. If you are angry, make sure she knows you are not angry with her, and you will help her. Let your child know how brave she is to tell you and that you understand how scared she feels. This is even more important if the child has been abused by a close and trusted relative or family friend.

2) **Take charge of the situation.** Protect the child from further abuse.

3) **Discuss the problem** with a pediatrician and a counselor who can provide support.

4) **Report abuse to the police or local child protection service agency.** Ask about crisis support help.

Can I deal with sexual abuse in my family without contacting the authorities?

Parents should not try to stop or treat sexual abuse themselves. If abuse is suspected, parents should follow the steps above and get help.

What will happen to the child and to the abuser if sexual abuse is reported?

Sexual abuse is against the law. It is a crime, no matter who the abuser is. Cases are investigated by the police, a social service agency, or both. With the help of a doctor, they will decide whether sexual abuse took place. Depending on the circumstances, the police may let social services manage the case, especially if the child is very young, shows no signs of physical injury, or the abuser is young or a family member. When a child is abused by a nonfamily member, the matter must be handled by the police.

After sexual abuse is reported, what happens next depends on the circumstances of the case. Preventing further abuse of the child is the first concern of the authorities. The abuser may be referred for treatment. The child and the entire family may also be referred to a treatment program. If the suspected abuser lives in the home and faces criminal charges, authorities will recommend that the suspected abuser leave the home. In any case, the child can usually stay in the home as long as her family will take the necessary steps to protect her from further abuse by asking the abuser to leave the home while the problem is investigated. Whatever the circumstances, the child and family will need a lot of support from relatives and friends.

What parents can do to prevent sexual abuse

The American Academy of Pediatrics encourages you to take the following steps:

- **Talk** to your child about sexual abuse. If your child's school sponsors a sexual abuse program, discuss what he learned.

- **Teach** your child which body parts are private (parts covered by a bathing suit) and the proper names of those parts. Let him know that his body belongs to him. Tell him to yell "no" or "stop" to anyone who may threaten him sexually.

- **Listen** when your child tries to tell you something, especially when it seems hard for him to talk about it. Make sure your child knows it's OK to tell you about any attempt to molest him or touch him in a way that made him feel uncomfortable, no matter who the abuser may be. Let him know he can trust you and that you will not be angry with him if he tells you.

- **Give** your child enough time and attention. Weekly family meetings can be used to talk about all good and bad experiences.

- **Know** the adults and children with whom your child is spending time. Be careful about allowing your child to spend time alone or in out-of-the-way places with other adults or older children. Make visits to your child's caregiver without notice. Ask your child about his visits to the caregiver or with child sitters.

- **Never** let your child enter a stranger's home without a parent or trusted adult. Door-to-door fund-raising is particularly risky for unsupervised children.

- **Check** to see if your child's school has an abuse prevention program for the teachers and children. If it doesn't, start one.

- **Tell** someone in authority if you suspect that your child or someone else's child is being abused.

Your child's teacher or school counselor can help you teach your child to avoid or report sexual abuse. They know how this can be done without upsetting or scaring your child. Your pediatrician also understands the importance of communication between parents and children. He or she is trained to detect the signs of child sexual abuse and is familiar with resources in the community. Ask your pediatrician for advice on how to protect your children.

For further information on child sexual abuse or other forms of abuse, please contact:

Prevent Child Abuse America
PO Box 2866
Chicago, IL 60690-9950
800/556-2722
Web site: http://www.childabuse.org

Talking with your child

Measures to protect your children from sexual abuse should begin early, since many child abuse cases involve preschoolers. The guidelines below offer topics to discuss with your children depending on their ages.

Age	Prevention Plan
18 months–3 years	Teach your child the proper names for body parts.
3–5 years	Teach your child about private parts of the body (parts covered by a bathing suit) and how to yell "no" to sexual advances. Use coloring books or reading books with examples. Give simple, easy-to-understand answers to questions about sex. Play the "What if…?" game. Ask your child what she would do in certain situations.
5–8 years	Discuss safety away from home and the difference between being touched in private parts of the body and other touching. Encourage your child to talk about scary experiences, including requests to touch someone else's private parts or look at pornography. Play the "What if…?" game. Ask your child what she would do in certain situations.
8–12 years	Stress personal safety and give examples of possible problem areas, such as video arcades, malls, locker rooms, and out-of-the-way places outdoors. Start to discuss rules of sexual conduct that are accepted by the family. Discuss basic facts about human reproduction.
12–18 years	Continue to stress personal safety and potential problem areas. Discuss the prevention of rape, date rape, sexually transmitted diseases, and unintended pregnancy. Talk about the effects of drugs and alcohol on sexual behavior.

The information contained in this publication should not be used as a substitute for the medical care and advice of your pediatrician. There may be variations in treatment that your pediatrician may recommend based on individual facts and circumstances.

American Academy of Pediatrics

DEDICATED TO THE HEALTH OF ALL CHILDREN™

The American Academy of Pediatrics is an organization of 60,000 primary care pediatricians, pediatric medical subspecialists, and pediatric surgical specialists dedicated to the health, safety, and well-being of infants, children, adolescents, and young adults.

American Academy of Pediatrics
Web site — www.aap.org

Copyright © 1990
American Academy of Pediatric, Updated 8/99

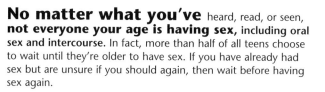

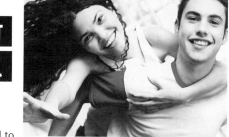

No matter what you've heard, read, or seen, **not everyone your age is having sex,** including oral sex and intercourse. In fact, more than half of all teens choose to wait until they're older to have sex. If you have already had sex but are unsure if you should again, then wait before having sex again.

New feelings

Being physically attracted to another person and trying to figure out how to deal with these feelings is perfectly normal. Kissing and hugging are often accompanied by really intense sexual feelings. These feelings may tempt you to "go all the way."

Before things go too far, **try asking yourself the following questions:**

- Do I really want to have sex?
- Is this person pressuring me to have sex?
- Am I ready to have sex?
- What will happen after I have sex with this person?

Remember, you can **show how you feel** about someone **without having sex** (being abstinent) with him or her.

Can you be **sexual without having** sex?

Yes. Being sexual can mean
- Spending romantic time together
- Holding hands, kissing, or cuddling

Are you **ready?**

Ask yourself the following questions:
- **How do you feel** when you are with this person?
- Is this person kind and caring?
- Does this person *respect* you and your opinions?
- Have you **talked together** about whether to have sex?
- Have you talked together about condoms and other **birth control?**
- Will you stay together even if one of you does not want to have sex?
- Do you know if your partner has *ever had sex with other people?*
- **Do you feel pressured** to have sex just to please your partner?

If you and your partner find it hard to talk about sex, it might be a sign that **you are not ready to have sex.** Open and honest communication is important in any relationship, especially one that involves sex.

Know **the risks**

It's normal for teens to be curious about sex, but deciding to have sex is a big step.

Sex does increase your chances of becoming pregnant, becoming a teen parent, and getting a sexually transmitted disease (STD), and it may affect the way you feel about yourself or how others feel about you.

Some things to think about before you have sex are
- What would *your parents* say if you had sex?
- Are you **ready to be a parent?**
- Could you handle being told that you have an STD?
- Do you know where to go for **birth control methods?**
- How would you feel if your partner tells you *it's over after you have sex?*
- How would you feel if your partner tells people at school the two of you had sex?
- How would you handle feeling **guilty, scared, or sad** because you had sex?

Set your limits

If you don't want to have sex, set **limits** before things get too serious. Never let anyone talk you into doing something you don't want to do. Boys and girls need to understand that **forcing someone to have sex is wrong.**

Stick by your decision

If you don't know what to say, here are some suggestions
- "I like you a lot, but I'm just not ready to have sex."
- "You're really fun to be with, and I wouldn't want to ruin our relationship with sex."
- "You're a great person, but sex isn't how I prove I like someone."
- "I'd like to wait until I'm older before I make the decision to have sex."

Remember, **"no" means "no"**—no matter how far you go. If you feel things are going too far sexually, tell your partner to stop.

Better safe than sorry

If you choose to wait to have sex, try to avoid

- **Being alone with your date too often.** Spending time with your other friends is important too.

- Giving your date the wrong idea. Stick to your limits. It's also not a good idea for you and your date to "make out" or go too far sexually if you don't really want to have sex.

- Using alcohol or drugs. Both of these *affect your judgment,* which may make it hard to stick to your decision not to have sex.

- **Giving in to the pressure.** It may be tempting to keep up with the crowd, but keep in mind that they may not be telling the truth.

Why wait?

People who **wait** until they are older to have sex usually find out that it's

- More *special*
- More satisfying
- **Less risky** to their health
- **Easier** to act responsibly and take precautions to avoid infections and pregnancy
- More accepted by others

Be patient. At some point, you will be ready for sex. **Move at your own pace, not someone else's.**

The information contained in this publication should not be used as a substitute for the medical care and advice of your pediatrician. There may be variations in treatment that your pediatrician may recommend based on individual facts and circumstances.

The persons whose photographs are depicted in this publication are professional models. They have no relation to the issues discussed. Any characters they are portraying are fiictional.

From your doctor

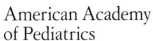

American Academy
of Pediatrics

DEDICATED TO THE HEALTH OF ALL CHILDREN™

The American Academy of Pediatrics is an organization of 60,000 primary care pediatricians, pediatric medical subspecialists, and pediatric surgical specialists dedicated to the health, safety, and well-being of infants, children, adolescents, and young adults.

American Academy of Pediatrics
Web site — www.aap.org

Copyright © 2005
American Academy of Pediatrics

making healthy decisions about sex

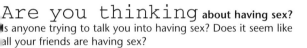

Are you thinking about having sex?

Is anyone trying to talk you into having sex? Does it seem like all your friends are having sex?

Before you make any decisions, or even if you have had sex but are unsure if you should again, read on for some **important information** about how to **stay healthy.** (And remember, if anyone has ever forced you to have sex, this is **WRONG** and not your fault! Tell someone you trust as soon as possible.)

It's OK to say NO Way!

Not everyone is having sex. **Half of all teens say "no" to sex.** There's nothing wrong if you decide to wait; in fact, it's a great idea. If you decide to wait, stick with your decision. Plan ahead how you are going to say "no" so that you are clearly understood. Stay away from situations that can lead to sex. Too many young people have sex without meaning to when they drink alcohol or use drugs. Not using alcohol and drugs will help you make clearer choices about sex. Whether you decide to have sex, it's important that you **know the facts** about birth control, diseases, and emotions.

Why wait?

- **Sex can lead to pregnancy. Are you ready** to be pregnant or a teen parent? *It's an awesome responsibility*—will your baby have food, clothes, and a safe place to live?
- **Sex has health risks.** You could become infected with one or more **sexually transmitted diseases (STDs)** like herpes, *Trichomonas,* or human immunodeficiency virus (HIV) (the virus that causes acquired immunodeficiency syndrome [AIDS]). One type of disease called human papillomavirus (HPV) may cause **cancer.**
- You may feel sad or angry if you let someone pressure you into having sex when you're not really ready.
- You also may feel sad or angry if you chose to have sex and then your partner leaves you. He may even tell other people that you had sex with him. **Can you handle that?**

If you don't want to get an STD, use condoms

If you're going to have sexual intercourse, using **condoms** is the best way to avoid getting STDs. Remember that **nothing will ever be 100% effective** in preventing diseases except abstinence (no sex). Use a **latex** condom every time you have sex—no matter what other type of birth control you and your partner also might use. To **protect** against getting a disease from having oral sex, use a condom, a dental dam, or non-microwavable plastic wrap. Your pediatrician can explain all these things to you. To make sure

you **stay healthy,** get regular medical checkups, urine testing for STDs, and a pelvic exam (if you're female).

Condoms are easy to use. They work best when you use them the right way. Here is *what you need to know.*

- **Use only latex or polyurethane condoms.** You also have a choice between a male condom or female condom. Never use these 2 types of condoms at the same time; they might tear. When buying male condoms, get the kind with a reservoir (nipple) at the tip to catch semen.
- **Follow the instructions** on the package to make sure you are using them the right way. Also, **check** the expiration date on the package. Don't buy or use expired condoms.
- **You can carry condoms with you at all times,** but do not store them where they will get hot (like in the glove compartment of a car). Heat can damage the condom. Also, you can carry them in a purse or wallet, but not for too long—this shortens their life.

If you don't want to get pregnant…

You need a **reliable form of birth control!**

- **Condoms** used the right way have a 90% chance of preventing pregnancy.
- "The pill" is the most popular type of birth control used by women. There are many brands of **the birth control pill.** For the pill to work, a woman must take it *every day.* When used correctly, the pill is 99% effective at preventing pregnancy.
- The birth control **patch** is similar to the pill and looks like an adhesive strip. The patch is placed on the skin and changed every week for 3 weeks. Side effects are similar to the pill.
- Depo-Provera is a **shot** that you get every 3 months. It is a popular choice for women who have trouble remembering to take the pill.

There may be **minor side effects** when using the pill, patch, or Depo-Provera like mild irregular bleeding, nausea, sore breasts, or weight gain. Your pediatrician will talk to you in detail about what to expect.

Other types of birth control

The following are **NOT recommended** for young people:

- **Withdrawal** (when the male "pulls out" of the female before he ejaculates or "cums") does not prevent pregnancy. If even a small amount of sperm enters a woman, pregnancy can occur.
- **Norplant.** It's no longer approved.

- **Diaphragms and spermicides.** These require some planning. The teen pregnancy rate using these methods is very high.
- The **"rhythm method."** This is when you avoid having sex during certain times of your monthly cycle. This method is not very effective at preventing pregnancy.
- The **intrauterine device (IUD),** unless you have had a baby and are at a low risk for STDs.

The choice to become sexually active is **your choice.** Choosing not to have sex is the *only* way to avoid all STDs and getting pregnant.

It's your choice!

Talk with your pediatrician about birth control—how safe and effective these methods are, what side effects they can cause, and how much they cost.

Note: Products are mentioned for informational purposes only and do not imply an endorsement by the American Academy of Pediatrics.

The information contained in this publication should not be used as a substitute for the medical care and advice of your pediatrician. There may be variations in treatment that your pediatrician may recommend based on individual facts and circumstances.

The persons whose photographs are depicted in this publication are professional models. They have no relation to the issues discussed. Any characters they are portraying are fiictional.

From your doctor

American Academy of Pediatrics

DEDICATED TO THE HEALTH OF ALL CHILDREN™

The American Academy of Pediatrics is an organization of 60,000 primary care pediatricians, pediatric medical subspecialists, and pediatric surgical specialists dedicated to the health, safety, and well-being of infants, children, adolescents, and young adults.

American Academy of Pediatrics
Web site — www.aap.org

Copyright © 2005
American Academy of Pediatrics

Talking With Your Teen About Sex

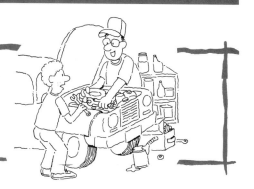

Children are exposed to sexual messages every day—on TV, on the Internet, in movies, in magazines, and in music. Sex in the media is so common that you might think that teens today already know all they need to know about sex. They may even claim to know it all, so sex is something you just don't talk about. Unfortunately, only a small amount of what is seen in the media shows responsible sexual behavior or gives correct information.

Your teen needs a reliable, honest source to turn to for answers—the best source is you. You may feel uneasy talking with your teen about sex, but your guidance is important. Beyond the basic facts about sex, your teen needs to hear from you about your family values and beliefs. This needs to be an ongoing discussion and not just one "big talk." The following information may help you talk with your teen about this important and sensitive subject.

Why should I talk to my teen about sex?

When it comes to something as important as sex and sexuality, nothing can replace your influence. You are the best person to teach your teen about relationships, love, commitment, and respect in what you say and by your own example.

Talk about sex should begin when your child first asks questions like "Where do babies come from?" If you wait until your children are teens to talk about sex, they will probably learn their first lessons about sex from other sources. Studies show that children who learn about sex from friends or through a program at school instead of their parents are more likely to have sex before marriage. Teens who talk with their parents about sex are sexually active at a later age than those who don't.

What should I tell my teen about sex?

Communication between parents and teens is very important. Your teen may not share the same values as you but that shouldn't stop you from talking about sex and sexuality.

Before your children reach their early teens, girls and boys should know about the following:

- Correct body names and functions of male and female sex organs
- Puberty and how the body changes
- Menstruation (periods)
- Sexual intercourse and the risk of getting pregnant and/or getting an STD, including HIV (the virus that causes AIDS)
- Your family values regarding dating, sexual activity, cigarettes, alcohol, and drugs

During the teen years, your talks about sex should focus more on the social and emotional aspects of sex, and your values. Be ready to answer questions like

- When can I start dating?
- When is it OK to kiss a boy (or a girl)?
- How far is too far?

Sex and the media

Media entertains, educates, and informs. But some messages may not be what we want children to learn.

American media today often portrays sexual images and suggestive sexual content. In fact, the average young viewer is exposed to more than 14,000 sexual references each year. Only a small amount of what is seen in the media shows responsible sexual behavior or gives correct information about abstinence (not having sex), birth control, or the risks of pregnancy and sexually transmitted diseases (STDs).

Media in any format can have a positive or negative effect on your teen. This makes it important for you to know what your teen is listening to or watching. Watch TV with your teen—it can be a great starting point for your next talk about sex.

- How will I know when I'm ready to have sex?
- Won't having sex help me keep my boyfriend (or girlfriend)?
- Do you think I should have sex before marriage?
- Is oral sex really sex?
- How do I say "No"?
- What do I do if someone tries to force me to have sex?

Answer your teen's questions based on your values—even if you think your values are old-fashioned. If you feel strongly that sex before marriage is wrong, share this with your teen and explain why you feel that way. If you explain the reasons for your beliefs, your teen is more likely to understand and adopt your values.

Other concerns include the following:

- **Peer pressure.** Teens face a lot of peer pressure to have sex. If they aren't ready to have sex, they may feel left out. But more than 50% of teens wait until after high school to have sex, and there are benefits of waiting. Abstinence from sex (oral, vaginal, and anal) provides 100% protection against STDs and pregnancy, and less emotional stress if there's a breakup.
- **STDs.** Teens need to know that having sex exposes them to the risk of STDs. Common STDs include chlamydia, gonorrhea, human papillomavirus, herpes, and trichomoniasis. AIDS is usually transmitted during sex and is a leading cause of death in young people aged 15 to 24. These young people were probably infected with HIV when they were teens.
- **Prevention.** The only sure way to prevent STDs is *not* to have sex.
- **Reducing the risk.** Condoms (male or female) are the safest method to prevent most STDs and should always be used. Also, postponing sex until later teen years or adulthood reduces the risk. If both partners are abstinent before marriage or a long-term, mature relationship, have never had an STD, and have sex with each other only, the risk is eliminated.

- **Birth control.** Girls *and* boys need to know about birth control whether they decide to have sex or not. If your teen doesn't know about birth control, an unplanned pregnancy might result. Ten percent of teen girls in the United States get pregnant each year. By the age of 20, 4 out of 10 girls become pregnant. Birth control pills, shots (trade name: Depo-Provera), and contraceptive patches only prevent pregnancy—they don't protect against STDs, including HIV/AIDS. Condoms and another reliable birth control method need to be used each time to help reduce the risk of STDs and pregnancy.
- **Date rape.** Date (or acquaintance) rape is a serious problem for teens. It happens when a person your teen knows (for example, a date, friend, or neighbor) forces her (or him) to have sex. Make sure your teen understands that "no always means no." Also, dating in groups instead of alone and avoiding drugs and alcohol may make date rape less likely to happen.
- **Sexuality.** This is a difficult topic for many parents, but your teen probably has many questions about heterosexuality, homosexuality, and bisexuality. Many young people go through a stage when they wonder "Am I gay?" It often happens when a teen is attracted to a friend of the same sex, or has a crush on a teacher of the same sex. This is common and doesn't necessarily mean your teen is gay, lesbian, or bisexual. Sexual identity may not be firmly set until adulthood. If your teen is gay, lesbian, or bisexual, your love and acceptance is important.
- **Masturbation.** Masturbation is a topic few people feel comfortable talking about. It's a normal and healthy part of human sexuality and shouldn't be discouraged. Discuss this in terms of your values. Talk with your pediatrician if your child can't limit masturbation to a private place (for example, bedroom or bathroom).

How do I talk with my teen?

Sex is a very personal and private matter. Many parents find it difficult to talk with their children about sex. Teens may be too embarrassed, not trust their parent's advice, or prefer not to talk with their parents about it. But sex is an important topic to talk about.

The following tips may help make talking with your teen easier:

- **Be prepared.** Read about the subject so your own questions are answered before talking with your teen. Practice what you plan to say with your spouse or partner, a friend, or another parent. This may make it easier to talk with your teen when the time comes. Speak calmly and clearly.
- **Be honest.** Let your teen know that talking about sex isn't easy for you but that you think it's important that information about sex comes from you. And even though you would prefer that your values be accepted, ultimately decisions about sex are up to your teen. If your teen disagrees with you or gets angry, take heart, you have been heard. These talks will help your teen develop a solid value system, even if it's different from your own.
- **Listen.** Give your teen a chance to talk and ask questions. It's important that you give your full attention.

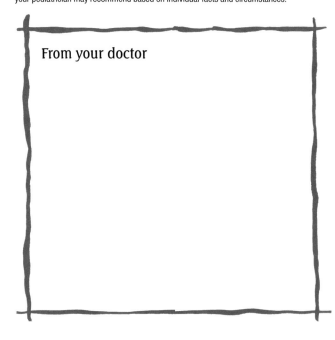

"Won't talking about sex with my children make them want to try it?"

Parents often fear that if they talk about sex, their children may want to try it. Teens are curious about sex, whether you talk to them about it or not. Studies show that teens whose parents talk openly about sex are actually *more* responsible in their sexual behavior.

Your guidance is important. It will help your teen make better-informed decisions about sex. Teens who don't have the facts about sex and look to friends and the media for answers are the most likely to get into trouble (such as getting STDs or becoming pregnant).

- **Try to strike a balance.** While teens need privacy, they also need information and guidance from parents. If your teen doesn't want to talk with you about sex and tells you that it's none of your business, be firm and say that it is your business. Your teen should know that you're asking out of love and concern, especially because there are potentially harmful situations. If your teen is quiet when you try to talk about sex, say what you have to say anyway. Your message may get through.
- **Ask for help.** If you just can't talk to your teen about sex, ask your pediatrician; a trusted aunt or uncle; or a minister, priest, or rabbi for help. Also, many parents find it useful to give their teens a book on human sexuality and say, "Take a look at this, and let's talk."

Note: Products are mentioned for informational purposes only and do not imply an endorsement by the American Academy of Pediatrics.

The information contained in this publication should not be used as a substitute for the medical care and advice of your pediatrician. There may be variations in treatment that your pediatrician may recommend based on individual facts and circumstances.

From your doctor

American Academy of Pediatrics

DEDICATED TO THE HEALTH OF ALL CHILDREN™

The American Academy of Pediatrics is an organization of 60,000 primary care pediatricians, pediatric medical subspecialists, and pediatric surgical specialists dedicated to the health, safety, and well-being of infants, children, adolescents, and young adults.

American Academy of Pediatrics
Web site—www.aap.org

Copyright © 2004
American Academy of Pediatrics

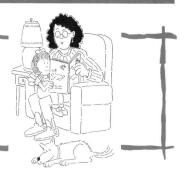

Talking With Your Young Child About Sex

As a parent, you know it's coming—that dreaded moment when your adorable, innocent little boy or girl suddenly glances up and asks, "Where do babies come from?"

Learning about sex begins as soon as your child is able to view, listen, and sense the world around her. Sexuality is part of every person's life, no matter what the age. As your child grows and develops, she may giggle with friends about "private parts," share "dirty" jokes, and scan through dictionaries looking up taboo words. Her curiosity is natural, and children of all ages have questions. When she is ready to ask you, as a parent you should be ready to answer.

Talking about sex and sexuality gives you a chance to share your values and beliefs with your child. Sometimes the topic or the questions may seem embarrassing, but your child needs to know there is always a reliable, honest source she can turn to for answers—you.

The best teacher

Your child will learn many things about the world from friends, movies, television, music, the Internet, and even advertisements. When it comes to something as important as sexuality, nothing can replace the influence of a parent. The best place for your child to learn about relationships, love, commitment, and respect is from you. When your child feels loved and respected by you, he is more likely to turn to you for answers and advice. Giving advice and teaching your child to make wise choices is one of your most important jobs as a parent.

Where to begin

Everyday events will give you plenty of chances to teach your child about topics related to sex. These are called *teachable moments*. For example, talking about body parts during bath time will be much more effective than talking about body parts during dinner. A pregnancy or birth in the family is a good time to discuss how babies are conceived and born. Watching television with your child may also be a good time to discuss sexuality issues.

Teachable moments can happen anywhere—while shopping, at the movies, or even at the park. Use them when they happen. You won't need to make a speech. First, find out what your child already knows. Let your child guide the talk with her questions. Some children may not ask for information if they think you might be uneasy with it. Others might test you by asking embarrassing questions. Talk openly, and let your child know she can ask you about anything.

When your child begins to ask questions, the following might make it easier for both of you:

- **Don't laugh or giggle,** even if the question is cute. Your child shouldn't be made to feel ashamed for her curiosity.
- **Try not to appear overly embarrassed or serious** about the matter.
- **Be brief.** Don't go into a long explanation. Answer in simple terms. Your 4-year old doesn't need to know the details of intercourse.

- **Be honest.** Use proper names for all body parts.
- **See if your child wants or needs to know more.** Follow up your answers with, "Does that answer your question?"
- **Listen** to your child's responses and reactions.
- **Be prepared to repeat yourself.**

If you are uneasy talking about sex or answering certain questions, be honest about that too. Consider asking a relative, close family friend, or your pediatrician to help talk to your child.

Questions, questions, questions

The questions your child asks and the answers that are appropriate to give will depend on your child's age and ability to understand. Following are some of the issues your child may ask about and what he should know at each stage:

Preschool children

"How did I get in your tummy?"
"Where was I before I got in your tummy?"
"How did I get out?"
"Where do babies come from?"
"How come girls don't have a penis?"

18 months to 3 years of age —Your child will begin to learn about his own body. It is important to teach your child the proper names for body parts. Making up names for body parts may give the idea that there is something bad about the proper name. Also, teach your child which parts are private (parts covered by a bathing suit).

4 to 5 years of age—Your child may begin to show an interest in basic sexuality, both her own and that of the opposite sex. She may ask where babies come from. She may want to know why boys' and girls' bodies are different. She may also touch her own genitals and may even show an interest in the genitals of other children. These are not adult sexual activities, but signs of normal interest. However, your child needs to learn what is all right to do and what is not. Setting limits to exploration is really a family matter. You may decide to teach your child the following:

- Interest in genital organs is healthy and natural.
- Nudity and sexual play in public are not all right.
- No other person, including even close friends and relatives, may touch her "private parts." The exceptions are doctors and nurses during physical exams and her own parents when they are trying to find the cause of any pain in the genital area.

  As your child approaches school-age, she should know the following:
- Proper names of body parts
- Functions of each
- Physical differences between boys and girls

School-age children

"How old do girls have to be before they can have a baby?"
"Why do boys get erections?"
"What is a period?"
"How do people have sexual intercourse?"
"Why do some men like other men?"

5 to 7 years of age—Your child is learning much more about how people get along with each other. He may become interested in what takes place sexually between adults. His questions will become more complex as he tries to understand the connection between sexuality and making babies. He may come up with his own explanations about how the body works or where babies come from. He may also turn to his friends for answers.

It is important to help your child understand sexuality in a healthy way. Lessons and values he learns at this age will stay with him as an adult. It will encourage meaningful adult relationships later.

8 to 9 years of age—Your child probably already has developed a sense of right and wrong. She is able to understand that sex is something that happens between two people who love each other. She may begin to become interested in how mom and dad met and fell in love. As questions about romance, love, and marriage arise, she may also ask about homosexual relationships. Use this time to discuss your family's thoughts about homosexuality. Explain that liking or loving someone does not depend on the person's gender and is different from liking someone sexually.

Media Matters

Most children can mimic a movie or TV character, sing an advertising jingle, or give other examples of what they have learned from media. Sadly, these examples may include naming a popular brand of beer, striking a "sexy" pose, or play fighting. Media offer entertainment, culture, news, sports, and education and are an important part of our lives. But some of what they teach may not be what we want children to learn.

American media today (TV, movies, videos, ads, computer games, as well as music lyrics and music videos), often contain sexual images and suggestive content. In fact, the average young viewer is exposed to over 14,000 sexual references each year. Only a small amount of what is seen in the media shows responsible sexual behavior or gives accurate information about birth control, abstinence, or the risks of pregnancy and sexually transmitted disease.

Whatever the form of media, messages can have a positive or negative effect on your child. Just as you would limit certain foods in your child's diet that may be unhealthy, you also should limit your child's media diet of messages.

At this age, your child will be going through many changes that will prepare her for puberty. As she becomes more and more aware of her sexuality, it is important that you talk to her about delaying sexual intercourse until she is older. You should also talk about contraception and sexually transmitted diseases (STDs), especially AIDS. Be sure she

understands how these diseases can spread and how she can protect herself from them and from pregnancy. Teaching your child to be sexually responsible is one of the most important lessons in her life.

A word about...masturbation

Masturbation is a part of childhood sexuality that many parents find difficult to discuss. Up to the age of 5 or 6, it is quite common. Around age 6, children become more socially aware and may feel embarrassed about touching themselves in public. Make sure your child understands that masturbation is a private activity, not a public one. Masturbation in private may continue and is normal.

There are times when frequent masturbation can point to a problem. It could be a sign that the child is under a lot of stress or not receiving enough attention at home. In rare cases, it could even be a tip-off to sexual abuse. Some sexually abused children become overly interested in their sexuality. If masturbation becomes a problem, talk to your pediatrician. For most children, masturbation is nothing to worry about. It is normal.

As your child approaches puberty, she should know about the following:

- The body parts related to sex and their functions
- How babies are conceived and born
- Puberty and how the body will change
- Menstruation (Both boys and girls can benefit from this information.)
- Sexual intercourse
- Birth control
- Sexually transmitted diseases (STDs) and how they are spread, including HIV and AIDS
- Masturbation
- Homosexuality
- Family and personal guidelines

For more information, visit the American Academy of Pediatrics (AAP) on the Web at www.aap.org or ask your pediatrician about other AAP brochures on sexuality. You also may want to look for books on talking to your child about sexuality from your local library or bookstore.

The information contained in this publication should not be used as a substitute for the medical care and advice of your pediatrician. There may be variations in treatment that your pediatrician may recommend based on individual facts and circumstances.

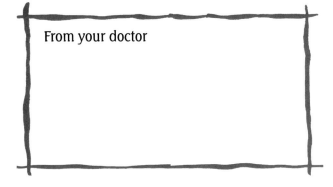

From your doctor

American Academy of Pediatrics

DEDICATED TO THE HEALTH OF ALL CHILDREN™

The American Academy of Pediatrics is an organization of 60,000 primary care pediatricians, pediatric medical subspecialists, and pediatric surgical specialists dedicated to the health, safety, and well-being of infants, children, adolescents, and young adults.

American Academy of Pediatrics
Web site—www.aap.org

Copyright © 2000
American Academy of Pediatrics

Testicular Self-Exam

Most people think that cancer is a disease that only old people get. Cancer of the testicles — the male reproductive glands — is different. It is one of the most common types of cancer in men 15 to 34 years old.

Most testicular cancers are found by young men themselves. By doing a regular exam of your testicles, you greatly increase your chance of finding testicular cancer early if it does occur. It takes only 3 minutes a month to do a simple check for lumps on your testicles.

Here's How:

1. Do the exam once a month, after a warm bath or shower when the scrotal skin is most relaxed.

2. Roll each testicle gently between the thumb and first two fingers of both hands. The testicles should be smooth, with the consistency of a hard-boiled egg without the shell.

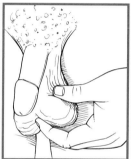

3. Feel for the small, comma-shaped cord, about the size of a pea, that is attached at the back of each testicle. This is a natural part of your testicles, and is called the epididymis. Learn what it feels like, so you will not confuse it with an abnormal lump.

4. Check each testicle for lumps. If you find a lump, tell your doctor about it right away. Not all lumps are cancerous, but only your doctor will be able to tell the difference. Don't let fear keep you from getting the medical help you need.

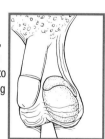

What Is Normal?

- Testicles hang in the scrotum, and are about the same size.
- The left testicle usually hangs down a little more in the scrotum than the right testicle.
- A rope-like structure called the spermatic cord runs from your scrotum up into your groin.

What Are Possible Signs of Cancer?

- A lump on one of the testicles, which usually doesn't hurt.
- One testicle that gets larger than the other.
- A dull ache in your groin that doesn't go away.
- Your testicles feel heavy, like they are dragging.

The information contained in this publication should not be used as a substitute for the medical care and advice of your pediatrician. There may be variations in treatment that your pediatrician may recommend based on individual facts and circumstances.

Illustrations by Lauren Shavell

From your doctor

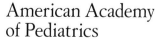

American Academy of Pediatrics

DEDICATED TO THE HEALTH OF ALL CHILDREN™

The American Academy of Pediatrics is an organization of 60,000 primary care pediatricians, pediatric medical subspecialists, and pediatric surgical specialists dedicated to the health, safety, and well-being of infants, children, adolescents, and young adults.

American Academy of Pediatrics
Web site — www.aap.org

Copyright © 1999
American Academy of Pediatrics

Substance Abuse Issues

Alcohol:
Your Child and Drugs

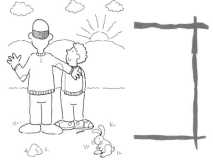

Children are challenged at younger ages than ever before to try drugs. Use of tobacco, marijuana, and cocaine are serious problems. However, one of the most abused drugs in our society is alcohol. Alcohol is a drug because it acts as a depressant on the nervous system and is very addictive. Though it's illegal for people under age 21 to drink, we all know that most teenagers are no strangers to alcohol. Many of them are introduced to alcohol during childhood.

Why parents should worry

- About 1 out of 5 fifth graders have been drunk.
- Four out of 10 sixth graders say there is pressure from other students to drink.
- Nearly 80% of high school seniors report having used alcohol.

Alcohol is often the first drug that young people try. Some parents may breathe a sigh of relief when they find out their teen is "only" drinking alcohol. Since alcohol is legal and found in most American homes, parents may think it isn't dangerous. Not true. Alcohol can be very harmful.

Childhood drinking begins early, often between 11 and 13 years of age, and sometimes even younger. When young people like the feeling they get from alcohol, they may be interested in trying other drugs later. This can lead to multiple drug use, which is very dangerous. The use of alcohol, by itself or with other drugs, can harm your child's normal growth and development.

Even if a teenager only drinks occasionally, intoxicated behavior can be lethal. Just one drink can impair decision making and slow down reaction time in any situation. Alcohol is linked with a variety of risky behaviors, such as:

- **Crime and serious violence.**
- **Early sexual activity, multiple partners, sexually transmitted diseases including AIDS, and unintended teenage pregnancy.**
- **Fetal Alcohol Syndrome.** Drinking during pregnancy can cause a baby to be born with major birth defects. No one knows exactly how much alcohol is too much during pregnancy, but the more a mother drinks, the greater the risk to her baby.
- **Drunk driving.** It is the leading cause of death for young adults, aged 15 to 24 years. In one study, an estimated 6% to 14% of drivers under 21 years of age who were stopped at roadside checkpoints had been drinking. This age-group makes up only one fifth of the licensed drivers in the United States, yet they are involved in almost half of all fatal car crashes.

Why young people drink

Young people drink alcohol for a variety of reasons.
1. Curiosity. They have heard that getting drunk is fun and they want to find out for themselves.
2. They see drinking as a "rite of passage" —something to be experienced on the way to adulthood.
3. To get drunk. This explains why they often drink until they are out of control. Binge drinking (consuming five or more drinks in a row for males, four for females) is alarmingly common. Sixteen percent of 8th graders, 25% of 10th graders, and 30% of seniors have reported binge drinking.
4. To fit in with friends who are already using alcohol.
5. To feel relaxed and to boost self-confidence.
6. To escape problems, such as depression, family conflict, trouble in school or with a boyfriend or girlfriend.

Stages of alcohol use

The same pattern of use and abuse exists for alcohol as with other drugs such as marijuana or cocaine. Experts have noted the following stages of alcohol use:

Stage 1: Experimenting with alcohol. There may be strong peer pressure to use alcohol "just for fun" and to be part of the group. Most use happens on weekends. There often is no change in behavior between uses.

Stage 2: Actively seeking alcohol. Alcohol is used to produce good feelings during times of stress. Usage occurs during the week. Schoolwork may suffer. Changes in behavior may include:
- an increase in time spent alone
- a decline in communication with family members, frequent arguing, and a high level of secretiveness
- changes in dress and grooming
- changes in choice of friends
- repeated or unexplained injuries or fights
- poor sleeping habits and a lack of energy
- irregular eating habits
- bloodshot eyes
- mood changes, including irritability and depression
- running away from home
- attempting suicide

Keep in mind that some of these symptoms occur from time to time in normal, nonalcohol-using teens, and none alone is proof of alcohol or drug use. However, a combination of any of the above symptoms may signal a problem.

Stage 3: Preoccupation with alcohol. There is an almost total loss of control over the use of alcohol. Attempts to limit alcohol use at this stage can cause withdrawal symptoms of depression, moodiness, and irritability. Alcoholic beverages may disappear from the home. There is a danger of turning to other drugs or stronger forms of liquor. Family possessions may also disappear as the alcohol user seeks money to support his habit. There may be trouble with the law for these same reasons.

Parents who drink

Parents who choose to use alcohol must be careful how it is used in the home. Having a drink should never be shown as a way to cope with problems. Don't drink in unsafe conditions—driving the car, mowing the lawn, using the stove, etc. Don't encourage your child to drink or to join you in having a drink. Never make jokes about getting drunk; make sure that your children understand that it is neither funny nor acceptable. Show your children that there are many ways to have fun without alcohol. Happy occasions and special events don't have to include drinking.

The good news

Most adolescents never move beyond the first stage of alcohol use. Whether they do or not depends for the most part on their personality, their family, and their community. For those who do move to the advanced stages, the entire process can take months or years. Many young people and adults receive help too late. This is why early detection is so important.

How to prevent alcohol use and abuse

As with any disease, prevention is the best treatment. Parents must learn the facts about teen alcohol use and abuse to help their children remain alcohol free.

Parents should set a good example at home by limiting their own use of alcohol and other drugs. Parents who don't drink should be aware that this alone will not guarantee their children and teenagers won't use alcohol. Parents who are alcoholics or problem drinkers place their children at increased risk of alcohol dependence. Studies suggest that alcoholism may run in the family. One out of 5 young adults with an alcoholic parent is likely to become an alcoholic too.

Education about alcohol should begin early. Parents can help their children resist alcohol use in these ways:
- **Give your child a sense of confidence.** This is the best defense against peer pressure. Build your child's self-esteem with praise and avoid frequent criticism.
- **Listen** to what your child says. Pay attention, and be helpful during periods of loneliness or doubt.

Alcohol and the media

Young people today are surrounded by messages in the media that drinking alcohol is normal, desirable, and harmless. Alcohol companies spend billions of dollars every year on advertising and promoting their products on TV, in movies and magazines, on billboards, and at sporting events. In fact, alcohol products are among the most advertised products in the nation. Young people are the primary targets of many of these ads.

Alcohol companies and advertisers never mention the dangers of alcoholism, drinking and driving, or Fetal Alcohol Syndrome. Most ads show drinkers as healthy, energetic, sexy, and successful. Help your teenager understand the difference between these misleading messages in advertising and the truth about the dangers of drinking.

- **Know who your child's friends are** and make a point to get to know them.
- **Provide parental supervision.** Don't allow your teen to attend parties where alcohol is being served. Insist that a parent be present at parties to supervise. Contact other parents to arrange alcohol-free social events.
- **Offer a "free call home."** Drinking and driving may lead to death. Make sure your child knows not to ride with a driver who has been drinking. Let him know that he can call home without fear of consequences that night. Discuss the incident the next day.
- **Help your child learn to handle strong emotions and feelings.** Model ways to control stress, pain, or tension.
- **Talk about things that are important issues for your child,** including alcohol, drugs, and the need for peer-group acceptance.
- **Encourage enjoyable and worthwhile outside things to do;** avoid turning leisure time into chores.
- **Join your child in learning all you can about preventing alcohol abuse.** Programs offered in schools, churches, and youth groups can help you both learn more about alcohol abuse.

What parents can do:
- Talk about ads with your child and help them to understand the real messages being conveyed.
- Teach your kids to be careful, questioning consumers.
- Make sure the TV shows and movies your child watches do not glamorize the use of alcohol.
- Do not allow your child to wear T-shirts, jackets, or hats that promote alcohol products.
- Talk to administrators at your teen's school about starting a media education program.

Your pediatrician understands that good communication between parents and children is one of the best ways to prevent alcohol use. If talking with your teenager about alcohol is difficult, your pediatrician may be able to help open the lines of communication. If you suspect your child is using alcohol or any other drug, ask your pediatrician for advice and help.

The information contained in this publication should not be used as a substitute for the medical care and advice of your pediatrician. There may be variations in treatment that your pediatrician may recommend based on individual facts and circumstances.

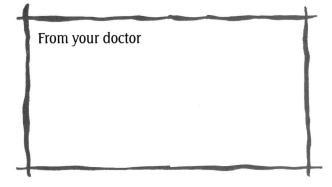

From your doctor

American Academy of Pediatrics

DEDICATED TO THE HEALTH OF ALL CHILDREN™

The American Academy of Pediatrics is an organization of 60,000 primary care pediatricians, pediatric medical subspecialists, and pediatric surgical specialists dedicated to the health, safety, and well-being of infants, children, adolescents, and young adults.
American Academy of Pediatrics
Web site—www.aap.org
Copyright © 1991
American Academy of Pediatrics, Updated 1998

Cocaine: Your Child and Drugs

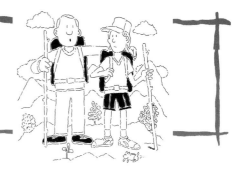

Cocaine use in the United States

Cocaine use by teens is a major problem and concern in America today. Many young people think that drugs are not all that harmful and that using cocaine is a symbol of status and success. They also think that trying cocaine is a step toward becoming an adult. The American Academy of Pediatrics has developed this information to help you learn about the dangers of cocaine use.

What is cocaine?

Cocaine is made from the leaves of the South American cocoa bush. The leaves are soaked in chemicals until they break down into cocaine crystals. These crystals are dried and crushed into a bitter, white powder.

How is cocaine used?

As a powder, cocaine is usually inhaled, or "snorted," through the nose. A less common method is to inject it directly into a vein. Cocaine can also be smoked in a pipe after it is hardened into a paste. This is called "free-basing."

Cocaine is also sold in a nugget form for as little as $5 to $15. This type of cocaine, called "crack," is also smoked. Users can make their own crack from a mixture of cocaine powder, baking soda, and water. Crack cocaine is much more powerful than cocaine in powder form.

The "high" from smoking crack cocaine is more intense and habit-forming than from snorting cocaine powder.

What are the effects of cocaine?

While most people know the effects of alcohol and marijuana, very few know the facts about cocaine. Cocaine is a powerful stimulant. It affects the nervous system and causes a user's heart rate and blood pressure to increase very quickly. Cocaine triggers pleasure centers in the brain and makes the user feel instantly alert. It also creates a false sense of joy (a "high"). But this "high" is short-lived—from 5 to 30 minutes, depending on how the drug is taken. As the drug's effects wear off, users may feel anxious, depressed, and tired. Marijuana, alcohol, sleeping pills, or "uppers" are sometimes used to ease cocaine's effects.

Is cocaine addictive?

The cocaine "high" tempts users to want more of the drug once its effects start to wear off. The more a person uses cocaine, the greater the desire to keep using it. The amount of cocaine needed to get high depends on how it is used, how long the person has been using it, and the strength (potency) of the drug. Cocaine is highly addictive. In laboratory tests, monkeys have starved or died because they chose cocaine instead of food and water. Smoking cocaine or crack increases the risk of addiction. When a person smokes cocaine, the lungs transfer the drug quickly into the bloodstream and it goes straight to the brain.

What are the dangers of cocaine?

Cocaine causes the user's heart rate and blood pressure to increase. The more cocaine used, the more intense this becomes. For some people, even small amounts of cocaine can cause dangerous increases in heart rate and abnormal heart rhythms. When this happens, the heart may not be able to pump enough blood to the brain, and a cocaine user can die.

In young people, cocaine can cause:
- Emotional problems
- School problems
- Low motivation
- Isolation from friends or family
- Family conflicts

Some cocaine users even turn to stealing or prostitution to support this costly drug habit. Pregnant women who use cocaine may have miscarriages, or their babies may be born with severe birth defects.

Stages of drug use

There are several stages of drug use. Be aware of any changes in your child's behavior that may indicate a problem with drugs.

Experimenting with drugs. In this stage, a person tries a drug such as cocaine in search of "fun." There is often strong peer pressure to enter this stage. Assuming there are no initial physical problems, there is usually no change in behavior, except for secret activities meant to hide the cocaine use.

Actively seeking drugs. In this stage, a person needs more cocaine to get the same feelings. This is called tolerance and is a sign of addiction. A person may use cocaine daily to get "high" and escape reality. Behavior begins to change and schoolwork may slip. Problems at home and school may lead the person to use more cocaine. Because cocaine is highly addictive, occasional users can quickly become frequent users.

Preoccupation with drugs. In this stage, there is a significant loss of control over drug use, and the user may become angry or isolated without cocaine. Heavy drug use is costly, and a user may lie and steal from family or friends to pay for cocaine. This may lead to trouble with the law.

Whether or not someone becomes a heavy user often depends on the reasons for trying cocaine in the first place. Recognizing the signs of abuse and getting help from family members, pediatricians, teachers, youth groups, or clergy are the first steps in helping your child recover from drug abuse or addiction.

How to help your child resist drugs

Sooner or later most youngsters will find themselves in a situation in which they must decide whether or not to take drugs. Follow these guidelines to help your child learn to resist this pressure:

- Build your child's self-esteem with plenty of praise and love.
- Avoid being overly critical when your child makes mistakes.
- Talk openly with your child about important topics like drugs and drug use.
- Help your child deal with peer pressure, strong emotions, and feelings.
- Encourage your child to get involved in hobbies, school clubs, and other activities.
- Spend leisure time with your child.

Remember, parents who use and abuse drugs place their children at higher risk for drug abuse. Make sure you set a good example at home by:

- Limiting your use of alcohol
- Not smoking cigarettes
- Using over-the-counter drugs sparingly and only according to directions on the label or from your physician

Despite your best efforts, your teen may still use or abuse drugs. Some warning signs of drug abuse include:

- Changes in choice of friends
- Changes in dress and appearance
- Frequent arguments and unexplained violent actions
- Changes in sleeping or eating habits
- Skipping school
- Falling grades
- Runaway and delinquent behavior
- Legal problems
- Suicide attempts

Positive, honest communication between you and your child is one of the best ways to help prevent drug use. If talking to your teen becomes a problem, your pediatrician may be able to help open the lines of communication. If you suspect your child is using cocaine or any other drug, talk to your pediatrician about how you can help.

The information contained in this publication should not be used as a substitute for the medical care and advice of your pediatrician. There may be variations in treatment that your pediatrician may recommend based on individual facts and circumstances.

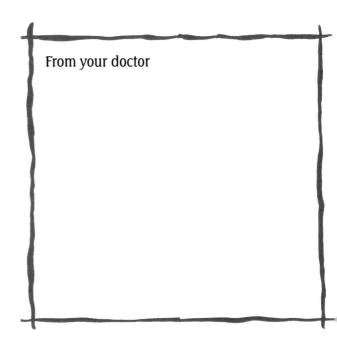

From your doctor

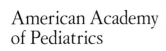

American Academy of Pediatrics

DEDICATED TO THE HEALTH OF ALL CHILDREN™

The American Academy of Pediatrics is an organization of 60,000 primary care pediatricians, pediatric medical subspecialists, and pediatric surgical specialists dedicated to the health, safety, and well-being of infants, children, adolescents, and young adults.

American Academy of Pediatrics
Web site — www.aap.org

Copyright © 1992
American Academy of Pediatrics, Updated 2/96

Testing Your Teen for Illicit Drugs: Information for Parents

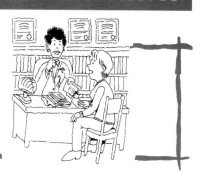

Despite some bright spots, national statistics on illicit drug use are alarming.

More than a third of US high school students have tried an inhalant or illicit drug by the time they are in eighth grade. More than half use an illegal drug by the time they finish high school. Eighty percent of today's high school students have used alcohol.

So if your teen suddenly becomes moody, is spending time with a different group of friends, or starts failing in school, you may wonder if drugs are to blame.

Medically testing your teen for drug use may seem like a straightforward way to get an answer. But it probably is not the best way.

Drug tests are not always reliable, and your teen may resent being tested. Other methods may be better. Through confidential interviews and questionnaires, your pediatrician can help assess whether your teen has a drug problem without resorting to lab tests.

If your teen does undergo a drug test, it should be voluntary. The American Academy of Pediatrics (AAP) opposes involuntary drug tests. Consult your pediatrician if you believe your teen should be tested for drug use.

Types of drug testing

Drug tests most commonly analyze urine. However, many body tissues and fluids can be tested for drug use. Hair, saliva, nails, and sweat are among them. Some of these alternatives show promise. For example, hair tests are difficult to fool and may reveal drug use months after it occurs.

But hair tests are fairly new and do not detect recent drug use. Hair color and type or secondhand marijuana smoke also may skew hair test results. Saliva, nail, and sweat testing need to be refined as well.

Limits of urine drug testing

A chemical analysis of urine—or urinalysis—is the most common drug test. But the test has limits and parents should consider the following pitfalls:

- Test may not detect all illicit drugs. Most routine urine tests do not catch LSD, ketamine, Ecstasy, inhalant, or anabolic steroid use. They also may not detect alcohol, the substance that teens are most likely to use.

- **Test results may be false negatives.** Other drugs are detectable for only a short time after they are used. Most drugs—other than marijuana—can be flushed from the user's system in as few as 12 hours. Within 2 or 3 days, these drugs are almost always undetectable.

  Teens also may try to "cheat" on a urine test. They might dilute their urine samples with tap or toilet water, or drink a lot of water before the test to flush drugs from their systems. Some users buy products designed to beat the test at nutritional supplement stores or through the Internet.

- **Test results may be false positives.** Urine tests that do detect drug use may be misleading and should be confirmed by more specific tests.

  For instance, routine urine test results may show marijuana use days—or even weeks—after your teen has quit using the drug. Some drug tests may mistake traces of legal painkillers containing ibuprofen or naproxen for signs of marijuana use.

Sinus or allergy medicines may show up as amphetamines in drug tests. Other common medicines can test as tranquilizers.

The poppy seeds baked into many foods can cause false positives for opiate use. Some antibiotics also may show up as opiates in tests.

Keep these possibilities in mind if your teen does take a drug test. Consider the test a preliminary screen. Most importantly, seek additional lab tests to confirm any positive results.

While further analysis can almost always pinpoint the cause of a positive drug test, it may take days or weeks to complete. Meanwhile, remember that your teen may be bearing the brunt of false suspicion—so try to avoid jumping to conclusions until all the results are in.

- **Testing may damage the pediatrician-patient relationship.** Involuntary drug testing may undermine your teen's trust in your pediatrician. Even results showing no drug use can be harmful if your teen feels coerced into the test. If your teen does use drugs, trust in your pediatrician is vital to successful substance abuse treatment.

When drug testing may be helpful

The court system or your teen's school may require a drug test. While still a controversial policy, many schools screen young athletes for drug use. Some private schools test all their students.

Urine tests also may help teens who are receiving drug treatment stay away from drugs.

If drug testing is called for, you and your pediatrician should work together to ensure you get reliable lab results. Make sure your teen's sample is carefully collected and handled by an experienced, certified laboratory. Guard against human error or false positives. Be certain the results are properly recorded and kept confidential.

Finally, remember that a lab test is just one measure of drug use. Your pediatrician also will take into account your teen's behavior as a whole.

Is home drug testing advisable?

You can buy home drug testing kits at pharmacies or through the Internet. But home test kits also may give false or deceptive results.

Accurate or not, the test can create hard feelings. Your teen may resent what seems to be a clear sign of distrust and become less open with you. Or anger could turn to rebellion. At the least, a resentful teen is less likely to turn to you for the emotional support that helps deter drug use.

Without a drug test, how can I tell if my teen is using drugs?

Certain symptoms and behaviors are red flags for drug use. But keep in mind they may also indicate other problems, such as depression.

Look for
- Alcohol, smoke, or other chemical odors on your teen's breath or clothing
- Obvious intoxication, dizziness, or bizarre behavior
- Changes in dress and grooming

- Changes in choice of friends
- Frequent arguments, sudden mood changes, and unexplained violent actions
- Changes in eating and sleeping patterns
- Loss of interest in activities
- Truancy
- Failing grades
- Runaway and delinquent behavior
- Suicide attempts

How your pediatrician can help

Your pediatrician may be able to identify drug use by interviewing your teen. Though you may want to participate, let the doctor talk to your teen alone and in strict confidence.

Privacy is crucial. One-on-one talks are most likely to produce the honest answers from your teen that you need.

Teens also want to know their answers to drug use questions will remain confidential. Your pediatrician will respect your child's privacy, but will tell both of you up front that a breach of confidentiality could occur if

- Your teen requires parental assistance.
- Your teen agrees to your request for information.
- Your teen lies to your pediatrician.
- Your pediatrician believes your teen may come to harm or harm someone else.

Do not worry that you will be kept in the dark about a serious problem. Your pediatrician will tell you if your teen is at immediate risk.

Resources

Below is a list of Internet sites that focus on substance abuse. This list is not comprehensive, but includes sites with links to other resources.

- National Institute on Drug Abuse, a division of the National Institutes of Health
  http://www.nida.nih.gov
- **For Real,** sponsored by the Center for Substance Abuse Prevention
  http://www.forreal.org/
- **Parenting is Prevention,** sponsored by the Center for Substance Abuse Prevention
  http://parentingisprevention.org/
- **American Council for Drug Education**
  http://www.acde.org/
- **National Clearinghouse for Alcohol and Drug Information,** sponsored by the Center for Substance Abuse Prevention
  http://www.health.org/
- **Medem,** founded by the American Academy of Pediatrics and other national medical societies
  http://www.medem.com/MedLB/articleslb.cfm?sub_cat=23

Remember

Some teens can stop using drugs based on a strong personal desire to change their lives, and little else. Others stop using drugs when they learn about the risks and potential costs of substance abuse. Many youths stop using alcohol or drugs as they reach late adolescence.

But sometimes teens need outside help to quit. Your pediatrician can help you find the right counseling and treatment. That may mean psychiatric treatment. Or it may mean a referral to a detoxification program.

Teen drug use is a serious problem. You do not have to handle it alone. Do not be afraid to seek professional help from your pediatrician, a counselor, support group, or treatment program. They can help you provide the support that is so crucial to the success of any treatment program.

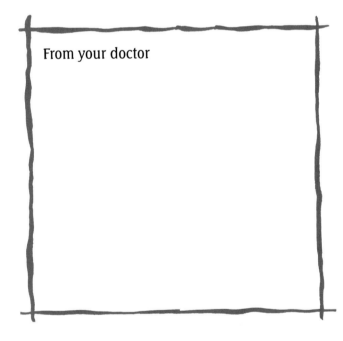

From your doctor

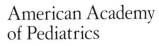

American Academy of Pediatrics

DEDICATED TO THE HEALTH OF ALL CHILDREN™

The American Academy of Pediatrics is an organization of 60,000 primary care pediatricians, pediatric medical subspecialists, and pediatric surgical specialists dedicated to the health, safety, and well-being of infants, children, adolescents, and young adults.

American Academy of Pediatrics
Web site—www.aap.org

Copyright © 2003
American Academy of Pediatrics

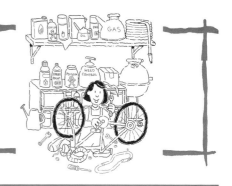

Inhalant Abuse:
Your Child and Drugs
Guidelines for Parents

When you think of young people using drugs, alcohol and marijuana probably come to mind first. Some young people do use those drugs, but each year more are abusing another group of substances that you may know little about. These are called inhalants. The abuse of inhalants is also called solvent abuse, huffing, sniffing, glue sniffing, or volatile substance abuse.

There are over 1,000 inhalants—common products most often found in the home, office, and classroom. These products are legal because they have a useful purpose. They are also safe when used for that purpose. But when young people misuse them by breathing them into their lungs, inhalants are poison. Over time, the abuse of inhalants can cause severe permanent damage to the body, especially the brain. **The scariest thing about inhalants is that your child could die from using them only once.**

Read this brochure to learn more about inhalants so that you can talk with your child about them. Educating young people about their dangers is an important step in preventing inhalant abuse. This brochure also describes the signs and symptoms of inhalant abuse. If you suspect your child is abusing inhalants, it is important to get help and, if necessary, treatment right away.

Common inhalants and how they are used

Hair spray. Gasoline. Spray paint. Glue. Typewriter correction fluid. You probably have at least one of these products in your home. These are just a few of the inhalants that are poisonous when children:

- Sniff or inhale them directly from the cans, bottles, or other containers they are in.
- Spray them into a bag, empty soft drink can, or other container and breathe them in. (Gases like nitrous oxide are often inhaled from balloons.)
- Spray or pour them onto a cloth or piece of clothing and inhale deeply from the fabric.

There are three general types of inhalants: solvents, gases, and nitrites.

- **Solvents** are usually liquid. They are found in household and industrial products, such as glues, paints, and polishes.
- **Gases** are found in many household and commercial products. Aerosol sprays like hair spray and spray paint, as well as medical gases like nitrous oxide, fall into this category. Almost all pressurized aerosol sprays can be abused.
- **Nitrites** are found in room deodorizers.

Inhalant abuse is on the rise

Inhalant abuse is a growing problem—one that deserves parents' attention. While the use of some drugs is declining, inhalant abuse is on the rise among children and teens. In the past decade it has nearly doubled. Adolescents 12 to 14 years of age are most likely to abuse inhalants, and almost 20% of eighth-graders have tried some form of them. Most young people who ever try inhalants do so before their second year of high school.

A household guide to inhalants

Here is a list of only a few of the common household products that are dangerous when inhaled:

Kitchen
Cooking spray
Typewriter correction fluid
Disinfectants
Fabric protectors
Felt-tip markers
Furniture polish and wax
Oven cleaners

Bathroom
Air fresheners
Spray deodorants
Hair sprays
Nail polish removers

Garage/Workshop
Pressurized aerosol sprays
Butane
Gasoline
Glues and adhesives
Paints and paint thinners
Refrigerants (freon)
Rust removers
Spray paints

Why do children abuse inhalants?

There are many reasons why inhalants appeal to children. They are cheap, easy to get, and easy to hide. For a few dollars, a can of butane offers a quick high. Or a child can sit in class and secretly sniff correction fluid. Because inhalants are legal, kids can easily make excuses if they are caught with them.

Another appeal of inhalants is the social part of using them. Kids enjoy abusing inhalants with other kids, and most inhalant abuse is thought to be done with friends.

Reasons why children use inhalants

- Low cost
- Way to rebel against parents
- Easy to get and hide

- Peer pressure or influence
- Not illegal to possess, so kids can make excuses if they are caught with inhalants
- Public is not aware of the dangers

Signs and symptoms of inhalant abuse

- Breath and clothing that smells like chemicals
- Spots or sores around the mouth
- Paint or stains on body or clothing
- Drunk, dazed, or glassy-eyed look
- Nausea, loss of appetite
- Anxiety, excitability, irritability

Prevention of inhalant abuse

Although some states have laws to try and deal with inhalant abuse, such laws are not always easy to enforce. Since inhalants are legal and kids can get them from so many different ways, it is not possible to make inhalants entirely off-limits. The best way to fight inhalant abuse is to educate your child about how harmful these products are. Explain how they can cause both short- and long-term health problems, further drug abuse, and death. It is important to start talking with children at a young age, because inhalant abuse often starts as young as 8 or 9 years old. Parents and teachers should also be able to recognize the warning signs of inhalant abuse.

Help prevent your child from turning to inhalants and other drugs by taking these steps:

Set a good example at home. As a parent, you are the best role model for your child. Parents who use drugs also place their children at higher risk for drug use.

Build self-esteem and confidence. Praise your child often. Encourage your son or daughter to set goals and make decisions to achieve them. With each success and your constant support, your child will become more confident in what he or she can do. Children with self-confidence feel good about themselves without needing drugs.

Help your child develop different interests. Encourage your child to read, have hobbies, play sports, or join clubs. These activities can keep your son or daughter from using drugs out of boredom or from having too much free time. Young people will find that they can have a lot of fun and feel good without drugs. Take an active interest in your child's interests and in his or her friends.

Help your child resist peer pressure. Being independent and self-confident can help your child resist pressure from friends to abuse inhalants. To foster independence, show confidence in your child's ability to make his or her own decisions. Encourage your child to make his or her own judgments, no matter what friends or others say or do.

Talk openly and often. Talk about things that are important to and relevant in your child's life. This includes discussing drugs and how some kids might use them to be accepted by their peers. Educating your pre-teen or teen about the dangers of drugs, including inhalant abuse, works best through talking rather than lecturing.

Treatment of inhalant abuse

When children are abusing inhalants, many times their parents do not find out until the abuse has already become a habit. Chronic inhalant abusers are hardest to treat because they often have many serious personal and social problems. They also have difficulty staying off inhalants and have very high rates of relapse. All of these reasons can keep chronic inhalant abusers from benefiting from many drug abuse treatment programs.

Toxic chemicals from inhalants stay in the body for weeks. Because of this, when chronic abusers stop using inhalants they may feel the effects of withdrawal for weeks. Withdrawal is the body's way of getting over its physical addiction to inhalants. During withdrawal from inhalants, a person may have:
- Hand tremors
- Excess sweating
- Constant headaches
- Nervousness

Treatment for inhalant abusers is usually long-term, sometimes as long as 2 years. It must address the many social problems most inhalant abusers have and involves:
- Support of the child's family
- Moving the child away from unhealthy friendships with other abusers
- Teaching and fostering better coping skills
- Building self-esteem and self-confidence
- Helping the child adjust to school or another learning setting

Inhalant abuse is a difficult form of substance abuse to treat. It is best to recognize and start treatment before the problem becomes a habit. Parents and educators need to be able to recognize the signs of inhalant abuse, especially because most abusers do not seek treatment on their own.

Parents also play the most important role in helping their children to resist abusing inhalants in the first place. The most effective prevention of inhalant abuse is through the education of parents, teachers, and school-aged children.

Information for you and your child

What are the effects of inhalants?

One thing that all inhalants have in common is that they contain chemicals that were never meant for people to consume. So why would anyone breathe toxic chemicals on purpose? Just like the users of other drugs, inhalant abusers try to get "high" from the chemicals.

The effects of inhalants usually last only a few minutes, unless users inhale repeatedly. At first, inhalants have a stimulating effect. Then if the users keep inhaling, they may feel dazed, dizzy, and have trouble walking. Sometimes users get aggressive or think they see things that are not there. Stronger chemicals or repeated inhaling can cause people to pass out. A user can also die suddenly from using inhalants.

When someone uses an inhalant, large amounts of toxic chemicals enter the lungs and pass from the bloodstream into the brain. There they damage and kill brain cells. The amount of fumes a young person inhales greatly exceeds what is considered safe even in a workplace setting. It takes at least 2 weeks for the body to get rid of some of the chemicals in inhalants. Inhalants exit the body mainly through exhaling, which is why an inhalant abuser's breath often smells like chemicals. Inhalants also pass out of the body through urine.

Short-term effects of inhalants are:

- Headaches, nausea, vomiting
- Loss of balance
- Dizziness
- Slurred and slow speech
- Mood changes
- Hallucinations

Over time, inhalants can cause more serious damage, such as:

- Loss of concentration
- Short-term memory loss
- Hearing loss
- Muscle spasms
- Permanent brain damage
- Death

How do inhalants kill?

No one can predict how much of an inhalant will kill. A young person can use a certain amount one time and seem fine, but his or her next use could be fatal.

The Texas Commission on Drugs and Alcohol Abuse reports the following ways that inhalants can kill:

- Asphyxia—Solvent gases can cause a person to stop breathing from a lack of oxygen.
- Choking—Users can choke on their own vomit.
- Suffocation—This is more common among users who inhale from plastic bags.
- Injuries—Inhalants can cause people to become careless or aggressive. This often leads to behaviors that can injure or kill, such as operating a motor vehicle dangerously or jumping from great heights. Teens also can get burned or even be killed if someone lights a cigarette while they are huffing butane, gasoline, or some other flammable substance.
- Suicides—Coming down from an inhalant high causes some people to feel depressed, which may lead them to take their own lives.
- Cardiac arrest—Chemicals from inhalants can make the heart beat very fast and irregularly, then suddenly stop beating. This is called cardiac arrest. One reason why this might happen is that inhalants somehow make the heart extra-sensitive to adrenaline. (Adrenaline is a hormone that the body produces, usually in response to fear, excitement, or surprise.) A sudden rush of adrenaline combined with inhalants can make the heart stop instantly. This "Sudden Sniffing Death," as it is called, is responsible for more than half of all deaths due to inhalant abuse.

Another very real danger of inhalants is that they often lead young people to try other drugs whose effects are even more intense and last longer.

The information contained in this publication should not be used as a substitute for the medical care and advice of your pediatrician. There may be variations in treatment that your pediatrician may recommend based on individual facts and circumstances.

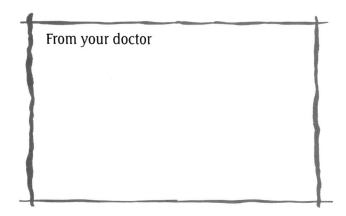

From your doctor

American Academy of Pediatrics

DEDICATED TO THE HEALTH OF ALL CHILDREN™

The American Academy of Pediatrics is an organization of 60,000 primary care pediatricians, pediatric medical subspecialists, and pediatric surgical specialists dedicated to the health, safety, and well-being of infants, children, adolescents, and young adults.

American Academy of Pediatrics
Web site—www.aap.org

Copyright © 1996
American Academy of Pediatrics

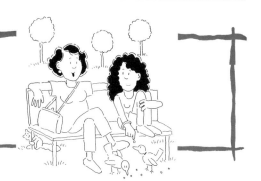

Marijuana:
Your Child and Drugs

Young people today can face strong peer pressure to try drugs. As a parent, you are your child's first and best protection against drug use. The first step is to become informed yourself. The American Academy of Pediatrics has developed this brochure to help you learn about marijuana and how you can help your child withstand pressure to use it.

Marijuana comes from the cannabis plant and looks like dried leaves. It is smoked either in a pipe or a hand-rolled cigarette, called a "joint." Other common names for marijuana are pot, weed, grass, herb, and reefer.

Marijuana is fairly easy for young people to get. It also tends to be the first illegal drug they try. After smoking marijuana, teens may go on to try "harder" drugs, such as cocaine and LSD.

Teens' use of marijuana has gone up in recent years. Among high school students, marijuana is one of the most widely abused drugs. A 1995 national survey of American high school seniors showed that:

- 41% have used marijuana at some time in their lives
- 21% used it in the past 30 days
- 4.6% use marijuana every day
- 88% said the drug is fairly easy or very easy to get

About one third of marijuana smokers start using the drug by sixth grade.

These statistics are cause for concern. Another concern is that marijuana today is about 25 times stronger than it was in the 1960s. THC, the main ingredient in marijuana, builds up in the body over time. The more a person smokes, the more THC builds up. It can take several weeks for the body to get rid of chemicals from just one marijuana cigarette. Besides THC, marijuana contains more than 400 other chemicals that can be health hazards.

Some short-term effects of smoking marijuana include:

- Calm, relaxed, sleepy feeling
- Increased appetite
- Dry, bloodshot eyes; dry throat and mouth
- Increased heart rate
- Slowed reaction time
- Poor short-term memory
- Anxiety, panic attacks, or paranoia

Why young people are at risk

Over time, marijuana may cause serious physical effects in teens who are still growing and maturing. These include:

- Lower sperm count and testosterone levels in males (Testosterone is a hormone that controls hair and penis growth, muscle mass, and voice changes during puberty.)
- Irregular menstrual periods and ovulation in females, which can lead to infertility
- Heart and lung damage
- Cancer

- Memory problems
- Psychological dependence on the drug

Marijuana can make it difficult for a person to think, listen, speak, remember things, solve problems, and form concepts. It can also affect how well your teen does in school. Heavy, chronic marijuana smokers often have less drive and ambition.

The effects of marijuana can make driving or playing sports risky. This is because marijuana impairs complex motor skills and the ability to judge speed and time. Using drugs like marijuana increases the risk of injury, such as from vehicle crashes.

In adolescence, sexual feelings are evolving and changing. Smoking marijuana can confuse these feelings and cause your teen to take sexual chances. This could lead to an unplanned pregnancy or a sexually transmitted disease (including HIV, the virus that causes AIDS).

Why do young people try marijuana?

There are many reasons why young people use drugs. Some of the most common reasons are:

- To fit in with their friends
- To avoid dealing with strong emotions or problems
- Because they are curious
- To rebel and be different
- For a quick way to feel good and have fun
- Because some media show drug use as "cool" or normal and not having any bad effects

Some teens may think using marijuana will make them "cool" or seem more adult-like. They need to know that marijuana use is not a normal step in growing up, despite what their peers may say.

Stages of marijuana use

There are three stages of drug use that can occur:

- **Casual use.** There is strong peer pressure to enter this stage, where a teen usually smokes marijuana to feel good and have fun. He or she still limits drug use in this stage.
- **Heavier use.** The user enters this stage when he or she starts to build a tolerance to marijuana. This is when a person needs more and more of a drug to get the same effects as before. You may notice behavior changes in this stage (see the box on this page). Your teen's schoolwork also may slip. Problems that develop at home and at school because of drug use may cause a teen to use even more drugs.
- **Dependency.** In this stage there is a real loss of control over drug use. The user now feels that he or she needs marijuana to get through the day. Without it, he or she may become angry or withdrawn. Because heavy use is costly, a teen may lie and steal from family and friends to be able to buy marijuana. This could lead to trouble with the law.

Whether or not someone becomes a heavy user will depend on his or her reasons for smoking marijuana in the first place. Being able to recognize the signs of abuse is the first step in getting help for your teen.

Signs your child may be using marijuana

Your child:

- Has red eyes; uses eye drops a lot
- Is hungry often and even gains weight
- Is less motivated and has an "I don't care" attitude
- Withdraws from the family; spends more time in his or her room or away from home
- Forgets things; has trouble paying attention or communicating
- Buys things like CDs and T-shirts with pro-marijuana messages or symbols
- Starts missing school or shows a drop in school grades
- Has new friends and interests; gives up old hobbies, sports, or other activities

How to help your child say "no" to marijuana

Talk with your teen about drugs: Young people who do not know the facts about drugs may try them just to see what they are like. After you become informed, talk with your teen about marijuana and its harmful effects. Try to get your teen to share any questions and concerns he or she has. Be sure to really listen to your teen; do not lecture or do all the talking.

Help your teen handle peer pressure: Peers and friends can strongly influence your teen to try marijuana. As a parent, your influence can be just as strong to help your teen be independent and resist peer pressure. Tell him or her that it is okay to say "no" to marijuana and mean it. Your teen might respond to friends by saying, "I tried marijuana and didn't like it," or "I would get in a lot of trouble if my parents ever found out." Practice these and other responses with your son or daughter. If a friend is offering the marijuana, it may be harder to say "no." Your teen can suggest other things to do with that friend. This shows that your teen is rejecting the drug, not the friend.

Help your teen deal with emotions: During the teen years, many young people face strong emotions for the first time. These new feelings can be hard to cope with, and your teen may sometimes get depressed or anxious. He or she may turn to marijuana to escape such feelings and forget problems. It is important to talk with your teen about any concerns and problems he or she is facing. Assure your teen that everything has an upside, and things do not stay "bad" for very long. Point out that even after using marijuana or other drugs, the same problems and hassles are still there.

Enhance your teen's self-confidence: Praise the positive qualities in your teen often. Encourage your son or daughter to set goals and make personal decisions to achieve them. With each success, your teen will gain more confidence. Applaud effort as well as success. As your teen becomes more responsible, you can still provide guidance, emotional support, and security when needed. Becoming responsible also means facing the results of one's

actions—good or bad. Making mistakes is a normal part of growing up; so try not to be too critical when your son or daughter makes a mistake.

Instill strong values in your teen. Teach your son or daughter the values that are important to your family. Also teach him or her to think of these values when deciding what is right and wrong. Explain that these are the standards your family lives by, despite what other people are doing.

Be a good role model: As a parent, you should avoid use of marijuana and other drugs. You are the best role model for your teen. Make a stand against drug issues—your teen will listen.

Encourage healthy ways to have fun: Young people are always looking for ways to have fun. They can also get bored easily. Drugs offer what seems to be a carefree "high" with little or no effort. Help your teen develop an interest in different hobbies, clubs, and activities. Look for healthy ways to reduce boredom and too much free time. Take an active interest in what is important to your teen.

Realize that not all young people will resist the lure of drugs. If your teen is using marijuana, he or she needs your help. Know the signs of marijuana use. Being able to recognize these signs is the first step in getting help for your teen. Pediatricians, family members, teachers, youth groups, mental health professionals, and clergy can provide support for your teen to stop smoking marijuana. If the problem is too much for you to handle on your own, get professional help. Your teen may need counseling, a support group, and/or a treatment program.

The information contained in this publication should not be used as a substitute for the medical care and advice of your pediatrician. There may be variations in treatment that your pediatrician may recommend based on individual facts and circumstances.

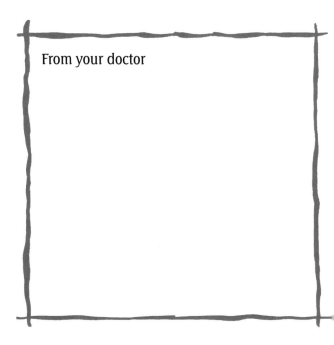

From your doctor

American Academy of Pediatrics

DEDICATED TO THE HEALTH OF ALL CHILDREN™

The American Academy of Pediatrics is an organization of 60,000 primary care pediatricians, pediatric medical subspecialists, and pediatric surgical specialists dedicated to the health, safety, and well-being of infants, children, adolescents, and young adults.

American Academy of Pediatrics
Web site—www.aap.org

Copyright © 1992
American Academy of Pediatrics, Updated 3/96

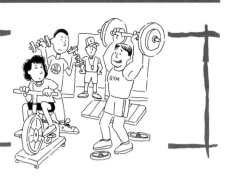

Steroids:
Play Safe, Play Fair

Athletes, whether they are young or old, professional or amateur, are always looking to gain an advantage over their opponents. The desire for an "edge" exists in all sports, at all levels of play. Successful athletes rely on practice and hard work to increase their skill, speed, power, and ability. However, some athletes resort to drugs to improve their performance on the field or the court.

Some high school and even middle school students are using steroids to gain an edge, improve their skill level, or become more athletic. Steroid use is not limited to males. More and more females are putting themselves at risk by using these drugs. It is important to know that using anabolic steroids not only is illegal, but it also can have serious side effects.

What are steroids?

You may have heard them called 'roids, juice, hype, or pump. Anabolic steroids are powerful drugs that many people take in high doses to boost athletic performance. Anabolic means "building body tissue." *Anabolic* steroids help build muscle tissue and increase body mass by acting like the body's natural male hormone, testosterone.

Lower doses of anabolic steroids sometimes are used to treat a handful of very serious medical conditions. They should not be confused with corticosteroids, which are used to treat common medical conditions such as asthma and arthritis. *Corticosteroids* are strong medications, but do not have muscle-building effects. Anabolic steroids are the ones abused by athletes and others who want a shortcut to becoming bigger and stronger.

Who uses steroids?

In the past, steroid use was seen mostly in college, Olympic, and professional sports. Today, steroids are being used by athletes as well as non-athletes, in high schools and middle schools. Most major professional and amateur athletic organizations have banned steroids for use by their athletes. These organizations include the International Olympic Committee, National Collegiate Athletic Association (NCAA), and the National Football League (NFL).

Most commonly, steroid use can be found among the following groups:
- Athletes involved in sports that rely on strength and size, like football, wrestling, or baseball
- Endurance athletes, such as those involved in track-and-field and swimming
- Athletes involved in weight training or bodybuilding
- Anyone interested in building and defining muscles

How are steroids used?

Steroids can be taken in the following two ways:
- By mouth (pills)
- Injected with a needle (Athletes who share needles to inject steroids also are at risk for serious infections including Hepatitis B and HIV, the AIDS virus.)

Some athletes take even higher doses, called "megadoses," to produce faster results. Others gradually increase the amount they take over time, which is called "pyramiding." Taking different kinds of anabolic steroids, possibly along with other drugs, is a particularly dangerous practice known as "stacking."

Will steroids make me a better athlete?

No. Steroids *cannot* improve an athlete's agility or skill. Many factors help determine athletic ability, including genetics, body size, age, sex, diet, and how hard the athlete trains. It is clear that the medical dangers of steroid use far outweigh the advantage of gains in strength or muscle mass.

What are the side effects of steroids?

Steroids can cause serious health problems. Many changes take place inside the body and may not be noticed until it is too late. Some of the effects will go away when steroid use stops, but some may not.

For both sexes

Possible side effects for males and females include the following:
- High blood pressure and heart disease
- Liver damage and cancers
- Stroke and blood clots
- Urinary and bowel problems, such as diarrhea
- Headaches, aching joints, and muscle cramps
- Nausea and vomiting
- Sleep problems
- Increased risk of ligament and tendon injuries
- Severe acne, especially on face and back
- Baldness

A special danger to adolescents

High school and middle school students and athletes need to be aware of the effect steroids have on growth. Anabolic steroids, even in small doses, have been shown to stop growth too soon. Adolescents also may be at risk for becoming dependent on steroids. Adolescents who use steroids are also more likely to use other addictive drugs and alcohol.

Males

One of the more disturbing effects of steroid use for males is that the body begins to produce less of its own testosterone. As a result, the testicles may begin to shrink. Following is a list of some of the other effects of steroid use for males:

- Reduced sperm count
- Impotence
- Increase in nipple and breast size (gynecomastia)
- Enlarged prostate (gland that mixes fluid with sperm to form semen)

Females

Since steroids act as a male hormone, females may experience the following side effects:

- Reduced breast size
- Enlarged clitoris (a very sensitive part of the genitals)
- Increase in facial and body hair
- Deepened voice
- Menstrual problems

A word about...supplements

Over-the-counter supplements such as creatine and androstenedione ("andro") are gaining popularity. Though these supplements are not steroids, manufacturers claim they can build muscles, and improve strength and stamina, without the side effects of steroids.

It is important to know that these substances are not regulated by the Food and Drug Administration (FDA) and are not held to the same strict standards as drugs. Like steroids, they are also banned by the NFL, NCAA, and International Olympic Committee.

Although both creatine and androstenedione occur naturally in foods, there are serious concerns about the long-term effects of using them as supplements. These products may be unsafe. Remember, there is no replacement for a healthy diet, proper training, and practice.

Emotional effects

Steroids also can have the following effects on the mind and behavior:

- "Roid rage"—severe, aggressive behavior that may result in violence, such as fighting or destroying property
- Severe mood swings
- Hallucinations—seeing or hearing things that are not really there
- Paranoia—extreme feelings of mistrust and fear
- Anxiety and panic attacks
- Depression and thoughts of suicide
- An angry, hostile, or irritable mood

Play safe, play fair

Success in sports takes talent, skill, and most of all, practice and hard work. Using steroids is a form of cheating and interferes with fair competition. More importantly, they are dangerous to your health. There are many healthy ways to increase your strength or improve your appearance. If you are serious about your sport and your health, keep the following tips in mind:

- Train safely, without using drugs.
- Eat a healthy diet.
- Get plenty of rest.
- Set realistic goals and be proud of yourself when you reach them.
- Seek out training supervision, coaching,and advice from a reliable professional.
- Avoid injuries by playing safely and using protective gear.
- Talk to your pediatrician about nutrition, your health, preventing injury, and safe ways to gain strength.

If you, your friends, or teammates are using steroids, get help. Share this information with friends and teammates. Take a stand against the use of steroids and other drugs. Truly successful athletes combine their natural abilities with hard work to win. There is no quick and easy way to become the best.

For more information, contact the following organizations:

National Institute on Drug Abuse (NIDA)
888/644-6432
Web site: http://www.nida.nih.gov/

National Clearinghouse for Alcohol and Drug Information (NCADI)
800/729-6686
Web site: http://www.health.org

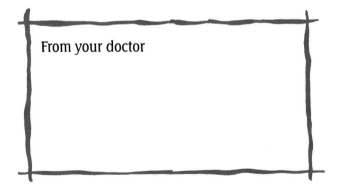

From your doctor

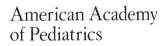

American Academy
of Pediatrics

DEDICATED TO THE HEALTH OF ALL CHILDREN™

The American Academy of Pediatrics is an organization of 60,000 primary care pediatricians, pediatric medical subspecialists, and pediatric surgical specialists dedicated to the health, safety, and well-being of infants, children, adolescents, and young adults.

American Academy of Pediatrics
Web site—www.aap.org

Copyright © 1999
American Academy of Pediatrics

Substance Abuse Prevention

Part I What Every Parent Needs To Know

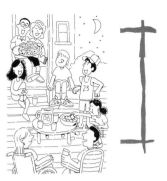

The use of tobacco, alcohol, and other drugs is one of the biggest problems facing young people today. This brochure is designed to help parents prevent some of these problems. Your pediatrician cares very much about your family, and wants to help if there are problems in any area—especially if you have concerns about substance abuse.

Prevention starts with parents

There are no guarantees that your child will not choose to use drugs, but as a parent, you can influence that decision by:

- not using drugs yourself
- providing guidance and clear rules about not using drugs
- spending time with your child sharing the good and the bad times

All of these are necessary to help your child grow up free from the problems of drug use.

Ask yourself a few questions

Much of what children learn about drugs comes from parents. Take a few minutes to answer the following questions about your feelings and behaviors about tobacco, alcohol, and other drugs.

- Do you usually offer alcoholic drinks to friends and family when they come to your home?
- Do you frequently take medicine for minor aches and pains or if you are feeling sad or nervous?
- Do you take sleeping pills to fall asleep?
- Do you use alcohol or any other drug in a way that you would not want your child to?
- Do you smoke cigarettes?
- Are you proud about how much you can drink?
- Do you make jokes about getting drunk or using drugs?
- Do you go to parties that involve a lot of drinking?
- Do you drink and drive or ride with drivers who have been drinking?
- Has your child ever seen you drunk?
- Do you let minors drink alcohol in your home?

Teach your child to say no

Tell your child exactly how you expect her to respond if someone offers her drugs:

- Ask questions ("What is it?" "Where did you get it?")
- Say no firmly.
- Give reasons ("No thanks, I'm not into that.")
- Suggest other things to do (go to a movie, the mall, or play a game)
- Leave (go home, go to class, join other friends)

Parents can also help their children choose not to use tobacco, alcohol, and other drugs in these ways:

- Build your child's self-esteem with praise and support for decisions. A strong sense of self-worth will help your child to say no to tobacco, alcohol, and other drugs and mean it.
- Gradually allow your child to make more decisions alone. Making a few mistakes is a normal part of growing up, so try not to be too critical when your child makes a mistake.
- Listen to what your child says. Pay attention, and be helpful during periods of loneliness or doubt.
- Offer advice about handling strong emotions and feelings. Help your child cope with emotions by letting her know that feelings will change. Explain that mood swings are not really bad, and they won't last forever. Model how to control mental pain or tension without the use of tobacco, alcohol, or other drugs.
- Plan to discuss a wide variety of topics with your child including alcohol, tobacco, and other drugs and the need for peer-group acceptance. Young people who don't know the facts about tobacco, alcohol, and other drugs are at greater risk of trying them.
- Encourage fun and worthwhile outside things to do; avoid turning too much of your child's leisure time into chores.
- Be a good role model by avoiding tobacco, alcohol, or other drugs yourself. You're the best role model for your child. Make a stand against drug issues—your child will listen.

Your pediatrician understands that good communication between parents and children is one of the best ways to prevent drug use. If talking to your child becomes a problem, your pediatrician may provide the key to opening the lines of communication.

Parents guide to teenage parties

If your teen is giving a party:

- **Plan in advance.** Go over party plans with your teen. Encourage your teen to plan some organized group activities or games.
- **Keep parties small.** 10 to 15 teens for each adult. Make sure at least one adult is present at all times. Ask other parents to come over to help you if you need it.
- **Set a guest list.** The party should be for invited guests only. No "crashers" allowed. This will help avoid the "open party" situation.
- **Set a time limit.** Set starting and ending times for the party. Check local curfew laws to determine an ending time.

- **Set party "rules."** Discuss them with your teen before the party. Rules should include the following:
  - ✓ No tobacco, alcohol, or other drugs.
  - ✓ No one can leave the party and then return.
  - ✓ Lights are left on at all times.
  - ✓ Certain rooms of the house are off-limits.
- **Know your responsibilities.** Remember, you are legally responsible for anything that happens to a minor who has been served alcohol or other drugs in your home. Help your child feel responsible for this as well. Guests who bring tobacco, alcohol, or other drugs to the party should be asked to leave. Be ready to call the parents of anyone who comes to the party intoxicated to make sure they get safely home.
- **Be there, but not square.** Pick out a spot where you can see what is going on without being in the way. You can also help serve snacks and beverages.

If your teen is going to a party:

- **Call the host's parent** to verify the party and offer any help. Make sure a parent will be at the party and that tobacco, alcohol, and other drugs will not be allowed.
- **Know where your child is going.** Have the phone number and address of the party. Ask your teen to call you if the location of the party changes. Be sure to let your child know where you will be during the party.
- **Make sure your teen has a way to get home from the party.** Make it easy for your child to leave a party by making it clear that he can call at any time for a ride home. Discuss why he might need to make such a call. Remind your teen NEVER to ride home with a driver who has been drinking.
- **Be up to greet your child when he comes home.** This can be a good way to check the time and talk about the evening.

Talk to your teen about safe partying

Maybe your teen has been to parties where there were tobacco, alcohol, and other drugs. Maybe he tried them. Maybe after using them your teen did something stupid, something he wouldn't normally do.

It's hard for people to stay safe when they aren't thinking clearly. How can teens keep a clear head and still have fun? Give them the following suggestions for staying safe while having a good time:

- Hang out with people who don't smoke, drink, or use other drugs.
- Plan not to smoke, drink, or use other drugs. Do whatever it takes to help you remember.
- Use the "buddy system"—team up with a friend. Use a code word to remind each other when it's time to leave a party.
- If your teen likes to meet new people, suggest trying some of the following activities instead of parties:

free concerts	dances
espresso bars	museums
extra-curricular "anythings"	community centers
libraries	sports events
religious activities	film festivals
athletic clubs	volunteer work

How can I tell if my child is doing drugs?

Despite your best efforts, your teen may still abuse drugs. Some warning signs of drug use are:

- Smell of alcohol, smoke, or other chemicals on your child's breath or clothing
- Obvious intoxication, dizziness, or bizarre behavior
- Change in dress, appearance, and grooming
- Change in choice of friends
- Frequent arguments, sudden mood changes, and unexplained violent actions
- Change in eating and sleeping patterns
- Skipping school
- Failing grades
- Runaway and delinquent behavior
- Suicide attempts

How parents can help

As you read this brochure, you may be worried that your child is using tobacco, alcohol, or other drugs. Before you confront your child, consider talking to friends, relatives, teachers, employers, and others who know your child. Get their impressions as to how she is doing. If others are concerned, this may make you more comfortable in your decision to talk to your child. Always choose a time when your child is awake, alert, and receptive to talking. Avoid interruptions, maintain privacy, and keep your wits about you. Go over the checklist with your child, highlighting those concerns that have you worried.

Send loving messages, for example:

- "I love you too much to let you hurt yourself."
- "I know other people your age use drugs, but I can't let you continue to behave this way."
- "We'll do anything we can to help you. If tobacco, alcohol, or other drugs are part of the problem, we must talk about it right away."
- "If you are sad, upset, or mad, we want to help you. But our family will not permit any use of tobacco, alcohol, or other drugs."

Don't be critical (avoid these statements):

- "There's only one reason you could be acting this way—you must be on drugs."
- "Don't think you are fooling me. I know what you are doing."
- "How could you be so stupid as to start using drugs and alcohol?"
- "How could you do this to our family?"
- "Where did I go wrong? What did I do to make you start using tobacco, alcohol, and other drugs?"

Remember, if your child is using drugs, she needs your help. Don't be afraid to be a strong parent! However, the problem could become too much for you to handle alone. Don't hesitate to seek professional help, such as your pediatrician, a counselor, support group, or treatment program.

The information contained in this publication should not be used as a substitute for the medical care and advice of your pediatrician. There may be variations in treatment that your pediatrician may recommend based on individual facts and circumstances.

American Academy of Pediatrics

DEDICATED TO THE HEALTH OF ALL CHILDREN™

The American Academy of Pediatrics is an organization of 60,000 primary care pediatricians, pediatric medical subspecialists, and pediatric surgical specialists dedicated to the health, safety, and well-being of infants, children, adolescents, and young adults.

American Academy of Pediatrics
Web site—www.aap.org

Copyright © 1999
American Academy of Pediatrics

Substance Abuse Prevention

Part II Additional Information

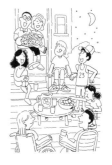

First a child needs roots to grow...then wings to fly

As a parent you can do a lot to prevent your child from using drugs. Use the following tips to help guide your child's thoughts and behaviors about drugs:

1. **Talk with your child honestly.** Don't wait to have "the drug talk" with your child. Make discussions about tobacco, alcohol, and other drugs part of your daily conversation. Know the facts about how drugs can harm your child. Clear up any wrong information, such as "everybody drinks" or "marijuana won't hurt you." Be clear about family rules for use of tobacco, alcohol, and other drugs.

2. **Really listen to your child.** Encourage your child to share questions and concerns about tobacco, alcohol, and other drugs. Do not do all the talking or give long lectures.

3. **Help your child develop self-confidence.** Look for all the good things in your child—and then tell your child how proud you are. If you need to correct your child, criticize the action, not your child. Praise your child's efforts as well as successes.

4. **Help your child develop strong values.** Talk about your family values. Teach your child how to make decisions based on these standards of right and wrong. Explain that these are the standards for your family, no matter what other families might decide.

5. **Be a good example.** Look at your own habits and thoughts about tobacco, alcohol, and other drugs. Your actions speak louder than words.

6. **Help your child deal with peer pressure and acceptance.** Discuss the importance of being an individual and the meaning of real friendships. Help your child to understand that he does not have to do something wrong just to feel accepted. Remind your child that a real friend won't care if he does not use tobacco, alcohol, and other drugs.

7. **Make family rules that help your child say "no."** Talk with your child about your expectation that he will say "no" to drugs. Spell out what will happen if he breaks these rules. (For example, "My parents said I can't use the car if I drink.") Be prepared to follow through, if necessary.

8. **Encourage healthy, creative activities.** Look for ways to get your child involved in athletics, hobbies, school clubs, and other activities that reduce boredom and excess free time. Encourage positive friendships and interests. Look for activities that you and your child can do together.

9. **Team up with other parents.** Work with other parents to build a drug-free environment for children. When parents join together against drug use, they are much more effective than when they act alone. One way is to form a parent group with the parents of your child's friends. The best way to stop a child from using drugs is to stop his friends from using them too.

10. **Know what to do if your child has a drug problem.** Realize that no child is immune to drugs. Learn the signs of drug use. Take seriously any concerns you hear from friends, teachers, or other kids about your child's possible drug use. Trust your instincts. If you truly feel that something is wrong with your child, it probably is. If there's a problem, seek professional help.

Tobacco, alcohol, and the media

A big influence on a teen's decision to use tobacco or alcohol is the media. Young people today are surrounded by messages in the media that smoking cigarettes, using smokeless tobacco, and drinking alcohol are normal, desirable, and harmless. Alcohol and tobacco companies spend billions of dollars every year promoting their products on TV, in movies and magazines, on billboards, and at sporting events. In fact, tobacco and alcohol products are among the most advertised products in the nation. Young people are the primary targets of many of these ads.

Ads for these products appeal to young people by suggesting that drinking alcohol and smoking cigarettes will make them more popular, sexy, and successful. Help your teenager understand the difference between the misleading messages in advertising and the truth about the dangers of using alcohol and tobacco products.

What parents can do:

- Talk about ads with your child. Help your child understand the real messages being conveyed.
- Teach your child to be a wary consumer.
- Make sure the TV shows and movies your child watches do not glamorize the use of tobacco, alcohol, and other drugs.
- Do not allow your child to wear T-shirts, jackets, or hats that promote alcohol or tobacco products.
- Talk to administrators at your teen's school about starting a media education program.

The information contained in this publication should not be used as a substitute for the medical care and advice of your pediatrician. There may be variations in treatment that your pediatrician may recommend based on individual facts and circumstances.

American Academy of Pediatrics

DEDICATED TO THE HEALTH OF ALL CHILDREN™

The American Academy of Pediatrics is an organization of 60,000 primary care pediatricians, pediatric medical subspecialists, and pediatric surgical specialists dedicated to the health, safety, and well-being of infants, children, adolescents, and young adults.
American Academy of Pediatrics
Web site—www.aap.org

Copyright © 1999
American Academy of Pediatrics

The Risks of Tobacco Use:
A Message to Parents and Teens

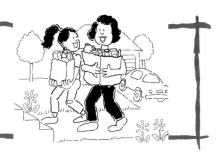

Many people think tobacco-related health problems affect only adults after a lifetime of smoking or tobacco use. Yet, children and teens suffer from tobacco-related health problems as well. The fact is tobacco use can affect every member of the family.

Infants and children

As a parent, you would never knowingly harm your child. Yet, if you are a smoker, the smoke from your cigarette, cigar, or pipe may be putting your child's health in danger. Environmental tobacco smoke, or ETS, is the smoke that is breathed out by a smoker. ETS also includes the smoke that comes from a burning cigarette, cigar, or pipe.

Exposure to ETS is a serious health threat to children. Children exposed to ETS have a greater risk of many health problems including:

- upper respiratory tract infections
- ear infections
- pneumonia
- bronchitis
- asthma
- long-term lung damage

Smoking and ETS are also dangerous to pregnant women and their unborn babies. They have been linked to low birth weight, delayed growth, miscarriage, and stillbirth. Recent studies have found that infants are at greater risk of dying from SIDS (sudden infant death syndrome) if exposed to ETS or if their mother was exposed to ETS during pregnancy.

For more information on ETS, ask your pediatrician about the brochure, *Environmental Tobacco Smoke: A Danger to Children* from the American Academy of Pediatrics.

Teenagers

Ninety percent of all smokers begin the habit during their teens. Over the past 10 years, the number of smokers has decreased in every age-group except teenagers. Among teens, the number of young women smokers has actually increased. Teenage smokers suffer from:

- addiction to nicotine
- long-term cough
- faster heart rate
- decreased lung function
- increased blood pressure
- decreased stamina
- increased risk of developing lung cancer
- increased respiratory tract infection

Smoking is a lifelong addiction that is often hard to break. It may also lead to other addictions and a poorer quality of life. Fighting the influence of the tobacco companies and convincing children not to use tobacco products is a tough task. Parents need to give teenagers the facts about the negative effects of smoking.

Smoking and the media

A big influence on a teen's decision to smoke is the media. Young people today are surrounded by images in the media that smoking is normal, desirable, and harmless. Tobacco companies spend billions of dollars every year promoting their products on TV, in movies and magazines, on billboards, and at sporting events. In fact, tobacco products are among the most advertised products in the nation. The tobacco companies hope to get back the profits they lose as older smokers die and as more and more adults quit smoking. As a result, young people are the primary targets of many of these ads.

Tobacco companies and advertisers never mention the harmful effects of smoking, such as bad breath, stained teeth, heart disease, and cancer. Most ads show smokers as healthy, energetic, sexy, and successful. Help your teenager understand the difference between these misleading messages in advertising and the truth about the dangers of smoking.

What parents can do:

- If you smoke or use tobacco, quit. Your actions will influence your child's behavior too.
- Talk about ads with your children. Help them to understand the real messages being conveyed.
- Teach your kids to be wary consumers.
- Make sure the TV shows and movies your child watches do not normalize or glamorize the use of tobacco.
- Do not allow your child to wear T-shirts, jackets, or hats that promote tobacco products.
- Talk to administrators at your teen's school about starting a media education program.

Adults

Smoking is the most preventable cause of death and disability in the United States. Consider the following facts:

- In this country, 350,000 deaths a year are related to tobacco use.
- One third of all deaths from cancer and heart disease are caused by smoking, chewing tobacco, or snuff.
- Three fourths of the deaths from chronic lung disease are related to tobacco.
- A nonsmoking spouse of a smoker has a 30% greater risk of lung cancer. This alone accounts for 2,000 deaths a year.
- Teenagers whose parents smoke are twice as likely to start smoking than children of nonsmokers.
- In 1964, 55% of adult Americans smoked cigarettes. By 1993, this percentage decreased to 25%. This shows that thousands of Americans have found a way to stop smoking. By doing so, they will live longer, feel better, and improve the health of their families.

Smokeless tobacco: not a safe choice!

The term "smokeless tobacco" refers to both chewing tobacco and snuff (also called "dip"). Chewing tobacco is a form of leaf tobacco. Snuff is finely ground tobacco. Both products lead to nicotine addiction because the nicotine is absorbed into the bloodstream. Smokeless tobacco products damage the lining of the mouth and throat and may cause mouth cancer, throat cancer, and gum disease.

Use of smokeless tobacco products also results in:

- stained teeth
- bad breath
- slow healing of mouth wounds
- lowered sense of taste and smell.

Tobacco companies have increased their advertising programs to promote smokeless tobacco products. Famous athletes often endorse these products, making them seem even more appealing to teenagers. As a result, the number of teenagers and young adults who are chewing tobacco is increasing. Parents need to oppose the use of smokeless tobacco. Inform your children of the serious side effects of its use. The facts on the health risks from smokeless tobacco make one thing very clear: IT IS NOT A SAFE CHOICE!

Break the habit

Would you like to join the growing numbers who have quit using tobacco? Have you tried in the past and failed, but would now like to try again? Why not ask your doctor for help? Your doctor may be just the person to help you find an effective stop-smoking program. For more information, contact any of the following organizations:

American Cancer Society:
1-800/ACS-2345
Web site: www.cancer.org

American Heart Association:
1-800/242-8721
Web site: www.americanheart.org

American Lung Association:
1-800/586-4872
Web site: www.lungusa.org

Your pediatrician understands that good communication between parents and children is one of the best ways to prevent drug use. If talking with your child about tobacco use is difficult, your pediatrician may be able to help open the lines of communication. If you suspect your child is smoking cigarettes or cigars, chewing tobacco, or using any other drug, rely on your pediatrician for advice and help.

The information contained in this publication should not be used as a substitute for the medical care and advice of your pediatrician. There may be variations in treatment that your pediatrician may recommend based on individual facts and circumstances.

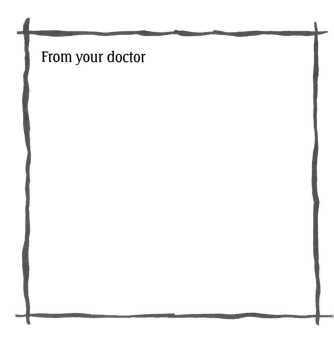

From your doctor

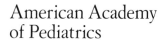

American Academy of Pediatrics

DEDICATED TO THE HEALTH OF ALL CHILDREN™

The American Academy of Pediatrics is an organization of 60,000 primary care pediatricians, pediatric medical subspecialists, and pediatric surgical specialists dedicated to the health, safety, and well-being of infants, children, adolescents, and young adults.

American Academy of Pediatrics
Web site—www.aap.org

Copyright © 1990
American Academy of Pediatrics, Updated 8/98

Smokeless Tobacco
Guidelines for Teens

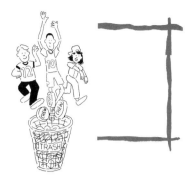

What is smokeless tobacco?

There are two forms of smokeless tobacco: chewing tobacco and snuff. Chewing tobacco is usually sold as leaf tobacco (packaged in a pouch) or plug tobacco (in brick form) that is put between the cheek and gum. Users keep chewing tobacco in their mouths for several hours to get a continuous buzz from the nicotine in the tobacco.

Snuff is a powdered tobacco (usually sold in cans) that is put between the lower lip and gum. Just a pinch is all that is needed to release the nicotine, which is then swiftly absorbed into the bloodstream, resulting in a quick high. Sounds harmless, right? Keep reading . . .

What is in smokeless tobacco?

Chemicals. Keep in mind that the smokeless tobacco you or your friends are using contains many chemicals that can be harmful to your health. Here are a few of the ingredients found in smokeless tobacco:

- Nicotine (addictive drug)
- Polonium 210 (nuclear waste)
- Cadmium (used in car batteries)
- N-Nitrosamines (cancer-causing)
- Lead (poison)
- Formaldehyde (embalming fluid)

The nicotine contained in smokeless tobacco is what gives the user a buzz. It also makes it very hard to quit. Why? Because every time you use smokeless tobacco your body gets used to the nicotine; it actually starts to crave it. Craving is one of the signs of addiction, or dependence.

Your body also adjusts to the amount of tobacco you need to chew to get a buzz. Pretty soon you will need a little more tobacco to get the same feeling. This process is called tolerance, which is another sign of addiction.

Some people say smokeless tobacco is okay because there is no smoke like a cigarette has. Do not believe them. It is not a safe alternative to smoking. You just move health problems from your lungs to your mouth.

Physical and mental effects of smokeless tobacco

If you use smokeless tobacco, here is what you might have to look forward to:

- **Cancer.** Cancer of the mouth (including the lip, tongue, and cheek) and throat. Cancers usually occur at the spot in the mouth where the tobacco is held. The surgery for cancer of the mouth could lead to removal of parts of your face, tongue, cheek, or lip.
- **Leukoplakia.** When you hold tobacco in one place in your mouth, your mouth becomes irritated by the tobacco juice. This causes a white, leathery-like patch to form, and this is called leukoplakia. These patches can be different in size, shape, and appearance. They are also considered precancerous: If you find one in your mouth, see your doctor immediately.

- **Heart Disease.** The constant flow of nicotine into your body causes many side effects including increased heart rate, increased blood pressure, and sometimes irregular heart beats. Nicotine in the body also causes constricted blood vessels that can slow down reaction time and cause dizziness—not a good move if you play sports.
- **Gum and Tooth Disease.** Smokeless tobacco permanently discolors teeth. Chewing tobacco causes halitosis (BAD BREATH). Its direct and repeated contact with the gums cause them to recede, which can cause your teeth to become loose. Smokeless tobacco contains a lot of sugar which, when mixed with the plaque on your teeth, forms acid that eats away at tooth enamel and causes cavities and chronic painful sores.
- **Social Effects.** Having really bad breath, discolored teeth, and gunk stuck in your teeth and constant spitting can have a very negative effect on your social life.

What if I want to quit?

You have just read the bad news, but here is the good news. Even though it is very difficult to quit chewing tobacco, it can be done. Read the following Tips to Quit for some helpful ideas to kick the habit. Remember, most people do not start chewing on their own, so do not try quitting on your own. Ask for help and positive reinforcement from your doctor, friends, parents, coaches, teachers, whomever . . .

Check for early warning signs of oral cancer

Check your mouth often, looking closely at the places where you hold the tobacco. See your doctor right away if you have any of the following:

- a sore that bleeds easily and does not heal
- a lump or thickening anywhere in your mouth or neck
- soreness or swelling that does not go away
- a red or white patch that does not go away
- trouble chewing, swallowing, or moving your tongue or jaw

Even if you do not find a problem today, if you are still using smokeless tobacco be sure to have your mouth checked at every routine doctor or dentist visit. Your chances for a cure are higher if oral cancer is found early.

Tips to Quit

Many smokeless tobacco users say it is even harder to quit smokeless tobacco than cigarettes. Chewing tobacco and snuff contain nicotine and are addictive. A recent study showed that the amount of nicotine in the bloodstream was actually twice as great for smokeless tobacco as for cigarettes. Trying to quit can be difficult, but not impossible. Here are some tips to spit it out and keep it out!

1. **Think of reasons why you want to quit.** You may want to quit because:
   - You do not like having bad breath after chewing and dipping.
   - You do not want stained teeth.
   - You do not want to risk getting cancer.
   - You do not like being addicted to nicotine.
   - You want to start leading a healthier life.
   - The people around you find it offensive.
   - You do not want to waste your money.

2. **Pick a quit date and throw out all your chewing tobacco and snuff.**

3. **Ask your friends, family, teachers, and coaches to help you kick the habit by giving you support and encouragement.** Tell friends not to offer you smokeless tobacco. You may want to ask a friend to quit with you.

4. **Ask your doctor about a tobacco quitting program.** These include nicotine chewing gum, a nicotine patch you wear on your arm (if you are old enough), and special support groups.

5. **Find alternatives to smokeless tobacco.** A few good examples are sugarless gum, pumpkin or sunflower seeds, or apple slices.

6. **Find activities to keep your mind off of smokeless tobacco.** You could work on a hobby, listen to music, or talk to a friend. Getting into exercise, such as bike riding, running, in-line skating, or cross-country skiing, also can help relieve any tension caused by quitting.

7. **Remember that everyone is different, so develop a personalized plan that works best for you.** Set realistic goals so you will be more likely to achieve them.

8. **Reward yourself.** You could save the money that would have been spent on smokeless tobacco and buy something nice for yourself.

The information contained in this publication should not be used as a substitute for the medical care and advice of your pediatrician. There may be variations in treatment that your pediatrician may recommend based on individual facts and circumstances.

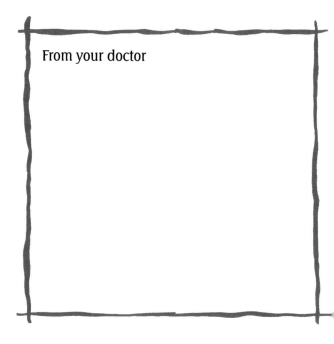

From your doctor

American Academy
of Pediatrics

DEDICATED TO THE HEALTH OF ALL CHILDREN™

The American Academy of Pediatrics is an organization of 60,000 primary care pediatricians, pediatric medical subspecialists, and pediatric surgical specialists dedicated to the health, safety, and well-being of infants, children, adolescents, and young adults.

American Academy of Pediatrics
Web site — www.aap.org

Copyright © 1995
American Academy of Pediatrics

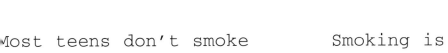

tobacco:
straight talk for teens

Most teens don't smoke

Did you know that about 80% of teens in the United States don't smoke? They've made a healthy choice.

But think about this:

One third of all new smokers will eventually die of smoking-related diseases.

And nearly 90% of all smokers started when they were teens.

This is what smoking does to your body

- Carbon monoxide in tobacco smoke takes oxygen from your body.
  Your lungs will turn gray and disgusting.
  Nicotine, a drug contained in tobacco, can cause your heart to beat faster and work less effectively.

Tobacco can kill

Each time you take a puff on a cigarette, you inhale **400 toxic chemicals like:**

- Nicotine (a drop of pure nicotine can **kill**)
- Cyanide (a deadly **poison**)
- Benzene (used in **making paints,** dyes, and plastics)
- Formaldehyde (used to **preserve dead bodies**)
- Acetylene (fuel used in **torches**)
- Ammonia (used in **fertilizers**)
- Carbon monoxide (**poisonous gas**)

Athletes who smoke can't run or swim as well as nonsmoking athletes because their bodies get less oxygen. This is why coaches tell athletes never to smoke.

Before you start smoking or if you're trying to quit...think about this:

It's a proven fact that the earlier a person starts smoking, the greater the risk of these diseases:

- Cancer
- Heart disease
- Chronic bronchitis—a serious disease of the airways to the lung
- Emphysema—a crippling lung disease

Smoking is addictive

Some of the chemicals in cigarettes cause people to become addicted very soon after they start smoking. If you are a smoker, you'll know you're addicted when

- You crave cigarettes.
- You feel nervous without cigarettes.
- You try to quit smoking and have trouble doing it.

Quitting can be hard, and it can take a long time. **The longer you smoke, the harder it is to stop.**

If you're already addicted, there's help available to you.

Smoking is ugly

- Smoking causes **bad breath** and **stained teeth.** Some teens say that kissing someone who smokes is like kissing an ashtray.
- Smoking often makes other people not want to be around you.
- Smoking stinks. If you smoke you may not smell smoke on you, but other people do.
- Studies show that most teens would rather date someone who doesn't smoke.

Smoking costs a lot of money

Do the math
One pack of cigarettes per day $3
Multiplied by the days in a year   x 365
Yearly cost for cigarettes   **$1,095**

That's more than **$1,000 a year** that you could be spending on CDs, clothes, a car, or college.

Chewing tobacco and snuff ("dip") are just as bad for you.

If you use smokeless tobacco you are at increased risk for illnesses that hurt your mouth, such as cancer and gum disease. You could lose some teeth. Also, you probably won't be able to taste or smell things as well as before.

Tobacco companies are targeting YOU

Tobacco companies spend billions of dollars every year promoting their products on TV, in movies and magazines, on billboards, and at sporting events. Teens are the main targets of many of these ads.

Most ads falsely show smokers as healthy, energetic, sexy, and successful.

The tobacco companies and advertisers don't mention the bad effects of smoking, like cancer, heart disease, bad breath, and stained teeth.

The fact is, tobacco companies need 3,000 new smokers every day to make up for the 400,000 people who die each year from tobacco-related diseases.

Think about it.

Quitting

If you smoke, quitting is the best thing you can do for yourself, your friends, and your family.

Myth

Many teens think they are not at risk from smoking. They tell themselves, "I won't smoke forever," or "I can quit any time."

Fact

If you ignore the warning signs and continue to smoke, your body will change. It will get used to the smoke. You won't cough or feel sick every time you puff on a cigarette, yet the damage to your body will get worse each time you smoke.

Deciding to stop smoking is up to you. Once you make the commitment to stop, get support from friends and family. You can get help from your pediatrician or school health office as well.

If you don't succeed at quitting the first time, keep trying.

From your doctor

For more information, visit the Web site of the American Academy of Pediatrics at **www.aap.org** or contact any of the following organizations:

Campaign for Tobacco-Free Kids
800/803-7178
www.tobaccofreekids.org

The truth: A campaign developed by teens
www.thetruth.com

American Cancer Society
800/ACS-2345 (800/227-2345)
www.cancer.org

American Heart Association
800/242-8721
www.americanheart.org

American Lung Association
800/586-4872
www.lungusa.org

Please note: Listing of resources does not imply an endorsement by the American Academy of Pediatrics (AAP). The AAP is not responsible for the content of the resources mentioned in this brochure. Phone numbers and Web site addresses are as current as possible, but may change at any time.

The information contained in this publication should not be used as a substitute for the medical care and advice of your pediatrician. There may be variations in treatment that your pediatrician may recommend based on individual facts and circumstances.

The persons whose photographs are depicted in this publication are professional models. They have no relation to the issues discussed. Any characters they are portraying are fictional.

American Academy
of Pediatrics

DEDICATED TO THE HEALTH OF ALL CHILDREN™

The American Academy of Pediatrics is an organization of 60,000 primary care pediatricians, pediatric medical subspecialists, and pediatric surgical specialists dedicated to the health, safety, and well-being of infants, children, adolescents, and young adults.

American Academy of Pediatrics
Web site—www.aap.org

Copyright © 2004
American Academy of Pediatrics

SECTION TEN

Immunization
Information

CHICKENPOX VACCINE

W H A T   Y O U   N E E D   T O   K N O W

1 | Why get vaccinated?

Chickenpox (also called varicella) is a common childhood disease. It is usually mild, but it can be serious, especially in young infants and adults.

The chickenpox virus can be spread from person to person through the air, or by contact with fluid from chickenpox blisters.

- It causes a rash, itching, fever, and tiredness.

- It can lead to severe skin infection, scars, pneumonia, brain damage, or death.

- A person who has had chickenpox can get a painful rash called shingles years later.

- About 12,000 people are hospitalized for chickenpox each year in the United States.

- About 100 people die each year in the United States as a result of chickenpox.

Chickenpox vaccine can prevent chickenpox.

Most people who get chickenpox vaccine will not get chickenpox. But if someone who has been vaccinated *does* get chickenpox, it is usually very mild. They will have fewer spots, are less likely to have a fever, and will recover faster.

2 | Who should get chickenpox vaccine and when?

✓ **Children should get 1 dose of chickenpox vaccine between 12 and 18 months of age**, or at any age after that if they have never had chickenpox.

People who do not get the vaccine until 13 years of age or older should get **2 doses**, 4-8 weeks apart.

Ask your doctor or nurse for details.

Chickenpox vaccine may be given at the same time as other vaccines.

3 | Some people should not get chickenpox vaccine or should wait

- People should not get chickenpox vaccine if they have ever had a life-threatening allergic reaction to **gelatin**, the antibiotic **neomycin**, or (for those needing a second dose) **a previous dose of chickenpox vaccine**.

- People who are moderately or severely ill at the time the shot is scheduled should usually wait until they recover before getting chickenpox vaccine.

- Pregnant women should wait to get chickenpox vaccine until after they have given birth. Women should not get pregnant for 1 month after getting chickenpox vaccine.

- Some people should check with their doctor about whether they should get chickenpox vaccine, including anyone who:
  - Has HIV/AIDS or another disease that affects the immune system
  - Is being treated with drugs that affect the immune system, such as steroids, for 2 weeks or longer
  - Has any kind of cancer
  - Is taking cancer treatment with x-rays or drugs

- People who recently had a transfusion or were given other blood products should ask their doctor when they may get chickenpox vaccine.

Ask your doctor or nurse for more information.

4 What are the risks from chickenpox vaccine?

A vaccine, like any medicine, is capable of causing serious problems, such as severe allergic reactions. The risk of chickenpox vaccine causing serious harm, or death, is extremely small.

Getting chickenpox vaccine is much safer than getting chickenpox disease.

Most people who get chickenpox vaccine do not have any problems with it.

Mild Problems
- Soreness or swelling where the shot was given (about 1 out of 5 children and up to 1 out of 3 adolescents and adults)
- Fever (1 person out of 10, or less)
- Mild rash, up to a month after vaccination (1 person out of 20, or less). It is possible for these people to infect other members of their household, but this is *extremely* rare.

Moderate Problems
- Seizure (jerking or staring) caused by fever (less than 1 person out of 1,000).

Severe Problems
- Pneumonia (very rare)

Other serious problems, including severe brain reactions and low blood count, have been reported after chickenpox vaccination. These happen so rarely experts cannot tell whether they are caused by the vaccine or not. If they are, it is extremely rare.

5 What if there is a moderate or severe reaction?

What should I look for?

Any unusual condition, such as a serious allergic reaction, high fever or behavior changes. Signs of a serious allergic reaction can include difficulty breathing, hoarseness or wheezing, hives, paleness, weakness, a fast heart beat or dizziness within a few minutes to a few hours after the shot. A high fever or seizure, if it occurs, would happen 1 to 6 weeks after the shot.

What should I do?

- **Call** a doctor, or get the person to a doctor right away.
- **Tell** your doctor what happened, the date and time it happened, and when the vaccination was given.
- **Ask** your doctor, nurse, or health department to report the reaction by filing a Vaccine Adverse Event Reporting System (VAERS) form.

  Or you can file this report through the VAERS web site at www.vaers.org, or by calling 1-800-822-7967.

  VAERS does not provide medical advice

6 The National Vaccine Injury Compensation Program

In the rare event that you or your child has a serious reaction to a vaccine, a federal program has been created to help you pay for the care of those who have been harmed.

For details about the National Vaccine Injury Compensation Program, call **1-800-338-2382** or visit the program's website at **http://www.hrsa.gov/osp/vicp**

7 How can I learn more?

- Ask your doctor or nurse. They can give you the vaccine package insert or suggest other sources of information.

- Call your local or state health department's immunization program.

- Contact the Centers for Disease Control and Prevention (CDC):
  - Call **1-800-232-4636 (1-800-CDC-INFO)**
  - Visit the National Immunization Program's website at **http://www.cdc.gov/nip**

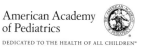

American Academy of Pediatrics
DEDICATED TO THE HEALTH OF ALL CHILDREN™

Reprinted by the American Academy of Pediatrics. Additional copies are available for purchase in pads of 100

To order, contact:
American Academy of Pediatrics
141 Northwest Point Blvd
Elk Grove Village, IL 60007-1098
Web site—http://www.aap.org
Minimum order 100

 U.S. DEPARTMENT OF HEALTH & HUMAN SERVICES
Centers for Disease Control and Prevention
National Immunization Program

Vaccine Information Statement
Varicella (12/16/98)   42 U.S.C. § 300aa-26

DIPHTHERIA TETANUS & PERTUSSIS VACCINES

WHAT YOU NEED TO KNOW

1 | Why get vaccinated?

Diphtheria, tetanus, and pertussis are serious diseases caused by bacteria. Diphtheria and pertussis are spread from person to person. Tetanus enters the body through cuts or wounds.

DIPHTHERIA causes a thick covering in the back of the throat.
• It can lead to breathing problems, paralysis, heart failure, and even death.

TETANUS (Lockjaw) causes painful tightening of the muscles, usually all over the body.
• It can lead to "locking" of the jaw so the victim cannot open his mouth or swallow. Tetanus leads to death in about 1 out of 10 cases.

PERTUSSIS (Whooping Cough) causes coughing spells so bad that it is hard for infants to eat, drink, or breathe. These spells can last for weeks.
• It can lead to pneumonia, seizures (jerking and staring spells), brain damage, and death.

Diphtheria, tetanus, and pertussis vaccine (DTaP) can help prevent these diseases. Most children who are vaccinated with DTaP will be protected throughout childhood. Many more children would get these diseases if we stopped vaccinating.

DTaP is a safer version of an older vaccine called DTP. DTP is no longer used in the United States.

2 | Who should get DTaP vaccine and when?

Children should get 5 doses of DTaP vaccine, one dose at each of the following ages:

✓ 2 months   ✓ 4 months   ✓ 6 months
    ✓15-18 months   ✓ 4-6 years

DTaP may be given at the same time as other vaccines.

3 | Some children should not get DTaP vaccine or should wait

• Children with minor illnesses, such as a cold, may be vaccinated. But children who are moderately or severely ill should usually wait until they recover before getting DTaP vaccine.

• Any child who had a life-threatening allergic reaction after a dose of DTaP should not get another dose.

• Any child who suffered a brain or nervous system disease within 7 days after a dose of DTaP should not get another dose.

• Talk with your doctor if your child:
- had a seizure or collapsed after a dose of DTaP,
- cried non-stop for 3 hours or more after a dose of DTaP,
- had a fever over 105°F after a dose of DTaP.

Ask your health care provider for more information. Some of these children should not get another dose of pertussis vaccine, but may get a vaccine without pertussis, called **DT**.

4 | Older children and adults

DTaP should not be given to anyone 7 years of age or older because pertussis vaccine is only licensed for children under 7.

But older children, adolescents, and adults still need protection from tetanus and diphtheria. A booster shot called **Td** is recommended at 11-12 years of age, and then every 10 years. There is a separate Vaccine Information Statement for Td vaccine.

Diphtheria/Tetanus/Pertussis   7/30/2001

5 What are the risks from DTaP vaccine?

Getting diphtheria, tetanus, or pertussis disease is much riskier than getting DTaP vaccine.

However, a vaccine, like any medicine, is capable of causing serious problems, such as severe allergic reactions. The risk of DTaP vaccine causing serious harm, or death, is extremely small.

Mild Problems (Common)

- Fever (up to about 1 child in 4)
- Redness or swelling where the shot was given (up to about 1 child in 4)
- Soreness or tenderness where the shot was given (up to about 1 child in 4)

These problems occur more often after the 4th and 5th doses of the DTaP series than after earlier doses. Sometimes the 4th or 5th dose of DTaP vaccine is followed by swelling of the entire arm or leg in which the shot was given, lasting 1-7 days (up to about 1 child in 30).

Other mild problems include:

- Fussiness (up to about 1 child in 3)
- Tiredness or poor appetite (up to about 1 child in 10)
- Vomiting (up to about 1 child in 50)

These problems generally occur 1-3 days after the shot.

Moderate Problems (Uncommon)

- Seizure (jerking or staring) (about 1 child out of 14,000)
- Non-stop crying, for 3 hours or more (up to about 1 child out of 1,000)
- High fever, over 105°F (about 1 child out of 16,000)

Severe Problems (Very Rare)

- Serious allergic reaction (less than 1 out of a million doses)
- Several other severe problems have been reported after DTaP vaccine. These include:
  - Long-term seizures, coma, or lowered consciousness
  - Permanent brain damage.

  These are so rare it is hard to tell if they are caused by the vaccine.

Controlling fever is especially important for children who have had seizures, for any reason. It is also important if another family member has had seizures. You can reduce fever and pain by giving your child an *aspirin-free* pain reliever when the shot is given, and for the next 24 hours, following the package instructions.

6 What if there is a moderate or severe reaction?

What should I look for?

Any unusual conditions, such as a serious allergic reaction, high fever or unusual behavior. Serious allergic reactions are extremely rare with any vaccine. If one were to occur, it would most likely be within a few minutes to a few hours after the shot. Signs can include difficulty breathing, hoarseness or wheezing, hives, paleness, weakness, a fast heart beat or dizziness. If a high fever or seizure were to occur, it would usually be within a week after the shot.

What should I do?

- **Call** a doctor, or get the person to a doctor right away.
- **Tell** your doctor what happened, the date and time it happened, and when the vaccination was given.
- **Ask** your doctor, nurse, or health department to report the reaction by filing a Vaccine Adverse Event Reporting System (VAERS) form.

Or you can file this report through the VAERS web site at www.vaers.org, or by calling 1-800-822-7967.
VAERS does not provide medical advice

7 The National Vaccine Injury Compensation Program

In the rare event that you or your child has a serious reaction to a vaccine, a federal program has been created to help pay for the care of those who have been harmed.

For details about the National Vaccine Injury Compensation Program, call **1-800-338-2382** or visit the program's website at **www.hrsa.gov/osp/vicp**

8 How can I learn more?

- Ask your health care provider. They can give you the vaccine package insert or suggest other sources of information.

- Call your local or state health department's immunization program.

- Contact the Centers for Disease Control and Prevention (CDC):
  - Call **1-800-232-4636 (1-800-CDC-INFO)**
  - Visit the National Immunization Program's website at **www.cdc.gov/nip**

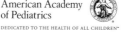

American Academy of Pediatrics
DEDICATED TO THE HEALTH OF ALL CHILDREN™

Reprinted by the American Academy of Pediatrics.
Additional copies are available for purchase in pads of 100.

To order, contact:
American Academy of Pediatrics
141 Northwest Point Blvd
Elk Grove Village, IL 60007-1098
Web site—http://www.aap.org
Minimum order 100

U.S. DEPARTMENT OF HEALTH & HUMAN SERVICES
Centers for Disease Control and Prevention
National Immunization Program

CDC

Vaccine Information Statement
DTaP (7/30/01)   42 U.S.C. § 300aa-2€

Haemophilus Influenzae Type b (Hib) Vaccine

W H A T   Y O U   N E E D   T O   K N O W

1 | What is Hib disease?

Haemophilus influenzae type b (Hib) disease is a serious disease caused by a bacteria. It usually strikes children under 5 years old.

Your child can get Hib disease by being around other children or adults who may have the bacteria and not know it. The germs spread from person to person. If the germs stay in the child's nose and throat, the child probably will not get sick. But sometimes the germs spread into the lungs or the bloodstream, and then Hib can cause serious problems.

Before Hib vaccine, Hib disease was the leading cause of bacterial meningitis among children under 5 years old in the United States. Meningitis is an infection of the brain and spinal cord coverings, which can lead to lasting brain damage and deafness. Hib disease can also cause:

- pneumonia
- severe swelling in the throat, making it hard to breathe
- infections of the blood, joints, bones, and covering of the heart
- death

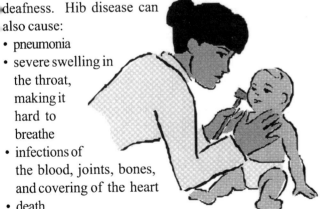

Before Hib vaccine, about 20,000 children in the United States under 5 years old got severe Hib disease each year and nearly 1,000 people died.

Hib vaccine can prevent Hib disease.

Many more children would get Hib disease if we stopped vaccinating.

2 | Who should get Hib vaccine and when?

Children should get Hib vaccine at:

- ✓ 2 months of age
- ✓ 4 months of age
- ✓ 6 months of age*
- ✓ 12-15 months of age

* Depending on what brand of Hib vaccine is used, your child might not need the dose at 6 months of age. Your doctor or nurse will tell you if this dose is needed.

If you miss a dose or get behind schedule, get the next dose as soon as you can. There is no need to start over.

Hib vaccine may be given at the same time as other vaccines.

Older Children and Adults

Children over 5 years old usually do not need Hib vaccine. But some older children or adults with special health conditions should get it. These conditions include sickle cell disease, HIV/AIDS, removal of the spleen, bone marrow transplant, or cancer treatment with drugs. Ask your doctor or nurse for details.

3 | Some people should not get Hib vaccine or should wait

- People who have ever had a life-threatening allergic reaction to a previous dose of Hib vaccine should not get another dose.

- Children less than 6 weeks of age should not get Hib vaccine.

- People who are moderately or severely ill at the time the shot is scheduled should usually wait until they recover before getting Hib vaccine.

Ask your doctor or nurse for more information.

4 · What are the risks from Hib vaccine?

A vaccine, like any medicine, is capable of causing serious problems, such as severe allergic reactions. The risk of Hib vaccine causing serious harm or death is extremely small.

Most people who get Hib vaccine do not have any problems with it.

Mild Problems

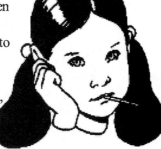

- Redness, warmth, or swelling where the shot was given (up to 1/4 of children)
- Fever over 101°F (up to 1 out of 20 children)

If these problems happen, they usually start within a day of vaccination. They may last 2-3 days.

5 · What if there is a moderate or severe reaction?

What should I look for?

Any unusual condition, such as a serious allergic reaction, high fever or behavior changes. Signs of a serious allergic reaction can include difficulty breathing, hoarseness or wheezing, hives, paleness, weakness, a fast heart beat, or dizziness within a few minutes to a few hours after the shot.

What should I do?

- **Call** a doctor, or get the person to a doctor right away.

- **Tell** your doctor what happened, the date and time it happened, and when the vaccination was given.

- **Ask** your doctor, nurse, or health department to report the reaction by filing a Vaccine Adverse Event Reporting System (VAERS) form.

Or you can file this report through the VAERS web site at www.vaers.org, or by calling 1-800-822-7967.

VAERS does not provide medical advice

6 · The National Vaccine Injury Compensation Program

In the rare event that you or your child has a serious reaction to a vaccine, a federal program has been created to help you pay for the care of those who have been harmed.

For details about the National Vaccine Injury Compensation Program, call **1-800-338-2382** or visit the program's website at **www.hrsa.gov/osp/vicp**

7 · How can I learn more?

- Ask your doctor or nurse. They can give you the vaccine package insert or suggest other sources of information.

- Call your local or state health department's immunization program.

- Contact the Centers for Disease Control and Prevention (CDC):
  - Call **1-800-232-4636 (1-800-CDC-INFO)**
  - Visit the National Immunization Program's website at **www.cdc.gov/nip**

American Academy of Pediatrics

DEDICATED TO THE HEALTH OF ALL CHILDREN™

Reprinted by the American Academy of Pediatrics. Additional copies are available for purchase in pads of

To order, contact:
American Academy of Pediatrics
141 Northwest Point Blvd
Elk Grove Village, IL 60007-1098
Web site—http://www.aap.org
Minimum order 100

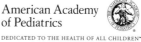 **U.S. DEPARTMENT OF HEALTH & HUMAN SERVICES**
Centers for Disease Control and Prevention
National Immunization Program

Vaccine Information Statement
Hib (12/16/98)   42 U.S.C. § 300aa-2●

HEPATITIS B VACCINE
W H A T   Y O U   N E E D   T O   K N O W

1 | Why get vaccinated?

Hepatitis B is a serious disease.
The hepatitis B virus (HBV) can cause short-term (acute) illness that leads to:
- loss of appetite • diarrhea and vomiting
- tiredness • jaundice (yellow skin or eyes)
- pain in muscles, joints, and stomach

It can also cause long-term (chronic) illness that leads to:
- liver damage (cirrhosis)
- liver cancer
- death

About 1.25 million people in the U.S. have chronic HBV infection.

Each year it is estimated that:
- 80,000 people, mostly young adults, get infected with HBV
- More than 11,000 people have to stay in the hospital because of hepatitis B
- 4,000 to 5,000 people die from chronic hepatitis B

Hepatitis B vaccine can prevent hepatitis B. It is the first anti-cancer vaccine because it can prevent a form of liver cancer.

2 | How is hepatitis B virus spread?

Hepatitis B virus is spread through contact with the blood and body fluids of an infected person. A person can get infected in several ways, such as:
- by having unprotected sex with an infected person
- by sharing needles when injecting illegal drugs
- by being stuck with a used needle on the job
- during birth when the virus passes from an infected mother to her baby

About 1/3 of people who are infected with hepatitis B in the United States don't know how they got it.

Hepatitis B	7/11/2001

3 | Who should get hepatitis B vaccine and when?

1) Everyone 18 years of age and younger
2) Adults over 18 who are at risk

Adults at risk for HBV infection include:
- people who have more than one sex partner in 6 months
- men who have sex with other men
- sex contacts of infected people
- people who inject illegal drugs
- health care and public safety workers who might be exposed to infected blood or body fluids
- household contacts of persons with chronic HBV infection
- hemodialysis patients

If you are not sure whether you are at risk, ask your doctor or nurse.

✓ **People should get 3 doses of hepatitis B vaccine according to the following schedule.** *If you miss a dose or get behind schedule, get the next dose as soon as you can. There is no need to start over.*

Hepatitis B Vaccination Schedule		WHO?		
		Infant whose mother is infected with HBV	Infant whose mother is *not* infected with HBV	Older child, adolescent, or adult
W H E N ?	**First Dose**	Within 12 hours of birth	Birth - 2 months of age	Any time
	Second Dose	1 -2 months of age	1 - 4 months of age (at least 1 month after first dose)	1 - 2 months after first dose
	Third Dose	6 months of age	6 - 18 months of age	4 - 6 months after first dose

- The second dose must be given at least 1 month after the first dose.
- The third dose must be given at least 2 months after the second dose and at least 4 months after the first.
- The third dose should *not* be given to infants under 6 months of age, because this could reduce long-term protection.

Adolescents 11 to 15 years of age may need only two doses of hepatitis B vaccine, separated by 4-6 months. Ask your health care provider for details.

Hepatitis B vaccine may be given at the same time as other vaccines.

4 — Some people should not get hepatitis B vaccine or should wait

People should not get hepatitis B vaccine if they have ever had a life-threatening allergic reaction to **baker's yeast** (the kind used for making bread) or to **a previous dose of hepatitis B vaccine**.

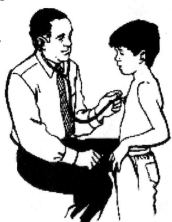

People who are moderately or severely ill at the time the shot is scheduled should usually wait until they recover before getting hepatitis B vaccine.

Ask your doctor or nurse for more information.

5 — What are the risks from hepatitis B vaccine?

A vaccine, like any medicine, is capable of causing serious problems, such as severe allergic reactions. The risk of hepatitis B vaccine causing serious harm, or death, is extremely small.

Getting hepatitis B vaccine is much safer than getting hepatitis B disease.

Most people who get hepatitis B vaccine do not have any problems with it.

Mild problems
- soreness where the shot was given, lasting a day or two (up to 1 out of 11 children and adolescents, and about 1 out of 4 adults)
- mild to moderate fever (up to 1 out of 14 children and adolescents and 1 out of 100 adults)

Severe problems
- serious allergic reaction (very rare)

6 — What if there is a moderate or severe reaction?

What should I look for?

Any unusual condition, such as a serious allergic reaction, high fever or unusual behavior. Serious allergic reactions are extremely rare with any vaccine. If one were to occur, it would be within a few minutes to a few hours after the shot. Signs can include difficulty breathing, hoarseness or wheezing, hives, paleness, weakness, a fast heart beat or dizziness.

What should I do?

- **Call** a doctor, or get the person to a doctor right away.

- **Tell** your doctor what happened, the date and time it happened, and when the vaccination was given.

- **Ask** your doctor, nurse, or health department to report the reaction by filing a Vaccine Adverse Event Reporting System (VAERS) form.

  Or you can file this report through the VAERS web site at www.vaers.org, or by calling 1-800-822-7967.

  VAERS does not provide medical advice

7 — The National Vaccine Injury Compensation Program

In the rare event that you or your child has a serious reaction to a vaccine, a federal program has been created to help you pay for the care of those who have been harmed.

For details about the National Vaccine Injury Compensation Program, call **1-800-338-2382** or visit the program's website at **www.hrsa.gov/osp/vicp**

8 — How can I learn more?

- Ask your doctor or nurse. They can give you the vaccine package insert or suggest other sources of information.

- Call your local or state health department's immunization program.

- Contact the Centers for Disease Control and Prevention (CDC):
  - Call **1-800-232-4636** (1-800-CDC-INFO) or **1-888-443-7232**
  - Visit the National Immunization Program's website at **www.cdc.gov/nip** or CDC's Division of Viral Hepatitis website at **www.cdc.gov/hepatitis**

American Academy of Pediatrics
DEDICATED TO THE HEALTH OF ALL CHILDREN™

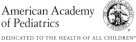

Reprinted by the American Academy of Pediatrics. Additional copies are available for purchase in pads of

To order, contact:
American Academy of Pediatrics
141 Northwest Point Blvd
Elk Grove Village, IL 60007-1098
Web site—http://www.aap.org
Minimum order 100

U.S. DEPARTMENT OF HEALTH & HUMAN SERVICES
Centers for Disease Control and Prevention
National Immunization Program

Vaccine Information Statement
Hepatitis B (7/11/01)   42 U.S.C. § 300aa-2

Recommended Immunization Schedule
for Children and Adolescents Who Start Late or Who Are More Than 1 Month Behind

UNITED STATES • 2006

The tables below give catch-up schedules and minimum intervals between doses for children who have delayed immunizations.
There is no need to restart a vaccine series regardless of the time that has elapsed between doses. Use the chart appropriate for the child's age.

CATCH-UP SCHEDULE FOR CHILDREN AGED 4 MONTHS THROUGH 6 YEARS

Vaccine	Minimum Age for Dose 1	Minimum Interval Between Doses			
		Dose 1 to Dose 2	Dose 2 to Dose 3	Dose 3 to Dose 4	Dose 4 to Dose 5
Diphtheria, Tetanus, Pertussis	6 wks	4 weeks	4 weeks	6 months	6 months[1]
Inactivated Poliovirus	6 wks	4 weeks	4 weeks	4 weeks[2]	
Hepatitis B[3]	Birth	4 weeks	8 weeks (and 16 weeks after first dose)		
Measles, Mumps, Rubella	12 mo	4 weeks[4]			
Varicella	12 mo				
Haemophilus influenzae type b[5]	6 wks	4 weeks if first dose given at age <12 months / 8 weeks (as final dose) if first dose given at age 12-14 months / No further doses needed if first dose given at age ≥15 months	4 weeks[6] if current age <12 months / 8 weeks (as final dose)[6] if current age ≥12 months and second dose given at age <15 months / No further doses needed if previous dose given at age ≥15 mo	8 weeks (as final dose) This dose only necessary for children aged 12 months–5 years who received 3 doses before age 12 months	
Pneumococcal[7]	6 wks	4 weeks if first dose given at age <12 months and current age <24 months / 8 weeks (as final dose) if first dose given at age ≥12 months or current age 24–59 months / No further doses needed for healthy children if first dose given at age ≥24 months	4 weeks if current age <12 months / 8 weeks (as final dose) if current age ≥12 months / No further doses needed for healthy children if previous dose given at age ≥24 months	8 weeks (as final dose) This dose only necessary for children aged 12 months–5 years who received 3 doses before age 12 months	

CATCH-UP SCHEDULE FOR CHILDREN AGED 7 YEARS THROUGH 18 YEARS

Vaccine	Minimum Interval Between Doses		
	Dose 1 to Dose 2	Dose 2 to Dose 3	Dose 3 to Booster Dose
Tetanus, Diphtheria[8]	4 weeks	6 months	6 months if first dose given at age <12 months and current age <11 years; otherwise 5 years
Inactivated Poliovirus[9]	4 weeks	4 weeks	IPV[2,9]
Hepatitis B	4 weeks	8 weeks (and 16 weeks after first dose)	
Measles, Mumps, Rubella	4 weeks		
Varicella[10]	4 weeks		

1. **DTaP.** The fifth dose is not necessary if the fourth dose was administered after the fourth birthday.

2. **IPV.** For children who received an all-IPV or all-oral poliovirus (OPV) series, a fourth dose is not necessary if third dose was administered at age ≥4 years. If both OPV and IPV were administered as part of a series, a total of 4 doses should be given, regardless of the child's current age.

3. **HepB.** Administer the 3-dose series to all children and adolescents <19 years of age if they were not previously vaccinated.

4. **MMR.** The second dose of MMR is recommended routinely at age 4–6 years but may be administered earlier if desired.

5. **Hib.** Vaccine is not generally recommended for children aged ≥5 years.

6. **Hib.** If current age <12 months and the first 2 doses were PRP-OMP (PedvaxHIB® or ComVax® [Merck]), the third (and final) dose should be administered at age 12–15 months and at least 8 weeks after the second dose.

7. **PCV.** Vaccine is not generally recommended for children aged ≥5 years.

8. **Td.** Adolescent tetanus, diphtheria, and pertussis vaccine (Tdap) may be substituted for any dose in a primary catch-up series or as a booster if age appropriate for Tdap. A five-year interval from the last Td dose is encouraged when Tdap is used as a booster dose. See ACIP recommendations for further information.

9. **IPV.** Vaccine is not generally recommended for persons aged ≥18 years.

10. **Varicella.** Administer the 2-dose series to all susceptible adolescents aged ≥13 years.

Report adverse reactions to vaccines through the federal Vaccine Adverse Event Reporting System. For information on reporting reactions following immunization, please visit www.vaers.hhs.gov or call the 24-hour national toll-free information line 800-822-7967. Report suspected cases of vaccine-preventable diseases to your state or local health department.

For additional information about vaccines, including precautions and contraindications for immunization and vaccine shortages, please visit the National Immunization Program Website at www.cdc.gov/nip or contact
800-CDC-INFO (800-232-4636)
(In English, En Español — 24/7)

DEPARTMENT OF HEALTH AND HUMAN SERVICES • CENTERS FOR DISEASE CONTROL AND PREVENTION

Recommended Childhood and Adolescent Immunization Schedule UNITED STATES • 2006

Vaccine ▼ / Age ▶	Birth	1 month	2 months	4 months	6 months	12 months	15 months	18 months	24 months	4–6 years	11–12 years	13–14 years	15 years	16–18 years
Hepatitis B[1]	HepB	HepB		HepB[1]	HepB						HepB Series			
Diphtheria, Tetanus, Pertussis[2]			DTaP	DTaP	DTaP		DTaP			DTaP	Tdap	Tdap		
Haemophilus influenzae type b[3]			Hib	Hib	Hib[3]	Hib								
Inactivated Poliovirus			IPV	IPV		IPV				IPV				
Measles, Mumps, Rubella[4]						MMR				MMR		MMR		
Varicella[5]						Varicella					Varicella			
Meningococcal[6]							Vaccines within broken line are for selected populations		MPSV4		MCV4	MCV4	MCV4	
Pneumococcal[7]			PCV	PCV	PCV	PCV				PCV	PPV			
Influenza[8]						Influenza (Yearly)				Influenza (Yearly)				
Hepatitis A[9]									HepA Series					

This schedule indicates the recommended ages for routine administration of currently licensed childhood vaccines, as of December 1, 2005, for children through age 18 years. Any dose not administered at the recommended age should be administered at any subsequent visit when indicated and feasible. ▒ Indicates age groups that warrant special effort to administer those vaccines not previously administered. Additional vaccines may be licensed and recommended during the year. Licensed combination vaccines may be used whenever any components of the combination are indicated and other components of the vaccine are not contraindicated and if approved by the Food and Drug Administration for that dose of the series. Providers should consult the respective ACIP statement for detailed recommendations. Clinically significant adverse events that follow immunization should be reported to the Vaccine Adverse Event Reporting System (VAERS). Guidance about how to obtain and complete a VAERS form is available at www.vaers.hhs.gov or by telephone, 800-822-7967.

▒ Range of recommended ages	▓ Catch-up immunization	▒ 11–12 year old assessment

1. **Hepatitis B vaccine (HepB).** *AT BIRTH:* **All newborns** should receive monovalent HepB soon after birth and before hospital discharge. **Infants born to mothers who are HBsAg-positive** should receive HepB and 0.5 mL of hepatitis B immune globulin (HBIG) within 12 hours of birth. **Infants born to mothers whose HBsAg status is unknown** should receive HepB within 12 hours of birth. The mother should have blood drawn as soon as possible to determine her HBsAg status; if HBsAg-positive, the infant should receive HBIG as soon as possible (no later than age 1 week). **For infants born to HBsAg-negative mothers,** the birth dose can be delayed in rare circumstances but only if a physician's order to withhold the vaccine and a copy of the mother's original HBsAg-negative laboratory report are documented in the infant's medical record. *FOLLOWING THE BIRTHDOSE:* The HepB series should be completed with either monovalent HepB or a combination vaccine containing HepB. The second dose should be administered at age 1–2 months. The final dose should be administered at age ≥24 weeks. It is permissible to administer 4 doses of HepB (e.g., when combination vaccines are given after the birth dose); however, if monovalent HepB is used, a dose at age 4 months is not needed. **Infants born to HBsAg-positive mothers** should be tested for HBsAg and antibody to HBsAg after completion of the HepB series, at age 9–18 months (generally at the next well-child visit after completion of the vaccine series).

2. **Diphtheria and tetanus toxoids and acellular pertussis vaccine (DTaP).** The fourth dose of DTaP may be administered as early as age 12 months, provided 6 months have elapsed since the third dose and the child is unlikely to return at age 15–18 months. The final dose in the series should be given at age ≥4 years. **Tetanus and diphtheria toxoids and acellular pertussis vaccine (Tdap – adolescent preparation)** is recommended at age 11–12 years for those who have completed the recommended childhood DTP/DTaP vaccination series and have not received a Td booster dose. Adolescents 13–18 years who missed the 11–12-year Td/Tdap booster dose should also receive a single dose of Tdap if they have completed the recommended childhood DTP/DTaP vaccination series. Subsequent **tetanus and diphtheria toxoids (Td)** are recommended every 10 years.

3. *Haemophilus influenzae* **type b conjugate vaccine (Hib).** Three Hib conjugate vaccines are licensed for infant use. If PRP-OMP (PedvaxHIB® or ComVax® [Merck]) is administered at ages 2 and 4 months, a dose at age 6 months is not required. DTaP/Hib combination products should not be used for primary immunization in infants at ages 2, 4 or 6 months but can be used as boosters after any Hib vaccine. The final dose in the series should be administered at age ≥12 months.

4. **Measles, mumps, and rubella vaccine (MMR).** The second dose of MMR is recommended routinely at age 4–6 years but may be administered during any visit, provided at least 4 weeks have elapsed since the first dose and both doses are administered beginning at or after age 12 months. Those who have not previously received the second dose should complete the schedule by age 11–12 years.

5. **Varicella vaccine.** Varicella vaccine is recommended at any visit at or after age 12 months for susceptible children (i.e., those who lack a reliable history of chickenpox). Susceptible persons aged ≥13 years should receive 2 doses administered at least 4 weeks apart.

6. **Meningococcal vaccine (MCV4).** Meningococcal conjugate vaccine (MCV4) should be given to all children at the 11–12 year old visit as well as to unvaccinated adolescents at high school entry (15 years of age). Other adolescents who wish to decrease their risk for meningococcal disease may also be vaccinated. All college freshmen living in dormitories should also be vaccinated, preferably with MCV4, although **meningococcal polysaccharide vaccine (MPSV4)** is an acceptable alternative. Vaccination against invasive meningococcal disease is recommended for children and adolescents aged ≥2 years with terminal complement deficiencies or anatomic or functional asplenia and certain other high risk groups (see *MMWR* 2005;54 [RR-7]:1-21); use MPSV4 for children aged 2–10 years and MCV4 for older children, although MPSV4 is an acceptable alternative.

7. **Pneumococcal vaccine.** The heptavalent **pneumococcal conjugate vaccine (PCV)** is recommended for all children aged 2–23 months and for certain children aged 24–59 months. The final dose in the series should be given at age ≥12 months. **Pneumococcal polysaccharide vaccine (PPV)** is recommended in addition to PCV for certain high-risk groups. See *MMWR* 2000; 49(RR-9):1-35.

8. **Influenza vaccine.** Influenza vaccine is recommended annually for children aged ≥6 months with certain risk factors (including, but not limited to, asthma, cardiac disease, sickle cell disease, human immunodeficiency virus [HIV], diabetes, and conditions that can compromise respiratory function or handling of respiratory secretions or that can increase the risk for aspiration), healthcare workers, and other persons (including household members) in close contact with persons in groups at high risk (see *MMWR* 2005;54[RR-8]:1-55). In addition, healthy children aged 6–23 months and close contacts of healthy children aged 0–5 months are recommended to receive influenza vaccine because children in this age group are at substantially increased risk for influenza-related hospitalizations. For healthy persons aged 5–49 years, the intranasally administered, live, attenuated influenza vaccine (LAIV) is an acceptable alternative to the intramuscular trivalent inactivated influenza vaccine (TIV). See *MMWR* 2005;54(RR-8):1-55. Children receiving TIV should be administered a dosage appropriate for their age (0.25 mL if aged 6–35 months or 0.5 mL if aged ≥3 years). Children aged ≤8 years who are receiving influenza vaccine for the first time should receive 2 doses (separated by at least 4 weeks for TIV and at least 6 weeks for LAIV).

9. **Hepatitis A vaccine (HepA).** HepA is recommended for all children at 1 year of age (i.e., 12–23 months). The 2 doses in the series should be administered at least 6 months apart. States, counties, and communities with existing HepA vaccination programs for children 2–18 years of age are encouraged to maintain these programs. In these areas, new efforts focused on routine vaccination of 1-year-old children should enhance, not replace, ongoing programs directed at a broader population of children. HepA is also recommended for certain high risk groups (see *MMWR* 1999; 48[RR-12]1-37).

The Childhood and Adolescent Immunization Schedule is approved by:
Advisory Committee on Immunization Practices www.cdc.gov/nip/acip • American Academy of Pediatrics www.aap.org • American Academy of Family Physicians www.aafp.org

Immunizations: What You Need To Know

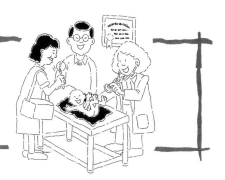

Immunizations have helped children remain healthy for more than 50 years. But many parents still ask, "Why does my child need to be immunized? Why does my child need to receive vaccinations or 'shots'?"

The following are common questions parents have about immunizations:

- Why are immunizations important?
- How well do vaccines work?
- What vaccines does my child need?
- How safe are vaccines?
- Where can I get more information?

Why are immunizations important?

Q: "Why are vaccines needed if the diseases they prevent are not as common anymore?"

A: Vaccines *are* still needed because the bacteria and viruses that cause these diseases still exist. Vaccines have protected children and continue to protect children from getting these diseases. In the United States many diseases are not as common or widespread as they used to be thanks to better nutrition, less crowded living conditions, better sanitation, antibiotics, and, most importantly, vaccines.

For example, the *Haemophilus influenzae* type b (Hib) vaccine protects children from serious childhood diseases that include meningitis, pneumonia, and infections of the blood, bones, joints, and throat. Before the Hib vaccine was developed in the 1980s, there were about 20,000 cases of Hib disease in the United States a year. Today there are fewer than 100 cases a year. Because the bacteria that causes Hib disease still exists, children younger than 5 years need the Hib vaccine to be protected.

Vaccines also are needed to protect children from diseases that may be brought into the United States from people who have visited or are visiting from other countries. Many vaccine-preventable diseases are still common in many parts of the world. Travelers may be carriers of these diseases without them knowing they are infected. Influenza is an example of a disease that is transmitted between countries every year.

Q: "Chickenpox is not a fatal disease, so why is the vaccine needed?"

A: Chickenpox is one of the most common childhood diseases. Although it is usually a mild disease, serious complications from chickenpox lead to the hospitalization of more than 7,000 children. About 1 child out of 500 who get chickenpox has to be hospitalized for severe bacterial infections of chickenpox sores (such as flesh-eating strep and staph toxic shock) and for brain inflammation. Four out of every 100,000 infants who get chickenpox die.

What vaccines does my child need?

Your child needs all of the following immunizations to stay healthy:

- **DTaP vaccine** protects against diphtheria, tetanus (lockjaw), and pertussis (whooping cough).
- **Hepatitis A vaccine** in selected areas protects against a serious liver disease.
- **Hepatitis B vaccine** protects against a virus that causes chronic liver disease and liver cancer.
- **Hib vaccine** protects against *Haemophilus influenzae* type b (a major cause of spinal meningitis).
- **Influenza vaccine** is recommended yearly for children older than 6 months with certain risk factors (such as lung, heart, and kidney disease). It is encouraged for all healthy children aged 6 to 23 months.
- **MMR vaccine** protects against measles, mumps, and rubella (German measles).
- **Pneumococcal vaccine** offers extra protection against bacterial meningitis and infections of the blood.
- **Polio vaccine** protects against crippling polio.
- **Varicella vaccine** protects against chickenpox and its many complications including flesh-eating strep, staph toxic shock, and encephalitis.

The chickenpox vaccine, licensed in 1995, is credited with the decline of cases of chickenpox and its frequent complications. Many studies show the vaccine is safe and effective. Research is being done to see how long the vaccine protects and if a person will need a booster shot in the future.

Q: "Does my baby need immunizations if I am breastfeeding?"

A: Breastfed babies still need immunizations. While breastfeeding can be considered a baby's first immunization and is the best nutrition for your baby, breastfeeding and immunizations work together to give your baby the best protection against serious illness. Studies show that some immunizations stimulate greater immune response in breastfed babies. Also, it is important to know that you can breastfeed right before and after your baby receives any immunization.

How well do vaccines work?

Q: "Do vaccines even work? Most of the people who get these diseases have been vaccinated."

A: Yes. Vaccines work extremely well. Millions of children have been protected from serious illnesses such as polio, whooping cough, measles, tetanus, and diphtheria because parents have had their children immunized.

Most childhood vaccines are 90% to 99% effective in preventing disease. They are even more effective in reducing disease severity. Occasionally a few children may not develop the desired protection after receiving a vaccine. But to *not* vaccinate your child gives them no protection from the possibility of getting one of these deadly diseases.

Q: "When should my child get immunized?"

A: Children should receive most of their shots during their first 2 years of life. Children need to be immunized when they are infants because vaccine-preventable diseases are deadliest in the very young. Some newborns receive their first shot (hepatitis B) at birth before leaving the hospital. Other shots are given before children go to school. Children who are behind on getting their shots are at great risk of getting many vaccine-preventable diseases. Also, children who are not immunized could spread diseases to others who have not been immunized. Talk with your child's pediatrician about getting your child back on schedule.

Older children and teens also need immunizations to continue to protect them throughout adolescence and early adulthood. Ask your child's pediatrician for the current recommended childhood immunization schedule to see when your child needs additional immunizations. Keep track of each vaccine your child receives and keep your child's immunization record with you at all times. Check with your child's pediatrician to make sure your child's immunizations are given on time and are up to date.

How safe are vaccines?

Q: "Is it safe to immunize a child who has a cold and fever?"

A: A child with a minor illness *can* safely be immunized. Examples of minor illnesses include the following: low-grade fever (<100.4°F), ear infection, cough, runny nose, or mild diarrhea in an otherwise healthy child.

Q: "I've heard that some children have serious side effects from vaccines. Are vaccines safe for my child?"

A: Vaccines *are* safe, and severe reactions to vaccines are very rare. Mild reactions to vaccines do occur, but they do not last long. There may be some swelling, redness, and discomfort where the shot was given. Your child may have a low-grade fever and be fussy afterward. Symptoms of more serious reactions are much less common. Call your child's pediatrician right away if your child has a
- Very high fever (>103°F)
- Generalized rash (including hives)
- Large amount of swelling around the shot or in the limb used for the shot
    Your child's pediatrician can decide whether your child should receive future doses of the same vaccine.

Children with certain health problems may need to avoid some vaccines or get them later. For example, children with cancer, those taking steroids for lung or kidney conditions, or those who have problems with their immune systems in most cases should not receive vaccines like the measles, mumps, and rubella (MMR) or chickenpox vaccine. These are not safe for children with these health problems because the vaccine is made with weakened live viruses. For children with seizures, the pertussis part of the diphtheria, tetanus, and pertussis (DTaP) vaccine may need to be delayed. Ask your child's pediatrician when the vaccine can be given.

Q: "Does the MMR vaccine cause autism?"

A: MMR *does not* cause autism. Many research studies have been done to address this issue. There is no scientific link between the MMR vaccine and autism. There may be confusion because autism is often identified in children from 18 to 30 months of age—around the same time the MMR vaccine is given. This has led some people to mistakenly assume the vaccine is the cause of autism. However, increasing evidence shows that autism starts before a baby is born.

Q: "Does the DTaP vaccine cause sudden infant death syndrome (SIDS)?"

A: Careful scientific studies have confirmed that the DTaP shot *does not* cause SIDS. This myth continues because the first dose of the vaccine is given at 2 months of age, and the greatest risk for SIDS is at 1 to 6 months of age. However, there is no link between the DTaP shot and SIDS.

Q: "I saw on the news that there are 'hot lots' of vaccines that are more dangerous than other lots. Is this true?"

A: No. More dangerous lots of vaccines have *never* been released. The federal government monitors every production lot of a vaccine before it is released. A database called the Vaccine Adverse Events Reporting System (VAERS) receives reports of reactions following a vaccination. People may think that if a number of VAERS reports result from a certain batch of vaccine, then this must be a "hot lot" that produces more side effects. No such vaccine lot has ever been released.

Keep in mind, the US Food and Drug Administration (FDA) licenses all vaccines. Vaccine manufacturing facilities are licensed and regularly inspected. Also, every vaccine lot is safety-tested by the manufacturer. The fact that a vaccine continues in use means that the FDA considers it safe.

Q: "What is thimerosal?"

A: Since the 1930s a preservative called thimerosal was added to vaccines to prevent bacterial contamination of vaccines packaged in multidose vials. However, since 2001 all routinely recommended vaccines for infants are made either thimerosal-free or contain only trace amounts of the preservative. Thimerosal contains very small amounts of mercury. The form of mercury in thimerosal has never been shown to cause health problems other than rare allergic reactions in some people. In amounts much larger than found in vaccines certain forms of mercury can cause brain and kidney damage. Because children can be exposed to mercury found in foods (such as fish and grains) and environmental sources (such as contaminated soils, water, and wastes) that cannot always be readily removed as an exposure threat, the US Public Health Service and the American Academy of Pediatrics (AAP) believe removing thimerosal from vaccines is one means of reducing mercury exposure.

Q: "Is it safe to give more than one immunization at a time?"

A: Many years of experience and careful research have shown that vaccines used for routine childhood immunizations can be given together safely and effectively. Side effects are not increased when multiple vaccines are given together when compared with vaccines given on separate occasions. Infants and children are able to handle the immunizations they receive during the typical well-baby office visit. Talk with your child's

> ### Remember
> Immunizations are an important part of your child's total health care. Immunize your child on time, and keep your child's immunization record up to date. Make sure you take your child to the pediatrician's office or a health clinic on a regular basis.

pediatrician if you are concerned that your child is scheduled to receive too many vaccines.

Q: "Don't shots hurt? How can I lessen the pain?"

A: Shots do hurt some, and your baby may cry for a few minutes. Your child's pediatrician may suggest ways to reduce the discomfort before and after your child receives his immunizations. Acetaminophen or ibuprofen can be used to help relieve some of the more common side effects, such as irritability and fever. Always check the dosage with your child's pediatrician.

If your child is old enough to understand, explain that immunizations help to keep him healthy. Distract your child as the vaccination is given. Comfort and play with your child after the immunization. Remember, protecting your child's long-term health and avoiding deadly vaccine-preventable diseases is worth a few tears.

Where can I find more information?

Q: "I want to learn more, where can I find more information?"

A: Be sure your information comes from reliable and accurate sources. You cannot trust everything you find on the Internet. Credible sources include

AAP Childhood Immunization Support Program
www.cispimmunize.org

Centers for Disease Control and Prevention's (CDC)
National Immunization Program
www.cdc.gov/nip

Immunization Action Coalition
www.immunize.org

Infectious Diseases Society of America
www.idsociety.org

National Network for Immunization Information
www.immunizationinfo.org

Vaccine Education Center
www.vaccine.chop.edu

Call your child's pediatrician, local public health department, or community health center if

- Your child is sick and is scheduled to receive an immunization.
- You need information about immunizations or your child's health care needs.

You can also call the CDC's National Immunization Information Hotline at
800/232-2522 (English)
800/232-0233 (Spanish)
800/243-7889 (TTY)

Please note: Listing of resources does not imply an endorsement by the American Academy of Pediatrics (AAP). The AAP is not responsible for the content of the resources mentioned in this brochure. Addresses, phone numbers, and Web site addresses are as current as possible, but may change at any time.

The information contained in this publication should not be used as a substitute for the medical care and advice of your pediatrician. There may be variations in treatment that your pediatrician may recommend based on individual facts and circumstances.

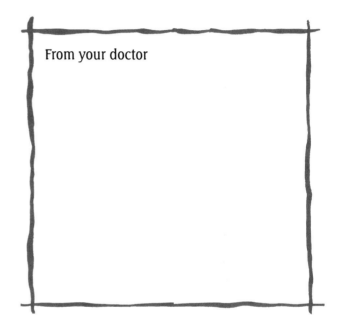

From your doctor

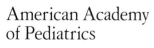

American Academy of Pediatrics

DEDICATED TO THE HEALTH OF ALL CHILDREN™

The American Academy of Pediatrics is an organization of 60,000 primary care pediatricians, pediatric medical subspecialists, and pediatric surgical specialists dedicated to the health, safety, and well-being of infants, children, adolescents, and young adults.

American Academy of Pediatrics
Web site—www.aap.org

Copyright © 2003
American Academy of Pediatrics, Updated 9/03

INACTIVATED INFLUENZA VACCINE

WHAT YOU NEED TO KNOW

1 | Why get vaccinated?

Influenza ("flu") is a very contagious disease.

It is caused by the influenza virus, which spreads from infected persons to the nose or throat of others.

Other illnesses can have the same symptoms and are often mistaken for influenza. But only an illness caused by the influenza virus is really influenza.

Anyone can get influenza. For most people, it lasts only a few days. It can cause:

- · fever   · sore throat   · chills   · fatigue
- · cough   · headache   · muscle aches

Some people get much sicker. Influenza can lead to pneumonia and can be dangerous for people with heart or breathing conditions. It can cause high fever and seizures in children. Influenza kills about 36,000 people each year in the United States, mostly among the elderly.

Influenza vaccine can prevent influenza.

2 | Inactivated Influenza vaccine

There are two types of influenza vaccine:

An **inactivated** (killed) vaccine, given as a shot, has been used in the United States for many years.

A **live**, weakened vaccine was licensed in 2003. It is sprayed into the nostrils. *This vaccine is described in a separate Vaccine Information Statement.*

Influenza viruses are constantly changing. Therefore, influenza vaccines are updated every year, and an annual vaccination is recommended.

For most people influenza vaccine prevents serious illness caused by the influenza virus. It will *not* prevent "influenza-like" illnesses caused by other viruses.

It takes about 2 weeks for protection to develop after the shot, and protection can last up to a year.

Inactivated influenza vaccine may be given at the same time as other vaccines, including pneumococcal vaccine.

Some inactivated influenza vaccine contains thimerosal, a preservative that contains mercury. Some people believe thimerosal may be related to developmental problems in children. In 2004 the Institute of Medicine published a report concluding that, based on scientific studies, there is no evidence of such a relationship. If you are concerned about thimerosal, ask your doctor about thimerosal-free influenza vaccine.

3 | Who should get inactivated influenza vaccine?

Influenza vaccine can be given to people 6 months of age and older. It is recommended for **people who are at risk of serious influenza or its complications**, and for **people who can spread influenza to those at high risk** (including all household members):

People at high risk for complications from influenza:

- **All children** 6-23 months of age.
- People **65 years of age and older**.
- Residents of **long-term care facilities** housing persons with chronic medical conditions.
- People who have **long-term health problems** with:
  - heart disease   - kidney disease
  - lung disease   - metabolic disease, such as diabetes
  - asthma   - anemia, and other blood disorders
- People with certain **muscle or nerve disorders** (such as seizure disorders or severe cerebral palsy) that can lead to breathing or swallowing problems.
- People with a **weakened immune system** due to:
  - HIV/AIDS or other diseases affecting the immune system
  - long-term treatment with drugs such as steroids
  - cancer treatment with x-rays or drugs
- People 6 months to 18 years of age on **long-term aspirin treatment** (these people could develop Reye Syndrome if they got influenza).
- Women who will be **pregnant** during influenza season.

People who can spread influenza to those at high risk:

- **Household contacts and out-of-home caretakers** of infants from 0-23 months of age.
- Physicians, nurses, family members, or anyone else in **close contact with people at risk** of serious influenza.

Influenza vaccine is also recommended for adults 50-64 years of age and anyone else who wants to **reduce their chance of catching influenza.**

An annual flu shot should be *considered* for:

- People who provide **essential community services.**
- People living in **dormitories** or under other crowded conditions, to prevent outbreaks.
- People at high risk of influenza complications who **travel** to the Southern hemisphere between April and September, or to the tropics or in organized tourist groups at any time.

4 When should I get influenza vaccine?

The best time to get influenza vaccine is in **October** or **November**.

Influenza season usually peaks in February, but it can peak any time from November through May. So getting the vaccine in December, or even later, can be beneficial in most years.

Some people should get their flu shot in *October* or earlier:
- people **50 years of age and older**,
- younger people at **high risk** from influenza and its complications (including **children 6 through 23 months of age**),
- **household contacts** of people at high risk,
- **healthcare workers**, and
- **children younger than 9 years of age** getting influenza vaccine for the first time.

Most people need one flu shot each year. **Children younger than 9 years of age getting influenza vaccine for the first time** should get 2 doses, given at least one month apart.

5 Some people should talk with a doctor before getting influenza vaccine

Some people should not get inactivated influenza vaccine or should wait before getting it.

- Tell your doctor if you have any **severe** (life-threatening) allergies. Allergic reactions to influenza vaccine are rare.
  - Influenza vaccine virus is grown in eggs. People with a severe egg allergy should not get the vaccine.
  - A severe allergy to any vaccine component is also a reason to not get the vaccine.
  - If you have had a severe reaction after a previous dose of influenza vaccine, tell your doctor.

- Tell your doctor if you ever had Guillain-Barré Syndrome (a severe paralytic illness, also called GBS). You may be able to get the vaccine, but your doctor should help you make the decision.

- People who are moderately or severely ill should usually wait until they recover before getting flu vaccine. If you are ill, talk to your doctor or nurse about whether to reschedule the vaccination. People with a **mild illness** can usually get the vaccine.

6 What are the risks from inactivated influenza vaccine?

A vaccine, like any medicine, could possibly cause serious problems, such as severe allergic reactions. The risk of a vaccine causing serious harm, or death, is extremely small.

Serious problems from influenza vaccine are very rare. The viruses in inactivated influenza vaccine have been killed, so you cannot get influenza from the vaccine.

Mild problems:
- soreness, redness, or swelling where the shot was given
- fever   • aches

If these problems occur, they usually begin soon after the shot and last 1-2 days.

Severe problems:
- Life-threatening allergic reactions from vaccines are very rare. If they do occur, it is within a few minutes to a few hours after the shot.

- In 1976, a certain type of influenza (swine flu) vaccine was associated with Guillain-Barré Syndrome (GBS). Since then, flu vaccines have not been clearly linked to GBS. However, if there is a risk of GBS from current flu vaccines, it would be no more than 1 or 2 cases per million people vaccinated. This is much lower than the risk of severe influenza, which can be prevented by vaccination.

7 What if there is a severe reaction?

What should I look for?
- Any unusual condition, such as a high fever or behavior changes. Signs of a serious allergic reaction can include difficulty breathing, hoarseness or wheezing, hives, paleness, weakness, a fast heart beat or dizziness.

What should I do?
- **Call** a doctor, or get the person to a doctor right away.

- **Tell** your doctor what happened, the date and time it happened, and when the vaccination was given.

- **Ask** your doctor, nurse, or health department to report the reaction by filing a Vaccine Adverse Event Reporting System (VAERS) form.
  Or you can file this report through the VAERS web site at www.vaers.hhs.gov, or by calling 1-800-822-7967.
  VAERS does not provide medical advice.

8 The National Vaccine Injury Compensation Program

In the event that you or your child has a serious reaction to a vaccine, a federal program has been created to help pay for the care of those who have been harmed.

For details about the National Vaccine Injury Compensation Program, call **1-800-338-2382** or visit their website at **www.hrsa.gov/osp/vicp**

9 How can I learn more?

- Ask your immunization provider. They can give you the vaccine package insert or suggest other sources of information.

- Call your local or state health department.

- Contact the Centers for Disease Control and Prevention (CDC):
  - Call **1-800-232-4636 (1-800-CDC-INFO)**
  - Visit CDC's website at **www.cdc.gov/flu**

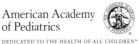

American Academy of Pediatrics
DEDICATED TO THE HEALTH OF ALL CHILDREN™

Reprinted by the American Academy of Pediatrics. Additional copies are available for purchase in pads of 1[?]

To order, contact:
American Academy of Pediatrics
141 Northwest Point Blvd
Elk Grove Village, IL 60007-1098
Web site—http://www.aap.org
Minimum order 100

Vaccine Information Statement
Inactivated Influenza Vaccine (10/20/05)   42 U.S.C. §300aa-26

U.S. DEPARTMENT OF HEALTH & HUMAN SERVICES
Centers for Disease Control and Prevention
National Immunization Program

© 2007 American Academy of Pediatrics

LIVE, INTRANASAL INFLUENZA VACCINE

WHAT YOU NEED TO KNOW

1 | Why get vaccinated?

Influenza ("flu") is a very contagious disease.

It is caused by the influenza virus, which spreads from infected persons to the nose or throat of others.

Other illnesses can have the same symptoms and are often mistaken for influenza. But only an illness caused by the influenza virus is really influenza.

Anyone can get influenza, but rates of infection are highest among children. For most people, it lasts only a few days. It can cause:

· fever	· sore throat	· chills	· fatigue
· cough	· headache	· muscle aches	

Some people get much sicker. Influenza can lead to pneumonia and can be dangerous for people with heart or breathing conditions. It can cause high fever and seizures in children. Influenza kills about 36,000 people each year in the United States.

Influenza vaccine can prevent influenza.

2 | Live, attenuated influenza vaccine (nasal spray)

There are two types of influenza vaccine:

Live, attenuated influenza vaccine (LAIV) was licensed in 2003. LAIV contains live but attenuated (weakened) influenza virus. It is sprayed into the nostrils rather than injected into the muscle. It is recommended for healthy children and adults from 5 through 49 years of age, who are not pregnant.

Inactivated influenza vaccine, sometimes called the "flu shot," has been used for many years and is given by injection. *This vaccine is described in a separate Vaccine Information Statement.*

Influenza viruses are constantly changing. Therefore, influenza vaccines are updated every year, and annual vaccination is recommended.

For most people influenza vaccine prevents serious illness caused by the influenza virus. It will *not* prevent "influenza-like" illnesses caused by other viruses.

It takes about 2 weeks for protection to develop after vaccination, and protection can last up to a year.

3 | Who can get LAIV?

Live, intranasal influenza vaccine is approved for **healthy children and adults from 5 through 49 years of age**, including those who can spread influenza to people at high risk, such as:

- **Household contacts and out-of-home care-takers** of infants from 0-23 months of age.

- Physicians and nurses, and family members or any one else in **close contact with people at risk** of serious influenza.

Influenza vaccine is also recommended for anyone else who wants to **reduce their chance of catching influenza**.

LAIV may be considered for:

- People who provide **essential community services.**

- People living in **dormitories** or under other crowded conditions, to prevent outbreaks.

4 | Who should *not* get LAIV?

LAIV is not licensed for everyone. The following people should check with their health-care provider about getting the **inactivated** vaccine.

- **Adults 50 years of age or older** or **children younger than 5**.

- People who have **long-term health problems** with:
  - heart disease
  - lung disease
  - asthma
  - kidney disease
  - metabolic disease, such as diabetes
  - anemia, and other blood disorders

- People with a **weakened immune system**.

- Children or adolescents on **long-term aspirin treatment**.

- **Pregnant women**.

- Anyone with a history of **Guillain-Barré syndrome** (a severe paralytic illness, also called GBS).

Inactivated influenza vaccine (the flu shot) is the preferred vaccine for people (including health-care workers, and family members) coming in **close contact with anyone who has a severely weakened immune system** (that is, anyone who requires care in a protected environment).

Some people should talk with a doctor before getting *either* influenza vaccine:

- Anyone who has ever had a <u>serious</u> allergic reaction to **eggs** or to a **previous dose** of influenza vaccine.

- People who are moderately or severely ill should usually wait until they recover before getting flu vaccine. If you are ill, talk to your doctor or nurse about whether to reschedule the vaccination. People with a **mild illness** can usually get the vaccine.

5 | When should I get influenza vaccine?

The best time to get influenza vaccine is in **October** or **November**, but LAIV may be given as soon as it is available. Influenza season usually peaks in February, but it can peak any time from November through May. So getting the vaccine in December, or even later, can be beneficial in most years.

Most people need one dose of influenza vaccine each year. **Children younger than 9 years of age getting influenza vaccine for the first time** should get 2 doses For LAIV, these doses should be given 6-10 weeks apart.

LAIV may be given at the same time as other vaccines.

6 | What are the risks from LAIV?

A vaccine, like any medicine, could possibly cause serious problems, such as severe allergic reactions. However, the risk of a vaccine causing serious harm, or death, is extremely small.

Live influenza vaccine viruses rarely spread from person to person. Even if they do, they are not likely to cause illness.

LAIV is made from weakened virus and does not cause influenza. The vaccine *can* cause mild symptoms in people who get it (see below).

Mild problems:
Some children and adolescents 5-17 years of age have reported mild reactions, including:
- runny nose, nasal congestion or cough
- headache and muscle aches   • fever
- abdominal pain or occasional vomiting or diarrhea

Some adults 18-49 years of age have reported:
- runny nose or nasal congestion   • sore throat
- cough, chills, tiredness/weakness   • headache

These symptoms did not last long and went away on their own. Although they can occur after vaccination, they may not have been caused by the vaccine.

Severe problems:
- Life-threatening allergic reactions from vaccines are very rare. If they do occur, it is within a few minutes to a few hours after the vaccination.

- If rare reactions occur with any new product, they may not be identified until thousands, or millions, of people have used it. Over two million doses of LAIV have been distributed since it was licensed, and no serious problems have been identified. Like all vaccines, LAIV will continue to be monitored for unusual or severe problems.

7 | What if there is a severe reaction?

What should I look for?
- Any unusual condition, such as a high fever or behavior changes. Signs of a serious allergic reaction can include difficulty breathing, hoarseness or wheezing, hives, paleness, weakness, a fast heart beat or dizziness.

What should I do?
- **Call** a doctor, or get the person to a doctor right away.
- **Tell** your doctor what happened, the date and time it happened, and when the vaccination was given.
- **Ask** your doctor, nurse, or health department to report the reaction by filing a Vaccine Adverse Event Reporting System (VAERS) form.

  Or you can file this report through the VAERS website at www.vaers.hhs.gov, or by calling 1-800-822-7967.

  VAERS does not provide medical advice.

8 | The National Vaccine Injury Compensation Program

In the event that you or your child has a serious reaction to a vaccine, a federal program has been created to help pay for the care of those who have been harmed.

For details about the National Vaccine Injury Compensation Program, call **1-800-338-2382** or visit their website at **www.hrsa.gov/osp/vicp**

9 | How can I learn more?

- Ask your immunization provider. They can give you the vaccine package insert or suggest other sources of information.

- Call your local or state health department.

- Contact the Centers for Disease Control and Prevention (CDC):
  - Call **1-800-232-4636 (1-800-CDC-INFO)**
  - Visit CDC's website at **www.cdc.gov/flu**

American Academy of Pediatrics
DEDICATED TO THE HEALTH OF ALL CHILDREN™

Reprinted by the American Academy of Pediatrics. Additional copies are available for purchase in pads of 1

To order, contact:
American Academy of Pediatrics
141 Northwest Point Blvd
Elk Grove Village, IL 60007-1098
Web site—http://www.aap.org
Minimum order 100

U.S. DEPARTMENT OF HEALTH & HUMAN SERVICES
Centers for Disease Control and Prevention
National Immunization Program

Vaccine Information Statement
Live, Attenuated Influenza Vaccine (10/20/05)   42 U.S.C. §300aa-26

MEASLES MUMPS & RUBELLA VACCINES

WHAT YOU NEED TO KNOW

1 Why get vaccinated?

Measles, mumps, and rubella are serious diseases.

Measles
- Measles virus causes rash, cough, runny nose, eye irritation, and fever.
- It can lead to ear infection, pneumonia, seizures (jerking and staring), brain damage, and death.

Mumps
- Mumps virus causes fever, headache, and swollen glands.
- It can lead to deafness, meningitis (infection of the brain and spinal cord covering), painful swelling of the testicles or ovaries, and, rarely, death.

Rubella (German Measles)
- Rubella virus causes rash, mild fever, and arthritis (mostly in women).
- If a woman gets rubella while she is pregnant, she could have a miscarriage or her baby could be born with serious birth defects.

You or your child could catch these diseases by being around someone who has them. They spread from person to person through the air.

Measles, mumps, and rubella (MMR) vaccine can prevent these diseases.

Most children who get their MMR shots will not get these diseases. Many more children would get them if we stopped vaccinating.

2 Who should get MMR vaccine and when?

Children should get 2 doses of MMR vaccine:

✓ The first at 12-15 months of age
✓ and the second at 4-6 years of age.

These are the recommended ages. But children can get the second dose at any age, as long as it is at least 28 days after the first dose.

Some adults should also get MMR vaccine: Generally, anyone 18 years of age or older, who was born after 1956, should get at least one dose of MMR vaccine, unless they can show that they have had either the vaccines or the diseases.

Ask your doctor or nurse for more information.

MMR vaccine may be given at the same time as other vaccines.

3 Some people should not get MMR vaccine or should wait

- People should not get MMR vaccine who have ever had a life-threatening allergic reaction to gelatin, the antibiotic neomycin, or to a previous dose of MMR vaccine.

- People who are moderately or severely ill at the time the shot is scheduled should usually wait until they recover before getting MMR vaccine.

- Pregnant women should wait to get MMR vaccine until after they have given birth. Women should avoid getting pregnant for 4 weeks after getting MMR vaccine.

- Some people should check with their doctor about whether they should get MMR vaccine, including anyone who:
  - Has HIV/AIDS, or another disease that affects the immune system
  - Is being treated with drugs that affect the immune system, such as steroids, for 2 weeks or longer.
  - Has any kind of cancer
  - Is taking cancer treatment with x-rays or drugs
  - Has ever had a low platelet count (a blood disorder)

Over . . .

- People who recently had a transfusion or were given other blood products should ask their doctor when they may get MMR vaccine

Ask your doctor or nurse for more information.

4 | What are the risks from MMR vaccine?

A vaccine, like any medicine, is capable of causing serious problems, such as severe allergic reactions. The risk of MMR vaccine causing serious harm, or death, is extremely small.

Getting MMR vaccine is much safer than getting any of these three diseases.

Most people who get MMR vaccine do not have any problems with it.

Mild Problems

- Fever (up to 1 person out of 6)
- Mild rash (about 1 person out of 20)
- Swelling of glands in the cheeks or neck (rare)

If these problems occur, it is usually within 7-12 days after the shot. They occur less often after the second dose.

Moderate Problems

- Seizure (jerking or staring) caused by fever (about 1 out of 3,000 doses)
- Temporary pain and stiffness in the joints, mostly in teenage or adult women (up to 1 out of 4)
- Temporary low platelet count, which can cause a bleeding disorder (about 1 out of 30,000 doses)

Severe Problems (Very Rare)

- Serious allergic reaction (less than 1 out of a million doses)
- Several other severe problems have been known to occur after a child gets MMR vaccine. But this happens so rarely, experts cannot be sure whether they are caused by the vaccine or not. These include:
  - Deafness
  - Long-term seizures, coma, or lowered consciousness
  - Permanent brain damage

5 | What if there is a moderate or severe reaction?

What should I look for?

Any unusual conditions, such as a serious allergic reaction, high fever or behavior changes. Signs of a serious allergic reaction include difficulty breathing, hoarseness or wheezing, hives, paleness, weakness, a fast heart beat or dizziness within a few minutes to a few hours after the shot. A high fever or seizure, if it occurs, would happen 1 or 2 weeks after the shot.

What should I do?

- **Call** a doctor, or get the person to a doctor right away.
- **Tell** your doctor what happened, the date and time it happened, and when the vaccination was given.
- **Ask** your doctor, nurse, or health department to report the reaction by filing a Vaccine Adverse Event Reporting System (VAERS) form. Or you can file this report through the VAERS web site at www.vaers.org, or by calling 1-800-822-7967.
  VAERS does not provide medical advice.

6 | The National Vaccine Injury Compensation Program

In the rare event that you or your child has a serious reaction to a vaccine, a federal program has been created to help you pay for the care of those who have been harmed.

For details about the National Vaccine Injury Compensation Program, call **1-800-338-2382** or visit the program's website at www.hrsa.gov/osp/vicp

7 | How can I learn more?

- Ask your doctor or nurse. They can give you the vaccine package insert or suggest other sources of information.

- Call your local or state health department's immunization program.

- Contact the Centers for Disease Control and Prevention (CDC):
  - Call **1-800-232-4636 (1-800-CDC-INFO)**
  - Visit the National Immunization Program's website at www.cdc.gov/nip

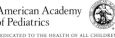

American Academy of Pediatrics
DEDICATED TO THE HEALTH OF ALL CHILDREN®

Reprinted by the American Academy of Pediatrics. Additional copies are available for purchase in pads of 100.

To order, contact:
American Academy of Pediatrics
141 Northwest Point Blvd
Elk Grove Village, IL 60007-1098
Web site—http://www.aap.org
Minimum order 100

U.S. DEPARTMENT OF HEALTH & HUMAN SERVICES
Centers for Disease Control and Prevention
National Immunization Program

Vaccine Information Statement
MMR (1/15/03)   42 U.S.C. § 300aa-26

MENINGOCOCCAL VACCINES

WHAT YOU NEED TO KNOW

1 | What is meningococcal disease?

Meningococcal disease is a serious illness, caused by a bacteria. It is a leading cause of bacterial meningitis in children 2-18 years old in the United States.

Meningitis is an infection of fluid surrounding the brain and the spinal cord. Meningococcal disease also causes blood infections.

About 2,600 people get meningococcal disease each year in the U.S. 10-15% of these people die, in spite of treatment with antibiotics. Of those who live, another 11-19% lose their arms or legs, become deaf, have problems with their nervous systems, become mentally retarded, or suffer seizures or strokes.

Anyone can get meningococcal disease. But it is most common in infants less than one year of age and people with certain medical conditions, such as lack of a spleen. College freshmen who live in dormitories have an increased risk of getting meningococcal disease.

Meningococcal infections can be treated with drugs such as penicillin. Still, about 1 out of every ten people who get the disease dies from it, and many others are affected for life. This is why *preventing* the disease through use of meningococcal vaccine is important for people at highest risk.

2 | Meningococcal vaccine

Two meningococcal vaccines are available in the U.S.:

- **Meningococcal polysaccharide vaccine (MPSV4)** has been available since the 1970s.
- **Meningococcal conjugate vaccine (MCV4)** was licensed in 2005.

Both vaccines can prevent **4 types** of meningococcal disease, including 2 of the 3 types most common in the United States and a type that causes epidemics in Africa. Meningococcal vaccines cannot prevent all types of the disease. But they do protect many people who might become sick if they didn't get the vaccine.

Both vaccines work well, and protect about 90% of those who get it. MCV4 is expected to give better, longer-lasting protection.

MCV4 should also be better at preventing the disease from spreading from person to person.

3 | Who should get meningococcal vaccine and when?

MCV4 is recommended for all children at their routine preadolescent visit (11-12 years of age). For those who have never gotten MCV4 previously, a dose is recommended at high school entry.

Other adolescents who want to decrease their risk of meningococcal disease can also get the vaccine.

Meningococcal vaccine is also recommended for other people at increased risk for meningococcal disease:

- College freshmen living in dormitories.
- Microbiologists who are routinely exposed to meningococcal bacteria.
- U.S. military recruits.
- Anyone traveling to, or living in, a part of the world where meningococcal disease is common, such as parts of Africa.
- Anyone who has a damaged spleen, or whose spleen has been removed.
- Anyone who has terminal complement component deficiency (an immune system disorder).
- People who might have been exposed to meningitis during an outbreak.

MCV4 is the preferred vaccine for people 11-55 years of age in these risk groups, but MPSV4 can be used if MCV4 is not available. MPSV4 should be used for children 2-10 years old, and adults over 55, who are at risk.

How Many Doses?

People 2 years of age and older should get 1 dose. (Sometimes an additional dose is recommended for people who remain at high risk. Ask your provider.)

MPSV4 may be recommended for children 3 months to 2 years of age under special circumstances. These children should get 2 doses, 3 months apart.

4 | Some people should not get meningococcal vaccine or should wait

- Anyone who has ever had a severe (life-threatening) **allergic reaction to a previous dose** of either meningococcal vaccine should not get another dose.

- Anyone who has a severe (life threatening) **allergy to any vaccine component** should not get the vaccine. Tell your doctor if you have any severe allergies.

- Anyone who is **moderately or severely ill** at the time the shot is scheduled should probably wait until they recover. Ask your doctor or nurse. People with a **mild illness** can usually get the vaccine.

- Anyone who has ever had **Guillain-Barré Syndrome** should talk with their doctor before getting MCV4.

- Meningococcal vaccines may be given to pregnant women. However, MCV4 is a new vaccine and has not been studied in pregnant women as much as MPSV4 has. It should be used only if clearly needed.

- Meningococcal vaccines may be given at the same time as other vaccines.

5 | What are the risks from meningococcal vaccines?

A vaccine, like any medicine, could possibly cause serious problems, such as severe allergic reactions. The risk of meningococcal vaccine causing serious harm, or death, is extremely small.

Mild problems

Up to about half of people who get meningococcal vaccines have mild side effects, such as redness or pain where the shot was given.

If these problems occur, they usually last for 1 or 2 days. They are more common after MCV4 than after MPSV4.

A small percentage of people who receive the vaccine develop a fever.

Severe problems

- Serious allergic reactions, within a few minutes to a few hours of the shot, are very rare.

- A few cases of Guillain-Barré Syndrome, a serious nervous system disorder, have been reported among people who got MCV4. There is not enough evidence yet to tell whether they were caused by the vaccine. This is being investigated by health officials.

6 | What if there is a moderate or severe reaction?

What should I look for?

- Any unusual condition, such as a high fever or behavior changes. Signs of a serious allergic reaction can include difficulty breathing, hoarseness or wheezing, hives, paleness, weakness, a fast heart beat or dizziness.

What should I do?

- **Call** a doctor, or get the person to a doctor right away.

- **Tell** your doctor what happened, the date and time it happened, and when the vaccination was given.

- **Ask** your doctor, nurse, or health department to report the reaction by filing a Vaccine Adverse Event Reporting System (VAERS) form.

  Or you can file this report through the VAERS web site at www.vaers.org, or by calling 1-800-822-7967.

  VAERS does not provide medical advice.

7 | How can I learn more?

- Ask your doctor or nurse. They can give you the vaccine package insert or suggest other sources of information.

- Call your local or state health department.

- Contact the Centers for Disease Control and Prevention (CDC):

  - Call **1-800-232-4636 (1-800-CDC-INFO)**

  - Visit CDC's National Immunization Program website at **www.cdc.gov/nip**

  - Visit CDC's meningococcal disease website at www.cdc.gov/ncidod/dbmd/diseaseinfo/meningococcal_g.htm

  - Visit CDC's Travelers' Health website at **www.cdc.gov/travel**

American Academy of Pediatrics

DEDICATED TO THE HEALTH OF ALL CHILDREN™

Reprinted by the American Academy of Pediatrics. Additional copies are available for purchase in pads of 100

To order, contact:
American Academy of Pediatrics
141 Northwest Point Blvd
Elk Grove Village, IL 60007-1098

Web site—http://www.aap.org
Minimum order 100

| Meningococcal | 10/7/05 | Vaccine Information Statement (Interim) |

U.S. DEPARTMENT OF HEALTH & HUMAN SERVICES
Centers for Disease Control and Prevention
National Immunization Program

© 2007 American Academy of Pediatrics

PNEUMOCOCCAL CONJUGATE VACCINE

W H A T   Y O U   N E E D   T O   K N O W

1 | Why get vaccinated?

Infection with *Streptococcus pneumoniae* bacteria can cause serious illness and death. Invasive pneumococcal disease is responsible for about 200 deaths each year among children under 5 years old. It is the leading cause of bacterial meningitis in the United States. (Meningitis is an infection of the covering of the brain).

Pneumococcal infection causes severe disease in children under five years old. Before a vaccine was available, each year pneumococcal infection caused:
- over 700 cases of meningitis,
- 13,000 blood infections, and
- about 5 million ear infections.

It can also lead to other health problems, including:
- pneumonia,
- deafness,
- brain damage.

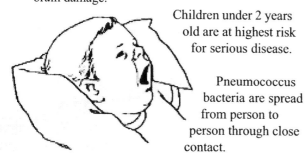

Children under 2 years old are at highest risk for serious disease.

Pneumococcus bacteria are spread from person to person through close contact.

Pneumococcal infections can be hard to treat because the bacteria have become resistant to some of the drugs that have been used to treat them. This makes **prevention** of pneumococcal infections even more important.

Pneumococcal conjugate vaccine can help prevent serious pneumococcal disease, such as meningitis and blood infections. It can also prevent some ear infections. But ear infections have many causes, and pneumococcal vaccine is effective against only some of them.

2 | Pneumococcal conjugate vaccine

Pneumococcal conjugate vaccine is approved for infants and toddlers. Children who are vaccinated when they are infants will be protected when they are at greatest risk for serious disease.

Some older children and adults may get a different vaccine called pneumococcal polysaccharide vaccine. There is a separate Vaccine Information Statement for people getting this vaccine.

3 | Who should get the vaccine and when?

- **Children Under 2 Years of Age**

The routine schedule for pneumococcal conjugate vaccine is 4 doses, one dose at each of these ages:
  - ✓ 2 months
  - ✓ 4 months
  - ✓ 6 months
  - ✓ 12-15 months

Children who weren't vaccinated at these ages can still get the vaccine. The number of doses needed depends on the child's age. Ask your health care provider for details.

- **Children Between 2 and 5 Years of Age**

Pneumococcal conjugate vaccine is also recommended for children between 2 and 5 years old who have not already gotten the vaccine and are at high risk of serious pneumococcal disease. This includes children who:
  § have sickle cell disease,
  § have a damaged spleen or no spleen,
  § have HIV/AIDS,
  § have other diseases that affect the immune system, such as diabetes, cancer, or liver disease, or who
  § take medications that affect the immune system, such as chemotherapy or steroids, or
  § have chronic heart or lung disease.

The vaccine should be considered for all other children under 5 years, especially those at higher risk of serious pneumococcal disease. This includes children who:
  § are under 3 years of age,
  § are of Alaska Native, American Indian or African American descent, or
  § attend group day care.

The number of doses needed depends on the child's age. Ask your health care provider for more details.

Pneumococcal conjugate vaccine may be given at the same time as other vaccines.

Pneumococcal Conjugate   9/30/2002

4 Some children should not get pneumococcal conjugate vaccine or should wait

Children should not get pneumococcal conjugate vaccine if they had a serious (life-threatening) allergic reaction to a previous dose of this vaccine, or have a severe allergy to a vaccine component. Tell your health-care provider if your child has ever had a severe reaction to any vaccine, or has any severe allergies.

Children with minor illnesses, such as a cold, may be vaccinated. But children who are moderately or severely ill should usually wait until they recover before getting the vaccine.

5 What are the risks from pneumococcal conjugate vaccine?

In studies (nearly 60,000 doses), pneumococcal conjugate vaccine was associated with only mild reactions:

- Up to about 1 infant out of 4 had redness, tenderness, or swelling where the shot was given.

- Up to about 1 out of 3 had a fever of over 100.4°F, and up to about 1 in 50 had a higher fever (over 102.2°F).

- Some children also became fussy or drowsy, or had a loss of appetite.

So far, no serious reactions have been associated with this vaccine. However, a vaccine, like any medicine, could cause serious problems, such as a severe allergic reaction. The risk of this vaccine causing serious harm, or death, is extremely small.

6 What if there is a moderate or severe reaction?

What should I look for?

Look for any unusual condition, such as a serious allergic reaction, high fever, or unusual behavior.

Serious allergic reactions are extremely rare with any vaccine. If one were to occur, it would most likely be within a few minutes to a few hours after the shot. Signs can include:

- difficulty breathing
- hoarseness or wheezing
- swelling of the throat
- weakness
- fast heart beat
- dizziness
- hives
- paleness

What should I do?

- **Call** a doctor, or get the person to a doctor right away.

- **Tell** your doctor what happened, the date and time it happened, and when the vaccination was given.

- **Ask** your doctor, nurse, or health department to report the reaction by filing a Vaccine Adverse Event Reporting System (VAERS) form.

  Or you can file this report through the VAERS web site at www.vaers.org, or by calling 1-800-822-7967.

VAERS does not provide medical advice.

7 The National Vaccine Injury Compensation Program

In the rare event that you or your child has a serious reaction to a vaccine, a federal program has been created to help pay for the care of those who have been harmed.

For details about the National Vaccine Injury Compensation Program, call **1-800-338-2382** or visit their website at **http://www.hrsa.gov/osp/vicp**

8 How can I learn more?

- Ask your health care provider. They can give you the vaccine package insert or suggest other sources of information.

- Call your local or state health department's immunization program.

- Contact the Centers for Disease Control and Prevention (CDC):
    - Call **1-800-232-4636** (**1-800-CDC-INFO**)
    - Visit the National Immunization Program's website at **http://www.cdc.gov/nip**

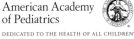

American Academy of Pediatrics

DEDICATED TO THE HEALTH OF ALL CHILDREN™

Reprinted by the American Academy of Pediatrics. Additional copies are available for purchase in pads of

To order, contact:
American Academy of Pediatrics
141 Northwest Point Blvd
Elk Grove Village, IL 60007-1098

Web site—http://www.aap.org
Minimum order 100

U.S. DEPARTMENT OF HEALTH & HUMAN SERVICES
Centers for Disease Control and Prevention
National Immunization Program

Vaccine Information Statement
Pneumococcal Conjugate Vaccine (9/30/02)   42 U.S.C. § 300aa-26

POLIO VACCINE
WHAT YOU NEED TO KNOW

1 | What is polio?

Polio is a disease caused by a virus. It enters a child's (or adult's) body through the mouth. Sometimes it does not cause serious illness. But sometimes it causes *paralysis* (can't move arm or leg). It can kill people who get it, usually by paralyzing the muscles that help them breathe.

Polio used to be very common in the United States. It paralyzed and killed thousands of people a year before we had a vaccine for it.

2 | Why get vaccinated?

Inactivated Polio Vaccine (IPV) can prevent polio.

History: A 1916 polio epidemic in the United States killed 6,000 people and paralyzed 27,000 more. In the early 1950's there were more than 20,000 cases of polio each year. **Polio vaccination was begun in 1955.** By 1960 the number of cases had dropped to about 3,000, and by 1979 there were only about 10. The success of polio vaccination in the U.S. and other countries sparked a world-wide effort to eliminate polio.

Today: No wild polio has been reported in the United States for over 20 years. But the disease is still common in some parts of the world. It would only take one case of polio from another country to bring the disease back if we were not protected by vaccine. If the effort to eliminate the disease from the world is successful, some day we won't need polio vaccine. Until then, we need to keep getting our children vaccinated.

3 | Who should get polio vaccine and when?

IPV is a shot, given in the leg or arm, depending on age. Polio vaccine may be given at the same time as other vaccines.

Children
Most people should get polio vaccine when they are children. Children get 4 doses of IPV, at these ages:
- ✓ A dose at 2 months
- ✓ A dose at 6-18 months
- ✓ A dose at 4 months
- ✓ A booster dose at 4-6 years

Adults
Most adults do not need polio vaccine because they were already vaccinated as children. But three groups of adults are at higher risk and *should* consider polio vaccination:
(1) people traveling to areas of the world where polio is common,
(2) laboratory workers who might handle polio virus, and
(3) health care workers treating patients who could have polio.

Adults in these three groups who **have never been vaccinated against polio** should get 3 doses of IPV:
- ✓ The first dose at any time,
- ✓ The second dose 1 to 2 months later,
- ✓ The third dose 6 to 12 months after the second.

Adults in these three groups who **have had 1 or 2 doses** of polio vaccine in the past should get the remaining 1 or 2 doses. It doesn't matter how long it has been since the earlier dose(s).

Adults in these three groups who **have had 3 or more doses** of polio vaccine (either IPV or OPV) in the past may get a booster dose of IPV.

Ask your health care provider for more information.

Oral Polio Vaccine: No longer recommended
There are two kinds of polio vaccine: **IPV**, which is the shot recommended in the United States today, and a live, oral polio vaccine (**OPV**), which is drops that are swallowed.

Until recently OPV was recommended for most children in the United States. OPV helped us rid the country of polio, and it is still used in many parts of the world.

Both vaccines give immunity to polio, but OPV is better at keeping the disease from spreading to other people. However, for a few people (about one in 2.4 million), OPV actually causes polio. Since the risk of getting polio in the United States is now extremely low, experts believe that using oral polio vaccine is no longer worth the slight risk, except in limited circumstances which your doctor can describe. The polio shot (IPV) does not cause polio. **If you or your child will be getting OPV, ask for a copy of the OPV supplemental Vaccine Information Statement.**

Polio - 1/1/2000

4 | Some people should not get IPV or should wait.

These people should not get IPV:

- Anyone who has ever had a life-threatening allergic reaction to the antibiotics **neomycin**, **streptomycin** or **polymyxin B** should not get the polio shot.

- Anyone who has a severe allergic reaction to a polio shot should not get another one.

These people should wait:

- Anyone who is moderately or severely ill at the time the shot is scheduled should usually wait until they recover before getting polio vaccine. People with minor illnesses, such as a cold, *may* be vaccinated.

Ask your health care provider for more information.

 5 | What are the risks from IPV?

Some people who get IPV get a sore spot where the shot was given. The vaccine used today has never been known to cause any serious problems, and most people don't have any problems at all with it.

However, a vaccine, like any medicine, could cause serious problems, such as a severe allergic reaction. *The risk of a polio shot causing serious harm, or death, is extremely small.*

 6 | What if there is a serious reaction?

What should I look for?
Look for any unusual condition, such as a serious allergic reaction, high fever, or unusual behavior.

If a serious allergic reaction occurred, it would happen within a few minutes to a few hours after the shot. Signs of a serious allergic reaction can include difficulty breathing, weakness, hoarseness or wheezing, a fast heart beat, hives, dizziness, paleness, or swelling of the throat

What should I do?
- **Call** a doctor, or get the person to a doctor right away.

- **Tell** your doctor what happened, the date and time it happened, and when the vaccination was given.

- **Ask** your doctor, nurse, or health department to report the reaction by filing a Vaccine Adverse Event Reporting System (VAERS) form.

  Or you can file this report through the VAERS website at www.vaers.org, or by calling 1-800-822-7967.

  VAERS does not provide medical advice.

Reporting reactions helps experts learn about possible problems with vaccines.

 7 | The National Vaccine Injury Compensation Program

In the rare event that you or your child has a serious reaction to a vaccine, there is a federal program that can help pay for the care of those who have been harmed.

For details about the National Vaccine Injury Compensation Program, call **1-800-338-2382** or visit the program's website at **http://www.hrsa.gov/osp/vicp**

8 | How can I learn more?

- Ask your doctor or nurse. They can give you the vaccine package insert or suggest other sources of information.

- Call your local or state health department's immunization program.

- Contact the Centers for Disease Control and Prevention (CDC):
  -Call **1-800-232-4636 (1-800-CDC-INFO)**
  -Visit the National Immunization Program's website at **http://www.cdc.gov/nip**

American Academy of Pediatrics
DEDICATED TO THE HEALTH OF ALL CHILDREN™

Reprinted by the American Academy of Pediatrics. Additional copies are available for purchase in pads of 100

To order, contact:
American Academy of Pediatrics
141 Northwest Point Blvd
Elk Grove Village, IL 60007-1098
Web site—http://www.aap.org
Minimum order 100

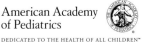 **U.S. DEPARTMENT OF HEALTH & HUMAN SERVICES**
Centers for Disease Control and Prevention
National Immunization Program

Vaccine Information Statement
Polio (1/1/2000)　　42 U.S.C. § 300aa-26

TETANUS AND DIPHTHERIA VACCINE (Td)

What you need to know before you or your child gets the vaccine

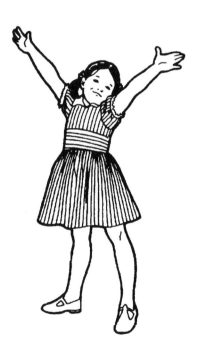

ABOUT THE DISEASES

Tetanus (lockjaw) and **diphtheria** are serious diseases. Tetanus is caused by a germ that enters the body through a cut or wound. Diphtheria spreads when germs pass from an infected person to the nose or throat of others.

Tetanus causes serious, painful spasms of all muscles	**Diphtheria causes** a thick coating in the nose, throat, or airway
It can lead to: - "locking" of the jaw so the patient cannot open his or her mouth or swallow	**It can lead to:** - breathing problems - heart failure - paralysis - death

ABOUT THE VACCINES

Benefits of the vaccines

Vaccination is the best way to protect against tetanus and diphtheria, Because of vaccination, there are many fewer cases of these **diseases**. Cases are rare in children because most get DTP (Diphtheria, Tetanus, and **Pertussis**), DTaP (Diphtheria, Tetanus, and acellular **Pertussis**), or DT (Diphtheria and Tetanus) vaccines. There would be many more cases if we stopped vaccinating people.

When should you get Td vaccine?

Td is made for people 7 years of age and older.

People who have not gotten at least 3 doses of any tetanus and diphtheria vaccine (**DTP**, DTaP or **DT**) during their lifetime should do so using Td. After a person gets the third dose, a Td dose is needed every 10 years ail through life.

Other vaccines may be given at the same time as Td.

Tell your doctor or nurse if the person getting the vaccine:

· ever had a serious allergic reaction or other problem with Td, or any other tetanus and diphtheria vaccine (**DTP**, DTaP or DT)

· now has a moderate or severe illness

· is pregnant

If you are not sure, ask your doctor or nurse.

What are the risks from Td vaccine?

As with any medicine, there are very small risks that serious problems, even death, could occur after getting a vaccine.

The risks from the vaccine are <u>much smaller</u> than the risks from the diseases if people stopped using vaccine.

Almost all people who get Td have no problems from it.

Mild problems

If these problems occur, they usually start within hours to a day or two after vaccination. They may last 1-2 days:

- soreness, redness, or swelling where the shot was given

These problems can be worse in adults who get Td vaccine very often.

Acetaminophen or ibuprofen (non-aspirin) may be used to reduce soreness.

Severe problems

These problems happen very rarely:

- serious allergic reaction

- deep, aching pain and muscle wasting in upper arm(s), This starts 2 days to 4 weeks after the shot, and may last many months.

What to do if there is a serious reaction:

☞ Call a doctor or get the person to a doctor right away,

☞ Write down what happened and the date and time it happened.

☞ Ask your doctor, nurse, or health department to file a Vaccine Adverse Event Report form or call:
    (800) 822-7967 (toll-free)

The **National Vaccine Injury Compensation Program** gives compensation (payment) for persons thought to be injured by vaccines. For details call:
    (800) 338-2382 (toll-free)

If you want to learn more, ask your doctor or nurse. She/he can give you the vaccine package insert or suggest other sources of information.

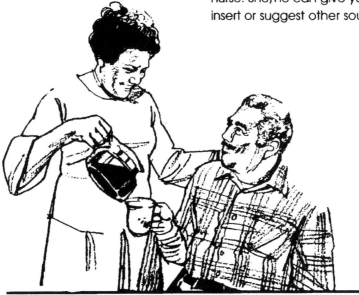

American Academy of Pediatrics

DEDICATED TO THE HEALTH OF ALL CHILDREN™

Reprinted by the American Academy of Pediatrics.
Additional copies are available for purchase in pads of 100.

To order, contact:
American Academy of Pediatrics
141 Northwest Point Blvd
Elk Grove Village, IL 60007-1098
Web site—http://www.aap.org
Minimum order 100

U.S. DEPARTMENT OF HEALTH & HUMAN SERVICES
Centers for Disease Control and Prevention
National Immunization Program

Td 6/10/94   42 U.S.C. § 300aa-26

Promoting Pediatric Care

How Special Is Your Child?

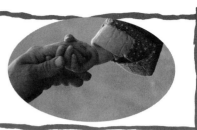

Special enough to be cared for by a doctor who only sees children and youth? Special enough to be cared for by a physician trained and experienced in the physical, mental, emotional, and social development of children and youth?

Special enough to be cared for as a child, not as a small adult?

Special enough to be cared for by a doctor who has had 3 to 6 years of pediatric training after medical school and has passed rigorous tests to be certified as a pediatrician?

Special enough to be treated with respect as an individual and as a person entitled to special care?

If you answered yes to all the above, WELCOME, You've come to the right place.

Your Child Deserves the Best in Pediatric Primary Care and Pediatric Subspecialty Care

Pediatricians spend as much as 3 to 6 years in pediatric training after medical school. That equals up to 24 times more training in the care of children than other physicians who receive an average of 3 additional months of pediatric training after medical school.

More Training in Caring for Children

36-72 Months Training—
Pediatricians/Pediatric
Subspecialists

3 Months Training—
Other Physicians

Cutting Edge Knowledge

Pediatricians see only children and youth. Constant changes in medicine can make it difficult to stay up to date. Pediatricians stay current by concentrating their efforts on changes in medicine affecting children.

Quality Primary Care

Pediatricians are trained to provide comprehensive care for children, includ-ing preventive care. Pediatricians often work in teams with other professionals, including nurse practitioners, to provide high-quality, cost-effective primary care. High-quality care leads to better outcomes for children and reduced costs for families and society.

Quality Pediatric Subspecialty Care

Pediatric subspecialists have an additional 24 to 36 months of in-depth fellowship training in addition to their 36 to 48 months of pediatric residency, concentrating on clinical and research aspects of specific areas of diseases of children and youth. A child's heart, lungs, kidneys, gastrointestinal system, and nervous system can have different problems than those organs of adults. Children with such problems may require referral by their pediatrician to pediatric medical and surgical subspecialists who have the training and knowledge to take care of these SPECIAL problems in the best manner possible.

Pediatricians Specialize in the Care of Children and Youth

Pediatricians are trained to:

- *Help* you determine healthy lifestyles for your child and useful ways to role model your choices.
- *Offer* advice to prevent illness and injuries.
- *Provide* early and appropriate care of acute illness to prevent its progression.
- *Treat* life-threatening childhood conditions requiring intensive care.
- *Guide* you in anticipating your child's needs from newborn to 21.

Experience

As part of their extensive training, pediatricians are experienced in the physical, emotional, and social development of children. Children may be too young or shy to talk so pediatricians understand the importance of listening carefully to your child, and to you. Pediatricians answer your questions, helping you to understand and promote your child's healthy development. Pediatricians also address issues affecting a child's family and home environment.

Pediatricians understand that children are not simply small adults.

They often present different symptoms from adults. They may need different prescriptions or treatments than adults. Pediatricians are specially trained to recognize the importance of these differences, especially with young children and newborns.

Pediatricians Are Great Advocates!

The American Academy of Pediatrics is highly respected for its child advocacy work. The Academy works to:

- Assure universal health care for all children from birth to 21 years and for all pregnant women.
- See that all immunizations are fully paid for by state and private insurance.
- Reduce the number of intentional and unintentional injuries, including those associated with alcohol and substance abuse.
- Promote healthy lifestyles for children and adolescents.
- Promote health education in schools.
- Increase access to health care for all children, including those with special needs and the homeless.
- Assure health and safety standards in child care settings.

By selecting a Board-Certified Pediatrician, you will have chosen the highest level of medical care for your child.

The information contained in this publication should not be used as a substitute for the medical care and advice of your pediatrician. There may be variations in treatment that your pediatrician may recommend based on individual facts and circumstances.

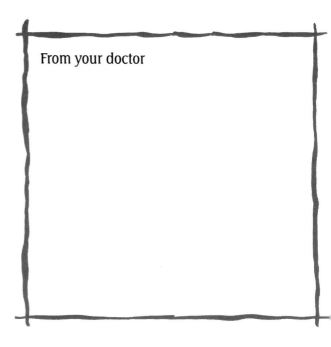

From your doctor

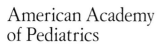

American Academy of Pediatrics

DEDICATED TO THE HEALTH OF ALL CHILDREN™

The American Academy of Pediatrics is an organization of 60,000 primary care pediatricians, pediatric medical subspecialists, and pediatric surgical specialists dedicated to the health, safety, and well-being of infants, children, adolescents, and young adults.

American Academy of Pediatrics
Web site — www.aap.org

Copyright © 1998
American Academy of Pediatrics

You and Your Pediatrician

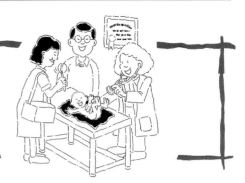

The American Academy of Pediatrics (AAP) has developed this information to help you

- Choose a pediatrician.
- Prepare for office visits with your pediatrician.
- Know what to do if you have a question or an emergency health problem.

In choosing a pediatrician, you can know that an expert in children's health is treating your child.

Why your child needs a pediatrician

Children have different health care needs than adults—both medical and emotional. Pediatricians are trained to prevent and manage health problems in infants, children, teens, and young adults. Older patients trust their pediatricians, because they have known one another for many years.

Training

To become trained in pediatrics, a doctor must take special courses for 3 or more years after medical school. This is called *residency*. After residency, a doctor usually takes a long, detailed test given by the American Board of Pediatrics. After passing the test, the doctor is a board-certified pediatrician. He or she gets a certificate that you may see displayed at the office. The doctor can then become a Fellow (or member) of the American Academy of Pediatrics (FAAP). All of this background prepares your pediatrician to manage your child's total health care needs, including the following:

- Growth and development
- Illnesses
- Nutrition
- Immunizations
- Injuries
- Physical fitness

Your pediatrician will also work with you on other issues, such as the following:

- Behavior
- Emotional or family problems
- Learning and other school problems
- Preventing and dealing with drug abuse
- Puberty and other teen concerns
- Television, the Internet, and other media

Pediatricians also work with teachers and other adults in child care centers, schools, and after-school programs. If your child has a very special or complex problem, your pediatrician can refer her to another specialist for further help, if needed.

In addition, your pediatrician can advise you about complementary and alternative medicine treatments and which treatments are safe for children. It is important that your pediatrician be aware of all uses of complementary and alternative medicines. Some can result in serious side effects when used along with conventional medicine.

Finding the right pediatrician for your child

Do not wait until your child is sick or needs a checkup to choose a pediatrician. Even if you recently moved, are changing insurance, or are having a baby, it is best to find a pediatrician as soon as you can. For recommendations about a pediatrician, ask other doctors you know, as well as family, friends, relatives, and coworkers. You may want to contact a nearby hospital, medical school, or your county medical society for a list of local pediatricians. Some health insurance plans may require you to choose a pediatrician from their approved network of doctors.

After you have a list of names, you may visit the pediatricians' offices to help you choose your child's doctor. While you are in the reception area, look around to see if it is clean. (But realize that children have been in it all day long.) Consider whether the office staff seems friendly and helpful.

Ask the office staff some questions, including the following:

- What are the office hours?
- Is emergency coverage available 24 hours a day, 7 days a week?
- Do nurses screen phone calls?
- If I cannot speak with the doctor, who will handle my questions?
- When is the best time to call with routine questions?
- Does the practice have an after-hours answering service?
- Is the after-hours phone service tied in with a university or children's hospital?
- Where are patients referred after hours?
- Is there access to specialists and intensive care if needed?
- Is payment due at the time of visit?
- How does the office handle billing?
- How are insurance claims handled?
- Is this pediatrician accepting new patients with my insurance or managed care plan?

Also prepare a list of questions to ask about the pediatrician including the following:

- What is his or her pediatric background?
- Does he or she have a subspecialty or area of pediatric interest? If so, what is it?
- To what hospital does he or she admit patients?
- Is he or she board certified through the American Board of Pediatrics?
- Is he or she a member of the American Academy of Pediatrics?
- Who are the physicians who will care for my child if my pediatrician is not available?
- Are they on staff at the same hospital? Are these physicians board certified?

These are just sample questions. Ask other questions about things that are important to you.

After your first visit with the pediatrician, ask yourself: Does this pediatrician listen, answer questions, and seem interested? Above all, ask yourself if you like and trust this person. If your instincts say "no," talk with the next pediatrician on your list.

When someone you know suggests a pediatrician, it is also helpful to ask that person some questions about the doctor, such as the following:

- Are all your questions answered by the pediatrician and the office staff?
- Do you think your children like the doctor?
- Does the pediatrician talk with and care about the children, and not just the parents?
- Does the pediatrician seem to know about current issues and advances in pediatric medicine?
- How helpful and friendly is the office staff?
- How well does the office staff manage your telephone calls?
- How does the office handle emergencies?
- Do you have to wait long before seeing the pediatrician?
- Is there anything about the pediatrician or the office that bothers you?

The American Academy of Pediatrics has an online pediatrician referral service for parents. For more information, please go to www.aap.org, click on "You and Your Family," and look for the "Pediatrician Referral Service" link.

Preparing for office visits

Regular visits to the pediatrician are a key part of preventive health care. At each visit, the pediatrician, pediatric nurse practitioner, or pediatric resident will fully examine your child. This checkup will give your child's pediatrician a chance to

- Make sure your child is eating well, growing well, and is healthy.
- Update immunizations.
- Track your child's growth and development.
- Find physical problems before they become serious.
- Help inform you on how to keep your child healthy and safe.
- Answer all of your questions.

Infants and children need frequent checkups during the first 24 months of life. After 2 years of age most children do not need regular visits as often. Your pediatrician will schedule visits based on your child's own needs. Ask your pediatrician how often your child needs a checkup.

Make sure you write down any questions you have before each office visit, so that you do not forget to ask them. Keep up-to-date records on your child's growth and immunizations. Bring this information with you to each visit.

Illnesses and injuries

All children get sick at one time or another. Minor illnesses like colds and coughs are common. This is especially true for children who are in child care or school, where they may be exposed to more infections from other children. It is also common for children to have many minor injuries, as well as other medical problems that will need your pediatrician's attention.

If you are not sure your child needs to see the pediatrician, always call his or her office. The office staff can often tell you over the phone if your child needs to be seen and, if so, can set up an appointment. The pediatrician or nursing staff may give medical advice over the phone if an office visit isnot needed.

Calling your child's pediatrician

You should *always* feel free to call your pediatrician's office, either during office hours for routine questions or at any time for an emergency. Call right away if you are worried about your child. Sometimes a parent feels

Recommended health care visits*

The American Academy of Pediatrics recommends regular health care visits at the following times:

- Before your baby is born (for first-time parents)
- Before your newborn is discharged from the hospital, and again within 48 to 72 hours for babies discharged before 2 full days of life
- During the first year of life—visits at about 2 to 4 weeks of age, and also at 2, 4, 6, 9, and 12 months of age
- During the second year of life—visits at 15, 18, and 24 months of age
- In early childhood—yearly visits from 2 through 5 years of age
- During the early school years—visits at 6, 8, and 10 years of age
- In adolescence and early adulthood—yearly visits from 11 through 21 years of age

*Your own pediatrician may recommend additional visits.

---

there is a problem before symptoms actually show up. Always call and get proper medical advice. Realize, though, that sometimes your pediatrician may not be able to answer your questions without seeing your child first. When you are not sure whether to call, trust your instincts.

Make the most of the phone. Your pediatrician may prefer that you call with general questions during office hours. Some offices even have special "phone-in" times. Before you call, have a pen and paper ready to write down any instructions and questions. You could easily forget some details, especially when you are worried about your child. Be prepared to provide information about your child's health.

- **Have your child near the phone,** if possible, to help you answer questions when you call your pediatrician. An older child may be able to tell you exactly where it hurts.
- **Take your child's temperature** before you call. If your child has a fever, write down the temperature and time you took it.
- **Remind the doctor about past medical problems.** Do not expect your pediatrician to always remember your child's medical condition. He or she cares for many children each day and may not remember that your child has asthma, seizures, or some other condition.
- **Be sure to mention medications.** If your child is taking any medication, including prescription or nonprescription drugs, inhalers, supplements, vitamins, herbal products, or home remedies, tell your pediatrician.
- **Keep immunization records at hand.** These are especially helpful if your child has an injury that may require a tetanus shot or if pertussis (whooping cough) is in your community.
- **Have your pharmacy phone number ready.**
  Unblock your telephone "call block," and keep phone lines open so that your pediatrician can return your call in a timely manner. Do not leave pager numbers. If you leave your cell phone number, be sure that you have your cell phone on and will be in an area where you can receive calls.

Routine and emergency calls

Routine calls include questions about medicines, minor illnesses, injuries, behavior, or parenting advice. You will usually not need urgent care for a simple cold or cough, mild diarrhea, constipation, temper tantrums, or sleep problems. For these cases you may just need proper medical advice

However, if your child has any of the following, call to find out if he needs to be seen:

- Vomiting and diarrhea that last for more than a few hours in a child of any age
- Rash, especially if there is also a fever
- Any cough or cold that does not get better in several days, or a cold that gets worse and is accompanied by a fever
- Cuts that might need stitches
- Limping or is not able to move an arm or leg
- Ear pain with fever, is unable to sleep or eat, is vomiting, has diarrhea, or is acting ill
- Drainage from an ear
- Sore throat or problems swallowing
- Sharp or persistent pains in the abdomen or stomach
- A rectal temperature of 100.4°F (38°C) or higher in a baby younger than 2 months of age
- Fever and vomiting at the same time
- Not eating for more than a day

Emergency calls require your pediatrician's prompt attention. But it is best to know what to do before a problem occurs. During a scheduled checkup, ask your pediatrician what to do and where to go should your child ever need emergency medical care. Learn basic first aid, including CPR (cardiopulmonary resuscitation). Keep emergency and poison center phone numbers posted by your telephone.

An infant or child needs emergency medical treatment **immediately** if he has any of the following:

- Bleeding that does not stop after applying pressure for 5 minutes
- Suspected poisoning
- Seizures (Rhythmic jerking and loss of consciousness)
- Increasing trouble with breathing
- Skin or lips that look blue, purple, or gray
- Neck stiffness or rash with fever
- Head injury with loss of consciousness, confusion, vomiting, or poor skin color
- Blood in the urine
- Bloody diarrhea or diarrhea that will not go away
- Sudden lack of energy or is not able to move
- Unconsciousness or lack of response
- Acting strangely or becoming more withdrawn and less alert
- Increasing or severe persistent pain
- A cut or burn that is large, deep, or involves the head, chest, or abdomen
- A burn that is large or involves the hands, groin, or face

Call 911 (or your emergency number) for any severely ill or injured child.

As your child grows

Your pediatrician can continue to be an important resource not only for illness or injury care, but for all sorts of health advice, including the following:

- Exercise
- Nutrition
- Being too thin or too heavy

- Emotional and behavioral problems
- Helping children cope with issues like divorce and death
- School or learning problems
- Family problems
- Media and Internet literacy
- Gun injury prevention

Your pediatrician can respond to your teen's special needs and can offer advice and counseling on

- Body changes during puberty
- Menstruation
- Growth and hygiene
- Coping and being happy with oneself and with others
- Substance abuse
- Dating and sexual issues
- Eating disorders
- Acne
- Birth control
- Violence and related problems
- Gang problems

Immunizations and your child's health

Many childhood diseases can be prevented with regular health care visits and up-to-date immunizations. Children need shots to protect them from diphtheria, tetanus, pertussis (whooping cough), measles, mumps, rubella (German measles), polio, hepatitis A, hepatitis B, *Haemophilus influenzae* type b, chickenpox, influenza, and pneumococcal infections.

Be sure your child is up-to-date with all needed vaccinations. It is the only way to protect your child against many serious diseases.

Your pediatrician can give you the latest information about new vaccines as they become available. At each checkup, ask your pediatrician if your child is fully immunized.

The information contained in this publication should not be used as a substitute for the medical care and advice of your pediatrician. There may be variations in treatment that your pediatrician may recommend based on individual facts and circumstances.

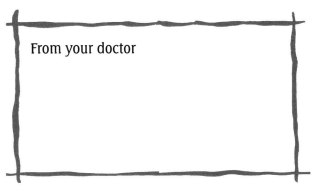

From your doctor

American Academy of Pediatrics

DEDICATED TO THE HEALTH OF ALL CHILDREN™

The American Academy of Pediatrics is an organization of 60,000 primary care pediatricians, pediatric medical subspecialists, and pediatric surgical specialists dedicated to the health, safety, and well-being of infants, children, adolescents, and young adults.

American Academy of Pediatrics
Web site — www.aap.org

Copyright © 2002
American Academy of Pediatrics

Pediatric Subspecialists

Part I: Surgical Subspecialists

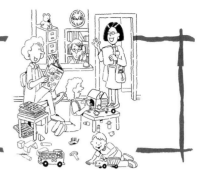

The American Academy of Pediatrics (AAP) has created a series of fact sheets about different surgical and medical pediatric subspecialists whom your children may be referred to. The fact sheets are available on the AAP Web site at http://www.aap.org/family/pedspecfactsheets.htm.

Following are excerpts from the surgical subspecialty series. If you have additional questions, please talk with your pediatrician.

If your child needs an operation, your pediatrician will refer your child to a pediatric surgical subspecialist. This type of doctor has had special training and is experienced in children's surgical needs from birth to young adulthood.

There are a variety of pediatric surgical subspecialists, including the following:

- Anesthesiologists
- General Surgeons (includes neonatal, prenatal, trauma, and cancer surgeons)
- Neurosurgeons (brain and spinal cord surgeons)
- Ophthalmologists (eye surgeons)
- Orthopedic Surgeons (bone surgeons)
- Otolaryngologists (ear, nose, and throat surgeons)
- Plastic Surgeons
- Urologists (kidney, bladder, and genital surgeons)

Pediatric surgical subspecialists are the best choice if your child needs any type of surgery because they have the most experience in treating children. This comes from their years of specialized training, which includes

- At least 4 years of medical school
- One year of a surgical or medical internship
- Three to 5 years of residency training in their specialized area of surgery
- One to 2 additional years of fellowship training in their *pediatric* surgical specialty

Pediatric Anesthesiologist

If your child has an illness, injury, or disease that requires surgery, a *Pediatric Anesthesiologist* has the experience and qualifications to assist in the treatment and to help ensure a successful surgery for your child.

A pediatric anesthesiologist is a fully trained anesthesiologist who has completed at least 1 year of specialized training in anesthesia care of infants and children. Most pediatric surgeons deliver care to children in the operating room along with a pediatric anesthesiologist. Many children who need surgery have complex medical problems that affect many parts of the body. The pediatric anesthesiologist is best qualified to evaluate these complex problems and plan a safe anesthetic for each child. Through special training and experience, pediatric anesthesiologists provide the safest care for infants and children undergoing anesthesia.

What types of treatments do pediatric anesthesiologists provide?

Pediatric anesthesiologists are primarily concerned with the anesthesia, sedation, and pain management needs of infants and children. Pediatric anesthesiologists generally provide the following services:

- Evaluation of complex medical problems in infants and children when surgery is necessary
- Planning and care for children before and after surgery
- A nonthreatening environment for children in the operating room
- Pain control, if needed, after surgery, either with intravenous (IV) medications or other anesthetic techniques
- Anesthesia and sedation for many procedures out of the operating room, such as magnetic resonance imaging (MRI), computed tomographic (CT) scan, and radiation therapy

Pediatric Surgeon

If your child has an illness, injury, or disease that requires surgery, a *Pediatric Surgeon* has the experience and qualifications to treat your child.

Surgical problems seen by pediatric surgeons are often quite different from those commonly seen by adult or general surgeons. Special training in pediatric surgery is important.

What types of treatments do pediatric surgeons provide?

Pediatric surgeons diagnose, treat, and manage all children's surgical needs, including the following:

- Surgical repair of birth defects
- Serious injuries that require surgery (liver lacerations, knife wounds, or gun shot wounds)
- Diagnosis and surgical care of tumors
- Transplantation operations
- Endoscopic procedures (bronchoscopy, esophagogastroduodenoscopy, colonoscopy)
- All other surgical procedures for children

Pediatric Neurosurgeon

If your child has problems involving the head, spine, or nervous system, a *Pediatric Neurosurgeon* has the experience and qualifications to treat your child.

Neurosurgical problems seen by pediatric neurosurgeons are often quite different from those commonly seen by adult or general neurosurgeons. Special training in pediatric diseases as they relate to pediatric neurosurgical diseases is important. Pediatric neurosurgical problems often are present for life. Pediatric neurosurgeons have a special and long-standing relationship with their patients. Children with nervous system problems frequently require ongoing and close follow-up throughout childhood and adolescence.

What types of treatments do pediatric neurosurgeons provide?

Pediatric neurosurgeons diagnose, treat, and manage all children's nervous system problems and head and spinal deformities, including the following:

- Problems and injuries of the brain, spine, or nerves
- Gait abnormalities (spasticity)
- Birth injuries (weakness of arms and legs)

Pediatric Ophthalmologist

If your child has an eye problem, is having difficulty with a vision screening exam, or needs surgery for an illness affecting the eyes, a *Pediatric Ophthalmologist* has the experience and qualifications to treat your child.

What types of treatments do pediatric ophthalmologists provide?

Pediatric ophthalmologists can diagnose, treat, and manage all children's eye problems. Pediatric ophthalmologists generally provide the following services:

- Perform eye exams.
- Prescribe eyeglasses and contact lenses.
- Perform surgery, microsurgery, and laser surgery of the eyes (for problems like weak eye muscles, crossed eyes, roving eyes, blocked tear ducts, and infections).
- Diagnose problems of the eye associated with diseases of the body, such as diabetes or juvenile rheumatoid arthritis (JRA).
- Diagnose visual processing disorders.
- Care for eye injuries.

Pediatric Orthopedic Surgeon

If your child has musculoskeletal (bone) problems, a *Pediatric Orthopedic Surgeon* has the experience and qualifications to treat your child.

What types of treatments do pediatric orthopedic surgeons provide?

Pediatric orthopedic surgeons diagnose, treat, and manage children's musculoskeletal problems, including the following:

- Limb and spine deformities (club foot, scoliosis)
- Gait abnormalities (limping)
- Bone and joint infections
- Broken bones

Pediatric Otolaryngologist

If your child needs surgical or complex medical treatment for illnesses or problems affecting the ear, nose, or throat, a *Pediatric Otolaryngologist* has the experience and qualifications to treat your child. Many general otolaryngologists provide surgical care for children. However, in many areas of the country, more specialized otolaryngology care is available for children.

What types of treatments do pediatric otolaryngologists provide?

Pediatric otolaryngologists are primarily concerned with medical and surgical treatment of ear, nose, and throat diseases in children. Pediatric otolaryngologists generally provide the following services:

- Diagnosis and treatment of ear, nose, and throat disorders, and head and neck diseases
- Surgery of the head and neck, including before- and after-surgery care
- Consultation with other doctors when ear, nose, or throat diseases are detected
- Assistance in the identification of communication disorders in children

Pediatric Plastic Surgeon

If your child needs surgery to fix a deformity caused by a birth defect, injury, illness, or tumor, a *Pediatric Plastic Surgeon* has the experience and qualifications to treat your child.

What types of treatments do pediatric plastic surgeons provide

Pediatric plastic surgeons generally provide treatment for the following:

- Birth defects of the face and skull (cleft lip and palate, misshapen skull)
- Birth defects of the ear (protruding or absent ear)
- Birth defects of the chest and limbs (misshapen breasts, webbed fingers)
- Injuries to the head, face, hands, arms, and legs
- Birthmarks and scars
- Burns
- Cosmetic surgery to improve a child's self-image

Pediatric Urologist

If your child has an illness or disease of the genitals or the urinary tract (kidneys, ureters, and bladder), a *Pediatric Urologist* has the experience and qualifications to treat your child.

A pediatric urologist usually devotes a minimum of 50% of his or her practice to the urologic problems of infants, children, and adolescents.

What types of treatments do pediatric urologists provide?

Pediatric urologists are surgeons who can diagnose, treat, and manage children's urinary and genital problems. Pediatric urologists generally provide the following services:

- Evaluation and management of voiding disorders, vesicoureteral reflux, and urinary tract infections that require surgery
- Surgical reconstruction of the urinary tract (kidneys, ureters, and bladder) including genital abnormalities, hypospadias, and intersex conditions
- Surgery for groin conditions in childhood and adolescence (undescended testes, hydrocele/hernia, varicocele)

Remember

To learn more about pediatric subspecialists, visit the AAP Web site at http://www.aap.org/family/pedspecfactsheets.htm.

From your doctor

American Academy of Pediatrics

DEDICATED TO THE HEALTH OF ALL CHILDREN™

The American Academy of Pediatrics is an organization of 60,000 primary care pediatricians, pediatric medical subspecialists, and pediatric surgical specialists dedicated to the health, safety, and well-being of infants, children, adolescents, and young adults.

American Academy of Pediatrics
Web site—www.aap.org

Copyright © 2003
American Academy of Pediatrics

Pediatric Subspecialists

Part II: Medical Subspecialists

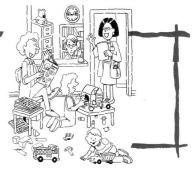

The American Academy of Pediatrics has created a series of fact sheets about different pediatric surgical and medical subspecialists whom your children may be referred to. The fact sheets are available on the AAP Web site at http://www.aap.org/family/pedspecfactsheets.htm.

Following are excerpts from the medical subspecialty series. If you have additional questions, please talk with your pediatrician.

There are a variety of pediatric medical subspecialists, including the following:

- Allergist/Immunologist
- Critical Care Specialist
- Dermatologist
- Endocrinologist
- Gastroenterologist
- Geneticist
- Hematologist/Oncologist
- Infectious Diseases Specialist
- Neonatologist
- Nephrologist
- Pulmonologist
- Radiologist
- Rheumatologist
- Sports Medicine Specialist

Pediatric Allergist/Immunologist

If your child suffers from allergies or other problems with his immune system, a *Pediatric Allergist/Immunologist* has special skills to treat your child.

What types of treatments do pediatric allergists/immunologists provide?

Pediatric allergists/immunologists generally provide treatment for the following:

- Asthma
- Hay fever (allergic rhinitis)
- Sinusitis
- Eczema (atopic dermatitis)
- Hives (urticaria, welts)
- Severe reactions to foods, insect stings, and medications (anaphylaxis)
- Immune disorders that lead to the following:
  — Frequent sinusitis, pneumonia, or diarrhea
  — Thrush and abscesses that keep coming back
  — Severe, unusual infections

Pediatric Critical Care Specialist

If your child has an illness or injury that results in your child being in an unstable critical condition, a hospital-based *Pediatric Critical Care*

Specialist (pediatric intensivist) can be called on to provide the special care that your child needs.

What types of treatments do pediatric critical care specialists provide?

Pediatric critical care specialists generally provide the following care to children who are critically ill:

- Diagnosis of children who have an unstable, life-threatening condition
- Thorough monitoring, medication, and treatment of children in a pediatric intensive care unit (PICU)
- Supervision of children on respirators
- Medical treatment for children with severe heart and lung disease
- Placement of special catheters in the blood vessels and heart
- Management of medications and treatments for children with brain trauma

Pediatric Dermatologist

If your child has skin conditions such as birthmarks, eczema, warts, or psoriasis, a *Pediatric Dermatologist* has the experience and qualifications to treat your child.

What types of treatments do pediatric dermatologists provide?

Pediatric dermatologists provide medical care for a variety of skin conditions. They generally provide the following services:

- Diagnosis and treatment of various skin conditions, including contact dermatitis, eczema, psoriasis, vitiligo, hives, warts, hemangiomas, birthmarks, and congenital skin disorders
- Prescription treatment of skin conditions
- Medical and/or surgical treatment of skin conditions such as warts and molluscum (pea-sized yellow or pink lumps)
- Surgical removal of molluscum, warts, and other small lumps in the skin (cysts)
- Skin biopsies

Pediatric Endocrinologist

If your child has problems with growth, puberty, diabetes, or other disorders related to the hormones and the glands that produce them, a *Pediatric Endocrinologist* may treat your child.

What types of treatments do pediatric endocrinologists provide?

Pediatric endocrinologists diagnose, treat, and manage hormonal disorders, including the following:

- Growth problems, such as short stature
- Early or delayed puberty
- Enlarged thyroid gland (goiter)
- Underactive or overactive thyroid gland
- Pituitary gland hypo/hyper function
- Adrenal gland hypo/hyper function

- Ambiguous genitals/intersex
- Ovarian and testicular dysfunction
- Diabetes
- Low blood sugar (hypoglycemia)
- Obesity
- Problems with vitamin D (rickets, hypocalcemia)

Pediatric Gastroenterologist

If your child has a digestive system, liver, or nutritional problem, a *Pediatric Gastroenterologist* has the expertise to treat your child.

What types of treatments do pediatric gastroenterologists provide?

Pediatric gastroenterologists generally provide treatment for the following:
- Bleeding from the gastrointestinal tract
- Lactose intolerance
- Food allergies or intolerances
- Severe or complicated gastroesophageal reflux disease (reflux or GERD)
- Inflammatory bowel disease
- Short bowel syndrome
- Liver disease
- Acute or chronic abdominal pain
- Vomiting
- Chronic constipation
- Chronic or severe diarrhea
- Pancreatic insufficiency (including cystic fibrosis) and pancreatitis
- Nutritional problems (including malnutrition, failure to thrive, and obesity)
- Feeding disorders

Pediatric Geneticist

Fortunately, most children are born healthy with no medical problems or birth defects. However, some children are born with differences in body structure, brain development, or body chemistry that can lead to problems with health, development, school performance, and/or social interaction. *Pediatric Geneticists* are trained to identify the causes and natural history of these disorders.

What types of treatments do pediatric geneticists provide?

Pediatric geneticists diagnose, counsel, and treat families with many different kinds of problems, including the following:
- Birth defects (physical differences present at birth causing a health problem)
- Conditions with one or more birth defects (Down syndrome, Williams syndrome, or achondroplasia)
- Conditions that can cause disabilities (fetal alcohol syndrome or fragile X syndrome)
- Inborn errors of metabolism (cystic fibrosis, phenylketonuria, or sickle cell disease)
- Familial or hereditary problems (congenital heart disease or hypercholesterolemia)
- Short or tall stature (height that is significantly below or above normal range)

Pediatric Hematologist/Oncologist

If your child or teen has a blood disease or cancer, a *Pediatric Hematologist/ Oncologist* has the experience and qualifications to evaluate and treat your child or teen.

What types of treatments do pediatric hematologists/oncologists provide?

Pediatric hematologists/oncologists diagnose, treat, and manage children and teens with the following:
- Cancers, including leukemias, lymphomas, brain tumors, bone tumors and solid tumors
- Diseases of blood cells, including disorders of white cells, red cells, and platelets
- Bleeding disorders

Pediatric Infectious Diseases Specialist

If your child has a recurring or persistent disease caused by an infectious agent such as bacteria, a fungus, a parasite, or other rare infection, a *Pediatric Infectious Diseases Specialist* has the experience and qualifications to help your physician diagnose and treat your child.

What types of treatments do pediatric infectious diseases specialists provide?

Pediatric infectious diseases specialists treat a wide range of infectious and immunologic diseases such as those caused by bacteria, viruses, fungi, and parasites. Other pediatric infectious diseases specialists are consulted for diseases that are complicated or atypical, including
- Illnesses that are of unclear cause, have prolonged fever, or are recurrent
- Respiratory infections
- Bone and joint infections
- Tuberculosis (TB)
- Acquired immunodeficiency syndrome (AIDS)
- Hepatitis
- Meningitis

Neonatologist

Although your pediatrician can solve most health problems of newborns, a *Neonatologist* is trained specifically to handle the most complex and high-risk situations.

What types of treatments do neonatologists provide?

Neonatologists generally provide the following care:
- Diagnose and treat newborns with conditions such as breathing disorders, infections, and birth defects.
- Coordinate care and medically manage newborns born premature, critically ill, or in need of surgery.
- Ensure that critically ill newborns receive the proper nutrition for healing and growth.
- Provide care to the newborn at a cesarean or other delivery that involves medical problems in the mother or baby that may compromise the infant's health and require medical intervention in the delivery room.
- Stabilize and treat newborns with any life-threatening medical problems
- Consult with obstetricians, pediatricians, and family physicians about conditions affecting newborns.

Pediatric Nephrologist

If your child has kidney or urinary tract disease, bladder problems, or high blood pressure, a *Pediatric Nephrologist* has the special skills and experience to treat your child. Pediatric nephrologists treat children from infancy through late adolescence.

What types of treatments do pediatric nephrologists provide?

Pediatric nephrologists diagnose, treat, and manage many disorders affecting the kidney and urinary tract, including kidney failure, high blood pressure, inherited kidney diseases, kidney stones, urinary tract infections, and abnormalities in the urine such as blood and protein. They also know how to evaluate and treat problems with growth and development that are specifically related to chronic kidney disease.

Pediatric nephrologists generally provide the following services:

Dialysis

Kidney transplantation

Kidney biopsies

Interpretation of x-ray studies of the kidney

Interpretation of laboratory studies related to kidney disease

Ambulatory blood pressure monitoring

Pediatric Pulmonologist

If your child has breathing problems, or a problem with his or her lungs, a *Pediatric Pulmonologist* has the experience and qualifications to treat your child.

What types of treatments do pediatric pulmonologists provide?

Pediatric pulmonologists often treat children with the following conditions:

Chronic cough

Difficulty breathing

Recurring pneumonia (infection of the lungs)

Asthma (chronic inflammation of the airways)

Cystic fibrosis (a genetic disease with pulmonary and nutritional symptoms)

Apnea (when a child's breathing stops for a prolonged time)

Chronic lung disease in premature infants

Noisy breathing

Conditions that require special equipment to monitor and/or help with breathing at home

Pediatric Radiologist

A *Pediatric Radiologist* is an expert in the diagnosis of illnesses, injuries, and diseases of infants, children, and adolescents, using imaging techniques and equipment.

What do pediatric radiologists do?

Pediatric radiologists are experts in selecting the best imaging techniques to diagnose medical and surgical problems. Examples of imaging techniques include x-ray, ultrasound, computed tomography (CT), magnetic resonance imaging (MRI), and nuclear medicine. Pediatric radiologists make sure that testing is performed properly and safely. They also interpret the results of the test and make an appropriate diagnosis.

Pediatric Rheumatologist

If your child has complaints of pain in the musculoskeletal system (joints, muscles, bones, or tendons), other symptoms of arthritis, or an autoimmune disorder, your pediatrician may recommend a *Pediatric Rheumatologist*.

What types of treatments do pediatric rheumatologists provide?

Pediatric rheumatologists work with pediatricians or family physicians to evaluate and treat a variety of joint, muscle, and bone disorders, including the following:

- Arthritis
- Autoimmune disorders, such as lupus; juvenile rheumatoid arthritis; scleroderma; Kawasaki disease; postinfectious arthritis; chronic vasculitis; and inflammatory disorders of the muscle, eye, or other organs
- Evaluation of prolonged fever
- Unexplained complaints of chronic musculoskeletal pain, weakness, poor appetite, fatigue, and/or loss of function or skills
- Unexplained symptoms, such as a rash, anemia, weight loss, or joint swelling
- Possible inflammatory disease

Pediatric Sports Medicine Specialist

If your child or teen has an injury or illness that affects sports performance, exercise, or activity, a *Pediatric Sports Medicine Specialist* has the expertise, experience, and qualifications to treat his or her youth-specific problems.

What types of treatments do pediatric sports medicine specialists provide?

Pediatric sports medicine specialists diagnose, treat, and manage the musculoskeletal and medical problems of children and teens, including the following:

- Sprains and strains
- Dislocations
- Ligament injuries
- Minor fractures and avulsions
- Apophysitis
- Tendinitis
- Overuse injuries
- Cartilage injuries
- Exercise-induced asthma
- Concussions
- Nutrition and supplement issues
- Diabetes
- Eating disorders
- Stress fractures
- Heat illness
- Unique conditions of the athlete with special needs

Remember

To learn more about pediatric subspecialists, visit the AAP Web site at http://www.aap.org/family/pedspecfactsheets.htm.

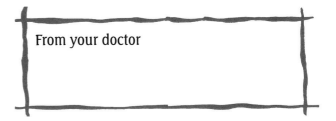

From your doctor

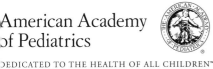

American Academy of Pediatrics

DEDICATED TO THE HEALTH OF ALL CHILDREN™

The American Academy of Pediatrics is an organization of 60,000 primary care pediatricians, pediatric medical subspecialists, and pediatric surgical specialists dedicated to the health, safety, and well-being of infants, children, adolescents, and young adults.

American Academy of Pediatrics
Web site—www.aap.org

Copyright © 2003
American Academy of Pediatrics

Index

Index

A

Abuse
alcohol, 358
child sexual, 343–344
inhalant, 363–364
substance, 334, 371–373
Acetaminophen, 20, 224
for fever, 41
Acne, 257
birth control pills and, 4
causes of, 3
hormones and, 3
management of, 3–4
Acquired immune deficiency syndrome (AIDS).
See also Human immunodeficiency
virus (HIV)
defined, 339
knowing facts about, 339–340
Active play, 173, 179
Acute epiglottitis, 30
Adapted vehicles for children with special needs, 112
Adenoid, 81
symptoms of enlarged, 81
Adolescent clinical psychologists, 309
Adolescent psychiatrists, 309
Adolescents
automobile driving by, 205–206
coping with depression and suicide, 279–280
gambling by, 295–297
gay, lesbian, and bisexual, 333–335
health services from pediatrician, 267–268
impact of media on, 305–307
need for pediatrician, 267
parents guide to parties of, 371–372
talking with, about sex, 349–350
testing for illicit drugs, 361–362
tips for parents of, 247–249
tobacco use by, 375
Adoption, 271–276
international, 275
of older child, 273–274
open, 275
single-parent, 317
Advertisers. *See also* Media
language of, 299–300
television, 321
Aerobic endurance, 183
Age, risk for ear infection and, 33
Age-appropriate toys, 237
AIDS. *See* Acquired immune deficiency syndrome
(AIDS); Human immunodeficiency
virus (HIV)
Air bags
safety of, 187
safety seats and, 100
Alcohol, 357–358. *See also* Substance abuse
adolescents and, 249
for college students, 253–254
media and, 358
preventing use and abuse of, 358
stages of use, 357
television and, 321
water safety and, 242
Allergens, 15
Allergic rhinitis, 11

Allergies, 11. *See also* Asthma; Hay fever
causes of, 11
common, 12
defined, 11
distinguishing between colds and, 11
food, 11, 12
milk, 12
need to see an allergist, 12
risk for ear infection and, 33
Allergist
need to see, 12
pediatric, 423
Amblyopia, 38
Anemia, 13–14
defined, 13
preventing, 14
signs and symptoms of, 13
treatment for, 13–14
types of, 13
Anesthesia, 189–191
after the procedure, 190–191
day of procedure, 190
illness of child prior to, 189
method of giving to child, 190
nausea and, 191
preparing for, 189
risks of, 189
vomiting and, 191
Anesthesiologist, pediatric, 189, 421
Anorexia
defined, 289
effect on body, 289
risk of developing, 289–290
Antibiotics, 193–194, 223. *See also* Medications
for acne, 3
for croup, 29
harmfulness of, 193
for meningococcal disease, 67
safe use of, 193
side effects of, 193
Anti-diarrhea medicines, 32
Antihistamines, 224
Apnea, 130
Appetite, 170
Asbestos, 207
Asperger syndrome, 148
Aspirin, 224
Asthma, 11, 12, 15–18. *See also* Allergies; Hay fever
defined, 15
devices to help deliver medications, 17
diagnosis of, 15
exercise and, 16
individuals with, 15
schools and, 17–18
symptoms of, 15
treatment of, 16–17
triggers of, 15–16
Atopic dermatitis, 12
Attention-deficit/hyperactivity disorder (ADHD), 5
behavior symptoms of, 5
causes of, 9
gender and, 9
homework and, 9
identifying, 9
medications for, 7–8
treatment for, 5
Auditory brainstem response (ABR), 127

Autism spectrum disorders (ASDs), 147–150
causes of, 148
diagnosis of, 149
differences in children with, 148–149
early signs of, 148
living with, 149–150
medical tests for, 149
symptoms of, 147
types of, 147–148
Autologous transfusion, 197
Automobiles, teen drivers and, 205–206

B

Babies
choking of, 200
crying by, 133–134
preparing children for new, 315–316
prevention of bronchiolitis in, 20
signs of infection in, 60
sleep problems in, 77
sun exposure and, 137–138
sunscreen for, 137–138
transportation of
in hip spica casts, 110
with tracheostomies, 110
Baby bottle tooth decay, 87
prevention of, 87
Babysitters, fire safety and, 212–213
Baby teeth, importance of, 87
Baby walkers, safety of, 89
Bacteremia, symptoms of, 69
Bacteria, resistant, 193
Bacterial infections, 194
Bacterial sinusitis
diagnosing, 73
distinguishing between cold and, 73
treating, 73–74
Basement
fire safety in, 212
poison-proofing, 229
Bathroom
poison-proofing, 229
safety checklist for, 217
Bedrooms
fire safety in, 211
safety checklist for, 217
Bedwetting, 80, 91–92
alarms for, 92
causes of, 91
managing, 91–92
Behavior, encouraging good, 281
Behavior therapy for attention-deficit/hyperactivity
disorder, 5
Benzoyl peroxide, for acne, 3
Bingeing, 290
Birth control, 350
condoms as, 347
emergency, 331–332
intrauterine device in, 348
need for reliable form of, 347–348
Birth control pills, acne and, 4
Birth order, siblings and, 313
Bisexuality, 333, 337
Bladder ultrasound, in following up on urinary tract
infections, 84
Blepharitis (swollen eyelids), 38
Blocked tear ducts, 38

Schools
asthma and, 17–18
learning to read in, 160
signs of good health program in, 261
Scratched cornea, 38
Seat belt adjusters, 99
Seat belts, 99
Secondhand smoke, 208, 233–234
long-term effects of, 233
Sedation, for imaging tests, 56
Seizures
epileptic, 39
febrile, 39, 41
headaches and, 47
Self-exam
breast, 329
testicular, 353
Separation, 317
Servings, child-size, 173
Sex
making healthy decisions about, 347–348
media and, 349
talking with teenager about, 349–350
talking with young children about, 351–352
television and, 321
Sex education, adolescents and, 248
Sexual abuse, child, 343–344
Sexual activity, deciding to wait, 345–346
Sexual health, for college students, 252
Sexually transmitted diseases (STDs), 347
sex and, 349
Sexual orientation, 333, 337
Shaken baby syndrome, 133–134
defined, 133
medical care for, 133
signs and symptoms, 133
Shingles, 24
Shock, treating for, 214
Shopping carts, car safety seats and, 100
Short-acting medications, and attention-deficit/
hyperactivity disorder, 7
Sibling relationships, 313–316
Sibling rivalry
role of parents in handling, 316
understanding, 313–314
Sickle-cell anemia, 13
Side air bags, safety seats and, 100
SIDS. See Sudden infant death syndrome (SIDS)
Single parenting, 317–320
adoption and, 317
child care and, 318
child custody and, 318
child support and, 320
dating and, 318
divorce and, 317
reducing stress, 319
separation and, 317
unplanned pregnancy, 317
Sinuses
fluid inside, 73
infections of, 15
Sinusitis, 73
diagnosing bacterial, 73
for pneumonia, 61
symptoms of, 69
treating bacterial, 73–74
Skin, poison on, 230
Skin cancer, 137

Skin products, 223
Sleep apnea, 75
causes of, 75
treatment of, 75
Sleep diary, keeping, 80
Sleep position for premature baby, 131
Sleep problems, 77
common, 79–80
infants, 77
in preschoolers, 78
in toddlers, 78
Sleep talking, 79
Sleepwalking, 79
Slides, playground safety and, 227
Smegma, 143
Smoke alarms, 211
Smoke-free environment, creating, 233–234
Smokeless tobacco, 376, 377–378
cancer and, 377
physical and mental effect of, 377
quitting, 378
Smoking
adolescents and, 248
defined, 233
media and, 375
quitting, 376
secondhand, 208
Snacks, 174
Snuff, 379
Social effects, smokeless tobacco and, 377
Solid foods, starting, 175–177
Sonography, 56
Spanking, 283
Spasmodic croup, 29
Speech and language disabilities, 158
Spermicides, 348
Sponging, 42
Sports, 181–182
age to start involvement, 181
desire to quit, 181
grades and participation in, 182
risks of injury, 181
Sports medicine specialist, pediatric, 425
Sports-related stress, 182
Sprains, for college students, 253
STDs. See Sexually transmitted diseases (STDs)
Step-siblings, 313
Steroids, 369–370
defined, 369
individuals using, 369
side effects of, 369–370
Stomach and intestinal problems, 225
Storage area, fire safety in, 212
Straight, 337
Strains, for college students, 253
Strep throat, 61
Stress
reducing, 319
sports-related, 182
Strong bones, calcium and, 163
Student health service, 251
Stuffy nose, relief from, 19
Stye (hordeolum), 38, 61
Substance abuse. See also Alcohol; Drugs
of cocaine, 359–360
for gay and lesbian youth, 334
of marijuana, 367–368
prevention of, 371–373

Sudden infant death syndrome (SIDS), 135
infant sleep positioning and, 77
Suicide, adolescent, 279–280
Sun, 210
Sunburn, dangers of, 137, 138
Sun exposure, baby and, 137–138
Sunscreen, for baby, 137–138
Surgeon, pediatric, 421
Surgery for tonsils, 82
Swimming lessons, 242
Swimming pools
safety checklist for, 218
water safety in, 241
Swings, playground safety and, 227
Swollen eyelids, 38
Syrup of ipecac, 225, 230
Systemic corticosteroids, 27

T
Tear ducts, blocked, 38
Teenagers. See Adolescents
Teeth. See also Dental health
cleaning child's, 203
Teeth grinding, 80
Television
family and, 321–323
rating of, 301–302
toppling, 323
Temperature
ear, 42
oral, 42
rectal, 42
taking, 42
underarm (axillary), 42
Temper tantrums, 325–326
causes of, 325
handling, 326
preventing, 325–326
as serious, 326
Testicular self-exam, 353
Tetanus and diphtheria vaccine (Td), 411–412
Tetanus (lockjaw), 385, 411
Tether straps, 110
Thalassemia, 13
Therapy, talking to child about, 310
Thimerosal, 396
Thumb sucking, 139, 203
Ticks, 66
removal of, 66
Tobacco
chewing, 379
risks of, 375–376
smokeless, 377–378
talking about, 379–380
television and, 321
Tobacco smoke, risk for ear infection and, 33
Toddlers
sleep problems in, 78
television for, 321
transportation of
in hip spica casts, 110
with tracheostomies, 110
Toilet training, 141–142
help from pediatricians, 142
readiness for, 142
teaching, 142–143